An Introduction to
Community Health

Seventh Edition

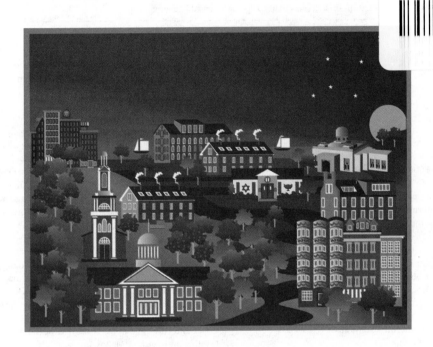

James F. McKenzie, PhD, MPH, CHES
Professor Emeritus

Robert R. Pinger, PhD
Professor Emeritus

Jerome E. Kotecki, HSD
Professor

Department of Physiology and Health Science
Ball State University

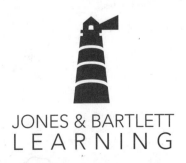

JONES & BARTLETT
LEARNING

World Headquarters

Jones & Bartlett Learning
40 Tall Pine Drive
Sudbury, MA 01776
978-443-5000
info@jblearning.com
www.jblearning.com

Jones & Bartlett Learning Canada
6339 Ormindale Way
Mississauga, Ontario L5V 1J2
Canada

Jones & Bartlett Learning International
Barb House, Barb Mews
London W6 7PA
United Kingdom

Jones & Bartlett Learning books and products are available through most bookstores and online booksellers. To contact Jones & Bartlett Learning directly, call 800-832-0034, fax 978-443-8000, or visit our website, www.jblearning.com.

Substantial discounts on bulk quantities of Jones & Bartlett Learning publications are available to corporations, professional associations, and other qualified organizations. For details and specific discount information, contact the special sales department at Jones & Bartlett Learning via the above contact information or send an email to specialsales@jblearning.com.

Copyright © 2012 by Jones & Bartlett Learning, LLC

All rights reserved. No part of the material protected by this copyright may be reproduced or utilized in any form, electronic or mechanical, including photocopying, recording, or by any information storage and retrieval system, without written permission from the copyright owner.

The authors, editor, and publisher have made every effort to provide accurate information. However, they are not responsible for errors, omissions, or for any outcomes related to the use of the contents of this book and take no responsibility for the use of the products and procedures described. Treatments and side effects described in this book may not be applicable to all people; likewise, some people may require a dose or experience a side effect that is not described herein. Drugs and medical devices are discussed that may have limited availability controlled by the Food and Drug Administration (FDA) for use only in a research study or clinical trial. Research, clinical practice, and government regulations often change the accepted standard in this field. When consideration is being given to use of any drug in the clinical setting, the health care provider or reader is responsible for determining FDA status of the drug, reading the package insert, and reviewing prescribing information for the most up-to-date recommendations on dose, precautions, and contraindications, and determining the appropriate usage for the product. This is especially important in the case of drugs that are new or seldom used.

Production Credits

Publisher, Higher Education: Cathleen Sether
Senior Acquisitions Editor: Shoshanna Goldberg
Senior Associate Editor: Amy L. Bloom
Editorial Assistant: Prima Bartlett
Production Manager: Julie Champagne Bolduc
Senior Production Editor: Katherine Crighton
Production Assistant: Sean Coombs
Associate Marketing Manager: Jody Sullivan

V.P., Manufacturing and Inventory Control: Therese Connell
Composition: Publishers' Design and Production Services, Inc.
Cover Design: Kate Ternullo
Photo Research and Permissions Supervisor: Christine Myaskovsky
Associate Photo Researcher: Sarah Cebulski
Cover and Title Page Image: Courtesy of Hannus Design Associates
Printing and Binding: Malloy, Inc.
Cover Printing: Malloy, Inc.

Library of Congress Cataloging-in-Publication Data

McKenzie, James F., 1948–
   An introduction to community health / James F. McKenzie, Robert R. Pinger,
Jerome E. Kotecki. — 7th ed.
      p. ; cm.
   Includes bibliographical references and index.
   ISBN 978-0-7637-9011-0
   1. Community health services—United States.   2. Public health—United
States.   3. Medical care—United States.   4. Environmental health—United
States.   I. Pinger, R. R.   II. Kotecki, Jerome Edward.   III. Title.
   [DNLM: 1. Community Health Services—United States.   2. Delivery of
Health Care—United States.   3. Environmental Health—United States.
4. Public Health—United States.   WA 546 AA1]
   RA445.M29 2011
   362.1—dc22
                                                                2011000582

6048

Printed in the United States of America
15   14   13   12   11   10   9   8   7   6   5   4   3   2

CONTENTS

PREFACE
for the Seventh Edition

As its title suggests, *An Introduction to Community Health* was written to introduce students to community health. It is a textbook that combines the power of today's electronic technology, via the Internet, with the traditional textbook presentation. We believe that your students will find *An Introduction to Community Health* easy to read, understand, and use. If they read the chapters carefully and make an honest effort to answer the review questions and to complete some of the activities, we are confident that students will gain a good understanding of the realm of community health. *An Introduction to Community Health* incorporates a variety of pedagogical elements that assist and encourage students to understand complex community health issues. Each chapter of the book includes:

- chapter objectives
- a scenario
- an introduction
- content
- marginal definitions of key terms
- a chapter summary
- a scenario analysis and response
- review questions
- activities
- information about Web activities
- references

In addition, many figures, tables, boxes, and photos have been presented to clarify and illustrate the concepts presented in the text. Select content in each chapter is dedicated to the *Healthy People 2020* goals and objectives. In the back of the book you will find four appendixes (calculation of an odds ratio, operational definitions used to classify federal data on race and ethnicity, and a self-assessment checklist for cultural diversity and cultural competency), a glossary of key terms used throughout the text, and a complete subject and person index.

Chapter Objectives

The chapter objectives identify the content and skills that should be mastered through reading the chapters, answering the end-of-chapter questions, and completing the activities. To use the objectives effectively, they should be reviewed before and after reading the chapters. This review will help your students focus on the major points in each chapter and facilitate answering the questions and completing the activities at the end of each chapter.

Scenarios

Short scenarios are presented at the beginning of each chapter. The purpose of these scenarios is to bridge the gap between your students' personal experiences and ideas discussed within the chapter. The chapter content will enable your students to propose solutions to the community health problem posed in the scenario.

Introduction

Each chapter begins with a brief introduction that informs the reader of the topics to be presented and explains how these topics relate to others in the book.

Marginal Definitions

Terms that are important to the understanding of the chapter are presented in boldface type and defined in the margin. Before reading the chapter, it is suggested that the student skim the chapters, paying particular attention to the key terms. This should provide greater understanding of the content. The boldfaced terms also appear in the glossary at the end of the book. In addition, some words in the textbook have been italicized for emphasis, and are often key terms that have been defined in another chapter.

Content

Although each chapter in the textbook could be expanded—indeed, there are entire books written on many of the topics we cover—we believe each chapter contains the essential material needed to introduce students to the issues related to community health. To enhance and facilitate learning, the chapters are organized in three units: Foundations of Community Health, The Nation's Health and Health Care Delivery, and Environmental Health and Safety.

Chapter Summary

At the end of each chapter, the reader will find several bulleted points that review the major concepts contained in each chapter.

Scenario: Analysis and Response

Following the chapter summary, students are provided with an opportunity to respond to the scenario presented earlier in the chapter. The content presented in the chapter will help the students to formulate their responses or solutions.

Review Questions

The purpose of the questions at the end of each chapter is to provide the readers with feedback regarding their mastery of the chapter's content. The questions reinforce the chapter objectives and key terms.

Activities

The activities at the end of each chapter provide an opportunity for students to apply their new knowledge in a meaningful way. The activities, which are presented in a variety of formats, should appeal to the varying learning styles of your students.

Community Health on the Web

The Internet contains a wealth of information about community and public health. The Web activities are presented to encourage students to further explore the chapter's content by visiting relevant Web sites. These activities recap three concepts or issues from the text in each chapter. The starting point for these activities is Jones & Bartlett's own exclusive Community Health Web page (http://health.jbpub.com/communityhealth/7e).

Once students have connected to the designated community health link through the Jones & Bartlett Community Health home page, they will be provided with activity instructions for further exploration of the Web site. Animated flashcards, an interactive glossary, and crossword puzzles are also available online. When more up-to-date information becomes available at an assigned site, the authors are able to immediately edit the exercise to reflect the most recent material.

The Web activities bring to life the content and theory presented in the text, thus giving students a real-world context for understanding community health concepts and issues. The intent of including Web activities in the textbook is to inspire the students, in real time, to authentically assess and to critically think about what they have just read in the text by asking them thought-provoking questions related to the assigned Web site. By integrating the Web into the text, we have created a dynamic learning environment that is as up-to-date as today's newspaper.

What Is New to This Edition?

Although the format of this edition is similar to previous editions, much has changed. First the content and statistics throughout the book have been reviewed and updated with the latest information. New tables, figures, boxes, and photographs have been added. In addition, we have included information and data from the recently released *Healthy People 2020*. Second, the book has been shortened. We have removed some tables and charts and combined several chapters. In the previous edition, we had two chapters each on health care and environmental health. In this edition, those four chapters have been reduced to two with one chapter on each topic. Third, when possible, we made the changes requested by the reviewers of the previous edition of this book:

Chapter 1 was shortened and some of the ancient history of community and public health is presented in an abbreviated form.

In Chapter 3 we added a discussion of the Criteria of Causation, while in Chapter 4 we included new discussions of the importance of immunizations and needle exchange programs in the prevention of communicable disease.

Chapter 5 starts with a new section on the social ecological approach and its importance to both community organizing/building and program planning.

The school health education chapter—Chapter 6—includes the latest information about school wellness polices and an overview of the Centers for Disease Control and Prevention's Health Education Curriculum Analysis Tool (HECAT) for curriculum review and development.

Chapter 8 has been revised using the most recent information from the Youth Risk Behavior Surveillance System (YRBSS), the Behavioral Risk Factor Surveillance System (BRFSS), and the National College Health Assessment (NCHA).

The revision of Chapter 11 includes new details on the causes of mental illness and the mental health needs of culturally diverse groups, and describes the nature of recovery from mental illness in the United States and in less-developed countries. Also included is a discussion of the relationship of mental illness to violent crime, and the use of mental health courts and other remedies to reduce the number of people with mental illness in jails and prisons. The chapter concludes with a new discussion of the social and economic challenges currently facing the mental health field.

New to Chapter 12 is the mention of the Family Smoking Prevention and Tobacco Control Act giving the FDA oversight of tobacco products. There is also discussion of the sharp rise in fatal unintentional poisonings (now the second leading cause of unintentional deaths) attributable to the use/abuse of nonmedically prescribed painkillers.

Chapter 13 is the newly combined chapter on health care delivery in the United States. In addition to the updating, the chapter also includes many of the details found in the Affordable Care Act, the health insurance reform law passed in March 2010.

Chapter 14, replacing Chapters 15 and 16 of the *Sixth Edition*, has been completely rewritten. Environmental threats to our air, water, and food resources, and the environmental health hazards associated with community living are succinctly described and explained. Governmental (regulatory) and nongovernmental approaches to reducing environmental health risks are discussed. The chapter concludes with a description of natural and human-generated environmental disasters and with a discussion of how communities respond to these disasters.

In Chapter 15 we removed several of the long tables providing state-by-state motorcycle helmet and safety belt regulations and moved them to the book's Web site for this edition. The chapter includes a new discussion of distracted driving, including texting and e-mailing while driving. Also there is mention of new court rulings concerning restriction of firearms on college campuses (Utah) and in cities (Chicago), and the ramifications for community safety.

Chapter 16 includes a new discussion of the plight of migrant farm workers and their children, including the 2010 Human Rights Watch report, "Fields of Peril: Child Labor in U.S. Agriculture." Updated material on the safety and health risks faced by miners is presented, including mention of the 2010 mine disaster at the Upper Big Branch Mine in West Virginia.

Accompanying Ancillaries

This edition is accompanied by an Instructor's ToolKit CD-ROM, which includes a lecture outline and PowerPoint presentation for each chapter as well as a computerized TestBank and Image Bank. These products are available free to adopters of the text. For more information about these ancillary products, please contact your sales representative at Jones & Bartlett Learning.

Acknowledgments

A project of this nature could not be completed without the assistance and understanding of a number of individuals. First, we would like to thank those individuals who have brought their expertise to the writing team: Elizabeth H. Chaney, PhD, CHES, Assistant Professor, Department of Health Education and Behavior, University of Florida, provided revisions for Chapter 2 (Organizations That Help Shape Community Health); Denise M. Seabert, PhD, CHES, Associate Professor, Department of Physiology and Health Science, Ball State University, completed revisions for Chapter 6 (The School Health Program: A Component of Community Health) and Chapter 8 (Adolescents, Young Adults, and Adults); David A. Haber, PhD, the John and Janice Fisher Distinguished Professor and Associate Director of the Fisher Institute for Wellness and Gerontology, Ball State University, was responsible for the revisions to Chapter 9 (Elders); and David V. Perkins, PhD, Professor, Department of Psychological Sciences, Ball State University, completed the revisions for Chapter 11 (Community Mental Health). Their expertise is both welcomed and appreciated.

Second, we would like to thank several colleagues for their contributions. They include Dale B. Hahn, PhD, Professor Emeritus, Department of Physiology and Health Science, Ball State University, for encouraging us to take on this project; the staff members of the High Library at Elizabethtown College, Elizabethtown, PA, for their assistance in making the project possible; and Billie Kennedy and Debbie Morris for their support and friendship.

Third, we would like to express our appreciation to those professionals who took the time and effort to review and provide feedback for this edition. They include:

- Elizabeth G. Calamidas, The Richard Stockton College of New Jersey
- Fran Henton, Nebraska Methodist College
- Harold Horn, Lincoln Land Community College
- John Janowiak, Appalachian State University
- Justine Pawlukewicz, New York City College of Technology
- Fred R. Pearson, Brigham Young University-Idaho
- Kerry J. Redican, Virginia Polytechnic Institute and State University
- Wanda Reygaert, Oakland University
- Patricia Rhynders, Touro University International and Texas Woman's University
- Joanne Sommers, Bowling Green State University
- Cynthia Stone, Indiana University
- Peter N. Tabbot, MPH, HO, Bloustein School of Planning and Public Policy, Rutgers, the State University
- and Maria Theresa Wessel, James Madison University.

Fourth, we would like to thank all of the employees of Jones & Bartlett Learning. Their hard work, support, guidance, and confidence in us has been most helpful in creating this and all previous editions of this text. Specifically, we would like to thank: Shoshanna Goldberg, Senior Acquisitions Editor; Julie Bolduc, Production Manager; Amy Bloom, Senior Associate Editor; Prima Bartlett, Editorial Assistant; Sarah Cebulski, Associate Photo Researcher; and Jody Sullivan, Associate Marketing Manager.

Finally, we would like to thank our families for their love, support, encouragement, and tolerance of all the time that writing takes away from family activities.

UNIT
ONE

FOUNDATIONS OF COMMUNITY HEALTH

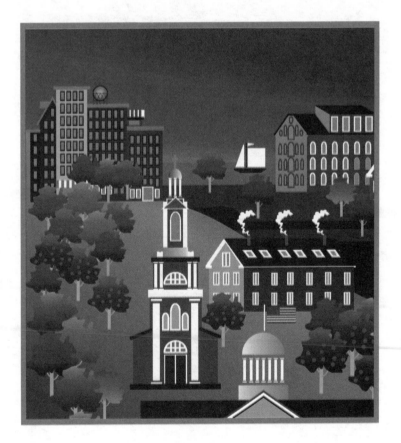

Chapter 1

Community Health: Yesterday, Today, and Tomorrow

Chapter Objectives

After studying this chapter, you will be able to:

1 Accurately define the terms *health, community,
community health, population health, public
health, public health system,* and *global health.*

2 Briefly describe the five major determinants of
health.

3 Explain the difference between personal and
community health activities.

4 List and discuss the factors that influence a
community's health.

5 Briefly relate the history of community/public
health, including the recent U.S. history of
community and public health in the twentieth and
early twenty-first centuries.

6 Provide a brief overview of the current health
status of Americans.

7 Describe the major community health problems
facing the United States today.

8 Describe the status of efforts to improve world
health and list some plans for the future.

9 Describe the purpose of the *Healthy People 2020*
goals and objectives as they apply to the planning
process of the health of Americans.

SCENARIO

Amy and Eric are a young working couple who are easing into a comfortable lifestyle. They have good-paying jobs, drive nice cars, are buying a home in a good neighborhood, and have two healthy preschool children. When Amy picked her children up from day care earlier in the day she learned from the head teacher that another parent had reported that his child was diagnosed with hepatitis. This news frightened Amy and made her begin to question the quality of the day care center. Amy told Eric of this situation when he got home from work. As the couple discussed whether or not they should take their children to day care as usual the following day, they discovered that they have many unanswered questions. How serious is hepatitis? What is the likelihood that their children will be at serious risk for getting the disease? What steps are being taken to control the outbreak? Is any state or local agency responsible for standardizing health practices at private day care centers in the community? Does the city, county, or state carry out any type of inspection when they license these facilities? And, if the children do not attend day care, which parent will stay home with them?

INTRODUCTION

In looking back over the last 100-plus years, it is easy to point to the tremendous progress that was made in the health and life expectancy of those in the United States (see Box 1.1) and of many people of the world. Infant mortality dropped, many of the infectious diseases have been brought under control, and better family planning became available. However, there is still room for improvement! Individual health behaviors, such as the use of tobacco, poor diet, and physical inactivity, have given rise to an unacceptable number of cases of illness and death from noninfectious diseases such as cancer, diabetes, and heart disease. New and emerging infectious diseases, such as the 2009 H1N1 flu and those caused by drug-resistant pathogens, are stretching resources available to control them. And events stemming from natural disasters such as floods and hurricanes, and humanmade disasters such as the Gulf oil spill and terrorism around the world have caused us to refocus our priorities. All of these events have severely disrupted Americans' sense of security[1] and sense of safety in the environment. In addition, many of these events revealed the vulnerability of the United States' ability to respond to such circumstances and highlighted the need for improvement in emergency response preparedness and infrastructure of the public health system.

Even with all that has happened in recent years in the United States and around the world, the achievement of good health remains a worldwide goal of the twenty-first century. Governments, private organizations, and individuals throughout the world are working to improve health. Although individual actions to improve one's own personal health certainly contribute to the overall health of the community, organized community actions are often necessary when health problems exceed the resources of any one individual. When such actions are not taken, the health of the entire community is at risk.

This chapter introduces the concepts and principles of community health, explains how community health differs from personal health, and provides a brief history of community health. Some of the key health problems facing Americans are also described, and an outlook for the twenty-first century is provided.

BOX
1.1
A Look Back on the Twentieth Century in the United States

As the twentieth century came to a close, the overall health status and life expectancy in the United States were at all-time highs. Since 1900, the average life span of people in the United States had lengthened by more than 30 years; 25 of these years have been attributed to advances in public health.[2] There were many public health achievements that can be linked to this gain in life expectancy, however. The Centers for Disease Control and Prevention (CDC), the U.S. government agency charged with protecting the public health of the nation, singled out the "Ten Great Public Health Achievements" in the United States between 1900 and 1999. Some of these achievements will be discussed in greater detail in other chapters of this book where they are more relevant to the content being presented. Here is the entire list:[3]

1. *Vaccination.* Vaccines are now available to protect children and adults against 15 life-threatening or debilitating diseases. Rates of all vaccine-preventable diseases are down more than 97% from peak levels before vaccines were available.[4]

2. *Motor vehicle safety.* A number of advances over the years, including safety belts, air bags, safer cars and roads, and enforcement of drunk driving and other laws, have saved many lives.[4]

3. *Safer workplaces.* A number of voluntary and mandatory practices in the workplace have created a much safer work environment. In the early 1900s, the work-related death rate was about 21 per 100,000. By the mid-1990s, that number had dropped to about 4 per 100,000.[5]

4. *Control of infectious diseases.* At the beginning of the twentieth century, the leading causes of death were infectious diseases, but by mid-century many of these diseases were under control. This control can be attributed to cleaner water, improved sanitation, and antibiotics.

5. *Decline of deaths from coronary heart disease and stroke.* Although these remain the leading causes of death, significant progress has been made in reducing the death rates since 1950. This progress can be attributed to the identification and modification of risk factors such as smoking and high blood pressure, and the improved access to early detection and better treatment.

6. *Safer and healthier foods.* Over the twentieth century much of the microbial contamination of food has been significantly reduced, and the nutritional value of foods has been greatly enhanced.

7. *Healthier mothers and babies.* Infant and maternal mortality rates have decreased 90% and 99%, respectively. This can be attributed to advances in hygiene, nutrition, antibiotics, medical technology, and access to health care.

8. *Family planning.* Advances in family planning and contraceptive services have provided for greater health benefits for mothers and babies and have reduced the transmission of several sexually transmitted diseases.

9. *Fluoridation of drinking water.* Though fluoridation of water only began in the mid-twentieth century, it has played an important role in the reduction of both tooth decay and tooth loss.

10. *Recognition of tobacco use as a health hazard.* Recognition of tobacco as the single most preventable cause of death in the United States has saved the lives and suffering of millions of people in this country.

Definitions

The word *health* means different things to different people. Similarly, there are other words that can be defined in various ways. Some basic terms we will use in this book are defined in the following paragraphs.

Health

The word *health* is derived from *hal,* which means "hale, sound, whole." When it comes to the health of people, the word *health* has been defined in a number of different ways—often in its social context, as when a parent describes the health of a child or when an avid fan defines the health of a professional athlete. The most widely quoted definition of health was the one created by the World Health Organization (WHO) in 1946. That definition states that

health
a dynamic state or condition of the human organism that is multidimensional in nature, a resource for living, and results from a person's interactions with and adaptations to his or her environment; therefore, it can exist in varying degrees and is specific to each individual and his or her situation

"health is a state of complete physical, mental, and social well-being and not merely the absence of disease and infirmity."[6] Further, the WHO has indicated that "health is a resource for everyday life, not the object of living, and is a positive concept emphasizing social and personal resources as well as physical capabilities."[6] Others have stated that health cannot be defined as a state because it is ever changing. Therefore, we have chosen to define **health** as a *dynamic* state or condition of the human organism that is multidimensional (i.e., physical, emotional, social, intellectual, spiritual, and occupational) in nature, a resource for living, and results from a person's interactions with and adaptations to his or her environment. Therefore, it can exist in varying degrees and is specific to each individual and his or her situation. "For example, a person can be healthy while dying, or a person who is a quadriplegic can be healthy in the sense that his or her mental and social well-being are high and physical health is as good as it can be."[7]

A person's health status is dynamic in part because of the many different factors that determine one's health. It is widely accepted that health status is determined by the interaction of five domains: gestational endowments (i.e., genetic makeup), social circumstances (e.g., education, employment, income, poverty, housing, crime, and social cohesion), environmental conditions where people live and work (i.e., toxic agents, microbial agents, and structural hazards), behavioral choices (e.g., diet, physical activity, substance use and abuse), and the availability of quality medical care.[8] "Ultimately, the health fate of each of us is determined by factors acting not mostly in isolation but by our experience where domains interconnect. Whether a gene is expressed can be determined by environmental exposures or behavioral patterns. The nature and consequences of behavioral choices are affected by social circumstances. Our genetic predispositions affect the health care we need, and our social circumstances affect the health care we receive."[9]

Community

community
a group of people who have common characteristics; communities can be defined by location, race, ethnicity, age, occupation, interest in particular problems or outcomes, or other common bonds

Traditionally, a community has been thought of as a geographic area with specific boundaries—for example, a neighborhood, city, county, or state. However, in the context of community health, a **community** is "a group of people who have common characteristics; communities can be defined by location, race, ethnicity, age, occupation, interest in particular problems or outcomes, or common bonds."[10] Today we can even talk about a cyber community.[11] Communities are characterized by the following elements:

(1) membership—a sense of identity and belonging; (2) common symbol systems—similar language, rituals, and ceremonies; (3) shared values and norms; (4) mutual influence—community members have influence and are influenced by each other; (5) shared needs and commitment to meeting them; and (6) shared emotional connection—members share common history, experiences, and mutual support.[12]

Examples of communities include the people of the city of Columbus (location), the Asian community of San Francisco (race), the Hispanic community of Miami (ethnicity), seniors in the church (age), the business or the banking communities (occupation), the homeless of Indiana (specific problem), those on welfare in Ohio (particular outcome), local union members (common bond), or those who are members of a social network (cyber). A community may be as small as the group of people who live on a residence hall floor at a university or as large as all of the individuals who make up a nation. "A healthy community is a place where people provide leadership in assessing their own resources and needs, where public health and social infrastructure and policies support health, and where essential public health services, including quality health care, are available."[13]

Public, Community, Population, and Global Health

Prior to defining the four terms *public health*, *community health*, *population health*, and *global health*, it is important to note that often the terms are used interchangeably by both laypeople and professionals who work in the various health fields. When the terms are used interchangeably, most people are referring to the collective health of those in society and the actions or activities taken to obtain and maintain that health. The definitions provided here for the four terms more precisely define the group of people in question and the origin of the actions or activities.

Of the four terms, *public health* is the most inclusive. The Institute of Medicine (IOM) defined **public health** in 1988 in its landmark report *The Future of Public Health* as "what we as a society do collectively to assure the conditions in which people can be healthy."[14] The **public health system**, which has been defined as "activities undertaken within the formal structure of government and the associated efforts of private and voluntary organizations and individuals,"[14] is the organizational mechanism for providing such conditions. Even with these formal definitions, some still see public health activities as only those efforts that originate in federal, state, and local governmental public health agencies such as the Centers for Disease Control and Prevention and local (i.e., city and county) health departments.

Community health refers to the health status of a defined group of people and the actions and conditions to promote, protect, and preserve their health. For example, the health status of the people of Muncie, Indiana, and the private and public actions taken to promote, protect, and preserve the health of these people would constitute community health.

The term *population health* is similar to *community health*. The primary difference between these two terms is the degree of organization or identity of the people. **Population health** refers to the health status of people who are not organized and have no identity as a group or locality and the actions and conditions to promote, protect, and preserve their health. Men younger than 50, adolescents, prisoners, and white-collar workers are all examples of populations.[15]

A term that has been used increasingly more in recent years is *global health*. The term "does not have one uniform definition. Several organizations have defined the term, and they generally use it in three different ways: (1) as a state or condition; (2) as a goal; and (3) as a field of study, research, and practice."[16] For our discussion here, and to keep it parallel with the terms we have already defined, we use a definition that defines it as a state or condition. Thus, **global health** is a term that describes "health problems, issues, and concerns that transcend national boundaries, may be influenced by circumstances or experiences in other countries, and are best addressed by cooperative actions and solutions."[17] Therefore, an issue such as the 2009 H1N1 flu pandemic can be viewed as a global health issue. Much of the rise in concern about global health problems comes from the speed of international travel and how easy it is for people who may be infected with a disease to cross borders into another country.

Personal Health versus Community Health

To further clarify the definitions presented in this chapter, it is important to distinguish between the terms *personal health activities* and *community health activities*.

Personal Health Activities

Personal health activities are individual actions and decision making that affect the health of an individual or his or her immediate family members or friends. These activities may be preventive or curative in nature but seldom directly affect the behavior of others. Choosing to eat

public health
actions that society takes collectively to ensure that the conditions in which people can be healthy can occur

public health system
the organizational mechanism of those activities undertaken within the formal structure of government and the associated efforts of private and voluntary organizations and individuals

community health
the health status of a defined group of people and the actions and conditions to promote, protect, and preserve their health

population health
the health status of people who are not organized and have no identity as a group or locality and the actions and conditions to promote, protect, and preserve their health

global health
describes health problems, issues, and concerns that transcend national boundaries, may be influenced by circumstances or experiences in other countries, and are best addressed by cooperative actions and solutions

wisely, to regularly wear a safety belt, and to visit the physician are all examples of personal health activities.

Community Health Activities

Community health activities are activities that are aimed at protecting or improving the health of a population or community. Maintenance of accurate birth and death records, protection of the food and water supply, and participating in fund drives for voluntary health organizations such as the American Lung Association are examples of community health activities.

Within this book, you are introduced to the many community health activities and to the organizations that are responsible for carrying them out. The following are some of the key topics that are covered in this text:

- Organizations that contribute to community health
- How communities measure health, disease, injury, and death
- Control of communicable and noncommunicable diseases
- How communities organize to solve health problems
- Community health in schools
- Community health needs of people at different stages of life
- Community health needs of special populations
- Community mental health
- Abuse of alcohol, tobacco, and other drugs
- The health care delivery system
- Environmental health problems
- Intentional and unintentional injuries
- Occupational safety and health

Factors That Affect the Health of a Community

There are a great many factors that affect the health of a community. As a result, the health status of each community is different. These factors may be physical, social, and/or cultural. They also include the ability of the community to organize and work together as a whole as well as the individual behaviors of those in the community (see Figure 1.1).

Physical Factors

Physical factors include the influences of geography, the environment, community size, and industrial development.

Geography

A community's health problems can be directly influenced by its altitude, latitude, and climate. In tropical countries where warm, humid temperatures and rain prevail throughout the year, parasitic and infectious diseases are a leading community health problem (see Figure 1.2). In many tropical countries, survival from these diseases is made more difficult because poor soil conditions result in inadequate food production and malnutrition. In temperate climates with fewer parasitic and infectious diseases and a more than adequate food supply, obesity and heart disease are important community health problems.

FIGURE 1.1

Factors that affect the health of a community.

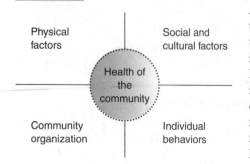

Environment

The quality of our environment is directly related to the quality of our stewardship of it. Many experts believe that if we continue to allow uncontrolled population growth and continue to deplete nonrenewable natural resources, succeeding generations will inhabit communities that are less desirable than ours. Many feel that we must accept responsibility for this stewardship and drastically reduce the rate at which we foul the soil, water, and air.

Community Size

The larger the community, the greater its range of health problems and the greater its number of health resources. For example, larger communities have more health professionals and better health facilities than smaller communities. These resources are often needed because communicable diseases can spread more quickly and environmental problems are often more severe in densely populated areas. For example, the amount of trash generated by the approximately 8.3 million people in New York City is many times greater than that generated by the entire state of Wyoming, with its population of about 544,270.

It is important to note that a community's size can have both a positive and negative impact on that community's health. The ability of a community to effectively plan, organize, and utilize its resources can determine whether its size can be used to good advantage.

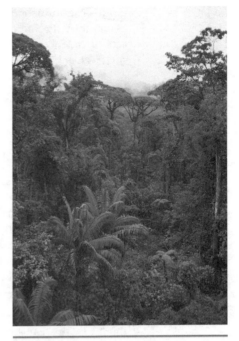

FIGURE 1.2

In tropical countries, parasitic and infectious diseases are leading community health problems.

Industrial Development

Industrial development, like size, can have either positive or negative effects on the health status of a community. Industrial development provides a community with added resources for community health programs, but it may bring with it environmental pollution and occupational injuries and illnesses. Communities that experience rapid industrial development must eventually regulate the way in which industries (1) obtain raw materials, (2) discharge by-products, (3) dispose of wastes, (4) treat and protect their employees, and (5) clean up environmental accidents. Unfortunately, many of these laws are usually passed only after these communities have suffered significant reductions in the quality of their life and health.

Social and Cultural Factors

Social factors are those that arise from the interaction of individuals or groups within the community. For example, people who live in urban communities, where life is fast-paced, experience higher rates of stress-related illnesses than those who live in rural communities, where life is more leisurely. On the other hand, those in rural areas may not have access to the same quality or selection of health care (i.e., hospitals or medical specialists) that is available to those who live in urban communities.

Cultural factors arise from guidelines (both explicit and implicit) that individuals "inherit" from being a part of a particular society. Culture "teaches us what to fear, what to respect, what to value, and what to regard as relevant in our lives."[18] Some of the factors that contribute to culture are discussed in the following sections.

Beliefs, Traditions, and Prejudices

The beliefs, traditions, and prejudices of community members can affect the health of the community. The beliefs of those in a community about such specific health behaviors as exercise and smoking can influence policy makers on whether or not they will spend money on bike trails and work toward no-smoking ordinances. The traditions of specific ethnic groups can influence the types of food, restaurants, retail outlets, and services available in a community. Prejudices of one specific ethnic or racial group against another can result in acts of violence and crime. Racial and ethnic disparities will continue to put certain groups, such as black Americans or certain religious groups, at greater risk.

Economy

Both national and local economies can affect the health of a community through reductions in health and social services. An economic downturn means lower tax revenues (fewer tax dollars) and fewer contributions to charitable groups. Such actions will result in fewer dollars being available for programs such as welfare, food stamps, community health care, and other community services. This occurs because revenue shortfalls cause agencies to experience budget cuts. With less money, these agencies often must alter their eligibility guidelines, thereby restricting aid to only the neediest individuals. Obviously, many people who had been eligible for assistance before the economic downturn become ineligible.

Employers usually find it increasingly difficult to provide health benefits for their employees as their income drops. The unemployed and underemployed face poverty and deteriorating health. Thus, the cumulative effect of an economic downturn significantly affects the health of the community.

Politics

Those who happen to be in political office can improve or jeopardize the health of their community by the decisions they make. In the most general terms, the argument is over greater or lesser governmental participation in health issues. For example, there has been a long-standing discussion in the United States on the extent to which the government should involve itself in health care. Historically, Democrats have been in favor of such action while Republicans have been against it. State and local politicians also influence the health of their communities each time they vote on health-related measures brought before them, such as a no-smoking ordinance.

Religion

A number of religions have taken a position on health care and health behaviors. For example, some religious communities limit the type of medical treatment their members may receive. Some do not permit immunizations; others do not permit their members to be treated by physicians. Still others prohibit certain foods. For example, Kosher dietary regulations permit Jews to eat the meat only of animals that chew cud and have cloven hooves and the flesh only of fish that have both gills and scales, while still others, like the Native American Church of the Morning Star, use peyote, a hallucinogen, as a sacrament.

Some religious communities actively address moral and ethical issues such as abortion, premarital intercourse, and homosexuality. Still other religions teach health-promoting codes of living to their members. Obviously, religion can affect a community's health positively or negatively (see Figure 1.3).

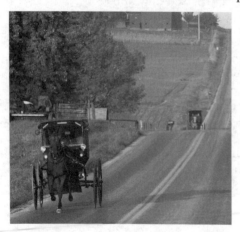

FIGURE 1.3

Religion can affect a community's health either positively or negatively.

Social Norms

The influence of social norms can be positive or negative and can change over time. Cigarette smoking is a good example. During the 1940s, 1950s, and 1960s, it was socially acceptable to smoke in most settings. As a matter of fact, in 1960, 53% of American men and 32% of American women smoked. Thus, in 1960 it was socially acceptable to be a smoker, especially if you were male. Now, early in the twenty-first century, those percentages have dropped to 23.1% (for males) and 18.3% (for females), and in most public places it has become socially unacceptable to smoke.[19] The lawsuits against tobacco companies by both the state attorneys general and private citizens provide further evidence that smoking has fallen from social acceptability. Because of this change in the social norm, there is less secondhand smoke in many public places, and in turn the health of the community has improved.

Unlike smoking, alcohol consumption represents a continuing negative social norm in America, especially on college campuses. The normal expectation seems to be that drinking is fun (and almost everyone wants to have fun). Despite the fact that most college students are too young to drink legally, approximately 60% of college students drink.[20] It seems fairly obvious that the American alcoholic-beverage industry has influenced our social norms.

Socioeconomic Status

Differences in socioeconomic status, whether "defined by education, employment, or income, both individual- and community-level socioeconomic status have independent effects on health."[21] "In the United States today, the health of poor people is threatened by the adverse environmental conditions of the inner cities, such as lead paint and air pollution, crime, and violence. Poor people also have poorer nutrition, less access to medical care, and more psychological stress."[1] In addition to health care access, higher incomes enable people to afford better housing, live in safer neighborhoods, and increase the opportunity to engage in health-promoting behaviors.[22]

Community Organizing

The way in which a community is able to organize its resources directly influences its ability to intervene and solve problems, including health problems. **Community organizing** "is a process through which communities are helped to identify common problems or goals, mobilize resources, and in other ways develop and implement strategies for reaching their goals they have collectively set."[23] It is not a science but an art of building consensus within a democratic process.[24] If a community can organize its resources effectively into a unified force, it "is likely to produce benefits in the form of increased effectiveness and productivity by reducing duplication of efforts and avoiding the imposition of solutions that are not congruent with the local culture and needs."[13] For example, many communities in the United States have faced community-wide drug problems. Some have been able to organize their resources to reduce or resolve these problems, whereas others have not. (See Chapter 5 for a full explanation of community organizing.)

community organizing
a process through which communities are helped to identify common problems or goals, mobilize resources, and in other ways develop and implement strategies for reaching their goals they have collectively set

Individual Behavior

The behavior of the individual community members contributes to the health of the entire community. It takes the concerted effort of many—if not most—of the individuals in a community to make a program work. For example, if each individual consciously recycles his or her trash each week, community recycling will be successful. Likewise, if each occupant would wear a safety belt, there could be a significant reduction in the number of facial injuries and deaths from car crashes for the entire community. In another example, the more individuals who become immunized against a specific disease, the slower the disease will spread and the fewer people will be exposed. This concept is known as **herd immunity**.

herd immunity
the resistance of a population to the spread of an infectious agent based on the immunity of a high proportion of individuals

A BRIEF HISTORY OF COMMUNITY AND PUBLIC HEALTH

The history of community and public health is almost as long as the history of civilization. This brief summary provides an account of some of the accomplishments and failures in

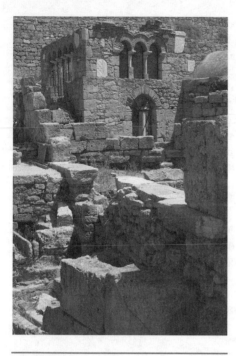

FIGURE 1.4

Archeological findings reveal community health practices of the past.

community and public health. It is hoped that a knowledge of the past will enable us to better prepare for future challenges to our community's health.

Earliest Civilizations

In all likelihood, the earliest community health practices went unrecorded. Perhaps these practices involved taboos against defecation within the tribal communal area or near the source of drinking water. Perhaps they involved rites associated with burial of the dead. Certainly, the use of herbs for the prevention and curing of diseases and communal assistance with childbirth are practices that predate archeological records.

Excavations at sites of some of the earliest known civilizations, dating from about 2000 B.C., have uncovered archeological evidence of community health activities (see Figure 1.4). A combination of additional archeological findings and written history provides much more evidence of community health activities through the seventeenth century. Box 1.2 provides a timeline and some of the highlights of that history for the Ancient Societies (before 500 B.C.), the Classical Cultures (500 B.C.–A.D. 500), the Middle Ages (A.D. 500–1500), and the period of Renaissance and Exploration (1500–1700)

The Eighteenth Century

The eighteenth century was characterized by industrial growth. Despite the beginnings of recognition of the nature of disease, living conditions were hardly conducive to good health. Cities were overcrowded, and water supplies were inadequate and often unsanitary. Streets were usually unpaved, filthy, and heaped with trash and garbage. Many homes had unsanitary dirt floors.

Workplaces were unsafe and unhealthy. A substantial portion of the workforce was made up of the poor, which included children, who were forced to work long hours as indentured servants. Many of these jobs were unsafe or involved working in unhealthy environments, such as textile factories and coal mines.

One medical advance made at the end of the eighteenth century deserves mention because of its significance for public health. In 1796, Dr. Edward Jenner successfully demonstrated the process of vaccination as a protection against smallpox. He did this by inoculating a boy with material from a cowpox (*Vaccinia*) pustule. When challenged later with material from a smallpox (*Variola*) pustule, the boy remained healthy.

Dr. Jenner's discovery remains as one of the great discoveries of all time for both medicine and for public health. Prior to Dr. Jenner's discovery, millions died or were severely disfigured by smallpox (see Figure 1.5). The only known prevention had been "variolation," inoculation with smallpox material itself. This was a risky procedure because people sometimes became quite ill with smallpox. Nonetheless, during the American Revolution, General George Washington ordered the Army of the American Colonies "variolated." He did this so that he could be sure an epidemic of smallpox would not wipe out his colonial forces.[27] Interestingly enough, the average age at death for one living in the United States during this time was 29 years.

Following the American Revolution, George Washington ordered the first U.S. census for the purpose of the apportionment of representation in the House of Representatives. The

BOX 1.2 **TIMELINE AND HIGHLIGHTS OF COMMUNITY AND PUBLIC HEALTH PRIOR TO 1700**

A. Early Civilizations
   1. Ancient Societies (before 500 B.C.)
      a. Prior to 2000 B.C.: Archeological findings provide evidence of sewage disposal and written medical prescriptions.
      b. Circa 1900 B.C.: Perhaps the earliest written record of public health was the Code of Hammurabi; included laws for physicians and health practices.[25]
      c. Circa 1500 B.C.: Bible's Book of Leviticus written; includes guidelines for personal cleanliness and sanitation.[25]
   2. Classical Cultures (500 B.C.–A.D. 500)
      a. Fifth and sixth centuries B.C.: Evidence that Greek men participated in games of strength and skill and swam in public facilities.[26]
      b. Greeks were involved in practice of community sanitation; involved in obtaining water from sources far away and not just local wells.[27]
      c. Romans were community minded; improved on community sanitation of Greeks; built aqueducts to transport water from miles away; built sewer systems; created regulation for building construction, refuse removal, and street cleaning and repair;[25] created hospitals as infirmaries for slaves.[28]
      d. Christians created hospitals as benevolent charitable organizations.[28]
      e. A.D. 476: Roman Empire fell and most public health activities ceased.
B. Middle Ages (A.D. 500–1500)
   a. A.D. 500–1000 (Dark Ages): Growing revulsion for Roman materialism and a growth of spirituality; health problems were considered to have both spiritual causes and spiritual solutions;[28] time referred to as the **spiritual era of public health**.

   b. Failure to take into account the role of the physical and biological environment in the causation of communicable diseases resulted in many unrelenting epidemics in which millions suffered and died.
      • Deadliest epidemics were from plague ("black death"); occurred in A.D. 543 and 1348 (this one killed 25 million; half of population of London lost and in some parts of France only 1 in 10 survived).[25]
      • A.D. 1200: More than 19,000 leper houses.
      • Other epidemics of period: Smallpox, diphtheria, measles, influenza, tuberculosis, anthrax, and trachoma.
      • A.D. 1492: Syphilis epidemic was last epidemic of the period.
C. Renaissance and Exploration (1500–1700)
   a. Rebirth of thinking about the nature of world and humankind.
   b. Belief that disease was caused by environmental, not spiritual, factors; for example, the term *malaria*, meaning bad air, is a direct reference to humid or swampy air.
   c. Observation of ill led to more accurate descriptions of symptoms and outcomes of diseases; observations led to first recognition of whooping cough, typhus, scarlet fever, and malaria as distinct and separate diseases.[27]
   d. Epidemics (e.g., smallpox, malaria, and plague) still rampant; plague epidemic killed 68,596 (15% of the population) in London in 1665.
   e. Explorers, conquerors, and merchants and their crews spread disease to colonists and indigenous people throughout the New World.

census, first taken in 1790, is still conducted every 10 years and serves as an invaluable source of information for community health planning.

As the eighteenth century came to a close, a young United States faced numerous disease problems, including continuing outbreaks of smallpox, cholera, typhoid fever, and yellow fever. Yellow fever outbreaks usually occurred in port cities such as Charleston, Baltimore, New York, and New Orleans, where ships arrived to dock from tropical America. The greatest single epidemic of yellow fever in America occurred in Philadelphia in 1793, where there were an estimated 23,000 cases, including 4,044 deaths in a population estimated at only 37,000.[29]

In response to these continuing epidemics and the need to address other mounting health problems, such as sanitation and protection of the water supply, several governmental

spiritual era of public health
a time during the Middle Ages when the causation of communicable disease was linked to spiritual forces

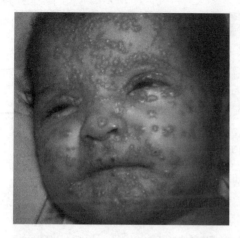

FIGURE 1.5

Prior to the elimination of smallpox, millions died or were severely disfigured by the disease.

health agencies were created. In 1798, the Marine Hospital Service (forerunner to the U.S. Public Health Service) was formed to deal with disease that was occurring onboard water vessels. By 1799, several of America's largest cities, including Boston, Philadelphia, New York, and Baltimore, also had founded municipal boards of health.

The Nineteenth Century

During the first half of the nineteenth century, few remarkable advancements in public health occurred. Living conditions in Europe and England remained unsanitary, and industrialization led to an even greater concentration of the population within cities. However, better agricultural methods led to improved nutrition for many.

During this period, America enjoyed westward expansion, characterized by a spirit of pioneering, self-sufficiency, and rugged individualism. The federal government's approach to health problems was characterized by the French term *laissez faire,* meaning noninterference. There were also few health regulations or health departments in rural areas. Health quackery thrived; this was truly a period when "buyer beware" was good advice.

Epidemics continued in major cities in both Europe and America. In 1854, another cholera epidemic struck London. Dr. John Snow studied the epidemic and hypothesized that the disease was being caused by the drinking water from the Broad Street pump. He obtained permission to remove the pump handle, and the epidemic was abated (see Figure 1.6). Snow's action was remarkable because it predated the discovery that microorganisms can cause disease. The predominant theory of contagious disease at the time was the "miasmas theory." According to this theory, vapors, or miasmas, were the source of many diseases. The miasmas theory remained popular throughout much of the nineteenth century.

In the United States in 1850, Lemuel Shattuck drew up a health report for the Commonwealth of Massachusetts that outlined the public health needs for the state. It included recommendations for the establishment of boards of health, the collection of vital statistics, the implementation of sanitary measures, and research on diseases. Shattuck also recommended health education and controlling exposure to alcohol, smoke, adulterated food, and nostrums (quack medicines).[25] Although some of his recommendations took years to implement (the Massachusetts Board of Health was not founded until 1869), the significance of Shattuck's report is such that 1850 is a key date in American public health; it marks the beginning of the **modern era of public health**.

modern era of public health the era of public health that began in 1850 and continues today

Real progress in the understanding of the causes of many communicable diseases occurred during the last quarter of the nineteenth century. One of the obstacles to progress was the theory of spontaneous generation, the idea that living organisms could arise from inorganic or nonliving matter. Akin to this idea was the thought that one type of contagious microbe could change into another type of organism.

In 1862, Louis Pasteur of France proposed his germ theory of disease. Throughout the 1860s and 1870s, he and others carried out experiments and made observations that supported this theory and disproved spontaneous generation. Pasteur is generally given credit for providing the death blow to the theory of spontaneous generation.

It was the German scientist Robert Koch who developed the criteria and procedures necessary to establish that a particular microbe, and no other, causes a particular disease. His first demonstration, with the anthrax bacillus, was in 1876. Between 1877 and the end of the century, the identity of numerous bacterial disease agents was established, including those that caused gonorrhea, typhoid fever, leprosy, tuberculosis, cholera, diphtheria, tetanus, pneumonia, plague, and dysentery. This period (1875-1900) has come to be known as the **bacteriological period of public health**.

Although most scientific discoveries in the late nineteenth century were made in Europe, there were significant public health achievements occurring in America as well. The first law prohibiting the adulteration of milk was passed in 1856, the first sanitary survey was carried out in New York City in 1864, and the American Public Health Association was founded in 1872. The Marine Hospital Service gained new powers of inspection and investigation under the Port Quarantine Act of 1878.[25] In 1890, the pasteurization of milk was introduced, and in 1891 meat inspection began. It was also during this time that nurses were first hired by industries (in 1895) and schools (in 1899). Also in 1895, septic tanks were introduced for sewage treatment. In 1900, Major Walter Reed of the U.S. Army announced that yellow fever was transmitted by mosquitoes.

The Twentieth Century

As the twentieth century began, life expectancy was still less than 50 years.[30] The leading causes of death were communicable diseases— influenza, pneumonia, tuberculosis, and infections of the gastrointestinal tract. Other communicable diseases, such as typhoid fever, malaria, and diphtheria, also killed many people.

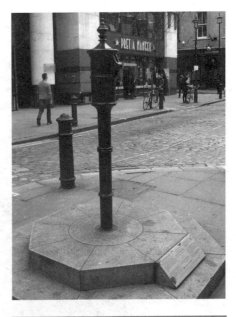

FIGURE 1.6

In London, England, 1854, John Snow helped interrupt a cholera epidemic by having the handle removed from this pump, located on Broad Street.

There were other health problems as well. Thousands of children were afflicted with conditions characterized by noninfectious diarrhea or by bone deformity. Although the symptoms of pellagra and rickets were known and described, the causes of these ailments remained a mystery at the turn of the century. Discovery that these conditions resulted from vitamin deficiencies was slow because some scientists were searching for bacterial causes.

bacteriological period of public health
the period of 1875–1900, during which the causes of many bacterial diseases were discovered

Vitamin deficiency diseases and one of their contributing conditions, poor dental health, were extremely common in the slum districts of both European and American cities. The unavailability of adequate prenatal and postnatal care meant that deaths associated with pregnancy and childbirth were also high.

Health Resources Development Period (1900–1960)

Much growth and development took place during the 60-year period from 1900 to 1960. Because of the growth of health care facilities and providers, this period of time is referred to as the **health resources development period**. This period can be further divided into the reform phase (1900-1920), the 1920s, the Great Depression and World War II, and the postwar years.

health resources development period
the years of 1900–1960, a time of great growth in health care facilities and providers

The Reform Phase (1900-1920)

By the beginning of the twentieth century, there was a growing concern about the many social problems in America. The remarkable discoveries in microbiology made in the previous years had not dramatically improved the health of the average citizen. By 1910, the urban population had grown to 45% of the total population (up from 19% in 1860). Much of the growth was the result of immigrants who came to America for the jobs created by new industries (see Figure 1.7). Northern cities were also swelling from the northward migration of black Americans from the southern states. Many of these workers had to accept poorly

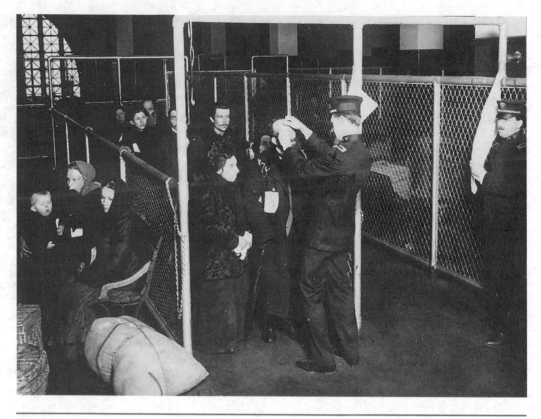

FIGURE 1.7

Ellis Island immigration between 1860 and 1910 resulted in dramatic increases in the urban population in America.

paying jobs involving hard labor and low wages. There was also a deepening chasm between the upper and lower classes, and social critics began to clamor for reform.

The years 1900 to 1920 have been called the **reform phase of public health**. The plight of the immigrants working in the meat packing industry was graphically depicted by Upton Sinclair in his book *The Jungle.* Sinclair's goal was to draw attention to unsafe working conditions. What he achieved was greater governmental regulation of the food industry through the passage of the Pure Food and Drugs Act of 1906.

The reform movement was broad, involving both social and moral as well as health issues. Edward T. Devine noted in 1909 that "Ill health is perhaps the most constant of the attendants of poverty."[30] The reform movement finally took hold when it became evident to the majority that neither the discoveries of the causes of many communicable diseases nor the continuing advancement of industrial production could overcome continuing disease and poverty. Even by 1917, the United States ranked fourteenth of 16 "progressive" nations in maternal death rate.[30]

Although the relationship between occupation and disease had been pointed out 200 years earlier in Europe, occupational health in America in 1900 was an unknown quantity. However, in 1910 the first International Congress on Occupational Diseases was held in Chicago.[31] That same year, the state of New York passed a tentative Workman's Compensation Act, and over the next 10 years most other states passed similar laws.[22] Also in 1910, the U.S. Bureau of Mines was created and the first clinic for occupational diseases was established in New York at Cornell Medical College.[30] By 1910, the movement for healthier conditions in the workplace was well established.

> **reform phase of public health**
> the years of 1900–1920, characterized by social movements to improve health conditions in cities and in the workplace

This period also saw the birth of the first national-level volunteer health agencies. The first of these agencies was the National Association for the Study and Prevention of Tuberculosis, which was formed in 1902. It arose from the first local voluntary health agency, the Pennsylvania Society for the Prevention of Tuberculosis, organized in 1892.[32] The American Cancer Society, Inc., was founded in 1913. That same year, the Rockefeller Foundation was established in New York. This philanthropic foundation has funded a great many public health projects, including work on hookworm and pellagra, and the development of a vaccine against yellow fever.

Another movement that began about this time was that of public health nursing. The first school nursing program was begun in New York City in 1902. In 1918, the first School of Public Health was established at Johns Hopkins University in Baltimore. This was followed by establishment of another school at Harvard University in 1923. Also in 1918 was the birth of school health instruction as we know it today.

These advances were matched with similar advances by governmental bodies. The Marine Hospital Service was renamed the Public Health and Marine Hospital Service in 1902 in keeping with its growing responsibilities. In 1912, it became the U.S. Public Health Service.[25]

By 1900, 38 states had state health departments. The rest followed during the first decades of the twentieth century. The first two local (county) health departments were established in 1911, one in Guilford County, North Carolina, and the other in Yakima County, Washington.

The 1920s

In comparison with the preceding period, the 1920s represented a decade of slow growth in public health, except for a few health projects funded by the Rockefeller and Millbank foundations. Prohibition resulted in a decline in the number of alcoholics and alcohol-related deaths. Although the number of county health departments had risen to 467 by 1929, 77% of the rural population still lived in areas with no health services.[32] However, it was during this period in 1922 that the first professional preparation program for health educators was begun at Columbia University by Thomas D. Wood, MD, whom many consider the father of health education. The life expectancy in 1930 had risen to 59.7 years.

The Great Depression and World War II

Until the Great Depression (1929–1935), individuals and families in need of social and medical services were dependent on friends and relatives, private charities, voluntary agencies, community chests, and churches. By 1933, after 3 years of economic depression, it became evident that private resources could never meet the needs of all the people who needed assistance. The drop in tax revenues during the Depression also reduced health department budgets and caused a virtual halt in the formation of new local health departments.[32]

Beginning in 1933, President Franklin D. Roosevelt created numerous agencies and programs for public works as part of his New Deal. Much of the money was used for public health, including the control of malaria, the building of hospitals and laboratories, and the construction of municipal water and sewer systems.

The Social Security Act of 1935 marked the beginning of the government's major involvement in social issues, including health. This act provided substantial support for state health departments and their programs, such as maternal and child health and sanitary facilities. As progress against the communicable diseases became visible, some turned their attention toward other health problems, such as cancer. The National Cancer Institute was formed in 1937.

America's involvement in World War II resulted in severe restrictions on resources available for public health programs. Immediately following the conclusion of the war, however, many of the medical discoveries made during wartime made their way into civilian medical practice. Two examples are the antibiotic penicillin, used for treating pneumonia, rheumatic fever, syphilis, and strep throat, and the insecticide DDT, used for killing insects that transmit diseases.

During World War II, the Communicable Disease Center was established in Atlanta, Georgia. Now called the Centers for Disease Control and Prevention (CDC), it has become the premier epidemiological center of the world.

The Postwar Years

Following the end of World War II, there was still concern about medical care and the adequacy of the facilities in which that care could be administered. In 1946, Congress passed the National Hospital Survey and Construction Act (the Hill-Burton Act). The goal of the legislation was to improve the distribution of medical care and to enhance the quality of hospitals. From 1946 through the 1960s, hospital construction occurred at a rapid rate with relatively little thought given to planning. Likewise, attempts to set national health priorities or to establish a national health agenda were virtually nonexistent.

The two major health events in the 1950s were the development of a vaccine to prevent polio and President Eisenhower's heart attack. The latter event helped America to focus on its number 1 killer, heart disease. When the president's physician suggested exercise, some Americans heeded his advice and began to exercise on a regular basis.

Period of Social Engineering (1960–1973)

The 1960s marked the beginning of a period when the federal government once again became active in health matters. The primary reason for this involvement was the growing realization that many Americans were still not reaping any of the benefits of 60 years of medical advances. These Americans, most of whom were poor or elderly, either lived in underserved areas or simply could not afford to purchase medical services.

Medicare
government health insurance for older adults and those with certain disabilities

In 1965, Congress passed the Medicare and Medicaid bills (amendments to the Social Security Act of 1935). **Medicare** assists in the payment of medical bills for older adults and certain people with disabilities, and **Medicaid** assists in the payment of medical bills for the poor. These pieces of legislation helped provide medical care for millions who would not otherwise have received it, and this legislation also improved standards in health care facilities. Unfortunately, the influx of federal dollars accelerated the rate of increase in the cost of health care for everyone. As a result, the 1970s, 1980s, and the 1990s saw repeated attempts and failures to bring the growing costs of health care under control.

Medicaid
government health insurance for the poor

Period of Health Promotion (1974– Present)

By the mid-1970s, it had become apparent that the greatest potential for saving lives and reducing health care costs in America was to be achieved through means other than health care.

> Most scholars, policymakers, and practitioners in health promotion would pick 1974 as the turning point that marks the beginning of health promotion as a significant component of national health policy in the twentieth century. That year Canada published its landmark policy statement, *A New Perspective on the Health of Canadians*.[33] In [1976] the United States, Congress passed PL 94-317, the Health Information and Health Promotion Act, which created the Office of Health Information and Health Promotion, later renamed the Office of Disease Prevention and Health Promotion.[34]

In the late 1970s, the Centers for Disease Control conducted a study that examined premature deaths (defined then as deaths prior to age 65, but now as deaths prior to age 75) in the United States in 1977. That study revealed that approximately 48% of all premature deaths could be traced to one's lifestyle or health behavior—choices that people make. Lifestyles characterized by a lack of exercise, unhealthy diets, smoking, uncontrolled hypertension, and the inability to control stress were found to be contributing factors to premature mortality.[35] This led the way for the U.S. government's publication *Healthy People: The*

Surgeon General's Report on Health Promotion and Disease Prevention.[36] "This document brought together much of what was known about the relationship of personal behavior and health status. The document also presented a 'personal responsibility' model that provided Americans with the prescription for reducing their health risks and increasing their chances for good health."[37]

Healthy People was then followed by the release of the first set of health goals and objectives for the nation, called *Promoting Health/Preventing Disease: Objectives for the Nation.*[38] At the time this edition of this book was going to press, the fourth edition of these goals and objectives, *Healthy People 2020*, was about to be released. Since their inception, these *Healthy People* documents have defined the nation's health agenda and guided its health policy since their inception (see Box 1.3).

BOX 1.3

TIMELINE AND HIGHLIGHTS OF COMMUNITY AND PUBLIC HEALTH FROM 1700–2000

A. Eighteenth Century (1700s)
  1. Period characterized by industrial growth; workplaces were unsafe and unhealthy
  2. 1790: first U.S. census
  3. 1793: yellow fever epidemic in Philadelphia
  4. 1796: Dr. Edward Jenner successfully demonstrated smallpox vaccination
  5. 1798: Marine Hospital Service (forerunner to U.S. Public Health Service) was formed
  6. By 1799: several of America's largest cities, including Boston, Philadelphia, New York, and Baltimore, had municipal boards of health

B. First Half of Nineteenth Century (1800–1848)
  1. U.S. government's approach to health was laissez faire
  2. 1813: first visiting nurse in United States

C. Second Half of 19th Century (1848–1900)
  1. 1849, 1854: London cholera epidemics
  2. 1850: Modern era of public health begins
  3. 1850: Shattuck's report
  4. 1854: Snow has pump handle removed from Broad Street pump
  5. 1863: Pasteur proposed germ theory
  6. 1872: American Public Health Association founded
  7. 1875–1900: Bacteriological period of public health
  8. 1876: Koch established relationship between a particular microbe and a particular disease
  9. 1900: Reed announced that yellow fever was transmitted by mosquitos

D. Twentieth Century
  1. Health Resources Development Period (1900–1960)
    a. The Reform Phase (1900–1920)
      • 1902: First national-level voluntary health agency created
      • 1906: Sinclair's *The Jungle* published
      • 1910: First International Congress on Occupational Diseases
      • 1910: 45% of U.S. population was in the cities
      • 1911: First local health department established

  • 1913: American Cancer Society founded
  • 1917: United States ranked 14th of 16 in maternal death rate
  • 1918: Birth of school health instruction
  • 1918: First school of public health established in United States
    2. 1920s
      a. 1922: Wood created first professional preparation program for health educators
      b. 1930: Life expectancy in the United States was 59.7 years
    3. The Great Depression and WWII
      a. 1933: New Deal; included unsuccessful attempt at national health care program
      b. 1935: Social Security Act passed
      c. 1937: National Cancer Institute formed
    4. Postwar Years
      a. 1946: National Hospital Survey and Construction (Hill-Burton) Act passed
      b. 1952: Development of polio vaccine
      c. 1955: Eisenhower's heart attack

E. Period of Social Engineering (1960–1973)
  1. 1965: Medicare and Medicaid bills passed

F. Period of Health Promotion (1974–present)
  1. 1974: Nixon's unsuccessful attempt at national health care program
  2. 1974: *A New Perspective on the Health of Canadians* published
  3. 1976: Health Information and Health Promotion Act passed
  4. 1979: *Healthy People* published
  5. 1980: *Promoting Health/Preventing Disease: Objectives of the Nation* published
  6. 1990: *Healthy People 2000* published
  7. 1997: Clinton's unsuccessful attempt at a national health care program
  8. 2000: *Healthy People 2010* published

Community Health in the Early 2000s

Early in the new millennium, it is widely agreed that although decisions about health are an individual's responsibility to a significant degree, society has an obligation to provide an environment in which the achievement of good health is possible and encouraged. Furthermore, many recognize that certain segments of our population whose disease and death rates exceed the general population may require additional resources, including education, to achieve good health.

The American people face a number of serious public health problems. These problems include the continuing rise in health care costs, growing environmental concerns, the ever-present lifestyle diseases, emerging and reemerging communicable diseases, serious substance abuse problems, and disasters, both natural and humanmade. In the paragraphs that follow, we have elaborated on each of these problems briefly because they seem to represent a significant portion of the community health agenda for the years ahead.

Health Care Delivery

In the previous edition of this book, in this section we wrote about the large number of Americans who were uninsured and the rising cost of health care and how these problems had detrimental effects on both the physical health of individuals and the economic health of the nation. In March 2010, significant changes were made to the U.S. health care system when President Barack Obama signed the Affordable Care Act (ACA) into law. Though the law has many components, the primary focus is to increase the number of Americans with health insurance (see Chapter 13 for a more in-depth discussion of the Affordable Health Care Act). The ACA does this, but by providing health insurance to an additional 32 million Americans, the costs will also go up, which will continue to make U.S. health care the most expensive in the world. In 2010, health expenditures were projected to be almost $2.6 trillion, consume 17.3% of the gross domestic product (GDP), and are expected to reach $4.5 trillion and 19.3% of the GDP by 2019.[39] America spends more per capita annually on health care (estimated at $8,290 in 2010)[39] than any other nation. The cost of health care is an issue that still needs to be addressed.

Environmental Problems

Millions of Americans live in communities where the air is unsafe to breathe, the water is unsafe to drink, or solid waste is disposed of improperly. With a few minor exceptions, the rate at which we pollute our environment continues to increase. Many Americans still believe that our natural resources are unlimited and that their individual contributions to the overall pollution are insignificant. In actuality, we must improve on our efforts in resource preservation and energy conservation if our children are to enjoy an environment as clean as ours. These environmental problems are compounded by the fact that the world population continues to grow; it is now more than 6.9 billion people and expected to reach 8 billion by the year 2026.[40]

Lifestyle Diseases

The leading causes of death in the United States today are not the communicable diseases that were so feared 100 years ago but chronic illnesses resulting from unwise lifestyle choices. The prevalence of obesity and diseases like diabetes is increasing. The four leading causes of death in the early 2000s are heart disease, cancer, chronic lower respiratory diseases, and stroke.[41] Although it is true that everyone has to die from some cause sometime, too many Americans die prematurely because of their unhealthy lifestyles. In the latter part of the twentieth century, it was known that better control of behavioral risk factors alone—such as lack of exercise, poor diet, use of tobacco and drugs, and alcohol abuse—could prevent between 40% and 70% of all premature deaths, one-third of all acute disabilities, and

Table 1.1
Comparison of Most Common Causes of Death and Actual Causes of Death

Most Common Causes of Death, United States, 2008	Actual Causes of Death, United States, 2000
1. Diseases of the heart	1. Tobacco
2. Malignant neoplasms (cancers)	2. Poor diet and physical inactivity
3. Chronic lower respiratory diseases	3. Alcohol consumption
4. Cerebrovascular diseases (stroke)	4. Microbial agents
5. Unintentional injuries (accidents)	5. Toxic agents
7. Alzheimer's disease	6. Motor vehicles
6. Diabetes mellitus	7. Firearms
8. Influenza and pneumonia	8. Sexual behavior
9. Nephritis, nephrotic syndrome, and nephrosis	9. Illicit drug use
10. Septicemia	

Sources: Miniño, A. M., J. Q. Xu, and K. D. Kochanek (2010). "Deaths: Preliminary Data for 2008." *National Vital Statistics Reports,* 59(2): Hyattsville, MD: National Center for Health Statistics; Mokdad, A. H., J. S. Marks, D. F. Stroup, and J. L. Gerberding (2004). "Actual Causes of Death, in the United States, 2000." *Journal of the American Medical Association,* 291(10): 1238–1245; and Mokdad, A. H., J. S. Marks, D. F. Stroup, and J. L. Gerberding (2005). "Correction: Actual Causes of Death, in the United States, 2000." *Journal of the American Medical Association,* 293(3): 293–294.

two-thirds of chronic disabilities.[42] Now into the twenty-first century, behavior patterns continue to "represent the single most prominent domain of influence over health prospects in the United States."[9] (See Table 1.1.)

Communicable Diseases

Although communicable (infectious) diseases no longer constitute the leading causes of death in the United States, they remain a concern for several reasons. First, they are the primary reason for days missed at school or at work. The success in reducing the life-threatening nature of these diseases has made many Americans complacent about obtaining vaccinations or taking other precautions against contracting these diseases. With the exception of smallpox, none of these diseases has been eradicated, although several should have been, such as measles.

Second, as new communicable diseases continue to appear, old ones such as tuberculosis reemerge, sometimes in drug-resistant forms, demonstrating that communicable diseases still represent a serious community health problem in America. Legionnaires' disease, toxic shock syndrome, Lyme disease, acquired immunodeficiency syndrome (AIDS), and severe acute respiratory syndrome (SARS) are diseases that were unknown only 30 years ago. The first cases of AIDS were reported in June 1981.[43] By August 1989, 100,000 cases had been reported,[44] and it took only an additional two years to report the second 100,000 cases.[45] By 2006, more than a million cases of the disease had been reported to the CDC.[46] (See Figure 1.8.) The total number of cases continues to grow with close to 40,000 new cases being diagnosed each year.[47] Also, diseases that were once only found in animals are now crossing over to human populations and causing much concern and action. Included in

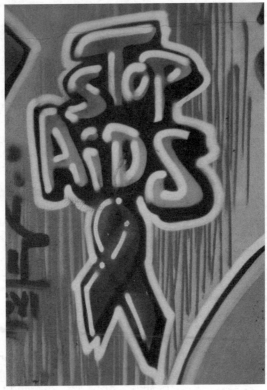

FIGURE 1.8
AIDS is one of the most feared communicable diseases today.

this group of diseases are avian flu, *Escherichia coli* O157:H7, hantavirus, mad cow disease, and SARS.[1]

Third, and maybe the most disturbing, is the use of communicable diseases for bioterrorism. **Bioterrorism** involves "the threatened or intentional release of biological agents (virus, bacteria, or their toxins) for the purpose of influencing the conduct of government or intimidating or coercing a civilian population to further political or social objectives. These agents can be released by way of the air (as aerosols) food, water or insects."[10] Concern in the United States over bioterrorism was heightened after 9/11 and the subsequent intentional distribution of *Bacillus anthracis* spores through the U.S. postal system (the anthrax mailings). The anthrax mailings resulted in 22 people developing anthrax, 5 of whom died. In addition, thousands more were psychologically affected, and between 10 thousand and 20 thousand people were advised to take postexposure prophylactic treatment because they were at known or potential risk for inhalational anthrax.[48]

bioterrorism
the threatened or intentional release of biological agents for the purpose of influencing the conduct of government or intimidating or coercing a civilian population to further political or social objectives

Alcohol and Other Drug Abuse

"Abuse of legal and illegal drugs has become a national problem that costs this country thousands of lives and billions of dollars each year. Alcohol and other drugs are often associated with unintentional injuries, domestic violence, and violent crimes."[49] Federal, state, and local governments as well as private agencies attempt to address the supply and demand problems associated with the abuse of alcohol and other drugs, but a significant challenge remains for America.

Health Disparities

health disparities
the difference in health among different populations

It has long been "recognized that some individuals are healthier than others and that some live longer than others do, and that often these differences are closely associated with social characteristics such as race, ethnicity, gender, location, and socioeconomic status."[50] These gaps between groups have been referred to as *health disparities* (also call health inequalities in some countries). More formally, **health disparities** has been defined as the difference in health among different populations. Health disparities are a problem in the United States in that many minority groups' health status, on many different measures, is not as good as the white population. Efforts have been put forth to eliminate the disparities, as evidenced by one of the *Healthy People 2020* overarching goals to "achieve health equity, eliminate disparities, and improve the health for all groups." Many experts think these differences have been caused by two *health inequities*—lack of access to health care, and/or when health care is received the quality has not been as good for those in minority groups. Whatever the reason, health disparities continue to be a problem and much more needs to be done.

Disasters

Disasters can be classified into two primary categories—natural (or conventional) and human-made (or technological disasters).[1] Whereas *natural disasters* are the result of the combination of the forces of nature (e.g., hurricane, flood, blizzard, tornado, earthquake, landslide) and human activities,[51] *humanmade disasters* result from either unintentional (e.g., spill of a toxic substance into the environment) or intentional (e.g., bioterrorism) human activities, often associated with the use or misuse of technology. Both types of disasters have the potential to cause injury, death, disease, and damage to property on a large scale.[1] In recent years, the United States has felt the large-scale impact of both types of disasters via the Gulf oil spill, Hurricanes Katrina and Rita, and the severe flooding in the middle of the country. All of these events showed us that the preparation for such disasters was not adequate and that each type of disaster required different resources and a different response.

Even though the causes of the two categories of disasters are different, preparedness for them has many common elements. It has been noted that preparedness for natural disasters is the foundation for preparedness for humanmade disasters.[52] That is, in preparing for natural disasters, the basic components of an adequate disaster response system have been defined, and the steps necessary to build disaster preparedness capacity have been established.[52] What needs to be added are specific steps to deal with the peculiarity of the humanmade disasters. An example of this would be the need for decontamination following exposure to a biological agent.

Even given the devastating consequences of natural disasters, such as Hurricanes Katrina and Rita, flooding, or the forest fires that consume many thousands of acres of woodlands each year (see Chapter 14 for more on natural disasters), it has been the intentional humanmade disasters—specifically terrorism—that have occupied much of our attention in recent years (see Figure 1.9).

Mention was made earlier of the use of a communicable disease as part of terrorism. However, in fact a number of agents could be used as part of terrorism. Since the anthrax mailings, community and public health professionals have focused on the possibility that future terrorism could include chemical, nuclear/radiological, and/or biological (CNB) agents, resulting in mass numbers of casualties. Such concern led to an evaluation of community and public health emergency preparedness and response. "Determining the level of state and local health departments' emergency preparedness and response capacities is crucial because public health officials are among those, along with firefighters, emergency medical personnel, and local law enforcement personnel, who serve on 'rapid response' teams when large-scale emergency situations arise."[13] Results of that evaluation showed that the public health infrastructure was not where it should be to handle large-scale emergencies, as well as a number of more common public health concerns.

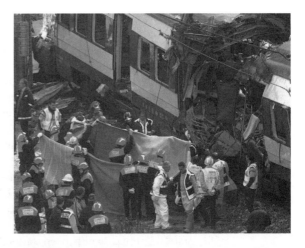

FIGURE 1.9

Terrorism has become a concern thoughout the world.

> The . . . public health infrastructure has suffered from political neglect and from the pressure of political agendas and public opinion that frequently override empirical evidence. Under the glare of a national crisis, policy makers and the public became aware of vulnerable and outdated health information systems and technologies, an insufficient and inadequately trained public health workforce, antiquated laboratory capacity, a lack of real-time surveillance and epidemiological systems, ineffective and fragmented communications networks, incomplete domestic preparedness and emergency response capabilities, and communities without access to essential public health services.[13]

Based on the results of several different evaluations that exposed many weaknesses in emergency preparedness in general and in the public health infrastructure more specifically, investment in public health preparedness has increased since September 11, 2001. Those federal departments that have been responsible for most of the effort have been the Departments of Homeland Security (DHS) and Health and Human Services (DHHS). The DHS has the responsibility of protecting America, whereas the DHHS, has taken the leadership for public health and medical preparedness. **Public health preparedness** has been defined as "the ability of the *public health system, community, and individuals* to prevent, protect against, quickly respond to, and recover from health emergencies, particularly those in which scale, timing, or unpredictability threatens to overwhelm routine capabilities,"[53] and **medical preparedness** has been defined as "the ability of the *health care system* to prevent, protect against, quickly respond to, and recover from health emergencies, particularly those whose scale, timing, or

public health preparedness the ability of the *public health system, community, and individuals* to prevent, protect against, quickly respond to, and recover from health emergencies, particularly those in which scale, timing, or unpredictability threatens to overwhelm routine capabilities

medical preparedness the ability of the *health care system* to prevent, protect against, quickly respond to, and recover from health emergencies, particularly those whose scale, timing, or unpredictability threatens to overwhelm routine capabilities

unpredictability threatens to overwhelm routine capabilities."[53] Information about emergency preparedness and response can be found on the Web sites of all DHHS agencies; however, those that have been most visible have been the Centers for Disease Control and Prevention (CDC), the Health Resources and Services Administration (HRSA), and the Agency for Healthcare Research and Quality (AHRQ).

Since 9/11, the federal government, through a variety of funding sources and programs, has worked to strengthen homeland security, emergency preparedness, and response at all levels. The funding has been used to create or enhance the various components needed in disaster situations (i.e., communication, coordination, and training for personnel). The funding also had to be used to bring much of the public health system up-to-date (i.e., laboratories, personnel, and surveillance) after many years of neglect.

Though the United States is better prepared than prior to 9/11, much still needs to be done. In December 2009, the Trust for America's Health (TFAH), a nonprofit, nonpartisan organization, and the Robert Wood Johnson Foundation released their seventh report on the state of public health preparedness in the United States.[54] The report, titled *Ready or Not 2009?: Protecting the Public's Health from Disease, Disasters, and Bioterrrorism*, contained preparedness scores for all 50 states and the District of Columbia based on 10 key indicators to assess health emergency preparedness capabilities. Much of the seventh report focuses on the H1N1 flu outbreak the previous flu season. The indicators were developed in consultation with leading public health experts based on data from publicly available sources or information provided by public officials. "Twenty states scored six or less out of 10 key indicators of public health emergency preparedness. Nearly two-thirds of states scored seven or less. Eight states tied for the highest score of nine out of 10: Arkansas, Delaware, New York, North Carolina, North Dakota, Oklahoma, Texas, and Vermont. Montana had the lowest score at three out of 10."[54] Some key findings from the report include the following:

- 27 states cut funding for public health from FY 2007–08 to 2008–09.

- 13 states have purchased less than 50 percent of their share of federally subsidized antiviral drugs to stockpile for use during an influenza pandemic.

- 14 states do not have the capacity in place to assure the timely pick-up and delivery of laboratory samples on a 24/7 basis to the Laboratory Response Network (LRN).

- 11 states and D.C. report not having enough laboratory staffing capacity to work five 12-hour days for six to eight weeks in response to an infectious disease outbreak, such as H1N1.[54]

Michelle Larkin, JD, Public Health Team Director and Senior Program Officer at the Robert Wood Johnson Foundation, commented on the report by saying, "State and local health departments around the country are being asked to do more with less during the H1N1 outbreak as budgets continue to be stretched beyond their limits. Public health provides essential prevention and preparedness services that help us lead healthier lives— without sustained and stable funding, Americans will continue to be needlessly at risk from the next public health threat."[55]

OUTLOOK FOR COMMUNITY HEALTH IN THE TWENTY-FIRST CENTURY

So far in this chapter we have discussed community health, past and present. Now we describe what community health leaders in the United States and elsewhere in the world hope to achieve in the coming years.

World Planning for the Twenty-First Century

World health leaders recognized the need to plan for the twenty-first century at the thirtieth World Health Assembly of the World Health Organization, held in 1977. At that assembly, delegations from governments around the world set as a target "that the level of health to be attained by the turn of the century should be that which will permit all people to lead a socially and economically productive life."[56] This target goal became known as "Health for All by the Year 2000." The following year in Alma-Ata, U.S.S.R., the joint WHO/UNICEF (United Nations Children's Fund) International Conference adopted a Declaration on Primary Health Care as the key to attaining the goal of Health for All by the Year 2000. At the thirty-fourth World Health Assembly in 1981, delegates from the member nations unanimously adopted a Global Strategy for Health for All by the Year 2000. That same year, the United Nations General Assembly endorsed the Global Strategy and urged other international organizations concerned with community health to collaborate with the WHO. The underlying concept of Health for All by the Year 2000 was that health resources should be distributed in such a way that essential health care services are accessible to everyone.

As we now know, the lofty goal of health for all around the world by the year 2000 was not reached. That does not mean that the goal was abandoned. With the passing into a new century, the program was renamed Health for All (HFA). HFA continues to seek "to create the conditions where people have, as a fundamental human right, the opportunity to reach and maintain the highest level of health. The vision of a renewed HFA policy builds on the WHO Constitution, the experience of the past and the needs for the future."[57]

As one might expect with all of the unrest worldwide, the progress to HFA is slow. Yet, some progress has been made. Life expectancy has increased by between 6 and 7 years globally in the last 30 years, due primarily to (1) social and economic development, (2) the wider provision of safe water and sanitation facilities, and (3) the expansion of national health services.[58] However, all do not share in this increased life expectancy. "There are widening health inequities between and within countries, between rich and poor, between men and women, and between different ethnic groups. More than a billion of the world's poorest people are not benefiting from the major advances in health care and several countries, particularly in sub-Saharan Africa, have seen a decline in life expectancy due in part to the HIV/AIDS epidemic."[58]

The work and the related tasks that face the WHO are enormous. The widening health gap is fueled by the impact of communicable diseases, global increases in noncommunicable diseases (especially from tobacco use, unhealthy diets, physical inactivity, and alcohol abuse), and unintentional injuries (primarily from road traffic crashes). What makes the work even more difficult is that "WHO operates in an increasingly complex and rapidly changing landscape. The boundaries of public health action have become blurred, extending into other sectors that influence health opportunities and outcomes. WHO responds to these challenges using a six-point agenda. The six points address two health objectives, two strategic needs, and two operational approaches."[59] These six points and a brief rationale for each are presented in Box 1.4.

As might be inferred from the stated priority areas in Box 1.4, much of the attention for improved world health in the twenty-first century is focused on the less developed and poorer countries of the world. The plan for tackling these global health challenges and other non-health-related global challenges of the twenty-first century is guided by the *United Nations Millennium Declaration*,[60] which was adopted at the United Nations' Millennium Summit in September 2000. More information about the declaration is presented in Chapter 2 in the section that discusses the WHO.

BOX 1.4

THE WHO AGENDA

1. *Promoting development.* During the past decade, health has achieved unprecedented prominence as a key driver of socioeconomic progress, and more resources than ever are being invested in health. Yet poverty continues to contribute to poor health, and poor health anchors large populations in poverty. Health development is directed by the ethical principle of equity: Access to life-saving or health-promoting interventions should not be denied for unfair reasons, including those with economic or social roots. Commitment to this principle ensures that WHO activities aimed at health development give priority to health outcomes in poor, disadvantaged, or vulnerable groups. Attainment of the health-related Millennium Development Goals, preventing and treating chronic diseases and addressing the neglected tropical diseases, are the cornerstones of the health and development agenda.

2. *Fostering health security.* Shared vulnerability to health security threats demands collective action. One of the greatest threats to international health security arises from outbreaks of emerging and epidemic-prone diseases. Such outbreaks are occurring in increasing numbers, fueled by such factors as rapid urbanization, environmental mismanagement, the way food is produced and traded, and the way antibiotics are used and misused. The world's ability to defend itself collectively against outbreaks has been strengthened since June 2007, when the revised International Health Regulations came into force.

3. *Strengthening health systems.* For health improvement to operate as a poverty-reduction strategy, health services must reach poor and underserved populations. Health systems in many parts of the world are unable to do so, making the strengthening of health systems a high priority for WHO. Areas being addressed include the provision of adequate numbers of appropriately trained staff, sufficient financing, suitable systems for collecting vital statistics, and access to appropriate technology including essential drugs.

4. *Harnessing research, information, and evidence.* Evidence provides the foundation for setting priorities, defining strategies, and measuring results. WHO generates authoritative health information, in consultation with leading experts, to set norms and standards, articulate evidence-based policy options, and monitor the evolving global heath situation.

5. *Enhancing partnerships.* WHO carries out its work with the support and collaboration of many partners, including UN agencies and other international organizations, donors, civil society, and the private sector. WHO uses the strategic power of evidence to encourage partners implementing programs within countries to align their activities with best technical guidelines and practices, as well as with the priorities established by countries.

6. *Improving performance.* WHO participates in ongoing reforms aimed at improving its efficiency and effectiveness, both at the international level and within countries. WHO aims to ensure that its strongest asset—its staff—works in an environment that is motivating and rewarding. WHO plans its budget and activities through results-based management, with clear expected results to measure performance at country, regional and international levels.

Source: Reprinted with permission of World Health Organization (2010). "The WHO Agenda." Available at http://www.who.int/about/agenda/en/index.html. Accessed October 28, 2010.

The United States' Planning for the Twenty-First Century

In addition to its participation in WHO's plans for the twenty-first century, the United States has created its own plans. The United States has decided to develop its planning process around 10-year blocks of time. The current plan is called *Healthy People 2020*.[61] As noted earlier in this chapter, *Healthy People 2020* and its three predecessor editions do in fact outline the health agenda of the nation. Some have referred to the *Healthy People* documents as the health blueprint of the nation. Each of these documents obviously is created on the best available data at the time, but all have been structured in a similar way. All four editions include several overarching goals and many supporting objectives for the nation's health. The goals provide a general focus and direction, while the objectives are used to measure progress within a specified period of time. Formal reviews (i.e., measured progress) of these objectives are conducted both at midcourse (i.e., halfway through the 10-year period) and again at the end of 10 years. The midcourse review provides an opportunity to update the document based on the events of the first half of the decade for which the objectives are written. For example, in *Healthy People 2010*, a number of objectives were changed, updated, or deleted because of the events of 9/11 and Hurricanes Katrina and Rita. Both the results of the midcourse and end reviews along with other available data are used to help create the next set of goals and objectives.

Healthy People 2020, which was released in December 2010, includes a vision statement, a mission statement, four overarching goals (see Table 1.2), and many objectives spread over 42 different topic areas (see Table 1.3). On the Healthy People.gov Web site each topic has its own Web page. At a minimum each page contains a concise goal statement, a brief overview of the topic that provides the background and context for the topic, a statement about the importance of the topic backed up by appropriate evidence, and references. There are two types of objectives—measurable and developmental. The measurable objectives provide direction for action and include national baseline data from which the 2020 target was set. The developmental objectives provide a vision for a desired outcome or health status, but national baseline data were not available when they were written. The purpose of developmental objectives is to identify areas of emerging importance and to drive the development of data systems to measure them.

The developers of *Healthy People 2020* think that the best way to implement the national objectives is with the framework referred to as MAP-IT (see Figure 1.10). MAP-IT stands for Mobilize, Assess, Plan, Implement, and Track. The Mobilize step of MAP-IT deals with bringing interested parties together within communities to deal with health issues. The second step, Assess, is used to find out who is affected by the health problem and examine what resources are available to deal with the problem. In the Plan step, goals and objectives are created and an intervention is planned that has the best chances of dealing with the health problem. The Implement step deals with putting the intervention into action. And the final step, Track, deals with evaluating the impact of the intervention on the health problem.[61]

Table 1.2
Healthy People 2020 Vision, Mission, and Goals

Vision

A society in which all people live long, healthy lives.

Mission

Healthy People 2020 strives to:
- Identify nationwide health improvement priorities
- Increase public awareness and understanding of the determinants of health, disease, and disability and the opportunities for progress
- Provide measurable objectives and goals that are applicable at the national, state, and local levels
- Engage multiple sectors to take actions to strengthen policies and improve practices that are driven by the best available evidence and knowledge
- Identify critical research, evaluation, and data collection needs

Overarching Goals
- Attain high-quality, longer lives free of preventable disease, disability, injury, and premature death.
- Achieve health equity, eliminate disparities, and improve the health of all groups.
- Create social and physical environments that promote good health for all.
- Promote quality of life, healthy development, and healthy behaviors across all life stages.

Source: U.S. Department of Health and Human Services (2010). *About Healthy People.* Available at http://www.healthypeople.gov/2020/about/default.aspx. Accessed December 13, 2010.

Table 1.3
Healthy People 2020 **Topic Areas**

1. Access to Health Services
2. Adolescent Health
3. Arthritis, Osteoporosis, and Chronic Back Conditions
4. Blood Disorders and Blood Safety
5. Cancer
6. Chronic Kidney Disease
7. Dementias, Including Alzheimer's Disease
8. Diabetes
9. Disability and Health
10. Early and Middle Childhood
11. Educational and Community-Based Programs
12. Environmental Health
13. Family Planning
14. Food Safety
15. Genomics
16. Global Health
17. Healthcare-Associated Infections
18. Health Communication and Health Information Technology
19. Health-Related Quality of Life and Well-Being
20. Hearing and Other Sensory or Communication Disorders
21. Heart Disease and Stroke
22. HIV
23. Immunization and Infectious Diseases
24. Injury and Violence Prevention
25. Lesbian, Gay, Bisexual, and Transgender Health
26. Maternal, Infant, and Child Health
27. Medical Product Safety
28. Mental Health and Mental Disorders
29. Nutrition and Weight Status
30. Occupational Safety and Health
31. Older Adults
32. Oral Health
33. Physical Activity
34. Preparedness
35. Public Health Infrastructure
36. Respiratory Diseases
37. Sexually Transmitted Diseases
38. Sleep Health
39. Social Determinants of Health
40. Substance Abuse
41. Tobacco Use
42. Vision

Source: U.S. Department of Health and Human Services (2010). *Topics & Objectives Index—Healthy People*. Available at http://www.healthypeople.gov/2020/topicsobjectives2020/default.aspx. Accessed December 13, 2010.

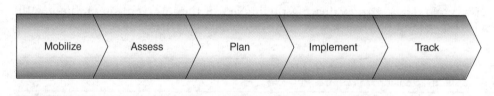

FIGURE 1.10

The Action Model to Achieve Healthy People Goals

Source: U.S. Department of Health and Human Services (2010). *Implementing Healthy People 2020*. Available at http://www.healthypeople.gov/2020/implementing/default.aspx. Accessed December 16, 2010.

As can be seen in the material presented in the last few pages, both the World Health Organization and the U.S. Department of Health and Human Services have much work ahead to improve the health of the people of the world and the United States in the twenty-first century. Because the planning to improve health is always changing, we urge all students of community and public health to stay up-to-date by regularly visiting both the World Health Organization and *Healthy People 2020* Web sites.

CHAPTER SUMMARY

- A number of key terms are associated with the study of community health, including *health, community, community health, population health, public health, public health system,* and *global health.*

- The four factors that affect the health of a community are physical (e.g., community size), social and cultural (e.g., religion), community organization, and individual behaviors (e.g., exercise and diet).

- It is important to be familiar with and understand the history of community health to be able to deal with the present and future community health issues.

- The earliest community health practices went unrecorded; however, archeological findings of ancient societies (before 500 B.C.) show evidence of concern for community health. There is evidence during the time of the classical cultures (500 B.C.–A.D. 500) that people were interested in physical strength, medicine, and sanitation.

- The belief of many living during the Middle Ages (A.D. 500–1500) was that health and disease were associated with spirituality. Many epidemics were seen during this period.

- During the Renaissance period (A.D. 1500–1700), there was a growing belief that disease was caused by the environment, not spiritual factors.

- The eighteenth century was characterized by industrial growth. Science was being used more in medicine and it was during this century that the first vaccine was discovered.

- The nineteenth century ushered in the modern era of public health. The germ theory was introduced during this time, and the last fourth of the century is known as the bacteriological period of public health.

- The twentieth century can be divided into several periods. The health resources development period (1900–1960) was a time when many public and private resources were used to improve health. The period of social engineering (1960–1973) saw the U.S. government's involvement in health insurance through Medicare and Medicaid. The health promotion period began in 1974 and continues today.

- Great concern still exists for health care, the environment, diseases caused by an impoverished lifestyle, the spread of communicable diseases (such as AIDS, Legionnaires' disease, toxic shock syndrome, and Lyme disease), the harm caused by alcohol and other drug abuse, and terrorism.

- Both the WHO and the U.S. government continue to plan for the health of humanity. The planning of the United States is reflected in the *Healthy People* documents, the health agenda for the nation.

SCENARIO: ANALYSIS AND RESPONSE

The Internet has many sources of information that could help Amy and Eric with the decisions that they will have to make about the continued use of the day care center for their children. Use a search engine (e.g., Google, Bing) and enter (a) hepatitis, and (b) hepatitis and day care centers. Print out the information that you find and use it in answering the following questions.

1. Based on the information you found on the Web, if you were Amy or Eric would you take your children to the day care center the next day? Why or why not?

2. Do you feel the hepatitis problem in day care centers is a personal health concern or a community health concern? Why?

3. Which of the factors noted in this chapter that affect the health of a community play a part in the hepatitis problem faced by Amy and Eric?

4. Why does the hepatitis problem remind us of the health problems faced by people in this country prior to 1900?

5. Under which of the focus areas in the *Healthy People 2020* would hepatitis fall? Why?

REVIEW QUESTIONS

1. How did the WHO define health in 1946? How has that definition been modified?

2. What is public health?

3. What are the differences among community health, population health, and global health?

4. What are the five major domains that determine a person's health?

5. What is the difference between personal health activities and community health activities?

6. Define the term *community*.

7. What are four major factors that affect the health of a community? Provide an example of each.

8. Identify some of the major events of community health in each of the following periods of time:

   Early civilizations (prior to A.D. 500)

   Middle Ages (A.D. 500–1500)

   Renaissance and Exploration (A.D. 1500–1700)

   The eighteenth century

   The nineteenth century

9. Provide a brief explanation of the origins from which the following twentieth-century periods get their names:

   Health resources development period

   Period of social engineering

   Period of health promotion

10. What are the major community health problems facing the United States in the twenty-first century?

11. What is included in the World Health Organization's Agenda?

12. What significance do the *Healthy People* documents have in community health development in recent years?

13. What significance do you think *Healthy People 2020* will have in the years ahead?

ACTIVITIES

1. Write your own definition for *health*.

2. In a two-page paper, explain how the five major determinants of health could interact to cause a disease such as cancer.

3. In a one-page paper, explain why heart disease can be both a personal health problem and a community health problem.

4. Select a community health problem that exists in your hometown; then, using the factors that affect the health of a community noted in this chapter, analyze and

discuss in a two-page paper at least three factors that contribute to the problem in your hometown.

5. Select one of the following individuals (all have been identified in this chapter), go to the library and do some additional reading or find two reliable Web sites, and then write a two-page paper on the person's contribution to community health.

   Edward Jenner

   John Snow

   Lemuel Shattuck

   Louis Pasteur

   Robert Koch

   Walter Reed

6. Review a copy of *Healthy People 2020* on the Web. Then, set up a time to talk with an administrator in your hometown health department. Find out which of the objectives the health department has been working on as priorities. Summarize in a paper what the objectives are, what the health department is doing about them, and what it hopes to accomplish by the year 2020.

COMMUNITY HEALTH ON THE WEB

The Internet contains a wealth of information about community and public health. Increase your knowledge of some of the topics presented in this chapter by accessing the Jones & Bartlett Learning Web site at **http://health .jbpub.com/book/communityhealth/7e** and follow the links to complete the following Web activities.

- *Healthy People 2020*
- Department of Homeland Security
- Global Health

REFERENCES

1. Schneider, M.-J. (2011). *Introduction to Public Health*, 3rd ed. Sudbury, MA: Jones and Bartlett.

2. Bunker, J. P., H. S. Frazier, and F. Mosteller (1994). "Improving Health: Measuring Effects of Medical Care." *Milbank Quarterly*, 72: 225–258.

3. Centers for Disease Control and Prevention (1999). "Ten Great Public Health Achievements—United States, 1900–1999." *Morbidity and Mortality Weekly Report*, 48(12): 241–243.

4. Koplan, J. (2000). *21st Century Health Challenges: Can We All Become Healthy, Wealthy, and Wise?* Available at http://www .pitt.edu/~super1/lecture/lec1361/origin.htm.

5. National Safety Council (1997). *Accident Facts, 1997 Edition*. Itasca, IL: Author.

6. World Health Organization (2010). *Glossary of Globalization, Trade, and Health Terms*. Geneva, Switzerland: Author. Available at http://www.who.int/trade/glossary/en/.

7. Hancock, T., and M. Minkler (2005). "Community Health Assessment or Healthy Community Assessment." In M. Minkler, ed., *Community Organizing and Community Building for Health*, 2nd ed. New Brunswick, NJ: Rutgers University Press, 138–157.

8. McGinnis, J. M. (2001). "United States." In C. E. Koop, ed., *Critical Issues in Global Health*. San Francisco: Jossey-Bass, 80–90.

9. McGinnis, J. M., P. Williams-Russo, and J. R. Knickman (2002). "The Case for More Active Policy Attention to Health Promotion." *Health Affairs*, 21(2): 78–93.

10. Turnock, B. J. (2009). *Public Health: What It Is and How It Works*, 4th ed. Sudbury, MA: Jones and Bartlett.

11. Minkler, M., N. Wallerstein, and N. Wilson (2008). "Improving Health Through Community Organizing and Community Building." In K. Glanz, B. K. Rimer, and K. Viswanath, eds., *Health Behavior and Health Education Practice: Theory, Research, and Practice*, 4th ed. San Francisco: Jossey-Bass, 287–312.

12. Israel, B. A., B. Checkoway, A. Schulz, and M. Zimmerman (1994). "Health Education and Community Empowerment: Conceptualizing and Measuring Perceptions of Individual, Organizational, and Community Control." *Health Education Quarterly*, 21(2): 149–170.

13. Institute of Medicine (2003). *The Future of the Public's Health in the 21st Century*. Washington, DC: National Academies Press.

14. Institute of Medicine (1988). *The Future of Public Health*. Washington, DC: National Academies Press.

15. Green, L. W., and J. F. McKenzie (2002). "Community and Population Health." In L. Breslow, ed., *Encyclopedia of Public Health*. New York: Macmillan Reference USA.

16. Kasier Family Foundation (2009). *Global Health: Background Brief*. Available at http://www.kaiseredu.org/topics_im.asp?imID=1&id=1033.

17. Institute of Medicine (1997). *America's Vital Interest in Global Health: Protecting Our People, Enhancing Our Economy, and Advancing Our International Interests*. Washington, DC: National Academy Press. Available at http://books.nap.edu/openbook.php?record_id=5717&page=R1.

18. Association for the Advancement of Health Education (1994). *Cultural Awareness and Sensitivity: Guidelines for Health Educators*. Reston, VA: Author.

19. U.S. Department of Health and Human Services, Centers for Disease Control and Prevention (2009). "Cigarette Smoking Among Adults and Trends in Smoking Cessation—United States, 2008." *Morbidity and Mortality Weekly Report*, 58(44): 1227–1232. Available at http://www.cdc.gov/mmwr/preview/mmwrhtml/mm5844a2.htm.

20. American College Health Association (2010). *American College Health Association—National College Health Assessment II (ACHA-NCHA II) Fall 2009: Reference Group Executive Summary*. Available at http://www.acha-ncha.org/reports_ACHA-NCHAII.html.

21. Shi, L., and D. A. Singh (2010). *Essentials of the US Health Care System*, 2nd ed. Sudbury, MA: Jones and Bartlett.

22. U.S. Department of Health and Human Services (2000). *Healthy People 2010*. Available at http://www.healthypeople.gov.

23. Minkler, M., and N. Wallerstein (2005). "Improving Health through Community Organizing and Community Building: A Health Education Perspective." In M. Minkler, ed., *Community Organizing and Community Building for Health*, 2nd ed. New Brunswick, NJ: Rutgers University Press, 26–50.

24. Ross, M. G. (1967). *Community Organization: Theory, Principles, and Practice*. New York: Harper & Row.

25. Pickett, G., and J. J. Hanlon (1990). *Public Health: Administration and Practice*, 9th ed. St. Louis, MO: Times Mirror/Mosby.

26. Legon, R. P. (1986). "Ancient Greece." *World Book Encyclopedia*. Chicago, IL: World Book.

27. Rosen, G. (1958). *A History of Public Health*. New York: MD Publications.

28. Burton, L. E., H. H. Smith, and A. W. Nichols (1980). *Public Health and Community Medicine*, 3rd ed. Baltimore: Williams & Wilkins.

29. Woodruff, A. W. (1977). "Benjamin Rush, His Work on Yellow Fever and His British Connections." *American Journal of Tropical Medicine and Hygiene*, 26(5): 1055–1059.

30. Rosen, G. (1975). *Preventive Medicine in the United States, 1900–1975*. New York: Science History Publications.

31. Smillie, W. G. (1955). *Public Health: Its Promise for the Future*. New York: Macmillan.

32. Duffy, J. (1990). *The Sanitarians: A History of American Public Health*. Chicago: University of Illinois Press.

33. Lalonde, M. (1974). *A New Perspective on the Health of Canadians: A Working Document*. Ottawa, Canada: Minister of Health.

34. Green, L. W. (1999). "Health Education's Contributions to the Twentieth Century: A Glimpse through Health Promotion's Rearview Mirror." In J. E. Fielding, L. B. Lave, and B. Starfield, eds., *Annual Review of Public Health*. Palo Alto, CA: Annual Reviews, 67–88.

35. U.S. Department of Health and Human Services, Public Health Service (1980). *Ten Leading Causes of Death in the United States, 1977*. Washington, DC: U.S. Government Printing Office.

36. U.S. Department of Health, Education, and Welfare (1979). *Healthy People: The Surgeon General's Report on Health Promotion and Disease Prevention* (DHEW pub. no. 79-55071). Washington, DC: U.S. Government Printing Office.

37. McKenzie, J. F., B. L. Neiger, and R. Thackeray (2009). *Planning, Implementing, and Evaluating Health Promotion Programs: A Primer*, 5th ed. San Francisco: Benjamin Cummings.

38. U.S. Department of Health and Human Services (1980). *Promoting Health/Preventing Disease: Objectives for the Nation*. Washington, DC: U.S. Government Printing Office.

39. U.S. Department of Health and Human Services, Centers for Medicare and Medicaid Services (2010). *National Health Expenditure Data*. Available at http://www.cms.gov/NationalHealthExpendData/01_Overview.asp#TopOfPage.

40. U.S. Census Bureau (2010). *World Population 1950–2050*. Available at http://www.census.gov/ipc/www/idb/worldpopgraph.php.

41. Miniño, A. M., J. Q. Xu, and K. D. Kochanek (2010). "Deaths: Preliminary Data for 2008." *National Vital Statistics Reports*, 59(2): Hyattsville, MD: National Center for Health Statistics..

42. U.S. Department of Health and Human Services (1990). *Prevention '89/'90*. Washington, DC: U.S. Government Printing Office.

43. Centers for Disease Control (1981). "Pneumocystis Pneumonia—Los Angeles." *Morbidity and Mortality Weekly Report*, 30: 250–252.

44. Centers for Disease Control (1989). "First 100,000 Cases of Acquired Immunodeficiency Syndrome—United States." *Morbidity and Mortality Weekly Report*, 38: 561–563.

45. Centers for Disease Control (1992). "The Second 100,000 Cases of Acquired Immunodeficiency Syndrome—United States, June 1981–December 1991." *Morbidity and Mortality Weekly Report*, 42(2): 28–29.

46. Centers for Disease Control and Prevention (2006). "Twenty-five Years of HIV/AIDS—United States, 1981-2006." *Morbidity and Mortality Weekly Report*, 55(21): 585–589.

47. Centers for Disease Control and Prevention (2010). *Diagnoses of HIV Infection and AIDS in the United States and Dependent Areas: 2008 HIV Surveillance Report*. Available at http://www.cdc.gov/hiv/surveillance/resources/reports/2008report/.

48. Gerberding, J. L., J. M. Hughes, and J. P. Koplan (2003). "Bioterrorism Preparedness and Response: Clinicians and Public Health Agencies as Essential Partners." In P. R. Lee and C. L. Estes, eds., *The Nation's Health*. Sudbury, MA: Jones and Bartlett, 305–309.

49. Pinger, R. R., W. A. Payne, D. B. Hahn, and E. J. Hahn (1998). *Drugs: Issues for Today*, 3rd ed. Boston: WCB McGraw-Hill.

50. King, N. (2009). "Health Inequalities and Health Inequities." In E. E. Morrison, ed., *Health Care Ethics: Critical Issues for the 21st Century*. Sudbury, MA: Jones and Bartlett, 339–354.

51. Federal Emergency Management Agency (2007). "Are You Ready? Natural Disaster." Available at http://www.fema.gov/areyouready/natural_hazards.shtm.

52. Agency for Healthcare Research and Quality (2004). *Bioterrorism and Health System Preparedness* (Issue Brief no. 2). Available at http://www.ahrq.gov/news/ulp/btbriefs/btbrief2.htm.

53. Centers for Disease Control and Prevention (2010). *Emergency Preparedness and Response: What CDC Is Doing*. Available at http://www.bt.cdc.gov/cdc/.

54. Trust for America's Health and the Robert Wood Johnson Foundation (2009). *Ready or Not 2009?: Protecting the Public's Health from Disease, Disasters, and Bioterrrorism*. Available at http://healthyamericans.org/reports/bioterror09/.

55. Trust for America's Health (2009). *New Report: H1N1 Reveals Gaps in Nation's Emergency Health Preparedness Efforts; Twenty States Score Six or Less Out of Ten Key Indicators*. Press release. Available at http://healthyamericans.org/newsroom/releases/?releaseid=201.

56. World Health Organization (1990). *Facts about WHO*. Geneva, Switzerland: Author.

57. World Health Organization (2003). *World Health Report 2003: Shaping the Future*. Geneva, Switzerland: Author.

58. World Healt=h Organization (2006). *Engaging in Health: Eleventh General Programme of Work 2006–2015*. Available at http://www.whyqlibdoc.who.int.hq/2006/GPW_ES_2006-2015_eng.pdf.

59. World Health Organization (2010). *The WHO Agenda*. Available at http://www.who.int/about/agenda/en/index.html.

60. United Nations (2000). *United Nations Millennium Declaration*. New York: Author.

61. U.S. Department of Health and Human Services (2010). *Implementing Healthy People 2020*. Available at http://www.healthypeople.gov/2020/implementing/default.aspx.

Chapter 2

Organizations That Help Shape Community Health

Chapter Outline

Chapter Objectives

After studying this chapter, you will be able to:

1 Explain the need for organizing to improve community health.

2 Explain what a governmental health organization is and give an example of one at each of the following levels—international, national, state, and local.

3 Explain the role the World Health Organization (WHO) plays in community health.

4 Briefly describe the structure and function of the United States Department of Health and Human Services (HHS).

5 State the three core functions of public health.

6 List the 10 essential public health services.

7 Explain the relationship between a state and local health department.

8 Explain what is meant by the term *coordinated school health program.*

9 Define the term *quasi-governmental* and explain why some health organizations are classified under this term.

10 List the four primary activities of most voluntary health organizations.

11 Explain the purpose of a professional health organization/association.

12 Explain how philanthropic foundations contribute to community health.

13 Discuss the role that service, social, and religious organizations play in community health.

14 Identify the major reason why corporations are involved in community health and describe some corporate activities that contribute to community health.

SCENARIO

Mary is a hardworking senior at the local university. She is majoring in physical education and looking forward to teaching elementary physical education after graduation. Mary has always been involved in team sports and has been a lifeguard at the local swimming pool for the past 4 years. Mary has a fair complexion with honey-blonde hair and blue eyes. She has always tanned easily, so, has not bothered very much with sunscreens. For the past few weeks, Mary has noticed a red, scaly, sharply outlined patch of skin on her forehead. She has put creams and ointments on it, but it will not go away and may be getting larger. Her roommate, Clare, sug-gests that she should make an appointment with the campus health services office. Mary lets it go another week and then decides to see the doctor.

After looking at the patch of skin, the doctor refers Mary to a specialist, Dr. Rice, who is a dermatologist. The dermatologist suggests a biopsy be taken of the lesion to test for skin cancer. The specialist tells Mary that if it is cancer, it is probably still in its early stages and so the prognosis is good.

A potential diagnosis of cancer often raises a lot of questions and concerns. Are there any resources in the community to which Mary can turn for help?

INTRODUCTION

As noted in Chapter 1, the history of community health dates to antiquity. For much of that history, community health issues were addressed only on an emergency basis. For example, if a community faced a drought or an epidemic, a town meeting would be called to deal with the problem. It has been only in the last 100 years or so that communities have taken explicit actions to deal aggressively with health issues on a continual basis.

Today's communities differ from those of the past in several important ways. Although individuals are better educated, more mobile, and more independent than in the past, communities are less autonomous and are more dependent on state and federal funding for support. Contemporary communities are too large and complex to respond effectively to sudden health emergencies or to make long-term improvements in public health without community organization and careful planning. Better community organizing and careful long-term planning are essential to ensure that a community makes the best use of its resources for health, both in times of emergency and over the long run.

top-down funding
a method of funding in which funds are transmitted from federal or state government to the local level

The ability of today's communities to respond effectively to their own problems is hindered by the following characteristics: (1) highly developed and centralized resources in our national institutions and organizations, (2) continuing concentration of wealth and population in the largest metropolitan areas, (3) rapid movement of information, resources, and people made possible by advanced communication and transportation technologies that eliminate the need for local offices where resources were once housed, (4) the globalization of health, (5) limited horizontal relationships between/among organizations, and (6) a system of **top-down funding** (money that comes from either the federal or state government to the local level) for many community programs.[1]

In this chapter, we discuss organizations that help to shape a community's ability to respond effectively to health-related issues by protecting and promoting the health of the community and its members. These community organizations can be classified as governmental, quasi-governmental, and nongovernmental—according to their sources of funding, responsibilities, and organizational structure.

GOVERNMENTAL HEALTH AGENCIES

Governmental health agencies are part of the governmental structure (federal, state, or local). They are funded primarily by tax dollars and managed by government officials. Each governmental health agency is designated as having authority over some geographic area. Such agencies exist at the four governmental levels—international, national, state, and local.

International Health Agencies

The most widely recognized international governmental health organization today is the **World Health Organization (WHO)** (see Figure 2.1). Its headquarters is located in Geneva, Switzerland, and there are six regional offices around the world. The names, acronyms, and cities and countries of location for WHO regional offices are as follows: Africa (AFRO), Brazzaville, Congo; Americas (PAHO), Washington, DC, United States; Eastern Mediterranean (EMRO), Cairo, Egypt; Europe (EURO), Copenhagen, Denmark; Southeast Asia (SEARO), New Delhi, India; and Western Pacific (WPRO), Manila, Philippines.[2]

Although the WHO is now the largest international health organization, it is not the oldest. Among the organizations (listed with their founding dates) that predate WHO are the following:

- International D'Hygiene Publique (1907), which was absorbed by the WHO;
- the Health Organization of the League of Nations (1919), which was dissolved when the WHO was created;
- the United Nations Relief and Rehabilitation Administration (1943) was dissolved in 1946, and its work is carried out today by the Office of the United Nations High Commissioner for Refugees (UNHCR) (1950);
- the United Nations Children's Fund (UNICEF) (1946) which was formerly known as the United Nations International Children's Emergency Fund;
- and the Pan American Health Organization (PAHO) (1902), which is still an independent organization but is integrated with WHO in a regional office.

Because the WHO is the largest and most visible international health agency, it is discussed at greater length in the following sections.

History of the World Health Organization

Planning for the WHO began when a charter of the United Nations was adopted at an international meeting in 1945. Contained in the charter was an article calling for the establishment of a health agency with wide powers. In 1946, at the International Health Conference, representatives from all of the countries in the United Nations succeeded in creating and ratifying the constitution of the WHO. However, it was not until April 7, 1948, that the constitution went into force and the organization officially began its work. In recognition of this beginning, April 7 is commemorated each year as World Health Day.[2] The sixtieth anniversary of the WHO was celebrated in 2008.

Organization of the World Health Organization

Membership in the WHO is open to any nation that has ratified the WHO constitution and receives a majority vote of the World Health Assembly. At the beginning of 2010, 193 countries were members.

governmental health agencies health agencies that are part of the governmental structure (federal, state, or local) and that are funded primarily by tax dollars

World Health Organization (WHO) the most widely recognized international governmental health organization

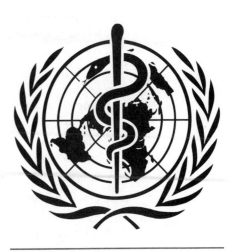

FIGURE 2.1
The emblem of the World Health Organization.

World Health Assembly
a body of delegates of the member nations of the WHO

The **World Health Assembly** comprises the delegates of the member nations. This assembly, which meets in general sessions annually and in special sessions when necessary, has the primary tasks of approving the WHO program and the budget for the following biennium and deciding major policy questions.[2]

The WHO is administered by a staff that includes a director-general, deputy director-general, and nine assistant directors-general. Great care is taken to ensure political balance in staffing WHO positions, particularly at the higher levels of administration.

Purpose and Work of the World Health Organization

The primary objective of the WHO, as stated in the constitution, is the attainment by all peoples of the highest possible level of health.[2] To achieve this objective, the WHO has 22 core functions:

- Act as the directing and coordinating authority on international health work
- Establish and maintain effective collaboration with the United Nations, specialized agencies, governmental health administrations, professional groups, and such other organizations as may be deemed appropriate
- Assist governments, upon request, in strengthening health services
- Furnish appropriate technical assistance and, in emergencies, necessary aid upon the request or acceptance of governments
- Provide or assist in providing, upon the request of the United Nations, health services and facilities to special groups, such as the peoples of trust territories
- Establish and maintain such administrative and technical services as may be required, including epidemiologic and statistical services
- Stimulate and advance work to eradicate epidemic, endemic, and other diseases
- Promote, in cooperation with other specialized agencies where necessary, the prevention of accidental injuries
- Promote, in cooperation with other specialized agencies where necessary, the improvement of nutrition, housing, sanitation, recreation, economic or working conditions, and other aspects of environmental hygiene
- Promote cooperation among scientific and professional groups that contribute to the advancement of health
- Propose conventions, agreements, and regulations and make recommendations with respect to international health matters and perform such duties as may be assigned thereby to the WHO that are consistent with its objective
- Promote maternal and child health and welfare and foster the ability to live harmoniously in a changing total environment
- Foster activities in the field of mental health, especially those affecting the harmony of human relations
- Promote and conduct research in the field of health
- Promote improved standards of teaching and training in the health, medical, and related professions
- Study and report on, in cooperation with other specialized agencies, where necessary, administrative and social techniques affecting public health and medical care from preventive and curative points of view, including hospital services and social security
- Provide information, counsel, and assistance in the field of health

- Assist in developing an informed public opinion among all peoples on matters of health
- Establish and revise as necessary international nomenclatures of diseases, of causes of death, and of public health practices
- Standardize diagnostic procedures as necessary
- Develop, establish, and promote international standards with respect to food, biological, pharmaceutical, and similar products
- Generally, take all necessary action to attain the objective of the organization[2]

The work of the WHO is financed by its member nations, each of which is assessed according to its ability to pay; the wealthiest countries contribute the greatest portion of the total budget.

Although the WHO has sponsored and continues to sponsor many worthwhile programs, an especially noteworthy one was the work of the WHO in helping to eradicate smallpox. In 1967, smallpox was active in 31 countries. During that year, 10 million to 15 million people contracted the disease, and of those, approximately 2 million died and many millions of others were permanently disfigured or blinded. The last known case of smallpox was diagnosed on October 26, 1977, in Somalia.[2] In 1979, the World Health Assembly declared the global eradication of this disease. Using the smallpox mortality figures from 1967, it can be estimated that more than 40 million lives have been saved since the eradication.

More recently, the WHO has made notable achievements in global public health. May 21, 2003, marked the unanimous decision by the World Health Assembly for the WHO to adopt the first global public health treaty to reduce tobacco-related deaths and diseases throughout the world. Additionally, in 2004, the WHO adopted the Global Strategy on Diet, Physical Activity, and Health.

As noted in Chapter 1, the current work of the WHO is guided by two documents—the *11th General Programme of Work*[2] and the United Nations Millennium Declaration, which was adopted at the Millennium Summit in 2003.[4] Because much of what is included in the *11th General Programme of Work* is summarized in Box 1.4 (The WHO Agenda) in Chapter 1, the discussion here focuses on the Millennium Declaration. The declaration set out principles and values in seven areas (peace, security, and disarmament; development and poverty eradication; protecting our common environment; human rights, democracy, and good governance; protecting the vulnerable; meeting special needs of Africa; and strengthening the United Nations) that should govern international relations in the twenty-first century.[4] Following the summit, the *Road Map* was prepared, which established goals and targets to be reached by 2015 in each of the seven areas.[5] The resulting eight goals in the area of development and poverty eradication are now referred to as the Millennium Development Goals (MDGs). More specifically, the MDGs are aimed at reducing poverty and hunger, tackling ill health, gender inequality, lack of education, lack of access to clean water, and environmental degradation.

As can be seen from this description, the MDGs are not exclusively aimed at health, but there are interactive processes between health and economic development that create a crucial link. That is, better health is "a prerequisite and major contributor to economic growth and social cohesion. Conversely, improvement in people's access to health technology is a good indicator of the success of other development processes."[3] As such, "three of the eight goals, eight of the 18 targets required to achieve them, and 18 of the 48 indicators of progress are health-related"[3] (see Table 2.1).

To date, progress has been made to achieve the MDGs by the target date of 2015; however, progress has been, to some extent, relatively slow. The midpoint progress data, evaluated and reported by the United Nations, suggest that some notable progress is being made

Table 2.1
Health-Related Millennium Development Goals, Targets, and Indicators

Goal: 1. Eradicate Extreme Poverty and Hunger
Target: 2. Halve, between 1990 and 2015, the proportion of people who suffer from hunger
    Indicator: 4. Prevalence of underweight children under five years of age
        5. Proportion of population below minimum level of dietary energy consumption[a]

Goal: 4. Reduce Child Mortality
Target: 5. Reduce by two-thirds, between 1990 and 2015, the under-five mortality rate
    Indicator: 13. Under-five mortality rate
        14. Infant mortality rate
        15. Proportion of 1-year-old children immunized against measles

Goal: 5. Improve Maternal Health
Target: 6. Reduce by three-quarters, between 1990 and 2015, the maternal mortality ratio
    Indicator: 16. Maternal mortality ratio
        17. Proportion of births attended by skilled health personnel

Goal: 6. Combat HIV/AIDS, Malaria, and Other Diseases
Target: 7. Have halted by 2015 and begun to reverse the spread of HIV/AIDS
    Indicator: 18. HIV prevalence among young people aged 15 to 24 years[b]
        19. Condom use rate of the contraceptive prevalence rate
        20. Number of children orphaned by HIV/AIDS
Target: 8. Have halted by 2015 and begun to reverse the incidence of malaria and other major diseases
    Indicator: 21. Prevalence and death rates associated with malaria
        22. Proportion of population in malaria-risk areas using effective malaria prevention and treatment measures
        23. Prevalence and death rates associated with tuberculosis
        24. Proportion of tuberculosis cases detected and cured under Directly Observed Treatment, Short-course (DOTS)

Goal: 7. Ensure Environmental Sustainability
Target: 9. Integrate the principles of sustainable development into country policies and programmes and reverse the loss of environmental resources
    Indicator: 29. Proportion of population using solid fuel
Target: 10. Halve by 2015 the proportion of people without sustainable access to safe drinking-water
    Indicator: 30. Proportion of population with sustainable access to an improved water source, urban and rural
Target: 11. By 2020 to have achieved a significant improvement in the lives of at least 100 million slum dwellers
    Indicator: 31. Proportion of urban population with access to improved sanitation

Goal: 8. Develop a Global Partnership for Development
Target: 17. In cooperation with pharmaceutical companies, provide access to affordable essential drugs in developing countries
    Indicator: 46. Proportion of population with access to affordable essential drugs on a sustainable basis

[a]Health-related indicator reported by the Food and Agriculture Organization only.
[b]Indicators from the MDG list reformulated by WHO and United Nations General Assembly Special Session on HIV/AIDS.

Source: World Health Organization (2003). *World Health Report 2003: Shaping the Future.* Geneva, Switzerland: Author, 28. Used with permission of the World Health Organization.

even in regions with the greatest challenges.[6] According to The *Millennium Development Goals Report 2007*, "the results achieved in the more successful cases demonstrate that success is possible in most countries, but that the MDGs will be attained only if concerted additional action is taken immediately and sustained until 2015."[6] The following is a summary of achievements documented in the 2007 midpoint progress report:

- Between 1990 and 2004, the proportion of individuals living in extreme poverty reduced from nearly a third to less than one-fifth.

- Since 2000, extreme poverty levels for the poor living in sub-Saharan Africa declined by nearly six percentage points; however, it should be noted that the region is not on track to meet the MDG of reducing poverty by half by the target date of 2015.

- Since 1991, primary school enrollment for children in developing countries increased by 8%.
- There has been a slight growth in women's political participation, even in countries where only men were allowed to run for political election. However, progress is very slow.
- Globally, the rate of child mortality has declined.
- Malaria interventions have been expanded.
- The tuberculosis epidemic is on the decline, but not at a rate to reach the 2015 MDG.[6]

Although much progress has been made, there is still much more work to be done. The following lists some of the key challenges, documented by the United Nations, that must be addressed to reach the 2015 MDGs for global health improvement:

- Preventable complications of pregnancy and childbirth take the lives of more than half a million women each year.
- As of 2007, trend projections indicate that the goal of halving the proportion of under-weight children will be missed by 30 million children.
- In 2006, AIDS deaths increased to 2.9 million because prevention methods are lacking in keeping pace with the epidemic growth.
- If the 2015 MDG to improve sanitation is to be met, an additional 1.6 billion people will need access to better sanitation (over the 2005–2015 time period).
- Unemployment rates of young people continue to rise.
- Climate change is projected to have serious impact on the progress made toward reaching the MDGs.[6]

Strategies for achieving large-scale and rapid progress toward meeting the MDGs involve strong government leadership and policies and strategies that meet the needs of the poor, combined with sufficient funding and technical support from the international community.[6]

Five major challenges to meeting the goals have been identified: (1) strengthening health systems, (2) ensuring health is recognized as a priority within development and economic policies, (3) developing appropriate strategies to address the diverse needs of the countries, (4) mobilizing more resources for health in the poor countries, and (5) improving the quality of health-related data to track progress toward the goals.[7,8] Much work lies ahead, by all people of the world, to improve the health of those most in need.

National Health Agencies

Each national government has a department or agency that has the primary responsibility for the protection of the health and welfare of its citizens. These national health agencies meet their responsibilities through the development of health policies, the enforcement of health regulations, the provision of health services and programs, the funding of research, and the support of their respective state and local health agencies.

In the United States, the primary national health agency is the Department of Health and Human Services (HHS). HHS "is the United States government's principal agency for protecting the health of all Americans and providing essential human services, especially for those who are least able to help themselves."[9] It is important to note, however, that other federal agencies also contribute to the betterment of our nation's health. For example, the Department of Agriculture inspects meat and dairy products and coordinates the Women, Infants, and Children (WIC) food assistance program; the Environmental Protection Agency (EPA) regulates hazardous wastes; the Department of Labor houses the Occupational

Safety and Health Administration (OSHA), which is concerned with safety and health in the workplace; the Department of Commerce, which includes the Bureau of the Census, collects much of the national data that drive our nation's health programs; and the Department of Homeland Security (DHS) deals with all aspects of terrorism within the United States. Whereas information about the DHS was presented in Chapter 1, each of these other departments or agencies is discussed in greater detail in later chapters. A detailed description of the Department of Health and Human Services follows.

Department of Health and Human Services

The HHS is headed by the Secretary of Health and Human Services, who is appointed by the president and is a member of his or her cabinet. The Department of Health and Human Services was formed in 1980 (during the administration of President Jimmy Carter), when the Department of Health, Education, and Welfare (HEW) was divided into two new departments, HHS and the Department of Education. HHS is the department most involved with the nation's human concerns. In one way or another it touches the lives of more Americans than any other federal agency. It is literally a department of people serving people, from newborn infants to persons requiring health services to our most elderly citizens. With an annual budget in excess of approximately $707 billion (representing about 25% of the federal budget), HHS is the largest department in the federal government, and it spends approximately $195 billion more per year than the Department of Defense.[9,10]

The fiscal year 2010 overview document of the United States government budget indicated that the approved HHS budget established a reserve fund of more than $630 billion, over a 10-year period, to fund health care system reform. According to the HHS budget document, "the reserve is funded half by new revenue and half by savings proposals that promote efficiency and accountability, align incentives toward quality, and encourage shared responsibility. In addition, the Budget calls for an effort beyond this down payment, to put the Nation on a path to health insurance coverage for all Americans."[10]

To date, some significant legislation has been passed that works toward fundamental health care reform, such as the American Recovery and Reinvestment Act of 2009, which includes $19 billion for health information technology, subsidies for those who are recently unemployed to maintain health insurance, and $1 billion for continued effectiveness research in health.[10] Moreover, in March 2010, a sweeping bill to overhaul the American medical system, put forth by President Barack Obama, was passed by a historic vote of 219 votes to 212. The new health care reform law provided a series of duties and responsibilities for the HHS. Among these were (1) the implementation of new provisions to assist families and small business owners in getting information to make the best choices for insurance coverage, in a "new open, competitive insurance market"; (2) working with states and additional partners to strengthen public programs, such as the children's health insurance plan (CHIP), Medicare, and Medicaid; (3) coordinating efforts with other departments to design and implement "a prevention and health promotion strategy" to promote prevention, wellness, and public health; (4) taking action to strengthen and support the primary care workforce; (5) taking on the new and improved authority to establish a transparent health care system to oversee that every dollar authorized to be spent in the act is done so in a wise and transparent manner; (6) the implementation of new provisions to decrease the costs of medications; (7) taking on authority to establish the Community Living Assistance Services and Supports Act (CLASS Act), which is a voluntary, self-funded long-term-care insurance option; and (8) the implementation of the Indian Health Care Improvement Act (ICHIA), which was reauthorized in the new health care law and provides modernized and improved health care services to Alaska Natives and American Indians.[11]

Since its formation, HHS has undergone several reorganizations. Some of the more recent changes have been the addition of the Center for Faith-Based and Community Initiatives and an Assistant Secretary for Public Health Emergency Preparedness. Currently, the HHS is organized into 11 operating agencies (see Figure 2.2) whose heads report directly to the Secretary. In addition, the HHS has 10 regional offices (see Table 2.2). These offices serve as representatives of the Secretary of HHS in direct, official dealings with the state and local governmental organizations. Eight of the 11 operating divisions of HHS (AHRQ, CDC, ATSDR, FDA, HRSA, IHS, NIH, and SAMSHA—see their descriptions below), along with Office of Global Health Affairs (OGHA), the Office of Public Health and Science (OPHS), and the Office

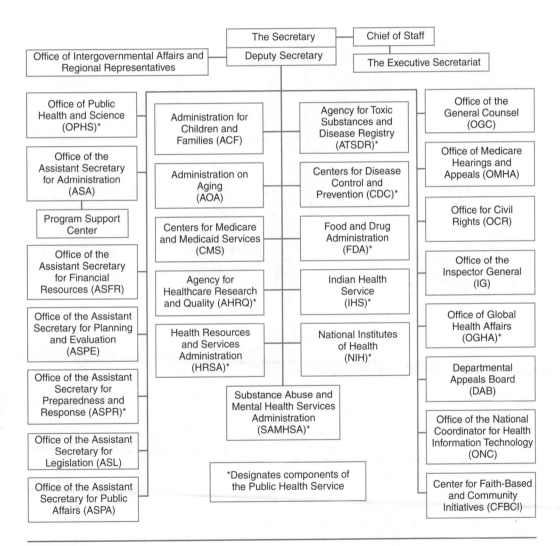

FIGURE 2.2

Organizational chart for the U.S. Department of Health and Human Services (HHS).

Source: U.S. Department of Health and Human Services (2010). U.S. Department of Health and Human Services Organizational Chart. Available at http://www.hhs.gov/about/orgchart.html. Accessed October 6, 2010.

Table 2.2
Regional Offices of the U.S. Department of Health and Human Services

Region/Areas Served	Office Address	Telephone Number
Region 1: CT, MA, ME, NH, RI, VT	John F. Kennedy Bldg. Government Center Boston, MA 02203	(617) 565-1500
Region 2: NJ, NY, Puerto Rico, Virgin Islands	Jacob K. Javits Federal Bldg. 26 Federal Plaza New York, NY 10278	(212) 264-4600
Region 3: DE, MD, PA, VA, WV, DC	Public Ledger Building 150 S. Independence Mall West Suite 436 Philadelphia, PA 19106	(215) 861-4633
Region 4: AL, FL, GA, KY, MS, NC, SC, TN	Sam Nunn, Atlanta Federal Center 61 Forsyth Street, SW Atlanta, GA 30303	(404) 562-7888
Region 5: IL, IN, MI, MN, OH, WI	233 N. Michigan Avenue Chicago, IL 60601	(312) 353-5160
Region 6: AR, LA, NM, OK, TX	1301 Young Street Dallas, TX 75202	(214) 767-3301
Region 7: IA, KS, MO, NE	Bolling Federal Building 601 East 12th Street Kansas City, MO 64106	(816) 426-2821
Region 8: CO, MT, ND, SD,UT, WY	Bryon G. Rogers Federal Office Building 1961 Stout Street Room 1076 Denver, CO 80294	(303) 844-3372
Region 9: AZ, CA, HI, NV, American Samoa, Guam, Commonwealth of the Northern Mariana Islands, Federated States of Micronesia, Republic of the Marshall Islands, Republic of Palau	Federal Office Building 50 United Nations Plaza San Francisco, CA 94102	(415) 437-8500
Region 10: AK, ID, OR, WA	Blanchard Plaza Bldg. 2201 6th Avenue Seattle, WA 98121	(206) 615-2010

Source: U.S. Department of Health and Human Services. HHS Region Map. Available at http://www.hhs.gov/about/regionmap.html. Accessed October 6, 2010.

of the Assistant Secretary for Preparedness and Response (ASPR) now constitute the Public Health Service (PHS). Another three operating divisions (CMS, ACF, and AoA) comprise the human services operating divisions.

Administration on Aging (AoA)

This division of the HHS is the principal agency designated to carry out the provisions of the Older Americans Act of 1965. (See Chapter 9 for more information on this act.) This agency tracks the characteristics, circumstances, and needs of older people; develops policies, plans, and programs to promote their welfare; administers grant programs to benefit older Americans; and administers training, research, demonstration programs, and protective services for older Americans. One exemplary program supported by the AoA is Meals on Wheels.

Administration for Children and Families (ACF)

The ACF is composed of a number of smaller agencies and is responsible for providing direction and leadership for all federal programs for needy children and families. One of the better-known programs originating from this division is Head Start, which serves more than 900,000 preschool children. Other programs are aimed at family assistance, refugee resettlement, and child support enforcement.

Agency for Healthcare Research and Quality (AHRQ)

Prior to 1999, this division of the HHS was called the Agency for Health Care Policy and Research, but its name was changed as part of the Healthcare Research and Quality Act of 1999. AHRQ is "the Nation's lead Federal agency for research on health care quality, costs, outcomes, and patient safety."[12] AHRQ sponsors and conducts research that provides evidence-based information on health care outcomes; quality; and cost, use, and access. The information helps health care decision makers—patients and clinicians, health system leaders, and policy makers—make more informed decisions and improve the quality of health care services.

Agency for Toxic Substances and Disease Registry (ATSDR)

This agency was created by the **Superfund legislation** (Comprehensive Environmental Response, Compensation, and Liability Act) in 1980. This legislation was enacted to deal with the cleanup of hazardous substances in the environment. ATSDR's mission is to "serve the public through responsive public health actions to promote healthy and safe environments and prevent harmful exposures."[13] To carry out its mission and to serve the needs of the American public, ATSDR evaluates information on hazardous substances released into the environment in order to assess the impact on public health; conducts and sponsors studies and other research related to hazardous substances and adverse human health effects; establishes and maintains registries of human exposure (for long-term follow-up) and complete listings of areas closed to the public or otherwise restricted in use due to contamination; summarizes and makes data available on the effects of hazardous substances; and provides consultations and training to ensure adequate response to public health emergencies. Although ATSDR has been responding to chemical emergencies in local communities across the country for the last 25 years, like many of the other federal health agencies its work has taken on new meaning since 9/11. For example, some of the projects the agency's staff have worked on or continue to work on include sampling dust in New York City residences after 9/11; working with New York health agencies to create a registry of people who lived or worked near the World Trade Center (WTC) on 9/11 to collect health information on those most heavily exposed to smoke, dust, and debris from the collapse of the WTC; conducting environmental sampling at anthrax-contaminated buildings; and disseminating critical information to agencies and organizations with a role in terrorism preparedness and response.[14]

> **Superfund legislation**
> legislation enacted to deal with the cleanup of hazardous substances in the environment

Centers for Disease Control and Prevention (CDC)

The CDC, located in Atlanta, Georgia (see Figure 2.3), "is the nation's premiere health promotion, prevention, and preparedness agency and global leader in public health."[15] The CDC serves as the national focus for developing and applying disease prevention (including bioterrorism) and control, environmental health, and health promotion and education activities designed to improve the health of the people of the United States.[15] Once known solely for its work to control communicable diseases, the CDC now also maintains records, analyzes disease trends, and publishes epidemiological reports on all types of diseases, including those that result from lifestyle, occupational, and environmental causes. Beyond its own specific responsibilities, the CDC also supports state and local health departments and cooperates with similar national health agencies from other WHO member nations.

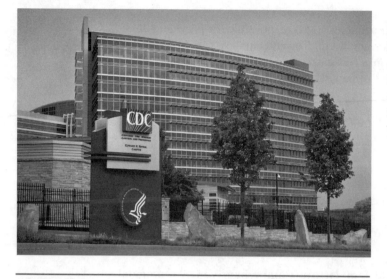

FIGURE 2.3

The Centers for Disease Control and Prevention (CDC) in Atlanta, Georgia, is one of the major operating agencies of the Department of Health and Human Services.

To better meet the challenges of public health for the twenty-first century, in 2003, the CDC began a strategic planning process called the *Futures Initiative*.[15] As a part of the Futures Initiative, the CDC adopted new overarching health protection goals and a new organizational structure. The goals that were adopted included the following:

- *Preparedness:* People in all communities will be protected from infectious, environmental, and terrorist threats.
- *Health promotion and prevention of disease, injury, and disability:* All people will achieve their optimal life span with the best possible quality of health in every stage of life.
- *Healthy places:* The places where people live, work, learn, and play should protect and promote human health and eliminate health disparities.

The reorganization of the CDC, as a result of the Futures Initiative, created a structure that included the Office of the Director, the National Institute for Occupational Safety and Health (NIOSH) (see Chapter 16 for a discussion of NIOSH), and six coordinating centers/offices. More recently, the CDC engaged in ongoing reorganization that changed the organizational structure of the agency. The CDC's Centers, Institutes, and Offices (CIOs) "allow the agency to be more responsive and effective when dealing with public health concerns. Each group implements the CDC's response in their areas of expertise, while also providing intra-agency support and resource-sharing for cross-cutting issues and specific health threats."[15] The CIOs, as of June 2010, include the following:

- *Center for Global Health:* Includes the Division of Global HIV/AIDS, Division of Parasitic Diseases and Malaria, Division of Global Disease Detection and Emergency Response, and the Division of Public Health Systems and Workforce Development
- *National Institute for Occupational Safety and Health (NIOSH):* Includes the Health Effects Laboratory Division; Education and Information Division; Division of Applied Research and Technology; Division of Respiratory Disease Studies; Division of Safety Research; Division of Surveillance, Hazard Evaluations and Field Studies; the National Personal Protective Technology Laboratory; the Office of Mine Safety and Health; and the Division of Compensation, Analysis and Support
- *Office of Infectious Diseases:* Includes the Influenza Coordination Unit; the National Center for Immunization and Respiratory Diseases; the National Center for HIV/AIDS, Viral Hepatitis, STD and TB Prevention; and the National Center for Emerging and Zoonotic Infectious Diseases
- *National Center for Immunization and Respiratory Diseases (NCIRD):* Includes the Influenza Division, Division of Viral Diseases, Division of Bacterial Diseases, Global Immunizations Division, and the Immunization Services Division
- *National Center for Emerging and Zoonotic Infectious Diseases (NCEZID):* (In 2010, NCEZID was a new center in transition; therefore, the following was updated April

2010.) Includes the Food Safety Office; the Division of Foodborne, Waterborne, and Environmental Diseases; the Division of Preparedness and Emerging Infections; the Division of Global Migration and Quarantine; the Division of Scientific Resources; the Division of Healthcare Quality Promotion; the Division of Vector-Borne Diseases; and the Division of High-Consequence Pathogens and Pathology

- *National Center for HIV/AIDS, Viral Hepatitis, STD, and TB Prevention (NCHHSTP):* Includes the Division of Sexually Transmitted Diseases Prevention, Division of HIV/AIDS Prevention, the Division of Viral Hepatitis, the Division of Tuberculosis Elimination, the Global AIDS Program (GAP)

- *Office of Noncommunicable Diseases, Injury and Environmental Health:* Includes the Division of Environmental Hazards and Health Effects, the Division of Emergency and Environmental Health Services, and the Division of Laboratory Sciences

- *National Center on Birth Defects and Developmental Disabilities:* Includes the Division of Human Development and Disability, the Division of Blood Disorders, and the Division of Birth Defects and Developmental Disabilities

- *National Center for Chronic Disease Prevention and Health Promotion:* Includes the Division of Adolescent and School Health; the Division of Adult and Community Health; the Division of Cancer Prevention and Control; the Division of Diabetes Translation; the Division of Nutrition, Physical Activity and Obesity; the Division of Oral Health; the Division of Reproductive Health; the Office on Smoking and Health; and the Division for Heart Disease and Stroke Prevention

- *National Center for Environmental Health/Agency for Toxic Substances and Disease Registry:* Includes the Division for Emergency and Environmental Health Services, the Division of Environmental Hazards and Health Effects, the Division of Laboratory Sciences, the Division of Health Assessment and Consultation, the Division of Health Studies, the Division of Regional Operations, and the Division of Toxicology and Environmental Medicine

- *National Center for Injury Prevention and Control:* Includes the Division of Injury Response, the Division of Unintentional Injury Prevention, and the Division of Violence Prevention

- *Office of Public Health Preparedness and Response:* Includes the Division of Emergency Operations, the Division of State and Local Readiness, the Division of Strategic National Stockpile, and the Division of Select Agents and Toxins

- *Office for State, Trial, Local and Territorial Support:* Includes the Division of Public Health Performance Improvement and the Division of Public Health Capacity Development

- *Office of Surveillance, Epidemiology, and Laboratory Services (OSELS is proposed for agency approval, as of June 2010, and will include the following, if approved):* Includes the National Center for Health Statistics; the National Office of Public Health Genomics; the Laboratory Science, Policy and Practice Program Office; the Public Health Informatics and Technology Program Office; the Public Health Surveillance Program Office; the Epidemiology and Analysis Program Office; and the Scientific Education and Professional Development Program Office

- *National Center for Health Statistics:* Includes the Classifications and Public Health Data Standards Staff, the Division of Health Examination Statistics, the Division of Health Care Surveys, the Division of Health Interview Statistics, the Division of Vital Statistics, the Office of Analysis and Epidemiology, and the Office of Research and Methodology[15]

Food and Drug Administration (FDA)

The FDA touches the lives of virtually every American every day. It "is charged with protecting the public health by ensuring the safety, efficacy, and security of human and veterinary drugs, biological products, and medical devices; ensuring the safety of foods, cosmetics, and radiation-emitting products; and regulating tobacco products."

Specifically, FDA is responsible for advancing the public health by:

- Helping to speed innovations that make medicines and foods safer and more effective
- Providing the public with the accurate, science-based information they need to use medicines and foods to improve their health
- Regulating the manufacture, marketing, and distribution of tobacco products to protect the public and reduce tobacco use by minors
- Addressing the nation's counterterrorism capability and ensuring the security of the supply of foods and medical products."[16]

Much of this work revolves around regulatory activities and the setting of health and safety standards as spelled out in the Federal Food, Drug, and Cosmetic Act and other related laws. However, because of the complex nature of its standards and the agency's limited resources, enforcement of many FDA regulations is left to other federal agencies and to state and local agencies. For example, the Department of Agriculture is responsible for the inspection of many foods, such as meat and dairy products. Restaurants, supermarkets, and other food outlets are inspected by state and local public health agencies.

Centers for Medicare and Medicaid Services (CMS)

Established as the Health Care Financing Administration (HFCA) in 1977, the CMS is responsible for overseeing the Medicare program (health care for the elderly and the disabled), the federal portion of the Medicaid program (health care for low-income individuals), and the related quality assurance activities. Both Medicare and Medicaid were created in 1965 to ensure that the special groups covered by these programs would not be deprived of health care because of cost. In 2008, about 99 million Americans were covered by these programs.[9] In 1997, the Children's Health Insurance Program (CHIP) also became the responsibility of the CMS. Medicare, Medicaid, and SCHIP are discussed in greater detail in Chapter 13.

Health Resources and Services Administration (HRSA)

The HRSA is the principal primary health care service agency of the federal government that provides access to essential health care services for people who are low-income, uninsured, or who live in rural areas or urban neighborhoods where health care is scarce.[9] It "is the primary federal agency for improving access to health care services for people who are underinsured, isolated, or medically vulnerable."[17] The cited mission of HRSA is "to improve health and achieve health equity through access to quality services, a skilled health workforce and innovative programs."[17] HRSA "maintains the National Health Service Corps and helps build the health care workforce through training and education programs."[9] The agency "administers a variety of programs to improve the health of mothers and children and serves people living with HIV/AIDS through the Ryan White CARE Act programs."[9] HRSA is also responsible for overseeing the nation's organ transplantation system.[9]

Indian Health Service (IHS)

The IHS "is responsible for providing federal health services to American Indians and Alaska Natives."[18] Currently, it "provides a comprehensive health service delivery system for approximately 1.9 million American Indians and Alaska Natives who belong to 564 federally recognized tribes in 35 states."[18] "The provision of health services to members of federally recognized tribes grew out of the special government-to-government relationship between the federal government and Indian tribes. This relationship, established in 1787, is based on Article I, Section 8 of the Constitution, and has been given form and substance by numerous treaties, laws, Supreme Court decisions, and Executive Orders. The IHS is the principal federal health care provider and health advocate for Indian people."[18] The mission of the IHS is "to raise the physical, mental, social, and spiritual health of American Indians and Alaska Natives to the highest level,"[18] while its goal is "to assure that comprehensive, culturally acceptable personal and public health services are available and accessible to American Indian and Alaska Native people."[18]

Though health services have been provided sporadically by the United States government since the early nineteenth century, it was not until 1989 that the IHS was elevated to an agency level; prior to that time it was a division in HRSA. (See Chapter 10 for more information on the IHS.)

National Institutes of Health (NIH)

Begun as a one-room Laboratory of Hygiene in 1887, the NIH today is one of the world's foremost medical research centers, and the federal focal point for medical research in the United States.[19] The mission of the NIH "is to seek fundamental knowledge about the nature and behavior of living systems and the application of that knowledge to enhance health, lengthen life, and reduce the burdens of illness and disability."[19] Although a significant amount of research is carried out by NIH scientists at NIH laboratories in Bethesda and elsewhere, a much larger portion of this research is conducted by scientists at public and private universities and other research institutions. These scientists receive NIH funding for their research proposals through a competitive, peer-review grant application process. Through this process of proposal review by qualified scientists, NIH seeks to ensure that federal research monies are spent on the best-conceived research projects. Table 2.3 provides a listing of all the institutes and centers located in NIH.

Table 2.3
Units within the National Institutes of Health (NIH)

National Cancer Institute (NCI)	National Institute on Drug Abuse (NIDA)
National Eye Institute (NEI)	National Institute of Environmental Health Sciences (NIEHS)
National Heart, Lung, and Blood Institute (NHLBI)	
National Human Genome Research Institute (NHGRI)	National Institute of General Medical Sciences (NIGMS)
National Institute on Aging (NIA)	National Institute of Mental Health (NIMH)
National Institute on Alcohol Abuse and Alcoholism (NIAAA)	National Institute of Neurological Disorders and Stroke (NINDS)
National Institute of Allergy and Infectious Diseases (NIAID)	National Institute of Nursing Research (NINR)
	National Library of Medicine (NLM)
National Institute of Arthritis and Musculoskeletal and Skin Diseases (NIAMS)	NIH Clinical Center (CC)
	Center for Information Technology (CIT)
National Institute of Biomedical Imaging and Bioengineering (NIBIB)	National Center for Complementary and Alternative Medicine (NCCAM)
Eunice Kennedy Shriver National Institute of Child Health and Human Development (NICHD)	National Center on Minority Health and Health Disparities (NCMHD)
National Institute on Deafness and Other Communication Disorders (NIDCD)	National Center for Research Resources (NCRR)
National Institute of Dental and Craniofacial Research (NIDCR)	John E. Fogarty International Center for Advanced Study in the Health Sciences (FIC)
	Center for Scientific Review (CSR)
National Institute of Diabetes and Digestive and Kidney Diseases (NIDDK)	

Source: National Institutes of Health (2010). "Institutes, Centers and Offices." Available at http://www.nih.gov/icd/. Accessed October 6, 2010.

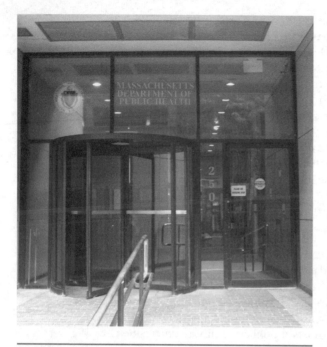

Substance Abuse and Mental Health Services Administration (SAMHSA)

The SAMHSA is the primary federal agency responsible for ensuring that up-to-date information and state-of-the-art practice are effectively used for the prevention and treatment of addictive and mental disorders. "SAMHSA's mission is to reduce the impact of substance abuse and mental illness on American's communities."[20] Within SAMHSA, there are three centers—the Center for Substance Abuse Treatment (CSAT), the Center for Substance Abuse Prevention (CSAP), and the Center for Mental Health Services (CMHS). Additionally, the agency houses one office, the Office of Applied Studies (OAS), which is responsible for "the collection, analysis and dissemination of behavioral health data."[20] Each of these centers has its own mission that contributes to the overall mission of SAMHSA (see Chapter 11 and Chapter 12 for more information on SAMHSA).

FIGURE 2.4
Each of the 50 states has its own health department.

State Health Agencies

All 50 states have their own state health departments (see Figure 2.4). Although the names of these departments may vary from state to state (e.g., Ohio Department of Health, Indiana State Department of Health), their purposes remain the same: to promote, protect, and maintain the health and welfare of their citizens. These purposes are represented in the **core functions of public health**, which include *assessment* of information on the health of the community, comprehensive public health *policy development*, and *assurance* that public health services are provided to the community.[21] These core functions have been defined further with the following 10 essential public health services.[22]

core functions of public health assessment, policy development, and assurance

1. Monitor health status to identify community health problems.
2. Diagnose and investigate health problems and health hazards in the community.
3. Inform, educate, and empower people about health issues.
4. Mobilize community partnerships to identify and solve health problems.
5. Develop policies and plans that support individual and community health efforts.
6. Enforce laws and regulations that protect health and ensure safety.
7. Link people to needed personal health services and assure the provision of health care when otherwise unavailable.
8. Ensure a competent public health and personal health care workforce.
9. Evaluate effectiveness, accessibility, and quality of personal- and population-based health services.
10. Research for new insights and innovative solutions to health problems (see Figure 2.5).

The head of the state health department is usually a medical doctor, appointed by the governor, who may carry the title of director, commissioner, or secretary. However, because of the political nature of the appointment, this individual may or may not have extensive experience in community or public health. Unfortunately, political influence sometimes reaches below the level of commissioner to the assistant commissioners and division chiefs; it is the commissioner, assistant commissioners, and division chiefs who set policy and provide direction for the state health department. Middle- and lower-level employees are usually hired through a merit system and may or may not be able to influence health department policy. These employees, who carry out the routine work of the state health department, are usually professionally trained health specialists such as microbiologists, engineers, sanitarians, epidemiologists, nurses, and health education specialist.

Most state health departments are organized into divisions or bureaus that provide certain standard services. Typical divisions include Administration, Communicable Disease Prevention and Control, Chronic Disease Prevention and Control, Vital and Health Statistics, Environmental Health, Health Education or Promotion, Health Services, Maternal and Child Health, Mental Health, Occupational and Industrial Health, Dental Health, Laboratory Services, Public Health Nursing, Veterinary Public Health, and most recently, a division of Public Health Preparedness to deal with bioterrorism issues.

In promoting, protecting, and maintaining the health and welfare of their citizens, state health departments play many different roles. They can establish and promulgate health regulations that have the force and effect of law throughout the state. The

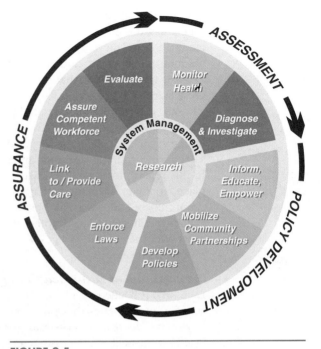

FIGURE 2.5

Core functions of public health and the 10 essential services.

Source: Public Health Functions Steering Committee, Members (July 1995). "Public Health in America." Available at http://web.health.gov/phfunctions/public.htm. Accessed October 28, 2010.

state health departments also provide an essential link between federal and local (city and county) public health agencies. As such, they serve as conduits for federal funds aimed at local health problems. Federal funds come to the states as block grants. Funds earmarked for particular health projects are distributed to local health departments by their respective state health departments in accordance with previously agreed upon priorities. State health departments may also link local needs with federal expertise. For example, epidemiologists from the CDC are sometimes made available to investigate local disease outbreaks at the request of the state health department. State health departments usually must approve appointments of local health officers and can also remove any local health officers who neglect their duties.

The resources and expertise of the state health department are also at the disposal of local health departments. One particular area where the state health departments can be helpful is laboratory services; many modern diagnostic tests are simply too expensive for local health departments. Another area is environmental health. Water and air pollution problems usually extend beyond local jurisdictions, and their detection and measurement often require equipment too expensive for local governments to afford. This equipment and expertise are often provided by the state health department.

Local Health Departments

Local-level governmental health organizations, referred to as local health departments (LHDs), are usually the responsibility of the city or county governments. In large metropolitan areas, community health needs are usually best served by a city health department. In smaller cities with populations of up to 75,000, people often come under the jurisdiction of a county health department. In some rural counties where most of the population is concentrated in a single city, a LHD may have jurisdiction over both city and county residents. In sparsely populated rural areas, it is not uncommon to find more than one county served by a single health department. In 2008, there were approximately 2,794 LHDs; of that number, 64% were located in nonmetropolitan areas and 36% were in metropolitan areas.[23]

It is through LHDs that health services are provided to the people of the community. A great many of these services are mandated by state laws, which also set standards for health and safety. Examples of mandated local health services include the inspection of restaurants, public buildings, and public transportation systems; the detection and reporting of certain diseases; and the collection of vital statistics such as births and deaths. Other programs such as safety belt programs and immunization clinics may be locally planned and implemented. In this regard, local health jurisdictions are permitted (unless preemptive legislation is in place) to enact ordinances that are stricter than those of the state, but these jurisdictions cannot enact codes that fall below state standards. It is at this level of governmental health agencies that sanitarians implement the environmental health programs, nurses and physicians offer the clinical services, and health education specialists present health education and promotion programs.

Organization of Local Health Departments

Each LHD is headed by a health officer/administrator/commissioner (see Figure 2.6). In most states, there are laws that prescribe who can hold such a position. Those often noted are physicians, dentists, veterinarians, or individuals with a master's or doctoral degree in public health. If the health officer is not a physician, then a physician is usually hired on a consulting basis to advise as needed. Usually, this health officer is appointed by a board of health, the members of which are themselves appointed by officials in the city or county government or, in some situations, elected by the general public. The health officer and administrative assistants may recommend which programs will be offered by the LHDs. However, they may need final approval from a board of health. Although it is desirable that those serving on the local board of health have some knowledge of community health programs, most states have no such requirement. Often, politics plays a role in deciding the makeup of the local board of health.

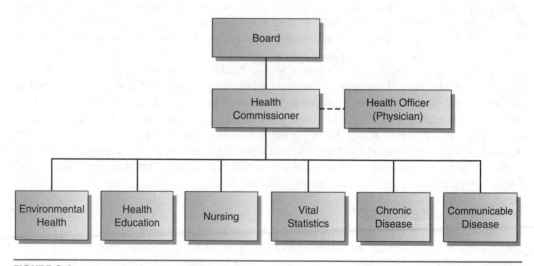

FIGURE 2.6
Organizational chart of a local public health agency.

The local health officer, like the state health commissioner, has far-reaching powers, including the power to arrest someone who refuses to undergo treatment for a communicable disease (tuberculosis, for example) and who thereby continues to spread disease in the community. The local health officer has the power to close a restaurant on the spot if it has serious health law violations or to impound a shipment of food if it is contaminated. Because many local health departments cannot afford to employ a full-time physician, the health officer is usually hired on a part-time basis. In such cases, the day-to-day activities of the LHD are carried out by an administrator trained in public health. The administrator is also hired by the board of health based upon qualifications and the recommendation of the health officer.

Local sources provide the greatest percentage of LHD revenues (25%), followed by state funds (20%) and federal pass-through funds (17%).[23] A limited number of LHD services are provided on a fee-for-service basis. For example, there is usually a fee charged for birth and death certificates issued by the LHD. Also, in some communities, minimal fees are charged to offset the cost of providing immunizations, lab work, or inspections. Seldom do these fees cover the actual cost of the services provided. Therefore, income from service fees usually makes up a very small portion of any LHD budget. And, it is not unusual to find that many LHDs use a **sliding scale** to determine the fee for a service.

sliding scale
the scale used to
determine the fee for
services based on
ability to pay

Coordinated School Health Programs

Few people think of public schools as governmental health agencies. Consider, however, that schools are funded by tax dollars, are under the supervision of an elected school board, and include as a part of their mission the improvement of the health of those in the school community. Because school attendance is required throughout the United States, the potential for school health programs to make a significant contribution to community health is enormous. In fact, Allensworth and Kolbe have stated that schools "could do more perhaps than any other single agency in society to help young people, and the adults they will become, to live healthier, longer, more satisfying, and more productive lives."[24] Yet coordinated school health programs have faced a number of barriers, including the following:[25]

1. Insufficient local administrative commitment
2. Inadequately prepared teachers
3. Too few school days to teach health in the school year
4. Inadequate funding
5. The lack of credibility of health education as an academic subject
6. Insufficient community/parental support
7. Concern for the teaching of controversial topics (i.e., sex education)

If communities were willing to work to overcome these barriers, the contribution of coordinated school health programs to community health could be almost unlimited.

What exactly is meant by coordinated school health? Prior to 1998, a coordinated school health program was commonly referred to as a *comprehensive school health program*. However, it was commonly confused with *comprehensive health education*. To eliminate this confusion, the term *coordinated* school health program is used. A coordinated school health program is defined as "an organized set of policies, procedures, and activities designed to protect, promote, and improve the health and well-being of students and staff, thus improving a student's ability to learn. It includes but is not limited to comprehensive school health education; school health services; a healthy school environment; school counseling; pyschological and social services; physical education; school nutrition services; family and community involvement in school health; and school-site health promotion for staff."[28]

Though all components of the coordinated school health program are important, there are three essential components: health education, a healthy school environment, and health services. Health instruction should be based on a well-conceived, carefully planned curriculum that has an appropriate scope (coverage of topics) and logical sequencing. Instructional units should include cognitive (knowledge), affective (attitudes), and psychomotor (behavioral) components. The healthy school environment should provide a learning environment that is both physically and mentally safe and healthy. Finally, each school's health program should provide the essential health services, from emergency care through health appraisals, to ensure that students will be healthy learners. These topics and others are discussed in much greater detail in Chapter 6.

QUASI-GOVERNMENTAL HEALTH ORGANIZATIONS

quasi-governmental health organizations organizations that have some responsibilities assigned by the government but operate more like voluntary agencies

The **quasi-governmental health organizations**—organizations that have some official health responsibilities but operate, in part, like voluntary health organizations—make important contributions to community health. Although they derive some of their funding and legitimacy from governments, and carry out tasks that may be normally thought of as government work, they operate independently of government supervision. In some cases, they also receive financial support from private sources. Examples of quasi-governmental agencies are the American Red Cross (ARC), the National Science Foundation, and the National Academy of Sciences.

The American Red Cross

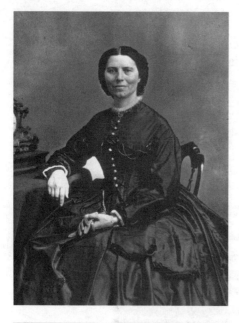

The ARC, founded in 1881 by Clara Barton (see Figure 2.7), is a prime example of an organization that has quasi-governmental status. Although it has certain "official" responsibilities placed on it by the federal government, it is funded by voluntary contributions. "Official" duties of the ARC include (1) providing relief to victims of natural disasters such as floods, tornadoes, hurricanes, and fires (Disaster Services) and (2) serving as the liaison between members of the active armed forces and their families during emergencies (Services to the Armed Forces and Veterans). In this latter capacity, the ARC can assist active-duty members of the armed services in contacting their families in case of an emergency, or vice versa.

In addition to these "official" duties, the ARC also engages in many nongovernmental services. These include blood drives, safety services (including water safety, first aid, CPR, and HIV/AIDS instruction), nursing and health services, youth services, community volunteer services, and international services.

The ARC was granted a charter by Congress in 1900, and the ARC and the federal government have had a special relationship ever since. The president of the United States is the honorary chairman of the ARC. The U.S. Attorney General and Secretary of the Treasury are honorary counselor and treasurer, respectively.

The Red Cross idea was not begun in the United States. It was begun in 1863 by five Swiss men in Geneva, Switzerland, who were concerned with the treatment provided to the wounded during

FIGURE 2.7

The American Red Cross was founded by Clara Barton in 1881.

times of war. The group, which was called the International Committee
for the Relief to the Wounded, was led by Henry Dunant. With the assistance of the Swiss government, the International Committee brought
together delegates from 16 nations in 1864 to the Geneva Convention
for the Amelioration of the Condition of the Wounded in Armies in the
Field (now known as the first Geneva Convention) to sign the Geneva
Treaty.

The efforts of Henry Dunant and the rest of the International
Committee led to the eventual establishment of the International
Committee of the Red Cross (ICRC). The ICRC, which still has its headquarters in Geneva and is still governed by the Swiss, continues to work
today during times of disaster and international conflict. It is the organization that visits prisoners of war to ensure they are being treated
humanely.[29,30]

Today, the international movement of the Red Cross comprises the
Geneva-based ICRC, the International Federation of Red Cross and Red
Crescent Societies (the red crescent emblem is used in Moslem countries),
and the over 180 National Red Cross and Red Crescent Societies.[29] There
are a number of other countries that believe in the principles of the Red
Cross Movement, but have not officially joined because the emblems used
by the movement are offensive. Thus, the ICRC has created a third
emblem that meets all the criteria for use as a protective device and at the
same time is free of any national, political, or religious connotations. The
design is composed of a red frame in the shape of a square on the edge of a white background.
The name chosen for this distinctive emblem was "red crystal," to signify purity. The emblem
was put into use on January 14, 2007 (see Figure 2.8).[30]

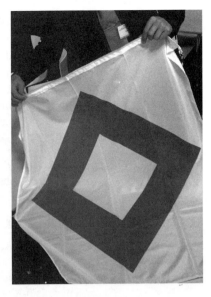

FIGURE 2.8

The red crystal: an additional emblem of the
ICRC.

Other Quasi-Governmental Organizations

Two other examples of quasi-governmental organizations in the United States are the
National Science Foundation (NSF) and the National Academy of Sciences (NAS). The purpose of NSF is the funding and promotion of scientific research and the development of individual scientists. NSF receives and disperses federal funds but operates independently of
governmental supervision. Chartered by Congress in 1863, the NAS acts as an advisor to the
government on questions of science and technology. Included in its membership are some of
America's most renowned scientists. Although neither of these agencies exists specifically to
address health problems, both organizations fund projects, publish reports, and take public
stands on health-related issues.

NONGOVERNMENTAL HEALTH AGENCIES

Nongovernmental health agencies are funded by private donations or, in some cases, by
membership dues. There are thousands of these organizations that all have one thing in
common: They arose because there was an unmet need. For the most part, the agencies
operate free from governmental interference as long as they meet Internal Revenue Service
guidelines with regard to their specific tax status. In the following sections, we discuss the
following types of nongovernmental health agencies—voluntary, professional, philanthropic,
service, social, religious, and corporate.

Voluntary Health Agencies

voluntary health agencies nonprofit organizations created by concerned citizens to deal with a health need not met by governmental health agencies

Voluntary health agencies are an American creation. Each of these agencies was created by one or more concerned citizens who felt that a specific health need was not being met by existing governmental agencies. In a sense, these new voluntary agencies arose by themselves, in much the same way as a "volunteer" tomato plant arises in a vegetable garden. New voluntary agencies continue to be born each year. Examples of recent additions to the perhaps 100,000 agencies already in existence are the Alzheimer's Association and the First Candle (formerly SIDS Alliance). A discussion of the commonalities of voluntary health agencies follows.

Organization of Voluntary Health Agencies

Most voluntary agencies exist at three levels—national, state, and local. At the national level, policies that guide the agency are formulated. A significant portion of the money raised locally is forwarded to the national office, where it is allocated according to the agency's budget. Much of the money is designated for research. By funding research, the agencies hope to discover the cause of and cure for a particular disease or health problem. There have been some major successes. The March of Dimes, for example, helped to eliminate polio as a major disease problem in the United States through its funding of immunization research.

There is not always a consensus of opinion about budget decisions made at the national level; some believe that less should be spent for research and more for treating those afflicted with the disease. Another common internal disagreement concerns how much of the funds raised at the local level should be sent to the national headquarters instead of being retained for local use. Those outside the agency sometimes complain that when an agency achieves success, as the March of Dimes did in its fight against polio, it should dissolve. This does not usually occur; instead, successful agencies often find a new health concern. The March of Dimes now fights birth defects; and when tuberculosis was under control, the Tuberculosis Society changed its name to the American Lung Association to fight all lung diseases.

The state-level offices of voluntary agencies are analogous to the state departments of health in the way that they link the national headquarters with local offices. The primary work at this level is to coordinate local efforts and to ensure that policies developed at the national headquarters are carried out. The state-level office may also provide training services for employees and volunteers of local-level offices and are usually available as consultants and problem solvers. In recent years, some voluntary agencies have been merging several state offices into one to help reduce overhead expenses.

The local-level office of each voluntary agency is usually managed by a paid staff worker who has been hired either by the state-level office or by a local board of directors. Members of the local board of directors usually serve in that capacity on a voluntary basis. Working under the manager of each agency are local volunteers, who are the backbone of voluntary agencies. It has been said that the local level is where the "rubber meets the road." In other words, this is where most of the money is raised, most of the education takes place, and most of the service is rendered. Volunteers are of two types, professional and lay. Professional volunteers have had training in a medical profession, while lay volunteers have had no medical training. The paid employees help facilitate the work of the volunteers with expertise, training, and other resources.

Purpose of Voluntary Health Agencies

Voluntary agencies share four basic objectives: (1) to raise money to fund their programs, with the majority of the money going to fund research, (2) to provide education both to professionals and to the public, (3) to provide service to those individuals and families that are afflicted with the disease or health problem, and (4) to advocate for beneficial policies, laws, and regulations that affect the work of the agency and in turn the people they are trying to help.

Fund-raising is a primary activity of many voluntary agencies. Whereas in the past this was accomplished primarily by door-to-door solicitations, today mass-mailing and telephone solicitation are more common. In addition, most agencies sponsor special events such as golf outings, dances, or dinners. One type of special event that is very popular today is the "a-thon" (see Figure 2.9). The term "a-thon" is derived from the name of the ancient Greek city Marathon and usually signified some kind of "endurance" event. Examples include bike-a-thons, rock-a-thons, telethons, skate-a-thons, and dance-a-thons. These money-making "a-thons" seem to be limited in scope only by the creativity of those planning them. In addition, some of these agencies have become United Way agencies and receive some funds derived from the annual United Way campaign, which conducts fund-raising efforts at worksites. The three largest voluntary agencies in the United States today (in terms of dollars raised) are the American Cancer Society (see Box 2.1), the American Heart Association, and the American Lung Association.

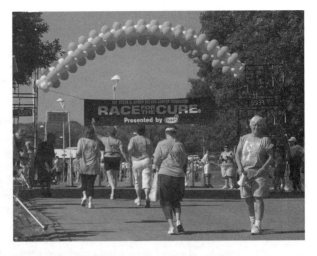

FIGURE 2.9
Most voluntary health agencies hold special events to raise money for their causes.

Over the years, the number of voluntary agencies formed to help meet special health needs has continually increased. Because of the growth in the number of new agencies, several consumer "watchdog" groups have taken a closer look into the practices of the agencies. A major concern of these consumer groups has been the amount of money that the voluntary agencies spend on the cause (e.g., cancer, heart disease, AIDS) and how much they spend on fund-raising and overhead (e.g., salaries, office furniture, leasing of office space). Well-run agencies will spend less than 15% of what they raise on fund-raising. Some of the not-so-well-run agencies spend as much as 80% to 90% on fund-raising. All consumers should ask agencies how they spend their money prior to contributing.

Professional Health Organizations/Associations

Professional health organizations and associations are made up of health professionals who have completed specialized education and training programs and have met the standards of registration, certification, and/or licensure for their respective fields. Their mission is to promote high standards of professional practice for their specific profession, thereby improving the health of society by improving the people in the profession. Professional organizations are funded primarily by membership dues. Examples of such organizations are the American Medical Association, the American Dental Association, the American Nursing Association, the American Public Health Association, the American Association for Health Education, and the Society for Public Health Education, Inc.

Although each professional organization is unique, most provide similar services to their members. These services include the certification of continuing-education programs for professional renewal, the hosting of annual conventions where members share research results and interact with colleagues, and the publication of professional journals and other reports. Some examples of journals published by professional health associations are the *Journal of the American Medical Association,* the *American Journal of Public Health,* and the *American Journal of Health Education.*

<table>
<tr><td>BOX
2.1</td><td>A Closer Look at One Voluntary Health Agency:
The American Cancer Society</td></tr>
</table>

The American Cancer Society (ACS) was founded in 1913 by 10 physicians and 5 laymen. At that time, it was known as the American Society for the Control of Cancer. Today, with offices throughout the country and approximately 2 million volunteers, ACS is one of our largest voluntary health organizations. In spite of its success, its mission has remained constant since its founding. It is "dedicated to eliminating cancer as a major health problem by preventing cancer, saving lives, and diminishing suffering from cancer, through research, education, advocacy and service."[31]

The mission of the ACS includes both short- and long-term goals. Its short-term goals are to save lives and diminish suffering. This is accomplished through education, advocacy, and service. Its long-term goal, the elimination of cancer, is being approached through the society's support of cancer research.

The American Cancer Society's educational programs are targeted at two different groups—the general public and the health professionals who treat cancer patients. The public education program promotes the following skills and concepts to people of all ages: (1) taking the necessary steps to prevent cancer, (2) knowing the seven warning signals, (3) understanding the value of regular checkups, and (4) coping with cancer. The society accomplishes this by offering free public education programs, supported by up-to-date literature and audiovisual materials, whenever and wherever they may be requested. These programs may be presented in homes, worksites, churches, clubs, organizations, and schools. A few of their better-known programs include I Can Cope, Reach to Recovery, and Man to Man.[31] From time to time, the society also prepares public service messages for broadcasting or televising.

The society's professional education program is aimed at the professionals who work with oncology patients. The objective of this program is to motivate physicians and other health care professionals "to maintain and improve their knowledge of cancer prevention, detection, diagnosis, treatment, and palliative care."[32] Such education is provided through professional publications, up-to-date audiovisual materials, conferences, and grants that fund specialized education experiences.

The ACS offers patient service and rehabilitation programs that ease the impact of cancer on those affected. The services offered include information and referral to appropriate professionals, home care supplies and equipment for the comfort of patients, transportation of patients to maintain their medical and continuing care programs, and specialized education programs for cancer patients to help them cope and feel better about themselves. There are also rehabilitation programs that provide social support for all cancer patients and specific programs for those who have had a mastectomy, laryngectomy, or ostomy.

The ACS is the largest source of private, not-for-profit cancer research funds in the United States, second only to the federal government in total dollars spent. Since 1946, when the ACS first started awarding grants, it has invested about $3.1 billion in cancer research. The research program consists of three components: extramural grants, intramural epidemiology and surveillance research, and the intramural behavioral research center.[31] The most recent addition to the work of the ACS is in the area of advocacy. Specifically, the ACS works to (1) support cancer research and programs to prevent, detect, and treat cancer; (2) expand access to quality cancer care, prevention, and awareness; (3) reduce cancer disparities in minority and medically underserved populations; and (4) reduce and prevent suffering from tobacco-related illnesses.[31]

All ACS programs—education, service, research, and advocacy—are planned primarily by the society's volunteers. However, the society does employ staff members to carry out the day-to-day operations and to help advise and support the work of the volunteers. This arrangement of volunteers and staff working together has created a very strong voluntary health agency.

Like voluntary health agencies, another important activity of some professional organizations is advocating on issues important to their membership. The American Medical Association, for example, has a powerful lobby nationally and in some state legislatures. Their purpose is to affect legislation in such a way as to benefit their membership and their profession. Many professional health organizations provide the opportunity for benefits, including group insurance and discount travel rates. There are hundreds of professional health organizations in the United States, and it would be difficult to describe them all here.

Philanthropic Foundations

Philanthropic foundations have made and continue to make significant contributions to community health in the United States and throughout the world. These foundations support community health by funding programs and research on the prevention, control, and treatment of many diseases. Foundation directors, sometimes in consultation with a review committee, determine the types of programs that will be funded. Some foundations fund an array of health projects, whereas others have a much narrower scope of interests. Some foundations, such as the Bill and Melinda Gates Foundation, fund international health projects, whereas others restrict their funding to domestic projects. The geographical scope of domestic foundations can be national, state, or local. Local foundations may restrict their funding to projects that only benefit local citizens.

The activities of these foundations differ from those of the voluntary health agencies in two important ways. First, foundations have money to give away, and therefore no effort is spent on fund-raising. Second, foundations can afford to fund long-term or innovative research projects, which might be too risky or expensive for voluntary or even government-funded agencies. The development of a vaccine for yellow fever by a scientist funded by the Rockefeller Foundation is an example of one such long-range project.

Some of the larger foundations, in addition to the Bill and Melinda Gates Foundation, that have made significant commitments to community health are the Commonwealth Fund, which has contributed to community health in rural communities, improved hospital facilities, and tried to strengthen mental health services; the Ford Foundation, which has contributed greatly to family-planning efforts throughout the world; the Robert Wood Johnson Foundation, which has worked to improve access to medical and dental care throughout the United States and lessen the impact of tobacco on health; the Henry J. Kaiser Family Foundation, which has supported the development of health maintenance organizations (HMOs) and community health promotion; the W. K. Kellogg Foundation, which has funded many diverse health programs that address human issues and provide a practical solution; and the Milbank Memorial Fund, which has primarily funded preventive-medicine projects.

Service, Social, and Religious Organizations

Service, social, and religious organizations have also played a part in community health over the years (see Figure 2.10). Examples of service and social groups involved in community health are the Jaycees, Kiwanis Club, Fraternal Order of Police, Rotary Club, Elks, Lions, Moose, Shriners, American Legion, and Veterans of Foreign Wars. Members of these groups enjoy social interactions with people of similar interests in addition to fulfilling the groups' primary reason for existence—service to others in their communities. Although health may not

> **philanthropic foundation** an endowed institution that donates money for the good of humankind

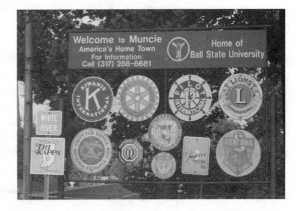

FIGURE 2.10

Community service groups contribute needed resources for the improvement of the health of the community.

be the specific focus of their mission, several of these groups make important contributions in that direction by raising money and funding health-related programs. Sometimes, their contributions are substantial. Examples of such programs include the Shriners' children's hospitals and burn centers; the Lions' contributions to pilot (lead) dog programs and other services for those who are visually impaired, such as the provision of eyeglasses for school-aged children unable to afford them; and the Lions' contributions to school health programs via the educational program named "Lions Quest."

The contributions of religious groups to community health have also been substantial. Such groups also have been effective avenues for promoting health programs because (1) they have had a history of volunteerism and preexisting reinforcement contingencies for volunteerism, (2) they can influence entire families, and (3) they have accessible meeting-room facilities.[33] One way in which these groups contribute is through donations of money for missions for the less fortunate. Examples of religious organizations that solicit donations from their members include the Protestants' One Great Hour of Sharing, the Catholics' Relief Fund, and the United Jewish Appeal. Other types of involvement in community health by religious groups include (1) the donation of space for voluntary health programs such as blood donations, Alcoholics Anonymous, and other support groups, (2) the sponsorship of food banks and shelters for the hungry, poor, and homeless, (3) the sharing of the doctrine of good personal health behavior, and (4) allowing community health professionals to deliver their programs through the congregations. This latter contribution has been especially useful in black American communities because of the importance of churches in the culture of this group of people.

In addition, it should be noted that some religious groups have hindered the work of community health workers. Almost every community in the country can provide an example where a religious organization has protested the offering of a school district's sex education program, picketed a public health clinic for providing reproductive information or services to women, or has spoken out against homosexuality.

Corporate Involvement in Community Health

From the way it treats the environment by its use of natural resources and the discharge of wastes, to the safety of the work environment, to the products and services it produces and provides, to the provision of health care benefits for its employees, corporate America is very much involved in community health. Though each of these aspects of community health is important to the overall health of a community, because of the concern for the "bottom line" in corporate America, it is the provision of health care benefits that often receives the most attention. In fact, many corporations today find that their single largest annual expenditure behind salaries and wages is for employee health care benefits. Consider, for example, the cost of manufacturing a new car. The cost of health benefits for those who build the car now exceeds the cost of the raw materials for the car itself.

In an effort to keep a healthy workforce and reduce the amount paid for health care benefits, many companies support health-related programs both at and away from the worksite. Worksite programs aimed at trimming employee medical bills have been expanded beyond the traditional safety awareness programs and first aid services to include such programs as substance abuse counseling, nutrition education, smoking cessation, stress management, physical fitness, and disease management. Many companies also are implementing health promotion policies and enforcing state and local laws that prohibit (or severely restrict) smoking on company grounds or that mandate the use of safety belts at all times in all company-owned vehicles. (See Chapter 16 for more on safety and health in the workplace.)

CHAPTER SUMMARY

- Contemporary society is too complex to respond effectively to community health problems on either an emergency or a long-term basis. This fact necessitates organizations and planning for health in our communities.

- The different types of organizations that contribute to the promotion, protection, and maintenance of health in a community can be classified into three groups according to their sources of funding and organizational structure—governmental, quasi-governmental, and nongovernmental.

- Governmental health agencies exist at the local, state, federal, and international levels and are funded primarily by tax dollars.

- WHO is the largest and most visible governmental health agency on the international level.

- The Department of Health and Human Services (HHS) is the U.S. government's principal agency for the protection of the health of all Americans and for providing essential human services, especially for those who are least able to help themselves.

- The core functions of public health include the assessment of information on the health of the community, comprehensive public health policy development, and assurance that public health services are provided to the community.

- Quasi-governmental agencies, such as the American Red Cross, share attributes with both governmental and nongovernmental agencies.

- Nongovernmental organizations include voluntary and professional associations, philanthropic foundations, and service, social, and religious groups.

- Corporate America has also become more involved in community health, both at the worksite and within the community.

REVIEW QUESTIONS

1. What characteristics of modern society necessitate planning and organization for community health?

2. What is a governmental health agency?

3. What is the World Health Organization (WHO), and what does it do?

4. What federal department in the United States is the government's principal agency for protecting the health of all Americans and for providing essential human services, especially to those who are least able to help themselves? What major services does this department provide?

5. What are the three core functions of public health?

6. What are the 10 essential public health services?

7. How do state and local health departments interface?

8. What is meant by the term *coordinated school health program*? What are the major components of it?

9. What is meant by the term *quasi-governmental agency*? Name one such agency.

10. Describe the characteristics of a nongovernmental health agency.

11. What are the major differences between a governmental health organization and a voluntary health agency?

12. What does a health professional gain from being a member of a professional health organization?

13. How do philanthropic foundations contribute to community health? List three well-known foundations.

SCENARIO: ANALYSIS AND RESPONSE

After having read this chapter, please respond to the following questions in reference to the scenario at the beginning of the chapter.

1. What type of health agency do you think will be of most help to Mary?

2. If this scenario were to happen to someone in your community, what recommendations would you give to him or her on seeking help from health agencies?

3. The Internet has many sources of information that could help Mary. Use a search engine (e.g., Google) and enter the word "cancer." Find the Web site of one governmental health agency at the national level and one voluntary health agency that might be able to help her. Explain how these agencies could be of help.

4. If Mary did not have Internet access, how would you suggest she find out about local health agencies in her area that could help her?

14. How do service, social, and religious groups contribute to the health of the community?

15. Why has corporate America become involved in community health?

ACTIVITIES

1. Using a local telephone book, list all the health-related organizations that service your community. Divide your list by the three major types of health organizations noted in this chapter.

2. Make an appointment to interview someone at one of the organizations identified in Activity 1. During your visit, find answers to the following questions:
   a. How did the organization begin?
   b. What is its mission?
   c. How is it funded?
   d. How many people (employees and volunteers) work for the organization, and what type of education/training do they have?
   e. What types of programs/services does the organization provide?

3. Obtain organizational charts from the U.S. Department of Health and Human Services (a copy is in this chapter), your state department of health, and your local health department. Compare and contrast these charts, and describe their similarities and differences.

4. Call a local voluntary health organization in your community and ask if you could volunteer to work 10 to 15 hours during this academic term. Then, volunteer those hours and keep a journal of your experience.

5. Carefully review your community newspaper each day for an entire week. Keep track of all articles or advertisements that make reference to local health organizations. Summarize your findings in a one-page paper. (If you do not subscribe to your local paper, copies are available in libraries.)

COMMUNITY HEALTH ON THE WEB

The Internet contains a wealth of information about community and public health. Increase your knowledge of some of the topics presented in this chapter by accessing the Jones & Bartlett Learning Web site at **http://health .jbpub.com/book/communityhealth/7e** and follow the links to complete the following Web activities.

- World Health Organization
- Department of Health and Human Services
- Association of State and Territorial Health Officials

REFERENCES

1. Green, L. W. (1990). "The Revival of Community and the Public Obligation of Academic Health Centers." In R. E. Bulger and S. J. Reiser, eds., *Integrity in Institutions: Humane Environments for Teaching, Inquiry and Health*. Iowa City: University of Iowa Press, 163–180.

2. World Health Organization (2010). "World Health Organization." Available at http://www.who.int/about/en/.

3. World Health Organization (2003). *World Health Report 2003: Shaping the Future*. Geneva, Switzerland: Author.

4. United Nations (2000). *United Nations Millennium Declaration*. New York: Author.

5. United Nations (2002). *Road Map Towards the Implementation of the United Nations Millennium Declaration*. New York: Author.

6. United Nations (2007). *The Millennium Development Goals Report*. New York: Author.

7. Dodd, R., and A. Cassels (2006). "Health, Development and the Millennium Development Goals." *Annals of Tropical Medicine and Parasitology,* 100(5/6): 379–387.

8. World Health Organization (2005). *Health and the Millennium Development Goals*. Geneva, Switzerland: Author.

9. U.S. Department of Health and Human Services (2010). "United States Department of Health and Human Services." Available at http://www.hhs.gov/about/whatwedo.html.

10. Government Printing Office Access (2010). *Budget of the United States Government: Browse Fiscal Year 2010*. Available at http://origin.www.gpoaccess.gov/usbudget/fy10/browse.html.

11. U.S. Department of Health and Human Services (2010). "Health Reform and the Department of Human Services." Available at http://www.healthreform.gov/health_reform_and_hhs.html.

12. Agency for Healthcare Research and Quality (2010). "What Is AHRQ?" Available at http://www.ahrq.gov/about/Whatis.htm.

13. Agency for Toxic Substances and Disease Registry (2006). "About the Agency for Toxic Substances and Disease Registry." Available at http://www.atsdr.cdc.gov/about.index.html.

14. Falk, H. (2003) "A Message from Dr. Henry Falk, ATSDR Assistant Administrator." *Public Health and the Environment*, 2(1/2): 1.

15. Centers for Disease Control and Prevention (2010). "Centers for Disease Control and Prevention." Available at http://www.cdc.gov/.

16. U.S. Food and Drug Administration (2010). "Strategic Priorities 2011–2015: Responding to the Public Health Challenges of the 21st Century, DRAFT 9/29/2010." Available at http://www.fda.gov/AboutFDA/ReportsManualsForms/Reports/ucm227527.htm#mission.

17. Health Resources and Services Administration (2006). "About HRSA." Available at http://www.hrsa.gov/about/default.htm.

18. Indian Health Service (2010). "Indian Health Service Introduction." Available at http://www.ihs.gov/PublicInfo/PublicAffairs/Welcome_Info/IHSintro.asp.

19. National Institutes for Health (2010). "Questions and Answers about NIH." Available at http://www.nih.gov/about/mission.htm.

20. Substance Abuse and Mental Health Services Administration (2010). "SAMSHA: Who Are We?" Available at http://www.samhsa.gov/about/background.aspx.

21. National Academy of Sciences, Institute of Medicine (1988). *The Future of Public Health*. Washington, DC: National Academy Press.

22. Office of Disease Prevention and Health Promotion (2008). "Public Health in America." Available at http://web.health.gov/phfunctions/public.htm.

23. National Association of County and City Health Officials (2009). *2008 National Profile of Local Health Departments*. Washington, DC: Author.

24. Allensworth, D. D., and L. J. Kolbe (1987). "The Comprehensive School Health Program: Exploring an Expanded Concept." *Journal of School Health*, 57(10): 409–412.

25. Butler, S. C. (1993). "Chief State School Officers Rank Barriers to Implementing Comprehensive School Health Education." *Journal of School Health*, 63(3): 130-132.

26. Clark, N. M. (2002). *A Letter from the Dean*. Ann Arbor, MI: University of Michigan, School of Public Health.

27. Institute of Medicine (2003). *The Future of the Public's Health*. Washington, DC: National Academies Press.

28. Joint Committee on Health Education and Promotion Terminology (2001). "Report of the 2000 Joint Committee on Health Education and Promotion Terminology." *American Journal of Health Education*, 32(2): 89-103.

29. American Red Cross (2010). "Red Cross History." Available at http://www.redcross.org/.

30. International Committee of the Red Cross (2006). "About the International Committee of the Red Cross—ICRC." Available at http://www.icrc.org.

31. American Cancer Society (2006). "About the American Cancer Society." Available at http://www.cancer.org/docroot/AA/AA_0.asp.

32. American Cancer Society (2006). "Continuing Medical Education." Available at http://www.cancer.org/docroot/PRO/content/PRO_2_Continuing_Medical_Education.asp.

33. Lasater, T. M., B. L. Wells, R. A. Carleton, and J. P. Elder (1986). "The Role of Churches in Disease Prevention Research Studies." *Public Health Report*, 101(2): 123-131.

Chapter 3

Epidemiology: The Study of Disease, Injury, and Death in the Community

Chapter Outline

Chapter Objectives

After studying this chapter, you will be able to:

1 Define the terms *epidemic, epidemiology,* and *epidemiologist,* and explain their importance in community health.

2 List some diseases that caused epidemics in the past and some that are causing epidemics today.

3 Discuss how the practice of epidemiology has changed since the days of Benjamin Rush and John Snow.

4 Explain why rates are important in epidemiology and list some of the commonly used rates.

5 Define incidence and prevalence rates and provide examples of each.

6 Calculate a variety of rates from the appropriate data.

7 Discuss the importance of disease reporting to a community's health and describe the reporting process.

8 Define the following standardized measurements of health status—life expectancy, years of potential life lost (YPLL), disability-adjusted life years (DALYs), and health-adjusted life expectancy (HALE).

9 Identify sources of standardized data used by epidemiologists, community health workers, and health officials and list the types of data available from each source.

10 List and describe the various types of epidemiological studies and explain the purpose of each.

SCENARIO

John thought about this afternoon's picnic. Everyone had a blast. For a while it had seemed almost too warm, but plenty of cold drinks were available, and by late afternoon it had become quite pleasant. The games were fun, too . . . Frisbee, soccer, softball, and volleyball. Then, there was the picnic itself—turkey, potato salad, bread and butter, milk, and dessert—served about noon.

It was now 8 P.M. that same night, and instead of studying as he had planned, John was lying on his bed with a bad stomachache. He was experiencing severe diarrhea and had made several hurried trips to the bathroom in the last half-hour.

The telephone rang, and it was Michael, John's roommate. He had gone to his girlfriend's house after the picnic to work on a class project with her. He and Caroline were both sick with stomach cramps and diarrhea, and Michael was calling to ask whether John was sick, too. As John was answering, he realized that he needed to run to the bathroom again. He quickly hung up, promising to call back soon. Moments later as he returned to his bedroom, John began to think about what a coincidence it was that all three of them were sick with the same symptoms at about the same time. Could they have become ill from food they ate at the picnic? There were about 50 people at the picnic; how many others might also be sick? Was it the heat? Was it the food? Was this an epidemic? A half-hour later, John called Michael back to tell him that he had decided to go to the campus health center.

Elsewhere . . .

This had turned out to be an interesting volunteer experience. As a requirement for her community health class, Kim had agreed to volunteer at the local health department. The spring semester was almost over now, and she was writing a final report of her activities. During the term, she had spent her Friday afternoons accompanying a sanitarian on his inspections of restaurants and retail food stores. She also had helped him complete his reports on substandard housing and malfunctioning septic tanks.

Dr. Turner, the health officer, had given Kim permission to use one of the department's personal computers for preparing her final report. Because it was Sunday evening, she was alone in the health department office when the telephone rang. She briefly considered not answering it but finally picked up the receiver. It was Dr. Lee from the University Health Center. He said he was calling in the hope that someone might be there because he needed to reach Dr. Turner immediately. He said that he had admitted six students to the infirmary with severe stomach cramps, vomiting, and diarrhea. The students had been at a picnic earlier, and he thought they could have food poisoning. He called to ask Dr. Turner to investigate this outbreak and asked Kim to try to reach him as soon as possible.

INTRODUCTION

When you become ill and visit a doctor, the first thing the physician does is take measurements and collect information. The measurements include your temperature, heart rate, and blood pressure. The information includes time of onset of your illness, where you have traveled, and what you might have eaten. Next, you may be given a physical examination and asked to provide a specimen such as urine or blood for laboratory examination. The information gathered helps the physician understand the nature of your illness and prescribe an appropriate treatment.

While a primary care physician is concerned with the course of disease in an individual patient, an epidemiologist is concerned with the course of disease in a population. When illness, injury, or death occur at unexpected or unacceptable levels in a community or population, epidemiologists seek to collect information about the disease status of the community. First, epidemiologists want to know *how many* people are sick. Second, they want to know *who* is sick—the old? the young? males? females? rich? poor? They also want to know *when* the people became sick, and finally, *where* the sick people live or have traveled. In summary, epidemiologists want to know what it is that the sick people have in common. For this reason, epidemiology is sometimes referred to as *population medicine*.

epidemiology
the study of the distribution and determinants of health-related states or events in specified populations

Epidemiology is one of the community health activities "aimed at protecting or improving the health of a population or community" discussed in Chapter 1. Information gathered from epidemiological studies assists community decision makers to make the best use of the community's human and financial health resources. Data gathered at local, state, and national levels can be used not only to prevent disease outbreaks or control those that are in progress, but also to assess whether an ongoing disease prevention program is effective.

Definition of Epidemiology

Before we discuss the types of questions an epidemiologist asks, we need to define the term *epidemiology*. **Epidemiology** is "the study of the distribution and determinants of health-related states or events in specified populations, and the application of this study to control health problems."[1] The term *epidemiology* is derived from Greek words that can be translated into the phrase "the study of that which is upon the people." The goal of epidemiology is to limit disease, injury, and death in a community by intervening to prevent or limit outbreaks or epidemics of disease and injury. This is accomplished by describing outbreaks and designing studies to analyze them and to validate new approaches to prevention, control, and treatment. Through these practices, epidemiologists contribute to our knowledge of how diseases begin and spread through populations, and how they can be prevented, controlled, and treated.

epidemic
an unexpectedly large number of cases of an illness, specific health-related behavior, or other health-related event in a particular population

The question might be asked, how many cases are required before a disease outbreak is considered an epidemic—10 cases? 100 cases? 1,000 cases? The answer is that it depends on the disease and the population, *but any unexpectedly large number of cases of an illness, specific health-related behavior, or other health-related event* in a particular population at a particular time and place can be considered an **epidemic**. Some recent epidemics in the United States are presented in Table 3.1.

endemic disease
a disease that occurs regularly in a population as a matter of course

The question might be asked, what are diseases called that occur regularly in a population but are not epidemic? These diseases are referred to as **endemic diseases**. Whether a disease is epidemic or endemic depends on the disease and the population. Heart disease is endemic in America, while in many regions of equatorial Africa, malaria is endemic.

epidemiologist
one who practices epidemiology

An **epidemiologist** is "an investigator who studies the occurrence of disease or other health-related conditions or events in defined populations."[1] Some epidemics begin as outbreaks of disease in animals, known as *epizootics*, and then spread to human populations. Examples are bubonic plague that first affects rodents, and West Nile fever virus that first affects birds. Occasionally, an epidemic will spread over a wide area, perhaps even across an entire continent or around the world. Such a widespread epidemic is termed a **pandemic**.

pandemic
an outbreak of disease over a wide geographical area such as a continent

The influenza pandemic of 1918 is an example (see Figure 3.1). This disease spread in Europe, Asia, and North America simultaneously.[2] An estimated 25 million people died over several years as a result of this pandemic. Could another influenza pandemic occur (see Box 3.1)? The

Table 3.1
Recent Epidemics in the United States

Disease	Cases in Previous Years	Epidemic Period	Number of Cases
St. Louis encephalitis	5–72	1975	1,815[4]
Legionnaires' disease	Unknown	1976	235[5]
Toxic shock syndrome	11–272	1980	877[6]
HIV/AIDS	Unknown (before 1975)	1981–2006	1,000,000+[7]
Lyme disease	Unknown (before 1975)	1992–2006	248,074[8]
West Nile virus	Unknown in United States	1999–2008	28,981[9]
Mumps	231–338	2006	6,584[10]
Mumps	231–338	2009	1,521[11]
Influenza A	2,585–10,609	2009–2010	66,589[12]

Source: Centers for Disease Control and Prevention.

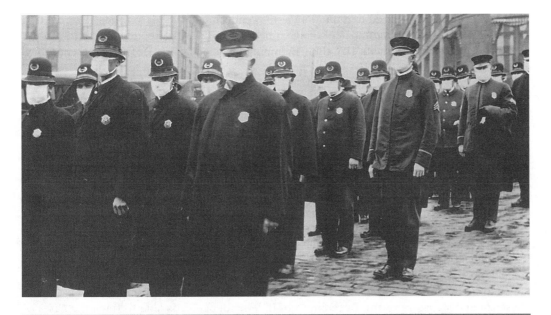

FIGURE 3.1

More than 25 million people died during the influenza pandemic of 1918–1919.

BOX
3.1

INFLUENZA: THE NEXT PANDEMIC?

In 1997, in Hong Kong, the first documented cases occurred in which avian influenza virus infected humans directly from birds. Previous human influenza virus infections had been traced to pig intermediaries. Because pigs can also be infected with human influenza virus, they are a host in which the two influenza virus strains can mix. A possible outcome of such mixing can be a strain that can be transmitted from human to human. In fact, this happens regularly, and new vaccines are introduced annually to combat the latest new strain or strains of influenza virus emanating from Asia.

The avian flu virus strain that infected people directly has been identified as the virulent H5N1 strain. Avian and human immunity to this strain is very low, so that most birds and people who become infected become very ill and many die. In December 2003, 19,000 of 25,000 chickens died on a farm in the Republic of Korea, and over the next several weeks more than a million chickens and ducks died. The virus next turned up in Vietnam and then Thailand, where human cases were reported. In these two countries there were 19 deaths among the 25 human cases in 2004. Since 2003, human H5N1 cases have been reported in Azerbaijan, Cambodia, China, Djibouti, Egypt, Indonesia, Iraq, and Turkey, according to the Centers for Disease Control and

Prevention (CDC). Since the first human case in 2003 through the middle of March 2010, 492 cases have been reported, with 291 deaths.

Health officials are concerned that the H5N1 strain could become pandemic because of the following reasons:

- It is especially virulent.
- It is being spread by migratory birds.
- It can be transmitted from birds to mammals and in some limited circumstances to humans.
- Like other influenza viruses, it continues to evolve.

The best source of information about avian influenza is the CDC Web site (http://pandemicflu.gov/). It provides scientific information about the flu virus, documents aimed at helping individuals and communities prepare for a possible flu pandemic, and links to state and local planning documents.

Another useful site is the World Health Organization's Web site (www.who.int/csr/disease/avian_influenza/en/), where you can read a history of the avian flu epidemic and get the latest information on the avian flu situation.

Sources: Centers for Disease Control and Prevention. "PandemicFlu.gov." Available at http://pandemicflu.gov/; and World Health Organization. "Avian Influenza." Available at http://www.who.int/csr/disease/avian_influenza/en/. Accessed October 1, 2010.

current outbreak of acquired immunodeficiency syndrome (AIDS) is another example of a pandemic. During 2007, an estimated 2 million people died of AIDS worldwide, and about 33 million people were living with HIV (human immunodeficiency virus).[3] This represents a leveling off or stabilization of the HIV/AIDS epidemic.

History of Epidemiology

If one searches diligently, it is possible to trace the roots of epidemiological thinking back to the "Father of Medicine," Hippocrates, who as early as 300 B.C. suggested a relationship between the occurrence of disease and the physical environment.[13] For example, cases of a disease fitting the description of malaria were found to occur in the vicinity of marshes and swamps.

With the fall of the classical civilizations of Greece and Rome and the return in Europe to a belief in spiritual causes of disease, few advances were made in the field of epidemiology. As a result, epidemics continued to occur. There were three waves of plague—one in 542-543, one in 1348-1349, and another in 1664-1665.[14] There were also epidemics of leprosy, smallpox, malaria, and, later, syphilis and yellow fever.

Epidemics occurred in the New World as well. One such epidemic of yellow fever struck Philadelphia in 1793, causing the death of 4,044 people. Yellow fever was epidemic again in Philadelphia in 1797, 1798, and in 1803.[15] Dr. Benjamin Rush, a prominent Philadelphia physician and signatory of the Declaration of Independence, was able to trace the cases of yellow fever to the docks where ships arrived from tropical ports. However, his conclusion that the disease was caused by vapors arising from decaying coffee beans in port warehouses was incorrect. He could not have known that yellow fever is caused by a virus and is carried by the yellow fever mosquito, *Aedes aegypti*. These facts were discovered by Major Walter Reed of the U.S. Army and his associates a century later.

cases
people afflicted with a disease

In 1849, some 50 years after the yellow fever outbreaks in Philadelphia, cholera became epidemic in London. A prominent physician, John Snow, investigated the outbreak by interviewing numerous victims and their families. He concluded that the source of the epidemic was probably water drawn from a particular communal well located on Broad Street. Snow extinguished the epidemic in 1854 when he removed the pump handle from the Broad Street pump, thus forcing people to obtain their water elsewhere.[16]

rate
the number of events that occur in a given population in a given period of time

John Snow's quashing of the London cholera epidemic in 1854 is a classic example of how epidemiological methods can be used to limit disease and deaths. His achievement was even more remarkable because it occurred 30 years before Louis Pasteur proposed his "germ theory of disease." It was not until 1883 that Robert Koch discovered the organism that causes cholera, *Vibrio cholerae*.

From its early use for the description and investigation of communicable diseases, epidemiology has developed into a sophisticated field of science. Epidemiological methods are used to evaluate everything from the effectiveness of vaccines to the possible causes of occupational illnesses and unintentional injury deaths.

natality (birth) rate
the number of live births divided by the total population

Knowledge of epidemiology is important to the community health worker who wishes to establish the presence of a set of needs or conditions for a particular health service or program or to justify a request for funding. Likewise, epidemiological methods are used to evaluate the effectiveness of programs already in existence and to plan to meet anticipated needs for facilities and personnel.

THE IMPORTANCE OF RATES

morbidity rate
the rate of illness in a population

Epidemiologists are concerned with numbers. Of prime importance is the number of health-related events, the number of **cases** (people who are sick), and, of course, the number of deaths. These numbers alone, however, are not enough to provide a description of the extent of the disease in a community. Epidemiologists must also know the total number in the susceptible population so that rates can be calculated. A **rate** is the number of events (births, cases of disease, or deaths) in a given population over a given period or at a given point in time. Three general categories of rates are **natality (birth) rates**, **morbidity** (sickness) **rates**, and **mortality or fatality (death) rates**.

Why are rates important? Why not simply enumerate the sick or dead? The answer is that rates enable one to compare outbreaks that occur at different times or in different places. For example, by using rates it is possible to determine whether there are more cases of gonorrhea per capita this year than there were last year or whether there are more homicides per capita in City A than in City B.

For example, suppose you wish to compare transportation deaths associated with travel by autos and airplanes. To examine this hypothetical situation, consider that for a given time period, 1,000 people died in auto crashes while 50 people died in airplane crashes. Without calculating rates, one might assume that auto travel is more dangerous than air travel. However, if you knew the population exposed (100,000 people for auto travel versus 1,000 people for air travel), you could calculate fatality rates, the number of deaths divided by the population, for each mode of travel.[17] (See Table 3.2.) These rates have greater meaning because they are based on the **population at risk**, those who are susceptible to disease or death from a particular cause. In this case, the fatality rates are 1/100 for autos and 5/100 for airplanes, thus indicating that in this hypothetical example air travel is five times more dangerous than auto travel.

Incidence, Prevalence, and Attack Rates

Three important types of morbidity rates are incidence rates, prevalence rates, and attack rates. An **incidence rate** is defined as the number of new health-related events or cases of a disease in a population exposed to that risk in a given time period—the number of *new* cases of influenza in a community over a week's time, for example. Those who became ill with influenza during the previous week and remain ill during the week in question are not counted in an incidence rate. Incidence rates are important in the study of **acute diseases**, diseases in which the peak severity of symptoms occurs and subsides within days or weeks. These diseases usually move quickly through a population. Examples of acute diseases are the common cold, influenza, chickenpox, measles, and mumps.

Prevalence rates are calculated by dividing *all* current cases of a disease (*old and new*) by the total population. Prevalence rates are useful for the study of **chronic disease**, diseases that usually last three months or longer. In these cases, it is more important to know how many people are currently suffering from a chronic disease—such as arthritis, heart disease, cancer, or diabetes—than it is to know when they became afflicted. Furthermore, with many chronic diseases, it is difficult or impossible to determine the date of onset of disease. Because a preponderance of health services and facilities are used for the treatment of persons with chronic diseases and conditions, prevalence rates are more useful than incidence rates for the planning of public health programs, personnel needs, and facilities.

mortality (fatality) rate the number of deaths in a population divided by the total population

population at risk those in the population who are susceptible to a particular disease or condition

incidence rate the number of new health-related events or cases of a disease in a population exposed to that risk during a particular period of time, divided by the total number in that same population

acute disease a disease that lasts three months or less

prevalence rate the number of new and old cases of a disease in a population in a given period of time, divided by the total number in that population

chronic disease a disease or health condition that lasts longer than 3 months

Table 3.2
Hypothetical Number of Deaths and Death Rates for Two Modes of Travel

	Source of Fatalities	
	Auto	**Airplane**
Number of fatalities per year	1,000	50
Number exposed to risk	100,000	1,000
Rate of fatality	0.01 (1/100)	0.05 (5/100)

Source: Mausner, J. S., and S. Kramer (1985). *Mausner and Bahn Epidemiology—An Introductory Text,* 2nd ed. Philadelphia, PA: W. B. Saunders Company, p. 5.

Table 3.3
Incidence Rates, Prevalence Rates, and Attack Rates

Name of Rate		Definition of Rate
Incidence rate	=	$\dfrac{\text{Number of new health-related events or cases of a disease}}{\text{Number of people exposed to risk during this period}}$
Prevalence rate	=	$\dfrac{\text{Total number of all individuals who have an attribute or disease at a time}}{\text{Population at risk of having the attribute or disease at this point or period of time}}$
Attack rate*	=	$\dfrac{\text{The cumulative incidence of infection in a group observed during an epidemic}}{\text{Number of people exposed}} \times 100$

*Attack rates are usually given as a percentage.

attack rate
an incidence rate calculated for a particular population for a single disease outbreak and expressed as a percentage

An **attack rate** is a special incidence rate calculated for a particular population for a single disease outbreak and expressed as a percentage (see Table 3.3). For example, suppose a number of people who traveled on the same airline flight developed a similar illness, and epidemiologists suspected that the cause of this illness was associated with the flight itself. An attack rate could be calculated for the passengers on that flight to express the percentage who became ill. Furthermore, attack rates could be calculated for various subpopulations, such as those seated at various locations in the plane, those who selected specific entrees from the menu, those of particular age groups, or those who boarded the flight at specific stops. Differences in attack rates for different subpopulations might indicate to the epidemiologists the source or cause of the illness.

crude rate
a rate in which the denominator includes the total population

Crude and Age-Adjusted Rates

crude birth rate
the number of live births per 1,000 in a population in a given period of time

Incidence and prevalence rates can be expressed in two forms—crude and specific. **Crude rates** are those in which the denominator includes the total population. The most important of these are the crude birth rate and the crude death rate. The **crude birth rate** is the number of live births in a given year, divided by the midyear population. The **crude death rate (CDR)** is the total number of deaths in a given year from all causes, divided by the midyear population (see Table 3.4). Crude rates are relatively easy to obtain and are useful when comparing similar populations. But they can be misleading when populations differ by age structure or by some other attribute. For example, crude birth rates are normally higher in younger populations, which have a higher proportion of people of reproductive age, than in populations with more elderly people. Conversely, CDRs are normally higher in older populations. This makes it difficult to use crude rates to compare the risk of death in different populations, such as those of the states of Florida and Alaska. To show what the level of mortality would be if the age composition of different populations were the same, epidemiologists use **age-adjusted rates**. For example, in 2008 because of its larger senior population, Florida had a higher crude death rate (931.2 per 100,000) compared with Alaska's (507.5 per 100,000), where the population is

crude death rate (CDR)
the number of deaths (from all causes) per 1,000 in a population in a given period of time

age-adjusted rate
rate used to make comparisons of relative risks across groups and over time when groups differ in age structure

Table 3.4
Crude Rates

Name of Rate		Definition of Rate		Multiplier
Crude birth rate	=	$\dfrac{\text{Number of live births}}{\text{Estimated midyear population}}$	×	1,000
Crude death rate	=	$\dfrac{\text{Number of deaths (all causes)}}{\text{Estimated midyear population}}$	×	100,000

Table 3.5
Crude and Age-Adjusted Mortality Rates for Alaska and Florida, 2008

State	Number of Deaths	Crude Death Rate*	Age-Adjusted Death Rate*
Alaska	3,483	507.5	739.6
Florida	170,668	931.2	679.0

*Deaths per 100,000 population.

Source: Miniño, A. M., J. Q. Xu, K. D. Kochanek. "Deaths: Preliminary Data for 2008." *National Vital Statistics Reports,* 59(2). Hyattsville, MD: National Center for Health Statistics. 2010. Available at http://www.cdc.gov/nchs/data/nvsr/nvsr59/nvsr59_02.pdf. Accessed December 16, 2010.

younger. However, when these death rates are adjusted for differences in the age structures of the populations of these two states, one can see that the death rate in Florida (679.0 per 100,000) compares favorably with the death rate in Alaska (739.6 per 100,000). See Table 3.5.[18] Methods for calculating age-adjusted rates can be found in standard epidemiology textbooks.

specific rate
a rate that measures morbidity or mortality for particular populations or diseases

Specific Rates

Specific rates measure morbidity and mortality for particular populations or for particular diseases. One could, for example, calculate the age-specific mortality rate for a population of 35- to 44-year-olds by dividing the number of deaths in that age group by the midyear population of 35- to 44-year-olds. Similarly, one could calculate race- and sex-specific mortality rates.

A very important specific rate is the **cause-specific mortality rate (CSMR)**, which measures the death rate for a specific disease. This rate can be calculated by dividing the number of deaths due to a particular disease by the total population. One could also calculate an age–specific, cause-specific mortality rate. Because fewer people can be expected to die from each cause than to die from all causes, CSMRs are usually reported per 100,000 population. Table 3.6 lists some important rates used in epidemiology, defines them, and gives an example of each.

cause-specific mortality rate (CSMR)
the death rate due to a particular disease

Table 3.6
Important Rates in Epidemiology

Rate		Definition		Multiplier	Examples (U.S. 2007)[18,19]
Crude birth rate	=	Number of live births / Estimated midyear population	×	1,000	14.0/1,000
Crude death rate	=	Number of deaths (all causes) / Estimated midyear population	×	100,000	760.9/100,000
Age-specific death rate	=	Number of deaths, 15–24 years / Estimated midyear population, 15–24 years	×	100,000	79.9/100,000
Infant mortality rate	=	Number of deaths under 1 year of age / Number of live births	×	1,000,000	674.9/100,000
Neonatal mortality rate	=	Number of deaths under 28 days of age / Number of live births	×	1,000	6.75/1,000
Cause-specific death rate	=	Number of deaths (diabetes mellitus) / Estimated midyear population	×	100,000	23.7/100,000
Age-specific, cause-specific death rate	=	Number of deaths, 15–24 years (motor vehicles) / Estimated midyear population	×	100,000	24.9/100,000

case fatality rate (CFR)
the percentage of cases of a particular disease that result in death

Two other important measures of disease are the **case fatality rate (CFR)** and the **proportionate mortality ratio (PMR)**. The CFR is simply the percentage of cases that result in death. It is a measure of the severity of a disease and is directly related to the virulence of the disease agent. It is calculated by dividing the number of deaths from a particular disease in a specified period of time by the number of cases of that same disease in the same time period. The resulting fraction is multiplied by 100 and is reported as a percentage. For example, if there were 200 cases of a severe illness and 10 of them resulted in death, the CFR would be $10 \div 200 \times 100 = 5\%$.

proportionate mortality ratio (PMR)
the percentage of overall mortality in a population that is attributable to a particular cause

The PMR describes the relationship between the number of deaths from a specific cause to the total number of deaths attributable to all causes. It is calculated by dividing the number of deaths attributed to a particular disease by the total number of deaths from all causes in the same population during the same period of time. This rate is also reported as a percentage. For example, in the United States, there were 617,527 deaths due to diseases of the heart in 2008, and 2,472,699 total deaths reported that same year.[18] Thus, the PMR for diseases of the heart can be calculated as follows: $617,527 \div 2,472,699 = 25\%$. In other words, in the United States, heart disease was responsible for one in four deaths in 2008.

REPORTING OF BIRTHS, DEATHS, AND DISEASES

notifiable diseases
infectious diseases for which health officials request or require reporting for public health reasons

It is important to epidemiologists that births, deaths, and cases of diseases be recorded promptly and accurately. Physicians, clinics, and hospitals are required by law to report all births and deaths as well as all cases of certain **notifiable diseases** to their local health departments. Notifiable diseases are infectious diseases that can become epidemic and for which health officials maintain weekly records. The Centers for Disease Control and Prevention (CDC) issues a list of notifiable diseases for which it requests reports from each state health department. This list is revised periodically. In 2008, the CDC designated more than 70 diseases as notifiable at the national level (see Table 3.7).[10] Several diseases caused by possible bioterrorism agents, such as anthrax and Q fever, were added. Individual states may require the reporting of additional diseases that are of local public health concern. Local health departments are required by their respective state health departments to summarize all records of births (see Figure 3.2), deaths, and notifiable diseases and to report them. State health departments summarize these reports and relay them to the CDC through the **National Electronic Telecommunications System (NETS)**. The reporting scheme for notifiable disease is shown in Figure 3.3.

National Electronic Telecommunications System (NETS)
the electronic reporting system used by state health departments and the CDC

The CDC summarizes state and territorial data and uses it to plan epidemiological research, conduct investigations, and issue reports. One series of reports, published weekly by the CDC, is called the *Morbidity and Mortality Weekly Report (MMWR)*. *MMWR*s are available to the public at the CDC Web site, www.cdc.gov/mmwr. Paper copies can usually be found in the government documents areas of certain larger libraries.

Unfortunately, the information reported is not always as good as it should be. One study estimated that local health departments may receive notification of only 35% of the cases of some communicable diseases and that many physicians are not familiar with the requirement of reporting. Clinics may not report each and every case of measles or gonorrhea. Doctors' offices and clinics may be understaffed or simply too busy to keep up with reporting. In other cases, patients recover—with or without treatment—before a diagnosis is confirmed. Also, changes in local and state government administration or other key personnel often interfere with the timely reporting of disease data. The accuracy of disease reporting also depends on the type of disease. In this regard, serious diseases are more likely to be reported than milder

Table 3.7
Infectious Diseases Designated as Notifiable at the National Level during 2008

Acquired immunodeficiency syndrome (AIDS)

Anthrax

Domestic arboviral diseases, neuroinvasive and
  nonneuroinvasive
  California serogroup virus
  Eastern equine encephalitis virus
  Powassan virus
  St. Louis encephalitis virus
  West Nile virus
  Western equine encephalitis virus

Botulism
  Foodborne
  Infant
  Other (wound and unspecified)

Brucellosis

Chancroid

Chlamydia trachomatis infections

Cholera

Coccidioidomycosis[a]

Cryptosporidiosis

Cyclosporiasis

Diphtheria

Ehrlichiosis/Anaplasmosis[a]
  Ehrlichia chaffeensis
  Ehrlichia ewingii
  Anaplasma phagocytophilum
  Undetermined

Giardiasis

Gonorrhea

Haemophilus influenzae, invasive disease

Hansen disease (Leprosy)

Hantavirus pulmonary syndrome

Hemolytic uremic syndrome, post-diarrheal

Hepatitis, viral, acute
  Hepatitis A, acute
  Hepatitis B, acute
  Hepatitis B virus, perinatal infection
  Hepatitis C, acute

Hepatitis, viral, chronic
  Chronic hepatitis B
  Hepatitis C virus infection (past or present)

Human immunodeficiency virus infection
  Adult (age ≥13 yrs)
  Pediatric (age <13 yrs)

Influenza-associated pediatric mortality

Legionellosis

Listeriosis

Lyme disease[a]

Malaria

Measles

Meningococcal disease

Mumps[a]

Novel influenza A virus infections

Pertussis

Plague

Poliomyelitis, paralytic

Poliovirus infection, nonparalytic

Psittacosis

Q fever[a]
  acute
  chronic

Rabies
  animal
  human

Rocky Mountain spotted fever[a]

Rubella

Rubella, congenital syndrome

Salmonellosis

Severe acute respiratory syndrome-associated
  coronavirus (SARS-CoV) disease

Shiga toxin-producing *Escherichia coli* (STEC)

Shigellosis

Smallpox

Streptococcal disease, invasive, Group A

Streptococcal toxic-shock syndrome

Streptococcus pneumoniae, drug resistant, all ages,
  invasive disease

Streptococcus pneumoniae, invasive disease non-drug
  resistant, in children aged <5 years

Syphilis

Syphilis, congenital

Tetanus

Toxic-shock syndrome (other than streptococcal)

Trichinellosis

Tuberculosis

Tularemia

Typhoid fever

Vancomycin-intermediate *Staphylococcus aureus*
  infection (VISA)

Vancomycin-resistant *Staphylococcus aureus* infection
  (VRSA)

Varicella (morbidity)

Varicella (mortality)

Vibriosis

Yellow fever

Note: Position Statements the Council of State and Territorial Epidemiologists approved in 2007 for national surveillance were implemented beginning in January 2008. No new conditions were added to the notifiable disease list in 2008.

[a]Revised national surveillance case definition.

Source: Centers for Disease Control and Prevention (2010). "Summary of Notifiable Diseases—United States, 2008." *Morbidity and Mortality Weekly Report*, 53(53): 1–82. Available at http://www.cdc.gov/mmwr/PDF/wk/mm5754.pdf. Accessed October 1, 2010.

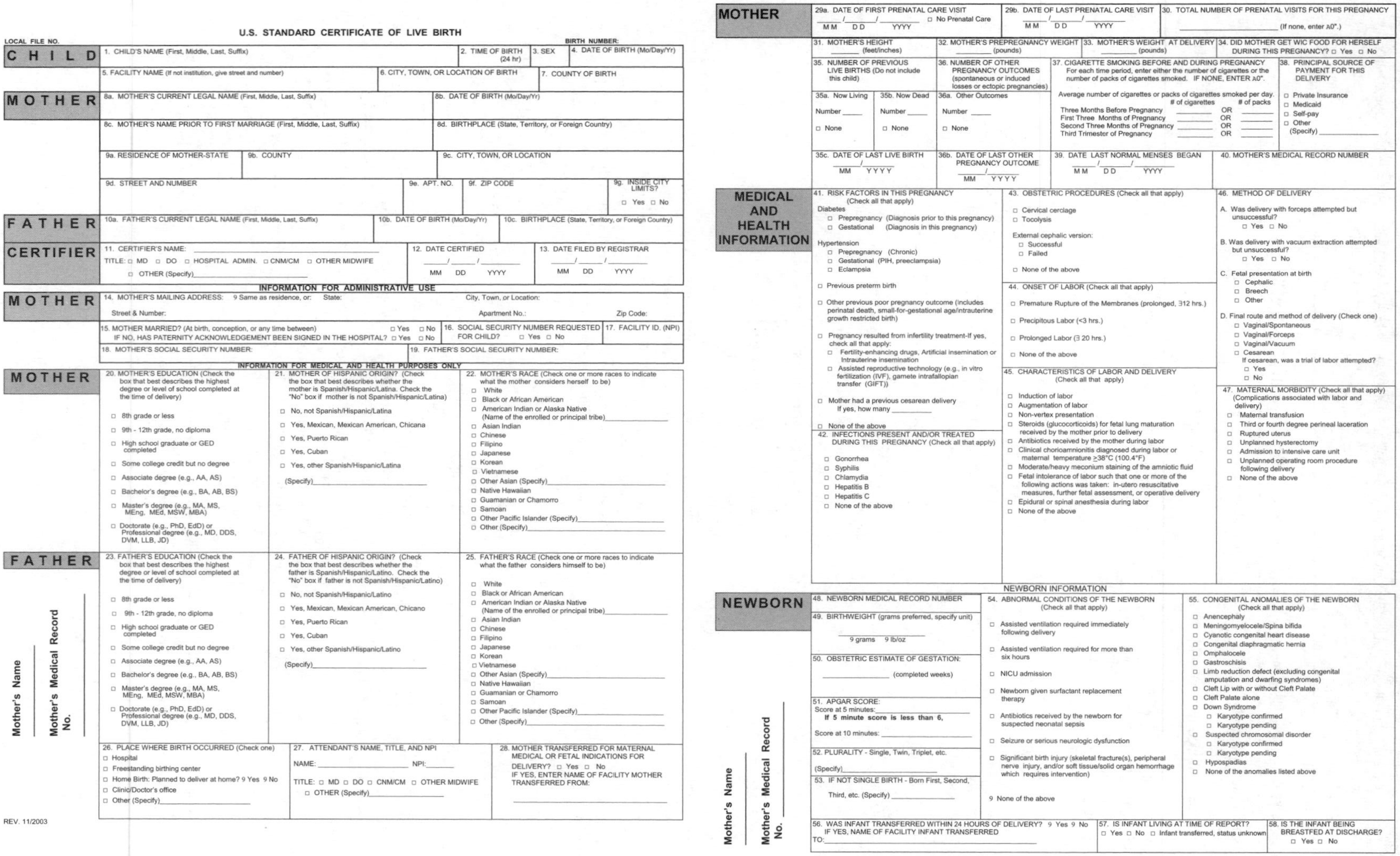
U.S. STANDARD CERTIFICATE OF LIVE BIRTH

LOCAL FILE NO.
BIRTH NUMBER:

CHILD
1. CHILD'S NAME (First, Middle, Last, Suffix)
2. TIME OF BIRTH (24 hr)
3. SEX
4. DATE OF BIRTH (Mo/Day/Yr)
5. FACILITY NAME (If not institution, give street and number)
6. CITY, TOWN, OR LOCATION OF BIRTH
7. COUNTY OF BIRTH

MOTHER
8a. MOTHER'S CURRENT LEGAL NAME (First, Middle, Last, Suffix)
8b. DATE OF BIRTH (Mo/Day/Yr)
8c. MOTHER'S NAME PRIOR TO FIRST MARRIAGE (First, Middle, Last, Suffix)
8d. BIRTHPLACE (State, Territory, or Foreign Country)
9a. RESIDENCE OF MOTHER-STATE
9b. COUNTY
9c. CITY, TOWN, OR LOCATION
9d. STREET AND NUMBER
9e. APT. NO.
9f. ZIP CODE
9g. INSIDE CITY LIMITS? □ Yes □ No

FATHER
10a. FATHER'S CURRENT LEGAL NAME (First, Middle, Last, Suffix)
10b. DATE OF BIRTH (Mo/Day/Yr)
10c. BIRTHPLACE (State, Territory, or Foreign Country)

CERTIFIER
11. CERTIFIER'S NAME: ____
TITLE: □ MD □ DO □ HOSPITAL ADMIN. □ CNM/CM □ OTHER MIDWIFE
□ OTHER (Specify)____
12. DATE CERTIFIED ___/___/___ MM DD YYYY
13. DATE FILED BY REGISTRAR ___/___/___ MM DD YYYY

INFORMATION FOR ADMINISTRATIVE USE

MOTHER
14. MOTHER'S MAILING ADDRESS: 9 Same as residence, or: State: City, Town, or Location:
Street & Number: Apartment No.: Zip Code:
15. MOTHER MARRIED? (At birth, conception, or any time between) □ Yes □ No
IF NO, HAS PATERNITY ACKNOWLEDGEMENT BEEN SIGNED IN THE HOSPITAL? □ Yes □ No
16. SOCIAL SECURITY NUMBER REQUESTED FOR CHILD? □ Yes □ No
17. FACILITY ID. (NPI)
18. MOTHER'S SOCIAL SECURITY NUMBER:
19. FATHER'S SOCIAL SECURITY NUMBER:

INFORMATION FOR MEDICAL AND HEALTH PURPOSES ONLY

MOTHER
20. MOTHER'S EDUCATION (Check the box that best describes the highest degree or level of school completed at the time of delivery)
□ 8th grade or less
□ 9th - 12th grade, no diploma
□ High school graduate or GED completed
□ Some college credit but no degree
□ Associate degree (e.g., AA, AS)
□ Bachelor's degree (e.g., BA, AB, BS)
□ Master's degree (e.g., MA, MS, MEng, MEd, MSW, MBA)
□ Doctorate (e.g., PhD, EdD) or Professional degree (e.g., MD, DDS, DVM, LLB, JD)
21. MOTHER OF HISPANIC ORIGIN? (Check the box that best describes whether the mother is Spanish/Hispanic/Latina. Check the "No" box if mother is not Spanish/Hispanic/Latina)
□ No, not Spanish/Hispanic/Latina
□ Yes, Mexican, Mexican American, Chicana
□ Yes, Puerto Rican
□ Yes, Cuban
□ Yes, other Spanish/Hispanic/Latina
(Specify)____
22. MOTHER'S RACE (Check one or more races to indicate what the mother considers herself to be)
□ White
□ Black or African American
□ American Indian or Alaska Native (Name of the enrolled or principal tribe)____
□ Asian Indian
□ Chinese
□ Filipino
□ Japanese
□ Korean
□ Vietnamese
□ Other Asian (Specify)____
□ Native Hawaiian
□ Guamanian or Chamorro
□ Samoan
□ Other Pacific Islander (Specify)____
□ Other (Specify)____

FATHER
23. FATHER'S EDUCATION (Check the box that best describes the highest degree or level of school completed at the time of delivery)
□ 8th grade or less
□ 9th - 12th grade, no diploma
□ High school graduate or GED completed
□ Some college credit but no degree
□ Associate degree (e.g., AA, AS)
□ Bachelor's degree (e.g., BA, AB, BS)
□ Master's degree (e.g., MA, MS, MEng, MEd, MSW, MBA)
□ Doctorate (e.g., PhD, EdD) or Professional degree (e.g., MD, DDS, DVM, LLB, JD)
24. FATHER OF HISPANIC ORIGIN? (Check the box that best describes whether the father is Spanish/Hispanic/Latino. Check the "No" box if father is not Spanish/Hispanic/Latino)
□ No, not Spanish/Hispanic/Latino
□ Yes, Mexican, Mexican American, Chicano
□ Yes, Puerto Rican
□ Yes, Cuban
□ Yes, other Spanish/Hispanic/Latino
(Specify)____
25. FATHER'S RACE (Check one or more races to indicate what the father considers himself to be)
□ White
□ Black or African American
□ American Indian or Alaska Native (Name of the enrolled or principal tribe)____
□ Asian Indian
□ Chinese
□ Filipino
□ Japanese
□ Korean
□ Vietnamese
□ Other Asian (Specify)____
□ Native Hawaiian
□ Guamanian or Chamorro
□ Samoan
□ Other Pacific Islander (Specify)____
□ Other (Specify)____

26. PLACE WHERE BIRTH OCCURRED (Check one)
□ Hospital
□ Freestanding birthing center
□ Home Birth: Planned to deliver at home? 9 Yes 9 No
□ Clinic/Doctor's office
□ Other (Specify)____
27. ATTENDANT'S NAME, TITLE, AND NPI
NAME: ____ NPI: ____
TITLE: □ MD □ DO □ CNM/CM □ OTHER MIDWIFE
□ OTHER (Specify)____
28. MOTHER TRANSFERRED FOR MATERNAL MEDICAL OR FETAL INDICATIONS FOR DELIVERY? □ Yes □ No
IF YES, ENTER NAME OF FACILITY MOTHER TRANSFERRED FROM:

Mother's Name
Mother's Medical Record No.

REV. 11/2003

MOTHER
29a. DATE OF FIRST PRENATAL CARE VISIT ___/___/___ MM DD YYYY □ No Prenatal Care
29b. DATE OF LAST PRENATAL CARE VISIT ___/___/___ MM DD YYYY
30. TOTAL NUMBER OF PRENATAL VISITS FOR THIS PREGNANCY ____ (If none, enter A0".)
31. MOTHER'S HEIGHT ____ (feet/inches)
32. MOTHER'S PREPREGNANCY WEIGHT ____ (pounds)
33. MOTHER'S WEIGHT AT DELIVERY ____ (pounds)
34. DID MOTHER GET WIC FOOD FOR HERSELF DURING THIS PREGNANCY? □ Yes □ No
35. NUMBER OF PREVIOUS LIVE BIRTHS (Do not include this child)
35a. Now Living Number ____ □ None
35b. Now Dead Number ____ □ None
36. NUMBER OF OTHER PREGNANCY OUTCOMES (spontaneous or induced losses or ectopic pregnancies)
36a. Other Outcomes Number ____ □ None
37. CIGARETTE SMOKING BEFORE AND DURING PREGNANCY
For each time period, enter either the number of cigarettes or the number of packs of cigarettes smoked. IF NONE, ENTER A0".
Average number of cigarettes or packs of cigarettes smoked per day.
# of cigarettes # of packs
Three Months Before Pregnancy ____ OR ____
First Three Months of Pregnancy ____ OR ____
Second Three Months of Pregnancy ____ OR ____
Third Trimester of Pregnancy ____ OR ____
38. PRINCIPAL SOURCE OF PAYMENT FOR THIS DELIVERY
□ Private Insurance
□ Medicaid
□ Self-pay
□ Other (Specify)____
35c. DATE OF LAST LIVE BIRTH ___/___ MM YYYY
36b. DATE OF LAST OTHER PREGNANCY OUTCOME ___/___ MM YYYY
39. DATE LAST NORMAL MENSES BEGAN ___/___/___ MM DD YYYY
40. MOTHER'S MEDICAL RECORD NUMBER

MEDICAL AND HEALTH INFORMATION
41. RISK FACTORS IN THIS PREGNANCY (Check all that apply)
Diabetes
□ Prepregnancy (Diagnosis prior to this pregnancy)
□ Gestational (Diagnosis in this pregnancy)
Hypertension
□ Prepregnancy (Chronic)
□ Gestational (PIH, preeclampsia)
□ Eclampsia
□ Previous preterm birth
□ Other previous poor pregnancy outcome (Includes perinatal death, small-for-gestational age/intrauterine growth restricted birth)
□ Pregnancy resulted from infertility treatment-If yes, check all that apply:
□ Fertility-enhancing drugs, Artificial insemination or Intrauterine insemination
□ Assisted reproductive technology (e.g., in vitro fertilization (IVF), gamete intrafallopian transfer (GIFT))
□ Mother had a previous cesarean delivery
If yes, how many ____
□ None of the above
42. INFECTIONS PRESENT AND/OR TREATED DURING THIS PREGNANCY (Check all that apply)
□ Gonorrhea
□ Syphilis
□ Chlamydia
□ Hepatitis B
□ Hepatitis C
□ None of the above
43. OBSTETRIC PROCEDURES (Check all that apply)
□ Cervical cerclage
□ Tocolysis
External cephalic version:
□ Successful
□ Failed
□ None of the above
44. ONSET OF LABOR (Check all that apply)
□ Premature Rupture of the Membranes (prolonged, 312 hrs.)
□ Precipitous Labor (<3 hrs.)
□ Prolonged Labor (3 20 hrs.)
□ None of the above
45. CHARACTERISTICS OF LABOR AND DELIVERY (Check all that apply)
□ Induction of labor
□ Augmentation of labor
□ Non-vertex presentation
□ Steroids (glucocorticoids) for fetal lung maturation received by the mother prior to delivery
□ Antibiotics received by the mother during labor
□ Clinical chorioamnionitis diagnosed during labor or maternal temperature ≥38°C (100.4°F)
□ Moderate/heavy meconium staining of the amniotic fluid
□ Fetal intolerance of labor such that one or more of the following actions was taken: in-utero resuscitative measures, further fetal assessment, or operative delivery
□ Epidural or spinal anesthesia during labor
□ None of the above
46. METHOD OF DELIVERY
A. Was delivery with forceps attempted but unsuccessful?
□ Yes □ No
B. Was delivery with vacuum extraction attempted but unsuccessful?
□ Yes □ No
C. Fetal presentation at birth
□ Cephalic
□ Breech
□ Other
D. Final route and method of delivery (Check one)
□ Vaginal/Spontaneous
□ Vaginal/Forceps
□ Vaginal/Vacuum
□ Cesarean
If cesarean, was a trial of labor attempted?
□ Yes
□ No
47. MATERNAL MORBIDITY (Check all that apply) (Complications associated with labor and delivery)
□ Maternal transfusion
□ Third or fourth degree perineal laceration
□ Ruptured uterus
□ Unplanned hysterectomy
□ Admission to intensive care unit
□ Unplanned operating room procedure following delivery
□ None of the above

NEWBORN INFORMATION

NEWBORN
48. NEWBORN MEDICAL RECORD NUMBER
49. BIRTHWEIGHT (grams preferred, specify unit)
____ 9 grams 9 lb/oz
50. OBSTETRIC ESTIMATE OF GESTATION:
____ (completed weeks)
51. APGAR SCORE:
Score at 5 minutes: ____
If 5 minute score is less than 6,
Score at 10 minutes: ____
52. PLURALITY - Single, Twin, Triplet, etc.
(Specify)____
53. IF NOT SINGLE BIRTH - Born First, Second, Third, etc. (Specify) ____
54. ABNORMAL CONDITIONS OF THE NEWBORN (Check all that apply)
□ Assisted ventilation required immediately following delivery
□ Assisted ventilation required for more than six hours
□ NICU admission
□ Newborn given surfactant replacement therapy
□ Antibiotics received by the newborn for suspected neonatal sepsis
□ Seizure or serious neurologic dysfunction
□ Significant birth injury (skeletal fracture(s), peripheral nerve injury, and/or soft tissue/solid organ hemorrhage which requires intervention)
9 None of the above
55. CONGENITAL ANOMALIES OF THE NEWBORN (Check all that apply)
□ Anencephaly
□ Meningomyelocele/Spina bifida
□ Cyanotic congenital heart disease
□ Congenital diaphragmatic hernia
□ Omphalocele
□ Gastroschisis
□ Limb reduction defect (excluding congenital amputation and dwarfing syndromes)
□ Cleft Lip with or without Cleft Palate
□ Cleft Palate alone
□ Down Syndrome
□ Karyotype confirmed
□ Karyotype pending
□ Suspected chromosomal disorder
□ Karyotype confirmed
□ Karyotype pending
□ Hypospadias
□ None of the anomalies listed above
56. WAS INFANT TRANSFERRED WITHIN 24 HOURS OF DELIVERY? 9 Yes 9 No
IF YES, NAME OF FACILITY INFANT TRANSFERRED TO:____
57. IS INFANT LIVING AT TIME OF REPORT? □ Yes □ No □ Infant transferred, status unknown
58. IS THE INFANT BEING BREASTFED AT DISCHARGE? □ Yes □ No

Mother's Name
Mother's Medical Record No.

FIGURE 3.2
Birth certificates are issued by local health departments that have jurisdiction where the birth occurred.
Source: Courtesy of Centers for Disease Control and Prevention.

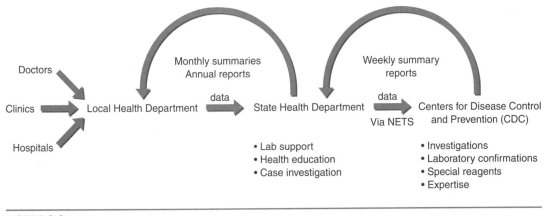

FIGURE 3.3
Scheme for the reporting of notifiable diseases.

ones. Rabies cases, for example, are almost 100% reported, whereas German measles cases may be only 80% to 90% reported. Therefore, morbidity data—although useful for reflecting disease trends—cannot always be considered to be precise counts of the actual number of cases of diseases.

STANDARDIZED MEASUREMENTS OF HEALTH STATUS OF POPULATIONS

It is often difficult to precisely measure the level of wellness or, for that matter, ill health. On the other hand, death can be clearly defined. For this reason, mortality statistics continue to be the single most reliable indicator of a population's health status. Although mortality statistics do not completely describe the health status of a population, they can be used to calculate other useful measurements; two of these are life expectancy and years of potential life lost. Finally, there are measurements of ill health that, although less precise than mortality, can nonetheless be meaningful. Such measurements are disability-adjusted life years and health-adjusted life expectancy.

Mortality Statistics

In 2008, 2,472,699 deaths were registered in the United States. The crude mortality rate was 813.3 per 100,000. The age-adjusted death rate, which eliminates the effects of the aging population, was 758.7 deaths per 100,000 U.S. standard population. This was a record low.[18] Age-adjusted death rates show what the level of mortality would be if no changes occurred in the age makeup of the population from year to year. Thus, they are a better indicator than are unadjusted (crude) death rates for examining changes in the risk of death over a period of time when the age distribution of the population is changing. Death rates and age-adjusted death rates for the 15 leading causes of death for the entire population in the United States in 2007 are presented in Table 3.8.[18] (Age-adjusted rates by race and ethnic group for 2008 were unavailable at press time.)

Naturally, morbidity and mortality rates vary greatly depending on age, sex, race, and ethnicity. For example, whereas heart disease is the leading cause of death for the general population and especially for older adults (those who have reached 65 years of age), cancer is the leading cause of death for the 45- to 64-years age group, and unintentional injuries are the leading cause of death for all age groups between 1 and 44. (In Chapters 7–10, we discuss the differences in the health statistics of people in different age, sex, and minority groups.)

Table 3.8

Deaths, Percentage of Total Deaths, and Death Rates for 2008 and Age-Adjusted Death Rates and Percent Changes in Age-Adjusted Rates from 2007 to 2008 for the 15 Leading Causes of Death: United States, Final 2007 and Preliminary 2008

Rank[1]	Cause of Death (Based on the *International Classification of Diseases, Tenth Revision, Second Edition, 2004*)	Number	Percentage of Total Deaths	Death Rate	Age-Adjusted Death Rate 2008	Age-Adjusted Death Rate 2007	Percent Change
. . .	All causes	2,472,699	100.0	813.2	758.6	760.2	–0.2
1	Diseases of heart (I00–I09, I11, I13, I20–I51)	617,527	25.0	203.1	186.7	190.9	–2.2
2	Malignant neoplasms (C00–C97)	566,137	22.9	186.2	175.5	178.4	–1.6
3	Chronic lower respiratory diseases (J40–J47)	141,075	5.7	46.4	44.0	40.8	7.8
4	Cerebrovascular diseases (I60–I69)	133,750	5.4	44.0	40.6	42.2	–3.8
5	Accidents (unintentional injuries) (V01–X59, Y85–Y86)[2]	122,207	4.9	39.9	38.6	40.0	–3.5
6	Alzheimer's disease (G30)	82,476	3.3	27.1	24.4	22.7	7.5
7	Diabetes mellitus (E10–E14)	70,601	2.9	23.2	21.8	22.5	–3.1
8	Influenza and pneumonia (J09–J18)[3]	56,335	2.3	18.5	17.0	16.2	4.9
9	Nephritis, nephrotic syndrome and nephrosis (N00–N07, N17–N19, N25–N27)	48,283	2.0	15.9	14.8	14.5	2.1
10	Septicemia (A40–A41)	35,961	1.5	11.8	11.1	11.0	0.9
11	Intentional self-harm (suicide) (*U03, X60–X84, Y87.0)[2]	35,933	1.5	11.8	11.6	11.3	2.7
12	Chronic liver disease and cirrhosis (K70, K73–K74)	29,963	1.2	9.9	9.2	9.1	1.1
13	Essential hypertension and hypertensive renal disease (I10, I12, I15)	25,823	1.0	8.5	7.7	7.4	4.1
14	Parkinson's disease (G20–G21)	20,507	0.8	6.7	6.4	6.4	0.0
15	Assault (homicide) (*U01–*U02, X85–Y09, Y87.1)[2]	17,837	0.7	5.9	5.9	6.1	–3.3
. . .	All other causes (Residual)	469,284	19.0	154.3	. . .	. . .	. . .

. . . Category not applicable.

[1]Rank based on number of deaths.

[2]For unintentional injuries, suicides, and homicides, preliminary and final data may differ significantly because of the truncated nature of the preliminary file.

[3]New code J09 (influenza due to identified avian influenza virus) was added to the category in 2007.

Note: Data are subject to sampling and random variation.

Data are based on a continuous file of records received from the states. Rates are per 100,000 population; age-adjusted rates per 100,000 U.S. standard population based on the year 2000 standard. Figures for 2008 are based on weighted data rounded to the nearest individual, so categories may not add to totals.

Source: : Miniño, A. M., J. Q. Xu, K. D. Kochanek (2010). "Deaths: Preliminary Data for 2008." *National Vital Statistics Reports,* 59(2). Hyattsville, MD: National Center for Health Statistics. Available at http://www.cdc.gov/nchs/data/nvsr/nvsr59/nvsr59_02.pdf. Accessed December 16, 2010.

A study of the mortality statistics for the twentieth century reveals a shift in the leading causes of death. When the century began, communicable diseases such as pneumonia, tuberculosis, and gastrointestinal infections were the leading causes of death.[20] However, a century of progress in public health practice and in biomedical research has resulted in a significant reduction in the proportion of deaths from communicable diseases so that the four leading causes of death today are noncommunicable diseases (see Table 3.9). At the beginning of the twenty-first century, the five leading causes of death in the United States—heart disease, cancer, chronic lower respiratory disease, stroke, and unintentional injuries (accidents and adverse effects)—account for about 65% of all deaths (see Table 3.9).[18]

This domination of annual mortality statistics by noncommunicable diseases masks the importance of communicable diseases as causes of deaths in certain age groups. For example, pneumonia and influenza still kill many older adults in this country each year. Also, HIV/AIDS, listed as the eighth overall leading cause of death for Americans as recently as 1996, kills more males than females. Thus, it is important to remember that viewing the leading causes of death for the entire population does not provide a clear picture of the health for any one segment of the population.

Table 3.9
Leading Causes of Death in the United States: 1900, 1940, 2008

1900

1.	Pneumonia, influenza
2.	Tuberculosis
3.	Diarrhea
4.	Diseases of the heart
5.	Cerebrovascular diseases (stroke)
6.	Nephritis
7.	Unintentional injuries (accidents)
8.	Malignant neoplasms (cancers)
9.	Senility
10.	Diphtheria

1940

1.	Diseases of the heart
2.	Malignant neoplasms (cancers)
3.	Cerebrovascular diseases (stroke)
4.	Nephritis
5.	Pneumonia, influenza
6.	Unintentional injuries (non-motor vehicle)
7.	Tuberculosis
8.	Diabetes mellitus
9.	Unintentional injuries (motor vehicle)
10.	Premature birth

2008

1.	Diseases of the heart
2.	Malignant neoplasms (cancers)
3.	Chronic lower respiratory diseases
4.	Cerebrovascular diseases (stroke)
5.	Unintentional injuries (all)
6.	Alzheimer's disease
7.	Diabetes mellitus
8.	Influenza and pneumonia
9.	Nephritis (kidney diseases)
10.	Septicemia

Sources: Miniño, A. M., J. Q. Xu, K. D. Kochanek. "Deaths: Preliminary Data for 2008." *National Vital Statistics Reports,* 59(2). Hyattsville, MD: National Center for Health Statistics. 2010. Available at http://www.cdc.gov/nchs/data/nvsr/nvsr59/nvsr59_02.pdf; and Centers for Disease Control and Prevention, National Center for Health Statistics (1998). Leading Causes of Death, 1900-1998. Available at http://www.cdc.gov/nchs/data/dvs/lead1900_98.pdf. Accessed December 16, 2010.

Life Expectancy

life expectancy
the average number
of years a person
from a specific cohort
is projected to live
from a given point in
time

Life expectancy is another standard measurement used to compare the health status of various populations. Also based on mortality, **life expectancy** is defined as the average number of years a person from a specific cohort is projected to live from a given point in time. Whereas life insurance companies are interested in life expectancy at every age, health statisticians are usually concerned with life expectancy at birth, at the age of 65 years, and, more recently, at age 75. It must be remembered that life expectancy is an average for an entire cohort (usually of a single birth year) and is not necessarily a useful prediction for any one individual. Moreover, it certainly cannot describe the quality of one's life. However, the ever-increasing life expectancy for Americans suggests that, as a country, we have managed to control some of those factors that contribute to early deaths.

Table 3.10 provides a summary of life expectancy figures for the United States from 1900 to 2006. The data presented indicate that the overall life expectancy at birth, at 65 years, and at 75 years has generally increased since 1900. Life expectancies at birth for both sexes rose from 47.3 years in 1900 to 77.5 years in 2006, when the life expectancy of a newborn baby girl was 80.2 years compared with a newborn baby boy—75.1 years.[21]

When compared with the life expectancy figures of other countries (see Table 3.11), the United States figures roughly correspond with those of other countries with well-developed economies. The highest life expectancy figures are reported in Japan (86 years for females); while the lowest are reported from countries in Africa.[21]

Years of Potential Life Lost

**years of potential
life lost (YPLL)**
the number of years
lost when death
occurs before the age
of 65 or 75

Whereas standard mortality statistics, such as leading causes of death, provide one measure of the importance of various diseases, **years of potential life lost (YPLL)** provides another, different measure. YPLL is calculated by subtracting a person's age at death from his or her life expectancy. Such calculations are difficult because each person may have a different life expectancy at any given time. Thus, the ages 65 years or 75 years are often used in these calculations. For a person who dies at age 59, the YPLL-75 is 16. For many years in the United States, a death prior to 65 years was considered a premature death, perhaps because 65 was the standard age of retirement and when full Social Security payments could begin. Now, how-

Table 3.10
Life Expectancy at Birth, at 65 Years of Age, and at 75 Years of Age According to Sex: In the United States, During the Selected Years 1900–2006

	At Birth			At 65 Years			At 75 Years		
Year	Both Sexes	Male	Female	Both Sexes	Male	Female	Both Sexes	Male	Female
1900	47.3	46.3	48.3	11.9	11.5	12.2	*	*	*
1950	68.2	65.6	71.1	13.9	12.8	15.0	*	*	*
1960	69.7	66.6	73.1	14.3	12.8	15.8	*	*	*
1970	70.8	67.1	74.7	15.2	13.1	17.0	*	*	*
1980	73.7	70.7	77.4	16.4	14.1	18.3	10.4	8.8	11.5
1990	75.4	71.8	78.8	17.2	15.1	18.9	10.9	9.4	12.0
2006	77.7	75.1	80.2	18.5	17.0	19.7	11.6	10.5	12.3

*Data not available.

Source: National Center for Health Statistics (2010). *Health, United States, 2009 with Special Feature on Medical Technology* [online]. (DHHS pub. no. 2010–1232). Hyattsville, MD: Author. Available at http://www.cdc.gov/nchs/hus.htm. Accessed October 1, 2010.

Table 3.11
Life Expectancy at Birth for Selected Countries by Sex in 2007

	Male	Female
Ethiopia	55	59
Malawi	49	51
India	63	65
Nicaragua	70	76
Ecuador	70	76
Congo	54	56
Thailand	67	73
Malaysia	70	75
South Africa	52	55
Brazil	70	76
Latvia	66	76
Republic of Korea	76	82
Greece	77	82
New Zealand	78	83
United Kingdom	77	82
United States	76	81
Sweden	79	83
Japan	79	86

Source: World Health Organization (2009). "World Health Statistics." Geneva, Switzerland: Author. Available at http://www.who.int/healthinfo/statistics/mortality/en. Accessed November 29, 2010.

ever, 75 years of age is increasingly being used to calculate YPLL because the life expectancy for a child born today is closer to 75 years (see Table 3.10). People are living longer, and many of us know people who continue to work beyond the age of 65; indeed, as of mid-July 2010, the median age in the U.S. Senate was 63 years. There were four senators in their 80s, 23 in their 70s, and 33 in their 60s.

YPLL weights deaths such that the death of a very young person counts more than the death of a very old person. Table 3.12 provides a summary of the age-adjusted YPLL before 75 (YPLL-75) for the 10 leading causes of death in the United States for 1990 and 2006.[21] In

Table 3.12
Age-Adjusted Years of Potential Life Lost Before 75 (YPLL-75) for the 10 Leading Causes of Death, United States, 1990 and 2006

	YPLL per 100,000 Population	
Cause	1990	2006
Diseases of the heart	1,617.7	1,138.0
Malignant neoplasms (cancer)	2,003.8	1,585.7
Cerebrovascular diseases (stroke)	259.6	199.3
Chronic lower respiratory diseases	187.4	181.4
Unintentional injuries	1,162.1	1,165.4
Influenza and pneumonia	141.5	78.8
Diabetes mellitus	155.9	186.6
Human immunodeficiency virus infection (HIV/AIDS)	383.8	124.5
Suicide	393.1	349.2
Homicide and legal intervention	417.4	281.0

Source: National Center for Health Statistics (2010). *Health, United States, 2009 with Special Feature on Medical Technology* [online]. (DHHS pub. no. 2010-1232). Hyattsville, MD: Author. Available at http://www.cdc.gov/nchs/hus.htm. Accessed October 1, 2010.

examining this table, note that the number of YPLL-75 per 100,000 population was higher for malignant neoplasms (cancer) than for heart disease. Also, YPLL resulting from unintentional injuries was the second highest. This is because unintentional injuries and malignant neoplasms (cancer) often kill people when they are young. These differences can also be seen in the two pie charts shown in Figure 3.4. Also, notice that the YPLL-75 per 100,000 population declined for most of the leading causes of death between 1990 and 2006. An important exception is for diabetes mellitus, a disease that is becoming epidemic in the United States.

YPLL from specific causes varies depending on the gender and face of the subpopulation under consideration. For example, the YPLL-75 per 100,000 population resulting from unintentional injuries is nearly three times as high for men as it is for women. The YPLL-75 per 100,000 for diseases of the heart for blacks is nearly twice that for whites, and for homicide, it is nearly six times greater.[21]

Disability-Adjusted Life Years

disability-adjusted life years (DALYs) a measure for the burden of disease that takes into account premature death and loss of healthy life resulting from disability

Mortality does not entirely express the burden of disease. For example, chronic depression and paralysis caused by polio are responsible for great loss of healthy life but are not reflected in mortality tables. Because of this, the World Health Organization (WHO) and the World Bank have developed a measure called the **disability-adjusted life years (DALYs)**.[23]

One DALY is one lost year of healthy life. Total DALYs for a given condition for a particular population can be calculated by estimating the total YPLL and the total years of life lived with disability, and then by summing these totals. As an example, the DALYs incurred through firearm injuries in the United States could be calculated by adding the total of YPLL incurred from fatal firearm injuries to the total years of life lived with disabilities by survivors of firearm injuries. Figure 3.5 illustrates the number of DALYs lost per 1,000 in 2004 from seven demographic regions of the world.[24]

Health-Adjusted Life Expectancy

health-adjusted life expectancy (HALE) the number of years of healthy life expected, on average, in a given population

Health-adjusted life expectancy (HALE), sometimes referred to as *healthy life expectancy*, is the number of years of healthy life expected, on average, in a given population or region of the world. The HALE indicator used by the WHO is similar to the disability-adjusted life expectancy (DALE) first reported in the original Global Burden of Disease study.[23] The methods used to calculate HALE are beyond the scope of this textbook, but have been described elsewhere.[25] Worldwide, HALE at birth in 2001 was 57.4 years, 7.5 years lower than overall life expectancy at birth. As with life expectancy, HALE in sub-Saharan Africa is very low—less than 40 years for males, compared with about 70 years for females in high-income countries (Figure 3.6).[26]

SOURCES OF STANDARDIZED DATA

Because demographic and epidemiological data are used in the planning of public health programs and facilities, students of community health should be aware of the sources of these standardized data. Students can obtain standardized data for use in community health work from the following sources: The U.S. Census, the *Statistical Abstract of the United States,* the *Monthly Vital Statistics Report, Morbidity and Mortality Weekly Report,* the National Health Interview Survey, the National Health and Nutrition Examination Survey, the Behavioral Risk Factor Surveillance System, the Youth Risk Behavior Surveillance System, the National Hospital Discharge Survey, and the National Hospital Ambulatory Medical Care Survey.

Each of these sources of national data has a specific value and usefulness to those in the public health field. Students interested in studying local health problems can obtain data from state and local health departments, hospitals, volunteer agencies, and disease registries. The

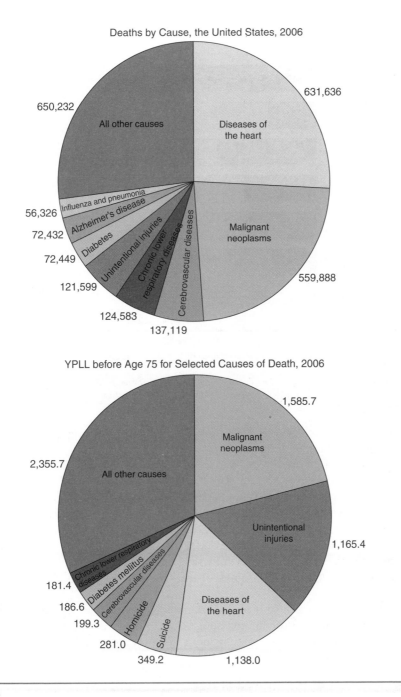

FIGURE 3.4

Deaths by cause in the United States, 2006, and the years of potential life lost before age 75 (YPLL-75) per 100,000 population for selected causes of death within the United States, 2006.

Sources: Heron, M. P., D. L. Hoyert, S. L. Murphy, J. Q. Xu, K. D. Kochanek, and B. Tejada-Vera (2009). "Deaths: Final Data for 2006." *National Vital Statistics Reports*, 57(14): 1–136; and National Center for Health Statistics (2010). *Health, United States, 2009 with Special Feature on Medical Technology* [online]. (DHHS pub. no. 2010-1232). Hyattsville, MD: Author. Available at http://www.cdc.gov/nchs/hus.htm. Accessed October 1, 2010.

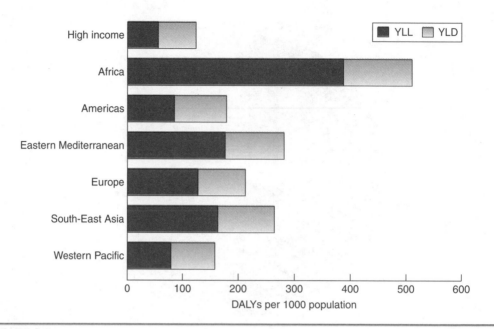

FIGURE 3.5

Burden of disease: years of life lost due to premature mortality (YLL) and years of life lived with a disability (YLD) per thousand by region, 2004. DALYs, disability-adjusted life years.

Source: World Health Organization. (2008). *The Global Burden of Disease: 2004 Update.* Available at http://www.who.int/ healthinfo/global_burden_disease/GBD_report_2004update_full.pdf. Accessed October 15, 2010.

study and analysis of these data provide a basis for planning appropriate health programs and facilities in your communities.

The U.S. Census

The **U.S. Census**, taken every 10 years, is an enumeration of the population living in the United States. George Washington ordered the first census in 1790 for the purpose of apportioning representation to the House of Representatives. Through the years, the census form has become much more complex than the one filled out more than 200 years earlier. Data are gathered about income, employment, family size, education, dwelling type, and many other social indicators (see Figure 3.7). Copies of the U.S. Census results are available in most libraries.

U.S. Census
the enumeration of the population of the United States that is conducted every 10 years

Census data are important to health workers because they are used for calculating disease and death rates and for program planning. The U.S. Census is carried out by the Bureau of the Census, located in the U.S. Department of Commerce. Information is available at www.census.gov.

Statistical Abstract of the United States

Another Bureau of the Census publication is the *Statistical Abstract of the United States* (SA). This book, published annually, is the standard summary of statistics on the social, political, and economic organization of the United States. Information is divided into sections under headings such as Population, Vital Statistics, Health and Nutrition, Education, Law Enforcement, Courts and Prisons, and many more. Data contained in the SA are extremely useful and are reasonably up-to-date. (A new edition is published every January and includes data from 2 years before the publication date.) The SA can be purchased from the Government Printing Office for about $50 and is available in most libraries. Information is also available at www.census.gov/compendia/statab/.

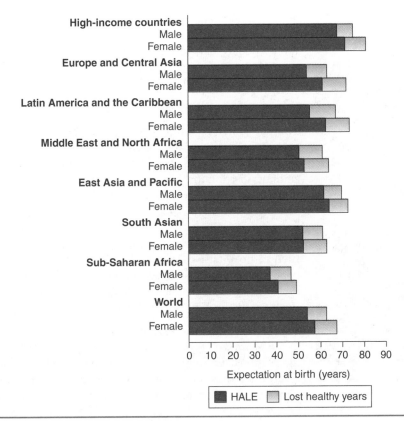

FIGURE 3.6

Life expectancy, health-adjusted life expectancy (HALE), and lost healthy years by region and sex, 2001.

Source: Lopez, A. D., C. D. Mathers, M. Ezzati, D. T. Jamison, and C. J. L. Murray, eds. (2006). *Global Burden of Disease and Risk Factors.* Washington, DC: World Bank and Oxford University Press. Used with permission of the International Bank for Reconstruction and Development/The World Bank.

Monthly Vital Statistics Report

The National Center for Health Statistics (NCHS), one of the Centers for Disease Control and Prevention, provides the most up-to-date national vital statistics available. These statistics appear in the *Monthly Vital Statistics Report,* published by the NCHS in Hyattsville, Maryland. **Vital statistics** are statistical summaries of vital records, that is, records of major life events. Listed are live births, deaths, marriages, divorces, and infant deaths. Death rates are also calculated by race and age and, in some issues, by cause. Selected issues also provide mortality data for specific causes (for example, diabetes, drug overdoses, and heart disease). Copies of this publication are available in government document areas of university and large public libraries, on the Web at www.cdc.gov/nchs/, or by writing directly to the NCHS (3311 Toledo Road, Suite 4113, Hyattsville, MD 20782).

vital statistics
statistical summaries
of records of major
life events such as
births, deaths,
marriages, divorces,
and infant deaths

Morbidity and Mortality Weekly Report

Reported cases of specified notifiable diseases are reported weekly in the *Morbidity and Mortality Weekly Report (MMWR),* which lists morbidity and mortality data by state and region of the country. The report is prepared by the CDC based on reports from state health departments. This report is printed and distributed through an agreement with the Massachusetts Medical Society, publishers of the *New England Journal of Medicine.* Each weekly issue also contains several reports of outbreaks of disease, environmental hazards, unusual cases, or

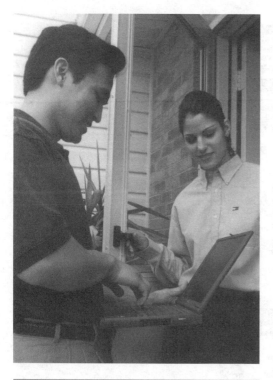

FIGURE 3.7

A census worker collects data used to calculate disease rates.

other public health problems. The *MMWR* and its annual summary reports are available in larger libraries, on the Web at www.cdc.gov/mmwr, and by subscription from the Massachusetts Medical Society (MMS Publications, C.S.P.O. Box 9120, Waltham, MA 02254).

National Health Surveys

Another source of standardized data is the National Health Surveys. These surveys are a result of the National Health Survey Act of 1956. This act authorized a continuing survey of the amount, distribution, and effects of illness and disability in the United States. The intent of this act is currently being fulfilled by three types of surveys: (1) health interviews of people; (2) clinical tests, measurements, and physical examinations of people; and (3) surveys of places where people receive medical care, such as hospitals, clinics, and doctors' offices. The following paragraphs describe these surveys. More information about these surveys and results is available at the National Center for Health Statistics Web site, www.cdc.gov/nchs.

National Health Interview Survey

In the *National Health Interview Survey* (NHIS), conducted by the National Center for Health Statistics (NCHS), people are asked numerous questions about their health. One of the questions asks respondents to describe their health status using one of five categories—excellent, very good, good, fair, or poor. Fewer than 1 in 10 of the respondents in 2008 described their health status as either fair or poor, while nearly 7 in 10 Americans believe they are in very good or excellent health. College graduates (38%) were about two times as likely as persons who had not graduated from high school (17%) to be in excellent health.

Persons with family incomes of $100,000 or more were almost twice as likely as those with incomes of less than $35,000 to be in excellent health (49% vs. 27%).[27]

It is important to remember that these data were generated by self-reported responses to NHIS questions and not by actual examinations objectively generated in a clinic. As such, respondents may overreport good health habits or underreport bad ones. Such reporting is often dependent on the respondent's perceived social stigma or support for a response and the degree to which people's responses are confidential or anonymous. Furthermore, people have widely divergent views on what constitutes poor or good health. For example, many sedentary, cigarette-smoking, high-stress people see themselves as being in good health, while "health nuts" feel their health is deteriorating when they miss a day of exercise. In general, the young assess their health better than the old do, males better than females, whites better than blacks, and those with large family incomes better than those with smaller ones.

National Health and Nutrition Examination Survey

Another of the National Health Surveys is the *National Health and Nutrition Examination Survey* (NHANES). The purpose of the NHANES is to assess the health and nutritional status of the general U.S. population. Using a mobile examination center (see Figure 3.8), the data are collected through direct physical examinations, clinical and laboratory testing, and related procedures on a representative group of Americans. These examinations result in the most authoritative source of standardized clinical, physical, and physiological data on the American people. Included in the data are the prevalence of specific conditions and diseases and data on

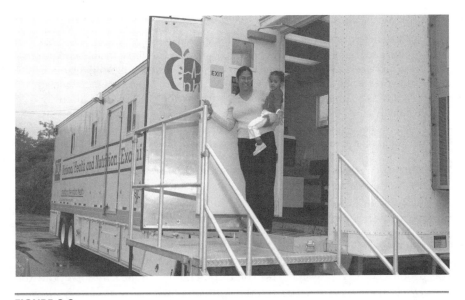

FIGURE 3.8

A *National Health and Nutrition Examination Survey* (NHANES) mobile examination center.

blood pressure, serum cholesterol, body measurements, nutritional status and deficiencies, and exposure to environmental toxins.

The first series of these surveys, known as *National Health Examination Surveys* (NHES), were carried out during the 1960s. Beginning in the 1970s, nutrition was added as a new focus, and the surveys became known as the *National Health and Nutrition Examination Survey* (NHANES). Three cycles of the NHANES were conducted by the National Center for Health Statistics, the third ending in 1994. The survey became a continuous program in 1999. The program's focus changes on a variety of health and nutrition measurements to meet emerging needs.

Results of NHANES benefit people in the United States in important ways. Facts about the distribution of health problems and risk factors in the population give researchers important clues to the causes of disease. Information collected from the current survey is compared with information collected in previous surveys. This allows health planners to detect the extent various health problems and risk factors have changed in the U.S. population over time. By identifying the health care needs of the population, government agencies and private sector organizations can establish policies and plan research, education, and health promotion programs that help improve present health status and will prevent future health problems.[28]

Each year, the survey examines a nationally representative sample of about 5,000 persons, located in 15 counties across the country using mobile examination centers.

Behavioral Risk Factor Surveillance System

The *Behavioral Risk Factor Surveillance System* (BRFSS) is a state-based telephone survey of the civilian, noninstitutional, adult population conducted by the Behavioral Surveillance Branch, a division of Adult and Community Health, National Center for Chronic Disease Prevention and Health Promotion at the CDC. This survey seeks to ascertain the prevalence of such high-risk behaviors as cigarette smoking, excessive alcohol consumption, and physical inactivity, and the lack of preventive health care such as screening for cancer. These results are published periodically as part of *MMWR*'s *CDC Surveillance Summaries* and are available wherever copies of the CDC *MMWR* are found. Information is also available at www.cdc.gov/brfss.

Youth Risk Behavior Surveillance System

The national Youth Risk Behavior Survey (YRBS) monitors six categories of priority health-risk behaviors among youth and young adults, including behaviors that contribute to unintentional injuries and violence; tobacco use; alcohol and other drug use; sexual behaviors that contribute to unintended pregnancy and sexually transmitted diseases (STDs), including human immunodeficiency virus (HIV) infection; unhealthy dietary behaviors; and physical inactivity. In addition, the national YRBS monitors the prevalence of obesity and asthma. The national YRBS is conducted every two years during the spring semester and provides data representative of 9th through 12th grade students in public and private schools in the United States.[29]

YRBS includes a national school-based survey conducted by the CDC, and state and local school-based surveys conducted by state and local education and health agencies. The YRBS is conducted by the CDC's National Center for Chronic Disease Prevention and Health Promotion. More information about YRBS is available at www.cdc.gov/healthyyouth/yrbs/.

National Health Care Survey

The *National Health Care Survey* (NHCS) comprises nine different national surveys that gather information on the nation's health care system. Two of the best-known health care surveys are the *National Hospital Discharge Survey* (NHDS) and the *National Hospital Ambulatory Medical Care Survey* (NHAMCS). The NHDS provides data on the characteristics of patients discharged from nonfederal, short-stay hospitals. These data can be used to examine a variety of important public health issues such as hospitalization rates for selected inpatient surgical procedures, infectious diseases, injuries, substance abuse, and other health problems. It can also be used to estimate costs for public health problems. The NHAMCS gathers and disseminates information about the health care provided by hospital outpatient departments and emergency departments. Summaries of the results of these surveys are published by the National Center for Health Statistics and are available at www.cdc.gov/nchs/nhcs.

EPIDEMIOLOGICAL STUDIES

When disease and/or death occurs in unexpected or unacceptable numbers, epidemiologists may carry out investigations. These investigations may be descriptive or analytic (observational or experimental/interventional) in nature, depending on the objectives of the specific study.

Descriptive Studies

descriptive study
an epidemiological study that describes an epidemic with respect to person, place, and time

epidemic curve
a graphic display of the cases of disease according to the time or date of onset of symptoms

Descriptive studies seek to describe the extent of disease in regard to person, time, and place. These studies are designed to answer the questions *who, when,* and *where*. To answer the first question, epidemiologists first take a "head count" to determine how many cases of a disease have occurred. At this time, they also try to determine who is ill—children, older adults, men, women, or both. The data they gather should permit them to develop a summary of cases by age, sex, race, marital status, occupation, and employer.

To answer the second question (*when*), epidemiologists must determine the time of the onset of illness for each case. The resulting data can be used to prepare an **epidemic curve**, a graphic display of the cases of disease by the time or date of the onset of their symptoms. Three types of epidemic curves are commonly used in descriptive studies—secular, seasonal, and single epidemic curves. The secular display of a disease shows the distribution of cases over many years (e.g., cases of paralytic poliomyelitis for the period 1972 to 2002; see Figure 3.9). Secular graphs illustrate the long-term trend of a disease. A graph of the case data by season or month is usually prepared to show cyclical changes in the numbers of cases of a disease. Cases of arthropodborne viral infections, for example, peak in the late summer months, following the seasonal rise in populations of the mosquitoes that transmit them (see Figure 3.10).

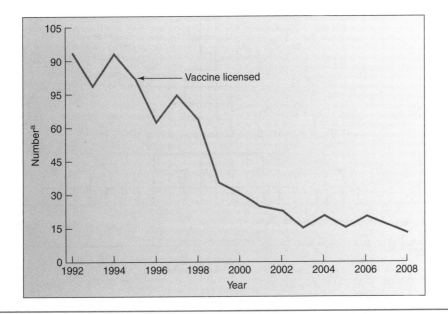

FIGURE 3.9

Varicella (Chickenpox). Number of reported cases—Illinois, Michigan, Texas, and West Virginia, 1992–2008.

Source: Centers for Disease Control and Prevention (2010). "Summary of Notifiable Diseases—United States, 2008." *Morbidity and Mortality Weekly Report*, 53(53): 1–82. Available at http://www.cdc.gov/mmwr/PDF/wk/mm5754.pdf. Accessed October 1, 2010.

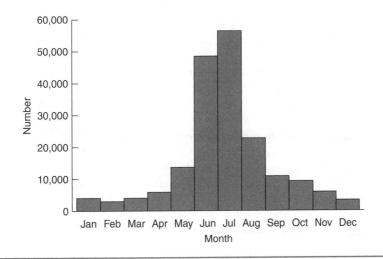

FIGURE 3.10

Number of reported Lyme disease cases, by month of illness onset—United States, 1992–2006.

Source: Centers for Disease Control and Prevention (2008). "Surveillance for Lyme Disease—United States, 1992–2006." *Surveillance Summaries, Morbidity and Mortality Weekly Report*, 57(SS-10): 1–10. Available at http://www.cdc.gov/mmwr.pdf/ss/ss5710.pdf. Accessed October 1, 2010.

Epidemic curves for single epidemics vary in appearance with each disease outbreak; however, two classic types exist. The first is the **point source epidemic curve** (see Figure 3.11). In a point source epidemic, each case can be traced to an exposure to the same source—spoiled food, for example. Because an epidemic curve shows cases of a disease by time or date of the

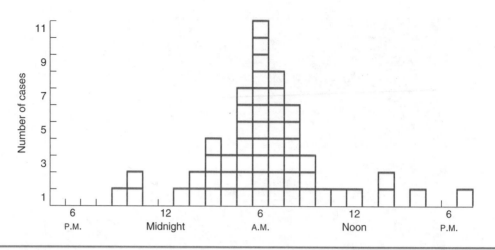

FIGURE 3.11

Point source epidemic curve: cases of gastroenteritis following ingestion of a common food source.

Source: Centers for Disease Control and Prevention.

point source epidemic curve
an epidemic curve depicting a distribution of cases that all can be traced to a single source of exposure

onset of their symptoms, the epidemic curve for a single epidemic can be used to calculate the **incubation period**, the period of time between exposure to an infectious agent and the onset of symptoms. The incubation period, together with the symptoms, can often help epidemiologists determine the cause of the disease.

The second type of epidemic curve for a solitary outbreak is a **propagated epidemic curve**. In this type of epidemic, primary cases appear first at the end of the incubation period following exposure to an infected source. *Secondary cases* arise after a second incubation period, and they represent exposure to the primary cases; *tertiary cases* appear even later as a result of exposure to secondary cases, and so on. Because new cases give rise to more new cases, this type of epidemic is termed a *propagated epidemic*. Epidemics of communicable diseases such as chickenpox follow this pattern (see Figure 3.12).

incubation period
the period between exposure to a disease and the onset of symptoms

Finally, epidemiologists must determine *where* the outbreak occurred. To determine where the illnesses may have originated, the residential address and travel history, including restaurants, schools, shopping trips, and vacations, of each case are recorded. This information provides a geographic distribution of cases and helps to delineate the extent of the outbreak. By plotting cases on a map, along with natural features such as streams and humanmade structures such as factories, it is sometimes possible to learn something about the source of the disease.

propagated epidemic curve
an epidemic curve depicting a distribution of cases traceable to multiple sources of exposure

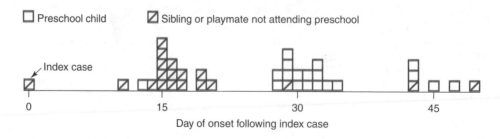

FIGURE 3.12

Propagated epidemic curve: cases of chickenpox during April through June.

Source: Centers for Disease Control and Prevention.

A descriptive study is usually the first epidemiological study carried out on a disease. Descriptive data provide valuable information to health care providers and administrators, enabling them to allocate resources efficiently and to plan effective prevention and education programs. Also, detectable patterns of cases may provide investigators with ideas that can lead to a hypothesis about the cause or source of the disease outbreak. This hypothesis can subsequently be tested in an analytic study.

As important and useful as they are, descriptive studies have some limitations. Results from descriptive studies are usually not applicable to outbreaks elsewhere. Also, the investigation of a single epidemic cannot provide information about disease trends. Last, with few exceptions, descriptive studies by themselves rarely identify with certainty the cause of an outbreak.

Analytic Studies

A second type of epidemiological study is the **analytic study**. The purpose of analytic studies is to test hypotheses about relationships between health problems and possible **risk factors**, factors that increase the probability of disease. Although front-line community health workers usually do not conduct analytic studies, it is important that students of community health understand how they are carried out and what kinds of data they generate. Only through such an understanding can those who work in community health interpret the findings of these studies to others in the community, who may then apply the knowledge to improve their own health and that of the community.

An example of an analytic study might be one designed to discover whether diabetes (health problem) is associated with obesity (possible risk factor), or whether lung cancer (health problem) is associated with cigarette smoking (possible risk factor). It is important to remember that the associations discovered through analytic epidemiological studies are not always cause-and-effect associations.

There are two types of analytic studies—observational and experimental (interventional). These differ in the role played by the investigator. In **observational studies** the investigator simply observes the natural course of events, taking note of who is exposed or unexposed and who has or has not developed the disease of interest. In experimental studies, the investigator actually allocates the exposure and subsequently follows the subjects for the development of disease.

Observational studies can be further divided into either case/control or cohort studies. The choice of which study to use when studying a particular disease-exposure relationship depends on the nature of the disease (rare or common) and the time and resources available. **Case/control studies** are analytic studies that compare people with disease (cases) to healthy people of similar age, sex, and background (controls) with respect to proportion of prior exposure to possible risk factors. These case/control studies are aimed at identifying familial, environmental, or behavioral factors that are more common or more pronounced in the case group than in the control group. Such factors could be associated with the disease under study. For example, epidemiologists might wish to study the factors associated with cervical cancer in women.

To carry out this study, epidemiologists would identify a number of women with cervical cancer (cases) and an equal or larger number of healthy women (controls). Medical histories for each group would be obtained and compared. In this hypothetical example, an examination of the histories suggests that cigarette smoking is more prevalent in the case group. If exposure to the possible risk factor (smoking) is significantly greater in the cases (of cervical cancer) than in the controls, an association is said to exist. Note that this association may or may not be one of cause and effect. Further studies are usually necessary to confirm initial findings. Case/control studies almost never prove causation by themselves. Instead, they usually indicate the direction for future studies.

analytic study
an epidemiological study aimed at testing hypotheses

risk factors
factors that increase the probability of disease, injury, or death

observational study
an analytic, epidemiological study in which the investigator observes the natural course of events, noting exposed and unexposed subjects and disease development

case/control study
a study that seeks to compare those diagnosed with a disease with those who do not have the disease for prior exposure to specific risk factors

cohort study
an epidemiological study in which a cohort is classified by exposure to one or more specific risk factors and observed to determine the rates at which disease develops in each class

cohort
a group of people who share some important demographic characteristic (year of birth, for example)

odds ratio
a probability statement about the association between a particular disease and a specific risk factor, resulting from a case/control study

relative risk
a statement of the relationship between the risk of acquiring a disease when a specific risk factor is present and the risk of acquiring that same disease when the risk factor is absent

experimental (interventional) studies
analytic studies in which the investigator allocates exposure or intervention and follows development of disease

placebo
a blank treatment

Cohort studies are epidemiological studies in which the researcher selects a **cohort**, a large number of healthy subjects who share a similar experience, such as year of birth or high school graduation. Subjects in this cohort are then classified on the basis of their exposure to one or more possible causative factors, such as cigarette smoking, dietary habits, or other factors. The entire cohort is then observed for a number of years to determine the rate at which disease develops in each subgroup that was classified by exposure factor.

It is important to note the difference in the type of results obtained from case/control and cohort studies and the advantages and disadvantages of each type of study. In case/control studies, results obtained are not true incidence rates because disease was already present at the beginning of the study; that is, there were cases and controls to begin with, rather than a population at risk. For this reason, case/control studies cannot calculate the incidence rate of development of disease. They can only provide a probability statement about the association between factor and disease. This probability statement can be stated mathematically as an odds ratio. The following is a hypothetical example of such a probability statement: Lung cancer patients have a probability of having smoked cigarettes that is 11 times greater than that of the control group. The **odds ratio** in this case is 11:1. (For a more detailed description of how to calculate an odds ratio and relative risk, see Appendix 1.)

In cohort studies, one begins with a population at risk, and therefore is able to calculate the incidence rate for developing disease associated with each exposure factor. This **relative risk** states the relationship between the rate of acquiring the disease in the presence of the risk factor to the rate of acquiring the disease in the absence of the risk factor. An example of a relative risk statement is as follows: Smokers are 11 times more likely to develop lung cancer than are nonsmokers.

Although cohort studies yield a relative risk, they have three distinct disadvantages: (1) they are expensive, (2) they usually take many years to complete, and (3) they are not very useful for studying rare diseases because the disease may not develop in the cohort. Case/control studies, on the other hand, are less expensive to carry out, can be completed more quickly, and are useful for studying rare diseases because one can select the cases. Unfortunately, they cannot yield a true risk for acquiring a disease.

Experimental studies are carried out to identify the cause of a disease or to determine the effectiveness of a vaccine, therapeutic drug, or surgical procedure. The central feature of experimental (interventional) studies is that the investigator can control the intervention or variable of interest. The subjects may be humans but more often are animals such as laboratory mice, rats, or monkeys. The use of research animals in experimental studies is necessary to determine the safety and effectiveness of new therapeutic agents or medical procedures with minimum risk to human health.

Whether animals or humans are used, every effort is made to reduce unwanted variability of factors other than the risk factors under study among the experimental subjects. In the case of animal studies, the variables over which the experimenter may wish to exert control include age, sex, diet, and environmental conditions. In addition to controlling variables, three other principles are essential to properly designed experimental studies—*control groups, randomization,* and *blinding.*

The use of *control groups* means that the experimental treatment (intervention), such as a drug, vaccine, smoke-free environment, or special diet, is withheld from a portion of the subjects. These subjects belong to the control group, which receives blank doses or treatments, called **placebos**. For a treatment regimen to be considered effective or for a factor to be considered causally related, it must significantly affect the *treatment group* differently (usually determined using a statistical test) from the control group.

Randomization refers to the practice of assigning subjects to treatments or control groups in a completely random manner. This can be accomplished by assigning numbers to subjects and then having numbers selected randomly. Numbers can be selected randomly from a table of random numbers, by drawing lots, or by using a computer-generated list of random numbers. Thus, each research subject, human or animal, has an equal chance of being placed in the treatment group.

Blinding refers to the practice in which the investigator(s) and/or subjects remain uninformed and unaware of the groups to which subjects are assigned throughout the period of experimentation and data gathering. This prevents the investigator(s) from looking favorably or unfavorably on the responses of any particular subject or group while gathering data during the experiment. Thus, the researcher can remain unbiased. When both the observer and subjects are kept ignorant, the study is referred to as a *double-blind trial*.

When studies involve human subjects, they often involve the use of a placebo, such as a saline (saltwater) injection or sugar pill. The use of a placebo prevents subjects from determining by observation whether or not they are receiving treatment. This is important because human thought processes are such that some people begin to feel better if they believe they have received a treatment. For a vaccine or therapeutic drug to be labeled as effective, it must consistently perform better than a placebo.

An example of just such an experiment was performed by Tonnesen and his colleagues, who studied the effectiveness of a 16-hour nicotine patch on smoking cessation.[30] They used a double-blind randomized design to compare the effects of a nicotine skin patch with those of a placebo skin patch. Subjects were assigned to the active treatment or the placebo according to computer-generated random numbers. There were 145 subjects who received a nicotine patch and 144 who received the placebo. Subjects were scheduled for visits 1, 3, 6, 12, 26, and 52 weeks after the first visit—the day smoking cessation was to begin. Table 3.13 presents the results of cessation for each group 6, 12, 26, and 52 weeks after the study began. The results of this study indicated that there was a significant difference between the effectiveness of the nicotine patch and the placebo patch with regard to smoking cessation.

Controlling variables, the use of treatment and control groups, randomization, and blinding are techniques aimed at ensuring objectivity and avoiding bias in experimental studies. Through strict adherence to these principles, investigators hope to achieve experimental results that accurately reflect what occurs in a natural setting.

By carrying out carefully planned descriptive studies, epidemiologists define outbreaks of disease, injury, and death in specific populations and develop hypotheses about the causes of these outbreaks. By designing and carrying out analytic and experimental studies, epidemiologists test these hypotheses.

Table 3.13
Percentage of Subjects Abstaining from Smoking 6, 12, 26, and 52 Weeks after the Start of the Program

Week Number	Percentage of People Remaining Abstinent	
	Nicotine Patch	Placebo Patch
6	53	17
12	41	10
26	24	5
52	17	4

Source: Tonnesen, P., J. Norregaard, K. Simonsen, and U. Sawe (1991). "A Double-Blind Trial of a 16-Hour Transdermal Nicotine Patch in Smoking Cessation." *New England Journal of Medicine,* 325(5): 311–315.

Criteria of Causation

Often, even after numerous epidemiologic studies have identified an association between exposure to a suspected risk factor (A) and the development of a specific disease (B), it may not be clear that A *causes* B in the same way we state that infection with the malaria parasite causes the disease malaria. In the study cited immediately previously, for example, researchers found an association between wearing a nicotine patch and abstaining from smoking. That is not quite the same as stating that wearing the nicotine patch *caused* smoking abstention. In 1965, this problem was addressed by Austin Bradford Hill, who laid out criteria that should be considered when deciding whether an association might be one of causation.[31] As he developed these criteria, he often cited the behavior of cigarette smoking and the development of lung cancer as examples. With minor modifications, Hill's criteria are outlined here:

Strength. How strong is the association between the exposure and the disease? Are those exposed 3, 5, 10, or 100 times more likely to develop disease than those who are not exposed? How many times more likely are cigarette smokers to get lung cancer than nonsmokers? Also, is there a dose-response relationship? Is it the case that the greater the exposure to a particular risk factor results in a higher rate of disease or death? Are those who smoke more heavily, more likely to develop lung cancer than lighter smokers are?

Consistency. Has the association been reported in a variety of people exposed in a variety of settings? Are the results repeatable by other researchers?

Specificity. Is the disease or health problem associated with the exposure the only one? When someone becomes ill after exposure is it always, or almost always, the same disease? When cigarette smokers become ill, is it always, or almost always lung cancer?

Temporality. Does A (the exposure) always precede B (the disease)? Does the behavior of cigarette smoking precede the onset of lung cancer, or do those with lung cancer take up the habit of smoking for some reason?

Biological plausibility. Does the suspected causation make sense with what we know about biology, physiology, and other medical knowledge? Does it make sense, in light of what we know about biology and physiology, that cigarette smoking could produce lung cancer?

Using these criteria together with analytic, epidemiological data, health researchers often can persuade legislatures and public officials to pass laws or alter public policies that promote health. In the next chapter, we examine how epidemiological studies can be used to prevent and control diseases and health problems in the community.

SCENARIO: ANALYSIS AND RESPONSE

Assume that you were Kim and you were able to reach Dr. Turner, the local health officer. He then asked whether you would like to help in the investigation of the foodborne outbreak mentioned in the scenario. You agreed to help. So far, you have learned that on Sunday, May 28, 49 people were at a picnic where they had eaten, beginning about noon. People began to report their illnesses later that night. Dr. Turner developed a foodborne outbreak investigation worksheet, which you helped to complete by making numerous phone calls and house visits with the public health nurse. The histories of people attending the picnic appear in Table 3.14.

Using Table 3.15, the Epidemic Curve Tally Sheet, you tally the cases by hour of onset of illness. Using the results of the tally, you establish the incubation period—the range of hours (after the meal) over which symptoms started. Next, you prepare a graph to illustrate the epidemic curve of the outbreak. Try to answer the following questions:

1. What is the incubation period?
2. Does the curve you prepared suggest a single- or multiple-exposure epidemic?
3. Based solely on the incubation period, can you make a guess as to the cause of the outbreak?

Table 3.14
Histories Obtained from Persons Eating Picnic Lunch

Person No.	Bread	Butter	Turkey	Potato Salad	Milk	Jell-O	Ill*	Not Ill
1			x	x	x		7:30	
2	x	x		x	x			x
3	x	x	x	x	x	x	8:00	
4			x		x	x		x
5			x	x	x		9:15	
6			x	x	x		7:40	
7	x	x		x	x			x
8	x	x	x	x	x	x	8:10	
9			x		x	x		x
10			x	x	x	x	10:15	
11	x			x	x			x
12	x	x	x	x	x	x	8:30	
13			x		x			x
14	x	x	x	x	x	x	9:30	
15	x	x		x	x			x
16	x			x	x			x
17	x	x	x	x	x	x	8:35	
18			x		x			x
19	x	x	x	x	x	x	10:05	
20	x	x		x	x	x		x
21			x		x	x	9:15	
22	x	x		x	x	x		x
23	x	x			x	x	8:30	
24	x	x			x	x		x
25	x	x	x	x	x	x	12:30 A.M.	
26			x		x	x	9:20	
27	x	x		x	x	x		x
28	x	x	x		x	x	8:40	
29	x	x			x	x		x
30	x	x	x	x	x		12:15 A.M.	
31			x	x	x		7:30	
32	x	x		x	x			x
33	x	x	x	x	x	x	8:00	
34			x		x	x		x
35			x	x	x		10:30	

(continues)

Table 3.14 (continued)

Person No.	Bread	Butter	Turkey	Potato Salad	Milk	Jell-O	Ill*	Not Ill
36			x	x	x		7:30	
37	x	x		x	x			x
38	x	x	x	x	x	x	8:05	
39			x		x	x		x
40			x	x	x	x	9:45	
41	x			x		x		x
42	x	x	x	x	x	x	8:30	
43			x		x			x
44	x	x	x	x	x	x	9:30	
45	x	x		x	x	x		x
46	x			x		x		x
47	x	x	x	x	x	x	8:30	
48		x			x	x		x
49	x	x	x	x	x	x	10:10	

*All time is p.m. unless otherwise indicated.

Table 3.15
Epidemic Curve Tally Sheet

Time of Onset	Tally	Number	Incubation Period
7:00–7:59			
8:00–8:59			
9:00–9:59			
10:00–10:59			
11:00–11:59			
12:00–12:59			

Unfortunately, by the time the investigation began, all the picnic food had been discarded, and no samples were available for laboratory testing. To determine which food at the picnic might have caused the outbreak, you need to calculate attack rates for people eating each food as well as for people not eating each food. Using Table 3.16, the Attack Rate Worksheet, calculate the attack rates for those who ate and did not eat each food served.

1. Which food would you most suspect of causing the illness?
2. Based on this information, what might the causative agent have been?
3. How could the Internet be of assistance to health department officials in this situation?

Table 3.16
Attack Rate Worksheet

Food	Persons Eating Food				Persons Not Eating Food			
	Total	Ill	Well	Attack Rate	Total	Ill	Well	Attack Rate
Bread								
Butter								
Turkey								
Potato salad								
Milk								
Jell-O								

CHAPTER SUMMARY

- Epidemiology is the study of the distribution and determinants of health-related states or events in specified populations, and the application of this study to control health problems.

- Rates of birth, death, injury, and disease are essential tools for epidemiologists.

- Incidence rates are a measurement of the number of new cases of disease, injury, or death in a population over a given period of time. Prevalence rates measure all cases. An attack rate is a special kind of incidence rate used for a single outbreak.

- Cases of certain diseases, called notifiable or reportable diseases, are reported by doctors, clinics, medical laboratories, and hospitals to local health agencies. These agencies then report them to state health agencies, who then forward the data to the CDC. These reports assist epidemiologists who study disease trends.

- The health status of a population or community can be measured in a number of different ways, including mortality statistics, life expectancy, years of potential life lost (YPLL), disability-adjusted life years (DALYs), and health-adjusted life expectancy (HALE).

- Epidemiologists also consult the data available from the U.S. Census, the *Statistical Abstract of the United States*, the *Monthly Vital Statistics Report*, the *Morbidity and Mortality Weekly Report*, and a variety of national health surveys.

- Epidemiologists conduct three general types of studies to learn about disease and injury in populations—descriptive studies, analytic studies, and experimental studies.

- Descriptive studies describe the extent of outbreaks in regard to person, place, and time.

- Analytic studies test hypotheses regarding associations between diseases and risk factors.

- Analytic studies can be either observational or experimental.

- Observational studies can be either case/control or cohort in design.

- Experimental studies examine the effects of specific factors under carefully controlled conditions.

- Criteria for judging whether an association identified in epidemiological studies represents a causal relationship include strength of association, consistency, specificity, temporal correctness, and biological plausibility.

- Epidemiological studies provide the data and information that enable public health officials and policy makers to make decisions and take actions to improve health.

REVIEW QUESTIONS

1. What is an epidemic? A pandemic? Name some diseases that caused epidemics in the past. Name some diseases that are epidemic today.

2. Why are epidemiologists sometimes interested in epizootics?

3. What does the term *endemic disease* mean? Give examples of such diseases.

4. What is the difference between natality, morbidity, and mortality?

5. Why are rates important in community health?

6. What is the difference between crude and specific rates?

7. Why are prevalence rates more useful than incidence rates for measuring chronic diseases?

8. What is an infant mortality rate? Why is it such an important rate in community health?

9. What are notifiable diseases? Give some examples.

10. In general, contrast the leading causes of death in the United States in 1900 with those in 2000. Comment on the differences.

11. At what ages is life expectancy calculated? What does it tell us about a population? Which country has the longest life expectancy?

12. What are years of potential life lost (YPLL)? How does calculating YPLL change the way we think about the leading causes of death?

13. How would you define disability-adjusted life years (DALYs)? How would you define health-adjusted life expectancy (HALE)?

14. What is the U.S. Census? How often is it conducted? What types of data does it gather?

15. What types of information can you find in the *Statistical Abstract of the United States*?

16. What kinds of data would you expect to find in the Centers for Disease Control and Prevention's *Morbidity and Mortality Weekly Report*?

17. List five important national health surveys that are valuable sources of data about the health and health care of our population.

18. What can be said about the reliability of self-reported health data?

19. What is the National Health Care Survey? Why is it carried out?

20. In a descriptive epidemiological study, what types of information does the epidemiologist gather?

21. What is the purpose of an analytic study? Contrast observational and experimental studies in regard to methodology and usefulness.

22. With regard to observational studies, how do case/control studies and cohort studies differ in design and in the kinds of results obtainable?

23. How do experimental studies differ from observational studies? What value do they have in epidemiology? To what principles must investigators adhere in order to properly carry out an experimental study?

24. What are Hill's criteria for judging whether an association between a risk factor and a disease can be considered causal?

Activities

1. When you hear the word *epidemic*, what disease comes to your mind first? Ask this question of 10 people you know, allowing them time to think and give you an answer. Try to find people of different ages as you complete your informal poll. List their answers on paper. Are there any answers that surprise you? Does your list include both classic and contemporary epidemic diseases?

2. Look at the data in Table 3.17. What conclusion can you draw about the risk for acquiring tuberculosis for populations in each age group? Write down your answer. Now examine Table 3.18. Which age groups exhibit the highest disease rates? Explain why it is important to calculate rates to report disease outbreaks accurately.

3. There are 346 students at Hillside School. During March and April, 56 pupils were absent with chickenpox. What is the attack rate for chickenpox at Hillside School? The 56 pupils who were absent had 88 brothers and sisters at home. Of the 88 siblings, 19 developed chickenpox. What was the attack rate among these children? Of the 75 total cases of chickenpox, one child died. Calculate the case fatality rate for chickenpox in this epidemic.

4. In an epidemic in Sample City (population 100,000—60,000 males and 40,000 females), there were 600 cases (350 males, 250 females) of a severe disease. There were 70 deaths (all males) resulting from this disease and 880 deaths resulting from causes other than the specific disease. Calculate the following—crude death rate, cause-specific mortality rate, case fatality rate, cause-specific morbidity rate for females, and case fatality rate for males.

5. Visit, call, or write your state or local health department. Ask for the total number of birth and death certificates issued for the latest year for which complete data are available. Assuming no migration into or out of your state or county occurred, what is the natural rate of population increase (number of births minus number of deaths)? Try to obtain an estimate of the total population of the state or county for that same year. Calculate a crude birth rate and a crude death rate (number of births and deaths) per 1,000 population.

6. Using the data presented in Table 3.10, estimate (as best you can) the life expectancy of your siblings, parents, and grandparents at birth. If your grandparents are older than 65, determine what their life expectancies were when they turned 65. If you were to fulfill your life expectancy exactly, in what year can you expect to die?

7. Visit your campus library and locate the *American Journal of Epidemiology*. Examine several recent issues, taking note of the different types of articles as they appear in the table of contents. Select six articles and read the abstracts. On a piece of paper, list the titles of these articles. Were these descriptive, analytic, or experimental studies? After each title that you have listed, put either the letter *D* (descriptive), *A* (analytic), or *E* (experimental) to denote the type of study that you examined.

Table 3.17
Reported Tuberculosis Cases, by Age Group, Low Socioeconomic Area, City of Dixon, 1960

Age Group in Years	Number of Cases	Age Group in Years	Number of Cases
0–4	7	35–44	6
5–14	7	45–54	9
15–24	6	55–64	8
25–34	10	65+	7

Source: Centers for Disease Control and Prevention.

Table 3.18
Reported Tuberculosis Cases and Incidence Rates per 100,000, Low Socioeconomic Area, City of Dixon, 1960

Age Group in Years	Number of Cases	Population of Age Group	Rate*
0–4	7	8,638	81.0
5–14	7	13,098	53.4
15–24	6	10,247	58.5
25–34	10	8,680	115.2
35–44	6	7,528	79.7
45–54	9	6,736	133.6
55–64	8	4,534	176.4
65+	7	4,075	171.8
Total	**60**	**63,536**	**94.4**

*Example: 7 cases ÷ 8,638 population × 100,000 = 81.0.

Source: Centers for Disease Control and Prevention.

COMMUNITY HEALTH ON THE WEB

The Internet contains a wealth of information about community and public health. Increase your knowledge of some of the topics presented in this chapter by accessing the Jones & Bartlett Learning Web site at **http://health.jbpub.com/book/communityhealth/7e** and follow the links to complete the following Web activities.

- Epidemiology Program Office
- *Morbidity and Mortality Weekly Report*
- National Center for Health Statistics

REFERENCES

1. Last, J. M., ed. (2001). *A Dictionary of Epidemiology*. New York: Oxford University Press.

2. Taubenberer, J. K., and D. M. Morens (2006). "1918 Influenza: The Mother of All Pandemics." *Emerging Infectious Diseases*, 12(1): 15-22.

3. United Nations Programme on HIV/AIDS (2009). *2008 Report on the Global AIDS Epidemic*. Available at http://www.unaids.org/en/KnowledgeCentre/HIVData/GlobalReport/2008/2008_Global_report.asp.

4. Monath, T. P. (1980). *St. Louis Encephalitis*. Washington, DC: American Public Health Association.

5. Centers for Disease Control and Prevention (2003). "Summary of Notifiable Diseases—United States, 2001." *Morbidity and Mortality Weekly Report*, 50(53): 1-108.

6. Centers for Disease Control and Prevention (1981). "Toxic Shock Syndrome—United States, 1970-1980." *Morbidity and Mortality Weekly Report*, 30(3): 25-33.

7. Centers for Disease Control and Prevention (2009). *HIV/AIDS Surveillance Report: Cases of HIV Infection and AIDS in the United States and Dependent Areas, 2007*. Available at http://www.cdc.gov/hiv/topics/surveillance/resources/reports/2007report/pdf/2007Surveillance Report.pdf.

8. Centers for Disease Control and Prevention (2008). "Surveillance for Lyme Disease—United States, 1992-2006." *Surveillance Summaries, Morbidity and Mortality Weekly Report*, 57(No. SS-10): 1-10. Available at http://www.cdc.gov/mmwr/pdf/ss/ss5710.pdf.

9. Centers for Disease Control and Prevention (2010). "Surveillance for Human West Nile Virus Disease—United States, 1999-2008." *Surveillance Summaries, Morbidity and Mortality Weekly Report*, 59(No. SS-2): 1-18. Available at http://www.cdc.gov/mmwr/pdf/ss/ss5902.pdf.

10. Centers for Disease Control and Prevention (2010). "Summary of Notifiable Diseases—United States, 2008." *Morbidity and Mortality Weekly Report*, 53(53): 1-82. Available at http://www.cdc.gov/mmwr/PDF/wk/mm5754.pdf.

11. Centers for Disease Control and Prevention (2010). "Update: Mumps Outbreak—New York and New Jersey, June 2009-January 2010." *Morbidity and Mortality Weekly Report*, 59(5): 125-129. Available at http://www.cdc.gov/mmwr/PDF/wk/mm5905.pdf.

12. Centers for Disease Control and Prevention (2010). "Update: Influenza Activity—United States, August 30, 2009-March 27, 2010, and Composition of the 2010-11 Influenza Vaccine." *Morbidity and Mortality Weekly Report*, 59(14): 423-430. Available at http://www.cdc.gov/mmwr/PDF/wk/mm5914.pdf.

13. Ibid.

14. Ibid.

15. Ibid.

16. Johnson, S. R. (2006). *The Ghost Map: The Story of London's Most Terrifying Epidemic—and How It Changed Science, Cities, and the Modern World*. New York: Riverhead Books.

17. Ibid.

18. Miniño, A. M., J. Q. Xu, K. D. Kochanek. "Deaths: Preliminary Data for 2008." *National Vital Statistics Reports*, 59(2). Hyattsville, MD: National Center for Health Statistics. 2010. Available at http://www.cdc.gov/nchs/data/nvsr/nvsr59/nvsr59_02.pdf.

19. Hamilton, B. E., J. A. Martin, and S. J. Ventura (2010). "Births: Preliminary Data for 2008." *National Vital Statistics Reports*, 58(16): 1-18. Available at http://www.cdc.gov/nchs/data/nvsr/nvsr58/nvsr58_16.pdf.

20. Centers for Disease Control and Prevention, National Center for Health Statistics (1998). "Leading Causes of Death, 1900-1998." Available at http://www.cdc.gov/nchs/data/dvs/lead1900_98.pdf.

21. National Center for Health Statistics (2010). *Health, United States, 2009 with Special Feature on Medical Technology* [online]. (DHHS pub. no. 2010-1232). Hyattsville, MD: Author. Available at http://www.cdc.gov/nchs/hus.htm.

22. World Health Organization (2009). "World Health Statistics." Geneva, Switzerland: Author. Available at http://www.who.int/healthinfo/statistics/mortality/en/.

23. Murray, D. J. L., and A. D. Lopez, eds. (1996). *The Global Burden of Disease: A Comprehensive Assessment of Mortality and Disability from Diseases, injuries and Risk Factors in 1990 and Projected to 2020*. Global Burden of Disease and Injury, Vol. 1. Cambridge, MA: Harvard School of Public Health on behalf of WHO.

24. World Health Organization (2008). "The Global Burden of Disease: 2004 Update." Available at http://www.who.int/healthinfo/global_burden_disease/GBD_report_2004update_full.pdf.

25. Mathers, C. C., R. Sdana, J. A. Salomon, C. J. L. Murray, and A. D. Lopez (2000). "Estimates of DALE for 191 Countries: Methods and Results." *Global Programme on Evidence for Health Policy Working Paper No. 16*. Geneva, Switzerland: World Health Organization. Available at http://www.who.int/healthinfo/paper16.pdf.

26. Lopez, A. S., C. D. Mathers, M. Ezzati, D. T. Jamison, and C. J. L. Murray, eds. (2006). *Global Burden of Disease and Risk Factors*. Washington, DC: World Bank and Oxford University Press.

27. Adams, P. F., K. M. Heyman, and J. L. Vickerie (2009). "Summary Health Statistics for the U.S. Population: National Health Interview Survey, 2008." *Vital and Health Statistics*, 10(243).

28. Centers for Disease Control and Prevention (2009). "National Health and Nutrition Examination Survey: About the National Health and Nutrition Examination Survey." Available at http://www.cdc.gov/nchs/nhanes/about_nhanes.htm.

29. Centers for Disease Control and Prevention (2010). "Youth Risk Behavior Surveillance—United States, 2009." *Surveillance Summaries*, 59(SS-5): *Morbidity and Mortality Weekly Report*, 1-148. Available at http://www.cdc.gov/mmwr/pdf/ss/ss5905.pdf.

30. Tonnesen, P., J. Norregaard, K. Simonsen, and U. Sawe (1991). "A Double-Blind Trial of a 16-Hour Transdermal Nicotine Patch in Smoking Cessation." *New England Journal of Medicine*, 325(5): 311-315.

31. Hill, A. B. (1965). "The Environment and Disease: Association or Causation?" *Proceedings of the Royal Society of Medicine*, 58: 295-300.

Chapter 4

Epidemiology: Prevention and Control of Diseases and Health Conditions

Chapter Outline

Chapter Objectives

After studying this chapter, you will be able to:

1 Explain the differences between communicable (infectious) and noncommunicable (noninfectious) diseases and between acute and chronic diseases and provide examples of each.

2 Describe and explain communicable and multicausation disease models.

3 Explain how communicable diseases are transmitted in a community using the "chain of infection" model and use a specific communicable disease to illustrate your explanation.

4 Explain why noncommunicable diseases are a community health concern and provide some examples of important noncommunicable diseases.

5 Explain the difference between primary, secondary, and tertiary prevention of disease and provide examples of each.

6 List and explain the various criteria that communities might use to prioritize their health problems in preparation for the allocation of prevention and control resources.

7 List and discuss important measures for preventing and controlling the spread of communicable diseases in a community.

8 List and discuss approaches to noncommunicable disease control in the community.

9 Define and explain the purpose and importance of *health screenings*.

10 Outline a chronic, noncommunicable disease control program that includes primary, secondary, and tertiary disease prevention components.

SCENARIO

Bob had always been an active and athletic person. He lettered in three sports in high school and played varsity tennis in college. Following graduation last May, he was lucky enough to land a job with one of the Fortune 500 companies in nearby Indianapolis. He shares an apartment with Chuck, a business colleague, and both work long hours in the hope that hard work will mean success and advancement. Neither seems to find time to exercise regularly, and both rely increasingly on fast-food restaurants. Bob's weight is now 12 pounds above his weight at graduation.

Bob is beginning to wonder whether he is compromising his health for financial success. When he first came to the company, he took the stairs between floors two at a time and was never winded, even after climbing several flights. Now he becomes tired after two flights. Also, Bob recently participated in a free serum cholesterol screening. Bob's cholesterol level was 259 mg/dL. Bob decided it was time to have a complete physical examination.

INTRODUCTION

In Chapter 3, we discussed the measurement and reporting of disease and the use of rates and ratios to describe disease incidence and prevalence. We then explained how epidemiologists describe disease outbreaks by person, place, and time, and how they search for causal associations through analytic and experimental studies.

In this chapter, we extend our discussion of epidemiology. We begin by describing the different ways to classify diseases and other health conditions. Then, we explain models of communicable and noncommunicable diseases, conceptual frameworks used by epidemiologists to develop prevention and control strategies. We also discuss criteria used by communities to prioritize their health problems and allocate health resources. Finally, we discuss some approaches to disease prevention and control; introduce the concepts of primary, secondary, and tertiary prevention; and provide examples of their application to a communicable and noncommunicable disease.

CLASSIFICATION OF DISEASES AND HEALTH PROBLEMS

Diseases and health problems can be classified in several meaningful ways. The public often classifies diseases by organ or organ system, such as kidney disease, heart disease, respiratory infection, and so on. Another method of classification is by causative agent—viral disease, chemical poisoning, physical injury, and so forth. In this scheme, causative agents may be biological, chemical, or physical. Biological agents include viruses, rickettsiae, bacteria, protozoa, fungi, and metazoa (multicellular organisms). Chemical agents include drugs, pesticides, industrial chemicals, food additives, air pollutants, and cigarette smoke. Physical agents that can cause injury or disease include various forms of energy such as heat, ultraviolet light, radiation, noise vibrations, and speeding or falling objects (see Table 4.1). In community health, diseases are usually classified as acute or chronic, or as communicable (infectious) or noncommunicable (noninfectious).

communicable (infectious) disease an illness caused by some specific biological agent or its toxic products that can be transmitted from an infected person, animal, or inanimate reservoir to a susceptible host

Communicable versus Noncommunicable Diseases

Another classification system divides diseases into communicable and noncommunicable diseases. **Communicable (infectious) diseases** are those diseases for which biological agents or their products are the cause and that are transmissible from one individual to another. The disease process begins when the agent is able to enter and grow or reproduce within the body of the host. The entrance and growth of microorganisms or viruses in the host are called *infections.*

noncommunicable (noninfectious) diseases or illnesses are those that cannot be transmitted from one person to another. Delineating the causes of noncommunicable diseases is often more difficult because several, or even many, factors may contribute to the development of a given noncommunicable health condition. These contributing factors may be genetic, environmental, or behavioral in nature. For this reason, many noncommunicable health conditions are called multicausation diseases; an example of such is heart disease. Genetics, environmental factors such as stress, and behavioral choices such as poor diet and lack of exercise can all contribute to heart disease.

noncommunicable disease (noninfectious disease)
a disease that cannot be transmitted from infected host to susceptible host

Acute versus Chronic Diseases and Illnesses

In the acute/chronic classification scheme, diseases are classified by their duration of symptoms. Acute diseases, as defined in Chapter 3, are diseases in which the peak severity of symptoms occurs and subsides within 3 months (usually sooner) and the recovery of those who survive is usually complete. Examples of acute communicable diseases include the common cold, influenza (flu), chickenpox, measles, mumps, Rocky Mountain spotted fever, and plague. Examples of acute noncommunicable illnesses are appendicitis, injuries from motor vehicle crashes, acute alcohol intoxication or drug overdose, and sprained ankles (see Table 4.2).

Chronic diseases or conditions are those in which symptoms continue longer than 3 months, and in some cases, for the remainder of one's life (see Figure 4.1). Recovery is slow and sometimes incomplete. These diseases can be either communicable or noncommunicable. Examples of chronic communicable diseases are AIDS, tuberculosis, herpes virus infections, syphilis, and Lyme disease. Chronic noncommunicable illnesses include hypertension, hypercholesterolemia, coronary heart disease, diabetes, and many types of arthritis and cancer.

Table 4.1
Causative Agents for Diseases and Injuries

Biological Agents	Chemical Agents	Physical Agents
Viruses	Pesticides	Heat
Rickettsiae	Food additives	Light
Bacteria	Pharmacologics	Radiation
Fungi	Industrial chemicals	Noise
Protozoa	Air pollutants	Vibration
Metazoa	Cigarette smoke	Speeding objects

Table 4.2
Classification of Diseases

Types of Diseases	Examples
Acute diseases	
Communicable	Common cold, pneumonia, mumps, measles, pertussis, typhoid fever, cholera
Noncommunicable	Appendicitis, poisoning, injury (due to motor vehicle crash, fire, gunshot, etc.)
Chronic diseases	
Communicable	AIDS, Lyme disease, tuberculosis, syphilis, rheumatic fever following streptococcal infections, hepatitis B
Noncommunicable	Diabetes, coronary heart disease, osteoarthritis, cirrhosis of the liver due to alcoholism

COMMUNICABLE DISEASES

Whereas **infectivity** refers to the ability of a biological agent to enter and grow in a host, the term **pathogenicity** refers to an infectious disease agent's ability to produce disease. Selected pathogenic agents and the diseases they cause are listed in Table 4.3. Under certain conditions, pathogenic biological agents can be transmitted from an infected individual in the community to an uninfected, susceptible one. Communicable disease agents may be further classified according to the manner in which they are transmitted.

The elements of a simplified **communicable disease model**—agent, host, and environment—are presented in Figure 4.2. These three factors are the minimal requirements for the occurrence and spread of communicable diseases in a population. In this model, the **agent** is the element that must be present for disease to occur. For example, the influenza virus must be present for a person to become ill with flu. The **host** is any susceptible organism—a single-celled organism, a plant, an animal, or a human—invaded by an infectious agent. The *environment* includes all other factors—physical, biological, or social—that inhibit or promote disease transmission. Communicable

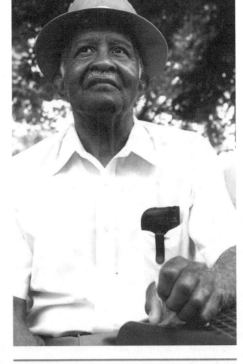

FIGURE 4.1
Arthritis is a noninfectious chronic condition that can persist for one's entire life.

infectivity
the ability of a biological agent to enter and grow in the host

pathogenicity
the capability of a communicable disease agent to cause disease in a susceptible host

communicable disease model
a visual representation of the interrelationships among causative agent, host, and environment

agent (pathogenic agent)
the cause of the disease or health problem

host
a person or other living organism that affords subsistence or lodgment to a communicable agent under natural conditions

Table 4.3
Biological Agents of Disease

Types of Agent	Name of Agent	Disease
Viruses	Varicella virus	Chickenpox
	Human immunodeficiency virus (HIV)	Acquired immune deficiency syndrome (AIDS)
	Rubella virus	German measles
Rickettsiae	*Rickettsia rickettsii*	Rocky Mountain spotted fever
Bacteria	*Vibrio cholerae*	Cholera
	Clostridium tetani	Tetanus
	Yersinia pestis	Plague
	Borrelia burgdorferi	Lyme disease
Protozoa	*Entamoeba histolytica*	Amebic dysentery
	Plasmodium falciparum	Malaria
	Trypanosoma gambiense	African sleeping sickness
Fungi and yeasts	*Tinea cruris*	Jock itch
	Tinea pedis	Athlete's foot
Nematoda (worms)	*Wuchereria bancrofti*	Filariasis (elephantiasis)
	Onchocerca volvulus	Onchocerciasis (river blindness)

chain of infection
a model to conceptualize the transmission of a communicable disease from its source to a susceptible host

case
a person who is sick with a disease

carrier
a person or animal that harbors a specific communicable agent in the absence of discernible clinical disease and serves as a potential source of infection to others

zoonosis
a communicable disease transmissible under natural conditions from vertebrate animals to humans

anthroponosis
a disease that infects only humans

disease transmission occurs when a susceptible host and a pathogenic agent exist in an environment conducive to disease transmission.

Chain of Infection

Communicable disease transmission is a complicated but well-studied process that is best understood through a conceptual model known as the **chain of infection** (see Figure 4.3). Using the chain of infection model, one can visualize the step-by-step process by which communicable diseases spread from an infected person to an uninfected person in the community. The *pathogenic* (disease-producing) agent

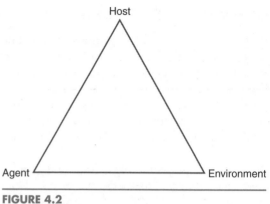

FIGURE 4.2
Communicable disease model.

leaves its *reservoir* (infected host) via a *portal of exit*. *Transmission* occurs in either a direct or indirect manner, and the pathogenic agent enters a susceptible host through a *portal of entry* to establish infection. For example, let us follow the common cold through the chain of infection. The agent (the cold virus) leaves its reservoir (the throat of an infected person), perhaps when the host sneezes. The portals of exit are the nose and mouth. Transmission may be direct if saliva droplets enter the respiratory tract of a susceptible host at close range, or it may be indirect if droplets dry and become airborne. The portal of entry could be the nose or mouth of a susceptible host. The agent enters, and a new infection is established.

There are many variations in the chain of infection, depending on the disease agent, environmental conditions, infectivity, and host susceptibility. For example, the reservoir for a disease may be a **case**—a person who has the disease—or a **carrier**—one who is well but infected and is capable of serving as a source of infection. A (disease) carrier could be one who is incubating the disease, such as a person who is HIV positive but has no signs of AIDS, or one who has recovered from the disease (is asymptomatic), as is sometimes the case in typhoid fever. For some diseases, the reservoir is not humans but animals. Diseases for which the reservoir resides in animal populations are called **zoonoses**. Plague, rabies, Rocky Mountain spotted fever, and Lyme disease are zoonoses. Diseases for which humans are the only known reservoir, like measles, are known as **anthroponoses**.

Portals of exit (see Figure 4.4) and entry vary from disease to disease. Natural portals of exit and examples of diseases that use them are the respiratory tract (cold, influenza, measles, tuberculosis, and whooping cough), urogenital tract (gonorrhea, syphilis, herpes, and AIDS), digestive tract (amebic dysentery, shigellosis, polio, typhoid fever, and cholera), and skin (ring-

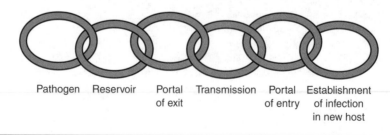

Pathogen Reservoir Portal of exit Transmission Portal of entry Establishment of infection in new host

FIGURE 4.3
Chain of infection.

worm and jock itch). The skin is actually a good barrier to infection, but it can be bypassed by a hypodermic needle or when there is an open wound. Blood-sucking insects and ticks make their own portals of entry with mouth parts that penetrate the skin. Finally, many pathogenic agents can cross the placenta from mother to fetus (for example, rubella virus, syphilis spirochetes, and hepatitis B virus).

Modes of Transmission

As noted in the previous paragraphs, communicable disease transmission may be direct or indirect. **Direct transmission** implies the immediate transfer of the disease agent between the infected and the susceptible individuals by direct contact "such as touching, biting, kissing, sexual intercourse, or by direct projection (droplet spread) of droplet spray onto the conjunctiva or onto the mucous membranes of the eye, nose or mouth during sneezing, coughing, spitting, singing or talking (usually limited to a distance of one meter or less)."[1] Examples of diseases for which transmission is usually direct are AIDS, syphilis, gonorrhea, rabies, and the common cold.

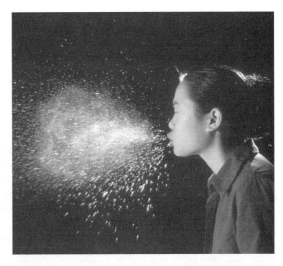

FIGURE 4.4

Portal of exit: The causative agents for many respiratory diseases leave their host via the mouth and nose.

Indirect transmission may be one of three types—airborne, vehicleborne, or vectorborne. *Airborne transmission* is the dissemination of microbial aerosols to a suitable portal of entry, usually the respiratory tract. Microbial aerosols are suspensions of dust or droplet nuclei made up wholly or in part of microorganisms. These particles may remain suspended and infective for long periods of time. Tuberculosis, influenza, histoplasmosis, and legionellosis are examples of airborne diseases.

In *vehicleborne transmission,* contaminated materials or objects (fomites) serve as **vehicles**—nonliving objects by which communicable agents are transferred to a susceptible host. The agent may or may not have multiplied or developed on the vehicle. Examples of vehicles include toys, handkerchiefs, soiled clothes, bedding, food service utensils, and surgical instruments. Also considered vehicles are water, milk, food, or biological products such as blood, serum, plasma, organs, and tissues. Almost any disease can be transmitted by vehicles, including those for which the primary mode of transmission is direct, such as dysentery and hepatitis.

Vectorborne transmission is the transfer of disease by a living organism such as a mosquito, fly, or tick. Transmission may be mechanical, via the contaminated mouth parts or feet of the **vector**, or biological, which involves multiplication or developmental changes of the agent in the vector before transmission occurs. In *mechanical transmission,* multiplication and development of the disease organism usually do not occur. For example, organisms that cause dysentery, polio, cholera, and typhoid fever have been isolated from insects such as cockroaches and houseflies and could presumably be deposited on food prepared for human consumption.

In *biological transmission,* multiplication and/or developmental changes of the disease agent occur in the vector before transmission occurs. Biological transmission is much more important than mechanical transmission in terms of its impact on community health. Examples of biological vectors include mosquitoes, fleas, lice, ticks, flies, and other insects. Mosquitoes are by far the most important vectors of human disease. They transmit the viruses that cause yellow fever and dengue fever as well as more than 200 other viruses, including West Nile fever virus. They also transmit malaria, which infects 100 million people

direct transmission
the immediate transfer of an infectious agent by direct contact between infected and susceptible individuals

indirect transmission
communicable disease transmission involving an intermediate step

vehicle
an inanimate material or object that can serve as a source of infection

vector
a living organism, usually an arthropod (e.g., mosquito, tick, louse, or flea), that can transmit a communicable agent to susceptible hosts

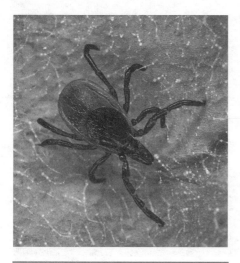

FIGURE 4.5

A female blacklegged tick, *Ixodes scapularis*, a vector of Lyme disease.

in the world each year (mostly in tropical areas), killing at least 1 million of them. Ticks, another important vector, transmit Rocky Mountain spotted fever, relapsing fever, and Lyme disease (see Figure 4.5). Other insect vectors (and the diseases they transmit) are flies (African sleeping sickness, onchocerciasis, loiasis, and leishmaniasis), fleas (plague and murine typhus), lice (epidemic typhus and trench fever), and kissing bugs (Chagas' disease).

NONCOMMUNICABLE DISEASES

Although communicable diseases remain an important concern for communities, certain noncommunicable diseases, such as heart disease, stroke, and cancer, now rank high among the nation's leading causes of death. Although these diseases are not infectious, they nonetheless can occur in epidemic proportions. Furthermore, the chronic nature of many of these diseases means that they can deplete a community's resources quite rapidly.

The complex **etiologies** (causes) of many of the noncommunicable diseases, such as coronary heart disease, are best illustrated by the **multicausation disease model** (see Figure 4.6). In this model, the human host is pictured in the center of the environment in which he or she lives. Within the host, there exists a unique genetic endowment that is inalterable. The host exists in a complex environment that includes exposures to a multitude of *risk factors* that can contribute to the disease process. These environmental risk factors may be physical, chemical, biological, or social in nature.

Physical factors include the latitude, climate, and physical geography of where one lives. The major health risks in the tropics—communicable and parasitic diseases—are different from those in temperate regions with cold winters—difficulty in finding food and remaining warm. Chemical factors include not only natural chemical hazards of polluted water and air but also the added pollutants of our modern, industrial society. Biological hazards include communicable disease agents such as pathogenic viruses, bacteria, and fungi. Social factors include one's occupation, recreational activities, and living arrangements. Poor choices in life can increase the number and severity of one's risk factors and be detrimental to one's health.

Diseases of the Heart and Blood Vessels

Diseases of the heart and blood vessels, cardiovascular diseases (CVDs), are a leading cause of death in the United States. **Coronary heart disease (CHD)** is the number 1 killer of Americans. In 2008 alone, more than 617,520 people died of heart disease in the United States, accounting for one in four deaths that year.[2] It is estimated that more than 74 million Americans have one or more types of CVD.[3]

The American Heart Association lists nine types of CVDs: CHD, stroke, high blood pressure, arrhythmias, diseases of the arteries, congestive heart failure, valvular heart disease, rheumatic fever/rheumatic heart disease, and congenital heart defects.[3] CHD causes more than half of all cardiovascular disease deaths. Sometimes called *coronary artery disease,* CHD is characterized by damage to the coronary arteries, the blood vessels that carry oxygen-rich blood to the heart muscle. Damage to the coronary arteries usually evolves from the condition known as *atherosclerosis,* a narrowing of the blood vessels. This narrowing usually results from the buildup of fatty deposits on the inner walls of arteries. When blood flow to the heart muscle is severely reduced or interrupted, a heart attack can occur. If heart damage is severe, the heart may stop beating—a condition known as cardiac arrest.

etiology
the cause of a disease

multicausation disease model
a visual representation of the host together with various internal and external factors that promote and protect against disease

coronary heart disease (CHD)
a chronic disease characterized by damage to the coronary arteries in the heart

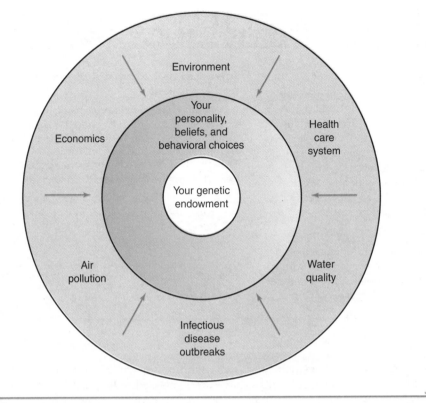

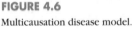

FIGURE 4.6
Multicausation disease model.

Over the past 50 years, a more complete understanding of the processes involved in CVDs has resulted in a 56% decline in deaths from heart disease and stroke (see Box 4.1). Numerous risk factors for coronary artery disease have been identified. Whereas some of these risk factors cannot be altered by changes in lifestyle or behavior, others can. Factors that cannot be altered include one's age, sex, race, and the genetic tendency toward developing the disease. Factors that can be modified include cigarette smoking, high blood pressure, high blood cholesterol, physical inactivity, obesity, diabetes, and stress.

Cerebrovascular disease (stroke) is the fourth leading cause of death in the United States. Strokes killed more than 133,137 people in 2008.[2] During a stroke, or cerebrovascular accident, the blood supply to the brain is interrupted.

The risk factors for developing cerebrovascular disease are similar to those for CHD and include hereditary, behavioral, and environmental factors. Hypertension and cigarette smoking are especially important risk factors for cerebrovascular disease.

cerebrovascular disease (stroke) a chronic disease characterized by damage to blood vessels of the brain resulting in disruption of circulation to the brain

Malignant Neoplasms (Cancer)

A total of 566,137 people died from malignant neoplasms (cancer) in 2008, making it the second leading cause of death in the United States.[2] **Malignant neoplasms** occur when cells lose control over their growth and division. Normal cells are inhibited from continual growth and division by virtue of their contact with adjacent cells. Malignant (cancerous) cells are not so inhibited; they continue to grow and divide, eventually piling up in a "new growth," a neoplasm or tumor. Early-stage tumors, sometimes called *in situ cancers,* are more treatable than are later-stage cancers. As tumor growth continues, parts of the neoplasm can break off

malignant neoplasm uncontrolled new tissue growth resulting from cells that have lost control over their growth and division

BOX 4.1

TEN GREAT PUBLIC HEALTH ACHIEVEMENTS, 1900–1999: DECLINE IN DEATHS FROM CORONARY HEART DISEASE AND STROKE

You Gotta Have Heart

Since 1921, heart disease has been the leading cause of death, and since 1938, stroke has been the third leading cause of death. However, since 1950, age-adjusted death rates from cardiovascular disease (CVD) have declined 60%, representing one of the most important public health achievements in the twentieth century. This decline was made possible through a better understanding of disease epidemiology and advances in prevention techniques, diagnoses, and treatment.

Disease Epidemiology

The risk-factor concept—the idea that particular biologic, lifestyle, and social conditions were associated with an increased risk for specific disease—developed as a result of population-based research into the causes of CVD.

Advances in Prevention, Diagnoses, and Treatment

Prevention efforts and improvements in early detection, treatment, and care have resulted in several beneficial trends that have likely contributed to declines in CVD.

Trends That Have Likely Contributed to Declines in Cardiovascular Disease

- A decline in cigarette smoking among adults
- A decrease in mean blood pressure levels
- A decrease in mean blood cholesterol levels

Source: Centers for Disease Control and Prevention. (1999). "Ten Great Public Health Achievements—United States, 1900-1999." *Morbidity and Mortality Weekly Report* 48(12): 241-242. Available at www.cdc.gov/mmwr/PDF/wk/mm4812.pdf. Acessed October 26, 2010.

---

metastasis
the spread of cancer cells to distant parts of the body by the circulatory or lymphatic system

and be carried to distant parts of the body, where they can lodge and continue to grow. When this occurs, the cancer is said to have **metastasized**. When malignant neoplasms have spread beyond the orginal cell layer where they developed, the cancer is said to be *invasive*.[4] The more the malignancy spreads, the more difficult it is to treat and the lower the survival rates. For more information on the staging of cancer, see Box 4.2.

Common cancer sites in order of frequency of reported cases and deaths for both men and women are shown in Figure 4.7. Cancer sites with the highest number of reported cases are the prostate gland (men) and breast (women), but cancer frequently occurs in other sites, including the lung, colon and rectum, pancreas, uterus, ovaries, mouth, bladder, and skin. Lung cancer is the leading cause of cancer deaths in both sexes. There were an estimated 222,520 new cases of lung cancer and an estimated 157,300 lung cancer deaths in 2010 alone. It has been estimated that 87% of these deaths can be attributed to smoking. Alcohol and smokeless tobacco contribute to cancers of the mouth, throat, larynx, esophagus, and liver.[4]

More than 1 million new cases of basal cell or squamous cell skin cancer are detected each year in the United States. Almost all of these cases are attributable to exposure to the sun, and yet many people continue to sunbathe or use tanning salons, believing that a tanned body is a healthy one. The number of cases of nonmelanoma skin cancer is expected to rise as long as the ozone layer in the atmosphere continues to be eroded (see Chapter 14). This is an example of how environmental policy affects public health.

Other Noncommunicable Disease Problems

Other noncommunicable diseases of major concern are (1) chronic obstructive pulmonary disease and allied conditions (the fourth leading cause of death), (2) diabetes mellitus (the seventh leading cause of death), and (3) chronic liver disease and cirrhosis (the tenth leading cause of death). Each of these chronic noncommunicable diseases and those listed in Table 4.4 place a burden not only on the afflicted individuals and their families but on the community's health resources as well.

BOX
4.2

HOW IS CANCER STAGED?

According to the American Cancer Society, "staging describes the extent or spread of the disease." A number of different staging systems exist. One of the most popular is the TNM staging system, which assesses tumors in three ways:

The extent of the primary tumor (T), absence or presence of regional lymph node involvement (N), and absence or presence of distant metastases (M). Once the T, N, and M are determined, a stage of I, II, III, or IV is assigned, with stage I being early stage and stage IV being advanced.

A different system of summary staging (in situ, local, regional, and distant) is used for descriptive and statistical analysis of tumor registry data. If cancer cells are present only in the layer of cells where they developed and have not spread, the stage is in situ. If the cancer has spread beyond the original layer of tissue, the cancer is invasive.

Source: Reprinted from American Cancer Society. *Cancer Facts and Figures 2010.* Atlanta: American Cancer Society, Inc. Available at www.cancer.org. Accessed October 15, 2010.

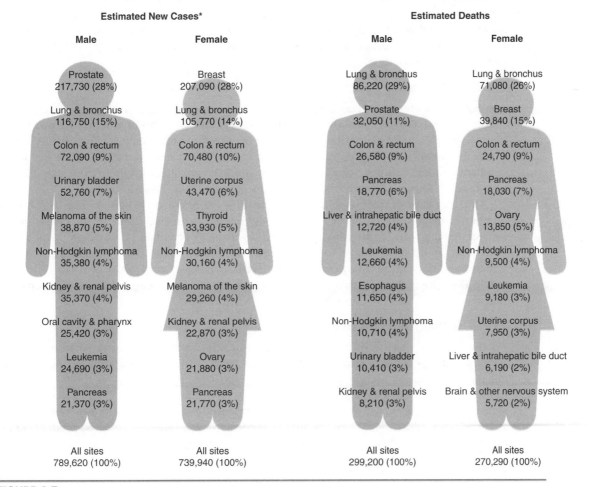

FIGURE 4.7

Leading sites of new cancer cases* and deaths—2006 estimates (percentages may not total 100% due to rounding).

*Excludes basal and squamous cell skin cancer and in situ carcinomas except urinary bladder.

Source: American Cancer Society. *Cancer Facts and Figures 2010.* Atlanta: American Cancer Society, Inc. Available at http://www.cancer.org. Accessed October 15, 2010.

Table 4.4
Some Noncommunicable Health Conditions That Affect Americans

Allergic disorders	Endogenous depression	Multiple sclerosis
Alzheimer's disease	Epilepsy	Osteoporosis
Arthritis	Fibrocystic breast condition	Premenstrual syndrome
Cerebral palsy	Lower back pain	Sickle cell trait and sickle cell disease

PRIORITIZING PREVENTION AND CONTROL EFFORTS

Communities are confronted with a multitude of health problems—communicable and non-communicable diseases, unintentional injuries, violence, substance abuse problems, and so on. How can health officials make logical and responsible choices about the allocation of community resources to prevent or control these problems? Which problems are indeed the most urgent? Which problems will benefit the most from a timely intervention? Several criteria are used to judge the importance of a particular disease to a community. Among these are (1) the number of people who die from a disease, (2) the number of years of potential life lost attributable to a particular cause, and (3) the economic costs associated with a particular disease or health condition.

Leading Causes of Death

The National Center for Health Statistics (NCHS) regularly publishes a list of the leading causes of death. For more than 80 years, the leading cause of death in America has been heart disease. Nearly one in every three deaths can be attributed to diseases of the heart. Cancers (malignant neoplasms) represent the second leading killer; nearly one in four deaths is the result of cancer. Chronic lower respiratory disease ranks third, cerebrovascular disease (stroke) rank fourth, and unintentional injuries rank fifth (see Table 3.8).[2]

One might prioritize expenditures of health care resources solely on the basis of the number of deaths, but in doing so one would spend about two-thirds of the entire health budget on the four leading health problems alone. Very little or perhaps none of the resources would be available for infant and childhood nutrition programs, for example, which have been shown to prevent more serious health care problems in later life. Nor would there be any funds available for the treatment of those with debilitating, but usually nonfatal, diseases such as chronic arthritis or mental illness.

Years of Potential Life Lost

Another approach to prioritizing a community's health care problems is by using the *years of potential life lost (YPLL)* statistic described in Chapter 3. Using this approach, diseases that kill people of all ages become as important as those that kill primarily older adults. Recall, for example, that malignant neoplasms (cancers) are the leading cause of YPLL-75 in the United States and account for 21.3% of all YPLL-75 compared with CVD, which accounts for only about 15.3%. Unintentional injuries are the second leading cause of YPLL-75, accounting for 15.7% of the total YPLL (refer to Table 3.12 and Figure 3.4).[6]

Economic Cost to Society

Still another way to evaluate the impact of a particular disease or health problem is to estimate the economic cost to the country or community. Economic cost data are hard to come by, and sometimes even experts cannot agree on the estimates obtained. An example of such an estimate is the cost to our federal, state, and local governments' spending resulting from the use and abuse of alcohol and other drugs, a whopping $467.7 billion annually, more than $1 billion per day.[7] This figure amounts to 10.7% of their entire $4.4 trillion budgets.

PREVENTION, INTERVENTION, CONTROL, AND ERADICATION OF DISEASES

The goals of epidemiology are to prevent, control, and in rare cases, to eradicate diseases and injuries. **Prevention** implies the planning for and taking of action to prevent or forestall the occurrence of an undesirable event, and is therefore more desirable than **intervention**, the taking of action during an event. For example, immunizing to prevent a disease is preferable to taking an antibiotic to cure one.

Control is a general term for the containment of a disease and can include both prevention and intervention measures. The term *control* is often used to mean the limiting of transmission of a communicable disease in a population. **Eradication** is the uprooting or total elimination of a disease from the human population. It is an elusive goal, one that is only rarely achieved in public health. Smallpox is the only communicable disease that has been eradicated (see Box 4.3). This was possible only because humans are the only reservoir.

LEVELS OF PREVENTION

There are three levels of application of preventive measures in disease control—primary, secondary, and tertiary. The purpose of **primary prevention** is to forestall the onset of illness or injury during the prepathogenesis period (before the disease process begins). Examples of primary prevention include health education and health promotion programs, safe-housing projects, and character-building and personality development programs. Other examples are the use of immunizations against specific diseases, the practice of personal hygiene such as hand washing, the use of rubber gloves, and the chlorination of the community's water supply. These are illustrated in Figure 4.8.

Unfortunately, disease or injury cannot always be avoided. Chronic diseases in particular sometimes cause considerable disability before they are detected and treated. In these cases, prompt *intervention* can prevent death or limit disability. **Secondary prevention** is the early diagnosis and prompt treatment of diseases before the disease becomes advanced and disability becomes severe.

One of the most important secondary prevention measures is *health screenings*. The goal of these screenings is not to prevent the onset of disease but rather to detect its presence during early pathogenesis, thus permitting early intervention (treatment) and limiting disability. It is important to note that the purpose of a health screening is not to diagnose disease. Instead, the purpose is to economically and efficiently sort those who are probably healthy from those who could possibly be positive for a disease (see Figure 4.9). Those who

prevention
the planning for and taking of action to forestall the onset of a disease or other health problem

intervention
efforts to control a disease in progress

eradication
the complete elimination or uprooting of a disease (e.g., smallpox eradication)

primary prevention
preventive measures that forestall the onset of illness or injury during the prepathogenesis period

secondary prevention
preventive measures that lead to an early diagnosis and prompt treatment of a disease or injury to limit disability and prevent more severe pathogenesis

---

BOX 4.3   COMMUNITY HEALTH IN YOUR WORLD: SMALLPOX ERADICATION

December 2007 marked 30 years since the last naturally acquired case of smallpox in the world. This last case occurred in Somalia in October 1977.[1] Although two cases of smallpox were reported in the United Kingdom in 1978, these were associated with a research laboratory and did not represent a natural recurrence.

Smallpox is caused by the variola virus. In its severest form, it is a disfiguring and deadly disease. Manifestations of the disease include fever, headache, malaise, and prostration. A rash appears and covers the body, and there is bleeding into the skin, mucous lin-

ings, and genital tract. The circulatory system is also severely affected. Between 15% and 40% of cases die, usually within 2 weeks. Survivors are terribly scarred for life and are sometimes blinded.

Mass vaccinations and case-finding measures by the World Health Organization (WHO), with financial support from the United States, led to the eradication of smallpox from the world. Why was it possible to eradicate smallpox? Why have we been unable to eradicate any other diseases since 1977? Do you think we will ever be able to do so? If so, what disease will be eliminated next?

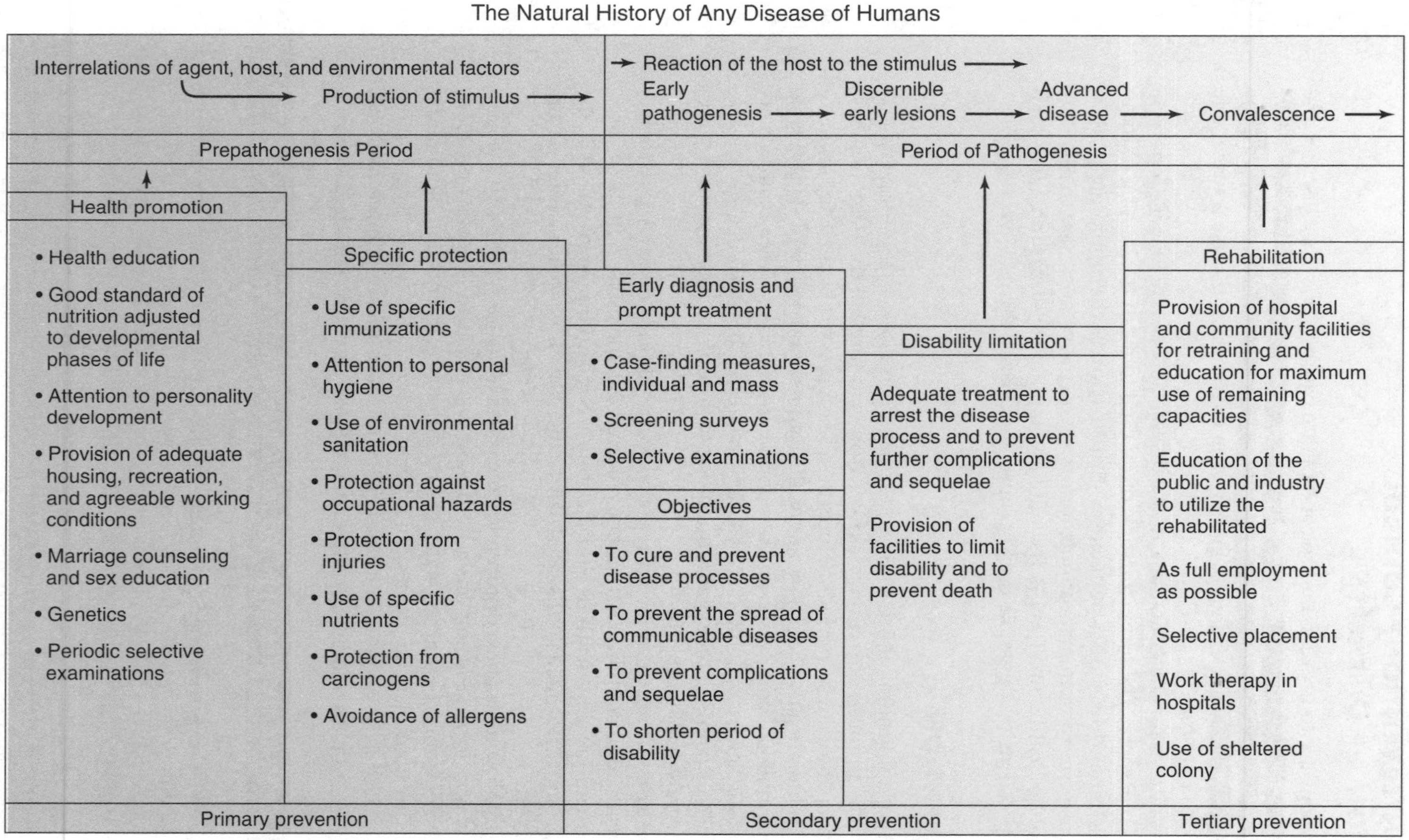

The Natural History of Any Disease of Humans
Interrelations of agent, host, and environmental factors
Production of stimulus
Reaction of the host to the stimulus
Early pathogenesis
Discernible early lesions
Advanced disease
Convalescence
Prepathogenesis Period
Period of Pathogenesis
Health promotion
• Health education
• Good standard of nutrition adjusted to developmental phases of life
• Attention to personality development
• Provision of adequate housing, recreation, and agreeable working conditions
• Marriage counseling and sex education
• Genetics
• Periodic selective examinations
Specific protection
• Use of specific immunizations
• Attention to personal hygiene
• Use of environmental sanitation
• Protection against occupational hazards
• Protection from injuries
• Use of specific nutrients
• Protection from carcinogens
• Avoidance of allergens
Early diagnosis and prompt treatment
• Case-finding measures, individual and mass
• Screening surveys
• Selective examinations
Objectives
• To cure and prevent disease processes
• To prevent the spread of communicable diseases
• To prevent complications and sequelae
• To shorten period of disability
Disability limitation
Adequate treatment to arrest the disease process and to prevent further complications and sequelae
Provision of facilities to limit disability and to prevent death
Rehabilitation
Provision of hospital and community facilities for retraining and education for maximum use of remaining capacities
Education of the public and industry to utilize the rehabilitated
As full employment as possible
Selective placement
Work therapy in hospitals
Use of sheltered colony
Primary prevention
Secondary prevention
Tertiary prevention

FIGURE 4.8
Applications of levels of prevention.

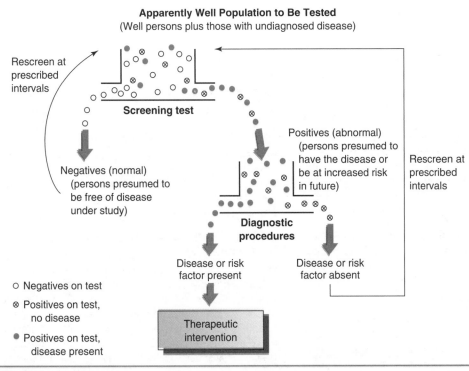

Apparently Well Population to Be Tested
(Well persons plus those with undiagnosed disease)

FIGURE 4.9

Flow diagram for a mass screening test.

Source: Mausner, J. S. and S. Kramer (1985). *Mausner and Bahn Epidemiology—An Introductory Text*, 2nd ed. Philadelphia, PA: W. B. Saunders Company, p. 216

screen positively can then be referred for more specific diagnostic procedures. Screenings for diabetes and high blood pressure are popular examples of health screenings, as are breast self-examination and testicular self-examination.

The goal of **tertiary prevention** is to retrain, re-educate, and rehabilitate the patient who has already incurred a disability. Tertiary preventive measures include those that are applied after significant pathogenesis has occurred. Therapy for a heart patient is an example of tertiary prevention.

> **tertiary prevention** measures aimed at rehabilitation following significant pathogenesis

Prevention of Communicable Diseases

Prevention and control efforts for communicable diseases include primary, secondary, and tertiary approaches. Successful application of these approaches, particularly primary prevention, resulting in unprecedented declines in morbidity and mortality from communicable diseases, has been one of the outstanding achievements in public health in this century (see Box 4.4).

Primary Prevention of Communicable Diseases

The primary prevention measures for communicable diseases can best be visualized using the chain of infection (see Figure 4.10). In this model, prevention strategies are evident at each link in the chain. Successful application of each strategy can be seen as weakening a link, with the ultimate goal of breaking the chain of infection, or interrupting the disease transmission cycle. Examples of community measures include chlorination of the water supply, the inspection of restaurants and retail food markets, immunization programs that reach all citizens, the

BOX
4.4

TEN GREAT PUBLIC HEALTH ACHIEVEMENTS, 1900–1999: CONTROL OF INFECTIOUS DISEASES

An Ounce of Prevention Is Worth a Century of Cure

Public health action to control infectious diseases in the twentieth century was founded on the late nineteenth century's discovery of microorganisms as causes of many diseases. Further scientific findings documented the interactions among humans, the environment, and microbes. Improvements in sanitation, hygiene, and food safety; the discovery of antibiotics; and the implementation of universal childhood vaccination programs resulted in the control of many fatal infectious diseases and the global eradication of one disease—smallpox. Scientific and technologic advances played a substantial role in these efforts. Today, those advances are the foundation for the disease surveillance and control systems that are used to combat all infectious diseases.

Sanitation and Hygiene

Early in the twentieth century, infections associated with overcrowding, poor housing, and contaminated water resulted in the transmission of tuberculosis, diphtheria, typhoid fever, and dysentery. Improvements in housing and public water supplies—including chlorination and filtration—and waste-disposal systems have resulted in swift progress in disease control.

Antibiotics and Other Antimicrobial Medicines

Antibiotics have been in common use since the 1940s and have saved the lives and health of persons with streptococcal and staphylococcal infections, gonorrhea, syphilis, and other infections. Penicillin was the first of many antibiotics that became widely available to cure previously untreatable bacterial diseases. Drugs also have been developed to treat viral, fungal, and parasitic diseases, but resistance to these miracle drugs is an ever-increasing challenge.

Emerging Diseases

For continued success in controlling infectious disease, the U.S. public health system must address such diverse challenges as the emergence of new infectious disease—for example, HIV and hantavirus—and the re-emergence of old diseases, sometimes in drug-resistant forms—for example, tuberculosis and malaria. Bioterrorism and pandemic influenza are also potential public health crises requiring advance preparedness.

Marvel of Medical Science, Miracle for Humankind

Sometimes a miracle happens and a disease is eradicated. Biomedical science and public health create this miracle when medicines and vaccines are developed that enable disease control and prevention. At the beginning of the twentieth century, few effective treatments and preventative measures existed to prevent infectious diseases. However, vaccines have been developed and are used to prevent many of the infectious diseases that threatened our parents, grandparents, and great-grandparents during the twentieth century.

Overall, U.S. vaccination coverage is at record high levels. Up-to-date training for the shot-givers and shot-callers is also at record high levels. Vaccines have the remarkable power to eradicate diseases. However, the combined effort of many partners is needed to achieve the full potential of these miraculous medicines.

Source: Centers for Disease Control and Prevention. (1999). "Ten Great Public Health Achievements—United States, 1900–1999." *Morbidity and Mortality Weekly Report* 48(12): 241-242. Available at www.cdc .gov/mmwr/PDF/wk/mm4812.pdf. Acessed October 26, 2010

maintenance of a well-functioning sewer system, the proper disposal of solid waste, and the control of vectors and rodents. To these can be added personal efforts at primary prevention, including hand washing, the proper cooking of food, adequate clothing and housing, the use of condoms, and obtaining all the available immunizations against specific diseases.

It is difficult to overstate the importance of vaccines or immunizations to community health. Vaccines prevent disease and save lives. They prevent disease in those who receive them and also protect those who come into contact with them. Many serious infectious diseases that were common as recently as the middle of the last century are rare now, including polio, measles, diphtheria, pertussis (whooping cough), rubella (German measles), mumps, tetanus, and *Haemophilus influenzae* type b (Hib).[8] Vaccines help the body fight off these diseases and help protect those members of the community who are unable to be vaccinated, namely, infants, those with certain diseases, such as childhood leukemia, and those unable to respond to an immunization. The Centers for Disease Control and Prevention issues recommendations for immunizations for children, for teens and college students, and for adults.

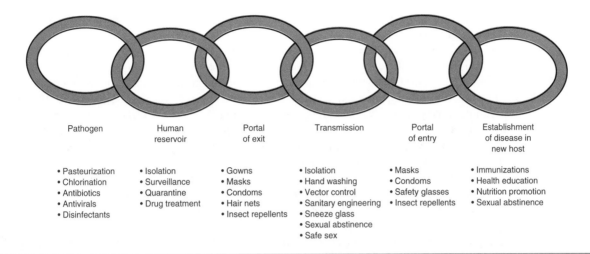

FIGURE 4.10

Chain of infection model showing disease prevention and control strategies.

These recommendations include immunizations for about 15 different disease agents and often indicate the need for a series of doses to acquire adequate protection. The current recommendations can be accessed through the Web site www.cdc.gov.[8]

Secondary Prevention of Communicable Diseases

Secondary preventive measures against communicable diseases for the individual involve either (1) self-diagnosis and self-treatment with nonprescription medications or home remedies, or (2) diagnosis and treatment with an antibiotic prescribed by a physician. Secondary preventive measures undertaken by the community against infectious diseases are usually aimed at controlling or limiting the extent of an epidemic. Examples include carefully maintaining records of cases and complying with the regulations requiring the reporting of notifiable diseases (see Chapter 3) and investigating cases and contacts—those who may have become infected through close contact with known cases.

Occasionally, secondary disease control measures may include isolation and quarantine. These two practices are quite different from one another and are often confused. **Isolation** is the separation, for the period of communicability, of infected persons or animals from others so as to prevent the direct or indirect transmission of the communicable agent to a susceptible person. **Quarantine** is the limitation of the freedom of movement of well persons or animals that have been exposed to a communicable disease until the incubation period has passed. Further control measures may include **disinfection**, the killing of communicable agents outside of the host, and mass treatment with antibiotics. Finally, public health education and health promotion should be used as both primary and secondary preventive measures.

Tertiary Prevention of Communicable Diseases

Tertiary preventive measures for the control of communicable diseases for the individual include convalescence from infection, recovery to full health, and return to normal activity. In some cases, such as paralytic poliomyelitis, return to normal activity may not be possible even after extensive physical therapy. At the community level, tertiary preventive measures are aimed at preventing the recurrence of an epidemic. The proper removal, embalming, and burial of the dead is an example. Tertiary prevention may involve the reapplication of primary and secondary measures in such a way as to prevent further cases. For example, in some countries, such as the Republic of Korea, people with colds or flu wear gauze masks in public to reduce the spread of disease.

isolation
the separation of infected persons from those who are susceptible

quarantine
limitation of freedom of movement of those who have been exposed to a disease and may be incubating it

disinfection
the killing of communicable disease agents outside the host, on countertops, for example

Application of Prevention Measures in the Control of a Communicable Disease: HIV Infection and AIDS

Acquired immune deficiency syndrome (AIDS) is the late stage of an infection with the human immunodeficiency virus (HIV). HIV destroys specific blood cells (CD4+ T cells) that are crucial in fighting diseases. People can become infected when they come in contact with the virus through unprotected sexual activity, intravenous drug use, or exposure to the blood of an infected person. "Within a few weeks of being infected with HIV, some people develop flu-like symptoms that last for a week or two, but others have no symptoms at all. People living with HIV may appear and feel healthy for several years. However, even if they feel healthy, HIV is still affecting their bodies."[9]

The late stage of HIV infection is AIDS. People with AIDS have a difficult time fighting other communicable diseases and certain cancers. In the past, it took only a few years for someone infected to develop AIDS. Now, with the development of advanced medications, people can live much longer, perhaps even decades, after acquiring an HIV infection.[9] Despite advances in the diagnosis and treatment, HIV infections and AIDS are still epidemic in the United States and in the world.

HIV is responsible for a pandemic of unprecedented size. The WHO estimates that 33 million people are living with HIV/AIDS worldwide. During 2007, 2.7 million people were newly infected with HIV and 2 million people died of AIDS.[10] In the United States, through December 2007, a cumulative total of 1,030,832 persons with AIDS were reported to the CDC by state and territorial health departments.[11] The reservoir for HIV is the infected human population; there are no known animal or insect reservoirs. Referring to the chain of infection, HIV normally leaves its infected host (reservoir) during sexual activity. The portal of exit is the urogenital tract. Transmission is direct and occurs when reproductive fluids or blood are exchanged with the susceptible host. In the case of injection drug users, however, transmission is indirect, by contaminated needles (vehicle). The portal of entry is usually either genital, oral, or anal in direct (sexual) transmission or transdermal in the case of injection drug users or blood transfusion recipients. Transmission can also occur during medical procedures if there is an accidental needlestick or some other type of contamination with blood or other potentially infectious material.

A closer examination of the chain of infection reveals that prevention or control measures can be identified for each link. The pathogen in the diseased host can be held in check by the appropriate drug. Outside the host, measures such as sterilizing needles and other possible vehicles and disinfecting surfaces readily kill the virus and reduce the likelihood of transmission by contamination. The infected host (reservoir) can be identified through blood tests and educated to take precautions against the careless transmission of live virus through unsafe sex and needle sharing. Portals of exit (and entry) can be protected by the use of condoms. One set of *Healthy People 2020* objectives focuses on reducing the rate of HIV transmission and, thus, the number of new cases of AIDS. One way to do this is to increase the proportion of sexually active persons using condoms. Another way is to increase the number of persons living with HIV who know their level of antibodies to HIV (their serostatus). Finally, one objective aims to increase the proportion of adolescents and adults who have been tested for HIV in the past 12 months (see Box 4.5).

For injection drug users, abstinence from such drug use would preclude transmission by needles and syringes. But a more realistic approach to reducing the transmission of HIV/AIDS in this population is a more reasonable syringe (and needle) exchange policy. Since 1988, Congress has banned the use of federal funding of needle exchange programs. In the interim, a number of research papers have provided evidence supporting the idea that syringe/needle exchange programs reduce the spread of HIV/AIDS, hepatitis, and other bloodborne diseases. More than 36 states and a variety of local governments have established their own syringe

---

BOX 4.5

HEALTHY PEOPLE 2020: OBJECTIVES

OBJECTIVES HIV-3, HIV-4, HIV-5, HIV-6, HIV-7, HIV-11, HIV-12, HIV 14.1, HIV-17.1, HIV-17.2. Reduce the number new AIDS cases, reduce the number of deaths from AIDS, increase survivorship of those diagnosed with AIDS, increase HIV testing, and increase condom use.

Target setting method: Consistent with the National HIV/AIDS Strategy; or 10% improvement

Data Sources: HIV Surveillance System, CDC, NCHHSTP

Targets and baselines:

Objective	2006 Baseline	2020 Target
HIV-3 Reduce the rate of HIV transmission among adolescents and adults	New infections per 100 persons living with HIV 5.0	3.5
HIV-4 Reduce the number of new AIDS cases among adolescents and adults	New cases of AIDS per 100,000 age 13 years and older 13	10
HIV-5 Reduce the number of new AIDS cases among heterosexual adolescents and adults	New cases of AIDS among heterosexuals 11,110	10,000
HIV-6 Reduce the number of new AIDS cases among adolescent and adult men who have sex with men	New cases of AIDS among males aged 13 years and older who have sex with men or with men and women 16,749	15,074
HIV-7 Reduce the number of new AIDS cases among adolescents and adults who inject drugs	New cases of AIDS among injection drug users 13 years and older 6,010	5,409
HIV-11 Increase the proportion of persons surviving more than 3 years after diagnosis with AIDS	Persons diagnosed with AIDS surviving more than 3 years after diagnosis 82% (diagnosed in 2002)	90.2%
HIV-12 Reduce deaths from HIV infection	Deaths from AIDS per 100,000 population 3.7	3.3
HIV-13 Increase the proportion of people living with HIV who know their serostatus	Persons 13 years and older living with HIV who are aware of their HIV infection 79.0% (in 2006)	90.0%
HIV-14.1 Increase the proportion of adolescents and adults who have been tested for HIV in the past 12 months	Persons 15–44 years of age reporting that they had an HIV test in the past 12 months (outside of blood donation) 15.4%	16.9%
HIV-17.1 Increase the proportion of sexually active females using condoms	Unmarried females aged 15–44 years 34.5%	38.0%
HIV-17.2 Increase the proportion of sexually active males using condoms	Unmarried males aged 15–44 years 55.2%	60.7%

For Further Thought

Reducing the rate of HIV transmission is the best way to reduce both the number of persons living with HIV infection and the number of new AIDS cases. Reducing the number of new AIDS cases reduces the number of deaths from AIDS. Unprotected sexual contact, whether homosexual or heterosexual, with a person infected with HIV is one of the most important ways HIV infections are transmitted. An important way to slow the rate of HIV transmission and the occurrence of new AIDS cases is to increase the proportion of sexually active females and males who use condoms. Can you think of ways to increase the rate of condom use in sexually active persons in your community?

Source: U.S. Department of Health and Human Services, Office of Disease Prevention and Health Promotion (2010). *Healthy People 2020.* Available at http://www.healthypeople.gov/2020/default.aspx. Accessed December 2, 2010.

---

exchange programs, distributing an estimated 30 million clean needles a year (see Figure 4.11).[12,13] In December 2009, the ban was lifted by Congress.[13] Although no federal funds were immediately forthcoming as a result of this action, AIDS activists regard the lifting of the ban a symbolic achievement.

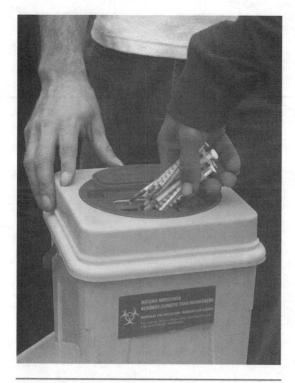

FIGURE 4.11

Distribution of clean needles and destruction of contaminated needles, reduces transmission of bloodborne pathogens such as human immunodeficiency virus (HIV).

For those working in the health professions, the risk of acquiring an HIV infection in the workplace is of particular concern. The Occupational Safety and Health Administration (OSHA) estimates that 5.6 million workers in the health care industry and related occupations are at risk of occupational exposure to **bloodborne pathogens**, including HIV, hepatitis B virus (HBV), hepatitis C virus (HCV), and others.[14] In 1991, OSHA, recognizing that workers in the health care industry were at risk of occupational exposure to bloodborne pathogens, issued the **Bloodborne Pathogens Standard**.

In November 2000, Congress, acknowledging the estimates of 600,000 to 800,000 needlestick and other percutaneous injuries occurring among health care workers annually, passed the Needlestick Safety and Prevention Act.[15] In 2001, in response to the Needlestick Safety and Prevention Act, OSHA revised its Bloodborne Pathogens Standard. This revised standard, currently in effect, "clarifies the need for employers to select safer needle devices and to involve employees in identifying and choosing these devices" and to maintain a log of injuries from contaminated sharps.[14] The goal of all of these regulations and standards is to reduce the number of HIV/AIDS cases, as well as cases of other bloodborne diseases, resulting from workplace exposure.

Prevention of Noncommunicable Diseases

Both the individual and the community can contribute substantially to the prevention and control of multicausation diseases. The community can provide a pro-health environment—physical, economic, and social—in which it becomes easier for individuals to achieve a high level of health.

Primary Prevention of Noncommunicable Diseases

Primary preventive measures for noncommunicable diseases include adequate food and energy supplies, good opportunities for education, employment, and housing, and efficient community services. Beyond this foundation, a community should provide health promotion and health education programs, health and medical services, and protection from environmental and occupational hazards.

Individuals can practice primary prevention by obtaining a high level of education that includes a knowledge about health and disease and the history of disease of others in one's family. In particular, the individual should take responsibility for eating properly, exercising adequately, maintaining appropriate weight, and avoiding the overuse of alcohol and other drugs. Individuals can also protect themselves from injury by adopting behaviors that reduce their risk of injuries. These behaviors include driving safely and wearing a safety belt at all times while traveling in a vehicle. Examples of primary prevention also include avoiding overexposure to the sun and limiting one's environmental pollutants that might cause cancer.

Secondary Prevention of Noncommunicable Diseases

Secondary preventive measures the community can take include the provision of mass screenings for chronic diseases (see Figure 4.12), case-finding measures, and the provision of adequate health personnel, equipment, and facilities for the community. Secondary prevention responsibilities of individual citizens include personal screenings such as self-examination of

bloodborne pathogens disease agents, such as HIV, that are transmissible in blood and other body fluids

Bloodborne Pathogens Standard a set of regulations promulgated by OSHA that sets forth the responsibilities of employers and employees with regard to precautions to be taken concerning bloodborne pathogens in the workplace

breasts or testes (for cancer of these organs), the Hemoccult test (for colorectal cancer), and medical screenings such as the Pap test (for cervical cancer), the PSA test for cancer of the prostate, mammography, and screenings for diabetes, glaucoma, or hypertension. Participating in such health screenings and having regular medical and dental checkups represent only the first step in the secondary prevention of noncommunicable diseases. This must be followed by the pursuit of definitive diagnosis and prompt treatment of any diseases detected.

Tertiary Prevention of Noncommunicable Diseases

Tertiary preventive measures for a community include adequate emergency medical personnel, services, and facilities to meet the needs of those citizens for whom primary and secondary preventive measures were unsuccessful. Examples include ambulance services, hospitals, physicians and surgeons, nurses, and other allied health professionals. Interestingly, most communities are doing a more-than-adequate job in tertiary prevention. Many experts feel that most communities in America need to reallocate resources from tertiary prevention to primary and secondary preventive measures.

Tertiary prevention for the individual often requires significant behavioral or lifestyle changes. Examples include strict adherence to prescribed medications, exercise programs, and diet. For example, a heart attack patient could receive nutrition education and counseling and be encouraged to participate in a supervised exercise program, thus maximizing the use of remaining capabilities. This could

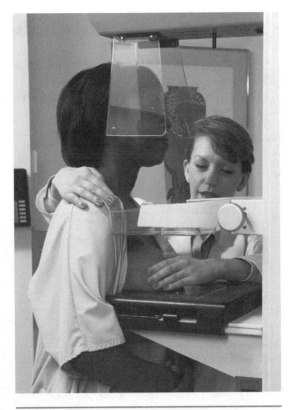

FIGURE 4.12

Mammography, used for screening and early detection of breast cancer, is an example of secondary prevention.

lead to a resumption of employment and the prevention of a second heart attack. For certain types of noncommunicable health problems, such as those involving substance abuse, regular attendance at support group meetings or counseling sessions may constitute an important part of a tertiary prevention program.

Application of Preventive Measures in the Control of a Noncommunicable Disease: CHD

One set of *Healthy People 2020* objectives aims at reducing risk factors and deaths from cardiovascular diseases including coronary heart disease (see Box 4.6). Many factors contribute to one's risk of developing this disease. Both the community and the individual can contribute to the prevention of CHD.

The Community's Role

The community must recognize the importance of preventing chronic disease; intervention following a crisis, such as a heart attack, is the least effective and most expensive way to provide help to a CHD patient. While individual behavioral changes hold the best prospects for reducing the prevalence of heart disease in this country, communities can provide a supporting environment for these behavioral changes. For example, the community can support restricting smoking areas and can provide a clear message to youth that smoking is damaging to health. Communities also can provide adequate opportunity for health screening for risk factors such as hypertension and serum cholesterol levels. In particular, schools can

BOX 4.6	HEALTHY PEOPLE 2020: OBJECTIVES

OBJECTIVES HDS-2, HDS-3, Reduce the heart disease and stroke death rates.

Target setting method: 20% improvement

Data Source: National Vital Statistics System—Mortality (NVSS—M), CDC, NCHS

Targets and baselines:

Objective	2006 Baseline	2020 Target
HDS-2 Reduce coronary heart disease deaths	Coronary heart disease deaths per 100,000 population	
	126.0	100.8
HDS-3 Reduce stroke deaths	Stroke deaths per 100,000 population	
	33.8	42.2

OBJECTIVES HDS-4 Increase the proportion of adults who have had their blood pressure measured.

Target setting method: 2% improvement

Data Source: National Health Interview Survey (NHIS), CDC, HCHS

Targets and baselines:

Objective	2008 Baseline	2020 Target
HDS-4 Increase the proportion of adults who have had their blood pressure measured within the preceding 2 years and can state whether it is normal or high	92%	94.9%

OBJECTIVES HDS-5.1, 5.2 Reduce the proportion of adults and children and adolescents with high blood pressure.

Target-Setting Method: 10%

Data Source: National Health and Nutrition Examination Survey (NHANES), CDC, NCHS

Targets and baselines:

Objective	2005–2008 Baseline	Target 2020
HDS-5.1 Reduce the proportion of adults with high blood pressure	Adults 18 years and older with high blood pressure	
	29.9%	26.9%
HDS-5.2 Reduce the proportion of children and adolescents with high blood pressure	Children and adolescents aged 8–17 years with high blood pressure	
	3.5%	3.2%

OBJECTIVE HDS-6 Increase the proportion of adults who have had their blood cholesterol checked within the preceding 5 years.

Target setting method: 10% improvement

Data Source: National Health Interview Survey (NHIS), CDC, HCHS

Targets and baselines:

Objective	2008 Baseline	2020 Target
HDS-6 Increase the proportion of adults who have had their cholesterol checked	Adults 18 years and older who had their blood cholesterol checked within the preceding 5 years	
	74.6%	82.1%

OBJECTIVE HDS-7 Reduce the proportion of adults with high total cholesterol.

Target-Setting Method: 10% improvement

Data Source: National Health and Nutrition Examination Survey (NHANES), CDC, NCHS

HEALTHY PEOPLE 2020: OBJECTIVES (CONTINUED)

Targets and baselines:

Objective	2005–2008 Baseline	2020 Target
HDS-7 Reduce the proportion of adults with high total cholesterol.	Percent of adults 20 years and older with total blood cholesterol levels of 240mg/dL or greater	
	15%	13.5%

OBJECTIVE HDS-8 Reduce the mean total cholesterol levels among adults.

Target-Setting Method: 10% improvement

Data Source: National Health and Nutrition Examination Survey (NHANES), CDC, NCHS

Targets and baselines:

Objective	2005–2008 Baseline	2020 Target
HDS-8 Reduce the mean total cholesterol levels among adults	Mean total blood cholesterol level for adults 20 years and older	
	197.7 mg/dl	177.9 mg/dl

For Further Thought

Cardiovascular diseases are the leading causes of deaths in the United States. While significant progress has been made in lowering the death from heart attack and stroke, further progress is certainly achievable. Important contributing factors are high blood pressure, high blood cholesterol, and obesity. What can individuals and communities do to reduce obesity, lower the average blood pressure and lower the mean level of cholesterol in the blood? Have you noticed efforts in your community to provide blood pressure screenings and cholesterol testing? If so, what agencies are offering these services?

Source: U.S. Department of Health and Human Services, Office of Disease Prevention and Health Promotion (2010). *Healthy People 2020.* Available at http://www.healthypeople.gov/2020/default.aspx. Accessed December 2, 2010.

---

permit the administration of Youth Risk Behavior Surveillance System surveys (see Chapter 3) and utilize these occasions as opportunities to teach students about the importance of healthy behavioral choices. Communities also can promote and assist in the development of areas for recreation and exercise, such as safe paths for jogging or cycling and lighted sidewalks for walking. Exercise reduces obesity and increases the high-density lipoproteins (HDLs) in the blood, thereby lowering risk for a heart attack. Finally, communities should promote sound nutrition throughout the life span, but particularly in schools.

The Individual's Role

The risk factors for CHD are multiple. Some of these risk factors are unmodifiable, whereas other risk factors can be modified (reduced) to improve one's health. Each person can increase his or her resistance to CHD by knowing the difference between the types of risk factors and by adopting behaviors that prevent or postpone the onset of CHD.

Each person is endowed with a unique genetic code. An individual's innate resistance or susceptibility to heart disease is encoded in the genes. **Unmodifiable risk factors** for CHD include one's race, gender, personality type, age, and basic metabolic rate. Also inherited is one's baseline serum cholesterol level. That is, children whose parents had high serum cholesterol levels are at risk for those same higher levels, independent of their diet.

Modifiable risk factors for CHD include environmental and behavioral factors over which an individual has some control. Modifiable risk factors that would increase the likeli-

unmodifiable risk factors
factors contributing to the development of a noncommunicable disease that cannot be altered by modifying one's behavior or environment

modifiable risk factors
factors contributing to the development of a noncommunicable disease that can be altered by modifying one's behavior or environment

hood of CHD include smoking, a diet too rich in fats, lack of exercise, obesity, uncontrolled hypertension, and too much stress. Although none of these factors alone is likely to cause a premature heart attack, each can contribute to the likelihood of CHD.

CHAPTER SUMMARY

- Diseases can be classified as communicable (infectious) or noncommunicable (noninfectious), and acute or chronic.

- Acute diseases last for less than three months, whereas chronic diseases continue longer than three months.

- Communicable diseases are caused by biological agents and are transmissible from a source of infection to a susceptible host.

- The process of communicable disease transmission is best understood by the chain of infection model, in which the interruption of disease transmission can be visualized as the breaking of one or more links in the chain.

- Noncommunicable diseases are often the result of multiple risk factors that can be genetic, behavioral, and environmental in origin.

- Several of the noncommunicable diseases rank among the leading causes of death in America.

- There are three levels of disease prevention—primary, secondary, and tertiary.

- Primary prevention includes measures that forestall the onset of disease or injury, while secondary prevention encompasses efforts aimed at early detection and intervention to limit disease and disability. Tertiary prevention includes measures aimed at re-education and rehabilitation after significant pathogenesis has occurred.

- Both the spread of communicable diseases and the prevalence of noncommunicable diseases can best be reduced by the appropriate application of primary, secondary, and tertiary preventive measures by the community and the individual.

- The prevention and control of noncommunicable diseases require both individual and community efforts.

REVIEW QUESTIONS

1. What are some of the ways in which diseases and health problems are classified in community health?

2. Contrast the terms *acute disease* and *chronic disease*. Provide three examples of each type of disease.

3. Contrast the terms *communicable disease* and *noncommunicable disease*. Provide three examples of each type of disease.

4. What is the difference between a communicable agent and a pathogenic agent?

5. What are the components of a simplified communicable disease model?

6. List some examples of environmental factors that can influence the occurrence and spread of disease.

7. Draw and explain the model for multicausation diseases.

8. What is the difference between prevention and intervention?

9. Explain the difference between primary, secondary, and tertiary prevention and provide an example of each.

10. What is the chain of infection model of disease transmission? Draw the model and label its parts.

11. Again referring to the chain of infection, indicate how prevention and control strategies could be implemented to interrupt the transmission of gonorrhea. Are most of these strategies primary, secondary, or tertiary prevention measures?

12. Define the following terms—*case, carrier, vector, vehicle.*

13. List five examples each of vectorborne diseases and nonvectorborne diseases.

14. Explain the difference between the public health practices of isolation and quarantine.

15. Explain the importance of vaccinations or immunizations in preventing diseases in the community.

16. Apply the principles of prevention and the examples given in this chapter to outline a prevention strategy for breast cancer that includes primary, secondary, and tertiary prevention components.

ACTIVITIES

1. Call your state health department and find out which are the top communicable (infectious) disease problems reported in your state. Which are the rarest? Is Lyme disease reportable?

2. List some of the infections you have had. How were these infections transmitted to you—directly, by vehicle, or by vector? Talk to someone who is very old about diseases they can recall from their youth and how these diseases affected them and their families. Take notes on the response, and hand them in or share them orally in class.

3. Look up the disease bubonic plague in an encyclopedia or on the Internet. After reading about the disease, see if you can complete a chain of infection model for plague. Identify the causative agent, the vector, the reservoir, and the mode of transmission.

SCENARIO: ANALYSIS AND RESPONSE

1. If Bob's roommate, Chuck, were to begin to show signs of the flu, what could Bob do to lessen his chances of becoming infected himself? (*Hint:* Think about the chain of infection.)

2. As an accountant, Bob spends most of his day behind a desk. To identify primary, secondary, and tertiary preventive measures Bob should take to reduce his risk for heart disease, visit one governmental and one nongovernmental Web site and find some information about prevention of heart disease. For each preventive measure you list, indicate whether it is primary, secondary, or tertiary prevention.

3. In what other health screenings should Bob and Chuck participate? Are there any health screenings available on the Internet?

4. What kinds of thoughts, behaviors, and conditions prevent people from participating in health screenings?

What types of prevention and control strategies were used in the past to stop the spread of this disease? What can be done differently today if there is an epidemic of plague?

4. Think about motor vehicle crashes. List some primary, secondary, and tertiary preventive measures that the community and you can take to reduce the number and seriousness of injuries caused by auto accidents.

COMMUNITY HEALTH ON THE WEB

The Internet contains a wealth of information about community and public health. Increase your knowledge of some of the topics presented in this chapter by accessing the Jones & Bartlett Learning Web site at **http://health.jbpub.com/book/communityhealth/7e** and follow the links to complete the following Web activities.

- National Center for Infectious Diseases
- National Center for Chronic Disease Prevention and Health Promotion
- Epidemic Intelligence Service

REFERENCES

1. Heymann, D. L., ed. (2008). *Control of Communicable Diseases Manual*, 19th ed. Washington, DC: American Public Health Association.

2. Miniño A. M., J. Q. Xu, K. D. Kochanek (2010). "Deaths: Preliminary Data for 2008." *National Vital Statistics Reports,* 59(2). Hyattsville, MD: National Center for Health Statistics. Available at http://www.cdc.gov/nchs/data/nvsr/nvsr59/nvsr59_02.pdf.

3. American Heart Association (2010). *Heart Disease and Stroke Statistics—2010 Update: A Report of the American Heart Association.* Dallas, TX: Author. Available at http://circ.ahajournals.org/.

4. American Cancer Society (2009). *Cancer Facts and Figures—2010.* Atlanta, GA: Author. Available at http://www.cancer.org/acs/groups/content/@nho/documents/document/acspc-024113.pdf.

5. Heron, M. P. (2010). "Deaths: Leading Causes for 2006." *National Vital Statistics Reports,* 58(14): 1–100.

6. National Center for Health Statistics (2010). *Health, United States, 2009 with Special Feature on Medical Technology* [online]. (DHHS pub. no. 2010-1232). Hyattsville, MD: Author. Available at http://www.cdc.gov/nchs/hus.htm.

7. National Center on Addiction and Substance Abuse at Columbia University (2009). *Shoveling Up II: The Impact of Substance Abuse on Federal, State and Local Budgets.* Available at http://www.casacolumbia.org/templates/Home.aspx?articleid=287&zoneid=32.

8. Centers for Disease Control and Prevention (2010). "Vaccines and Immunizations." Available at http://www.cdc.gov/vaccines/.

9. Centers for Disease Control and Prevention (2010). "Basic Information About HIV and AIDS." Available at http://www.cdc.gov/hiv/topics/basic/index.htm.

10. World Health Organization (2009). *AIDS Epidemic Update: December 2009.* Available at http://www.who.int/hiv/data/en/.

11. Centers for Disease Control and Prevention (2009). "HIV/AIDS Surveillance Report, 2007." *Basic Statistics*, 19: 1–63. Available at http://www.cdc.gov/hiv/topics/surveillance/resources/reports/2007report/default.htm.

12. Centers for Disease Control and Prevention (2005). "Update: Syringe Exchange Programs—United States, 2002." *Morbidity and Mortality Weekly Report*, 54(27): 673–676.

13. Sharon, S. (2009). "Ban Lifted on Federal Funding for Needle Exchange." NPR News. Available at http://www.npr.org/search/index.php?searchinput=Needle+Exchange.

14. Occupational Safety and Health Administration (2009). "Bloodborne Pathogens and Needlestick Prevention: Hazard Recognition." U.S. Department of Labor. Available at http://www.osha.gov/SLTC/bloodbornepathogens/index.html.

15. U.S. Congress (2000, October 3). "An Act to Require Changes in the Bloodborne Pathogens Standard in Effect under the Occupational Safety and Health Act of 1970." *Congressional Record*, 146.

Chapter 5

Community Organizing/ Building and Health Promotion Programming

Chapter Objectives

After studying this chapter, you will be able to:

1 Define *community organizing, community capacity, community participation,* and *empowered community.*

2 Identify the assumptions that underlie the process of community organization.

3 Briefly explain the difference between locality development, social planning, and social action approaches to community organization.

4 Explain the difference between needs-based and strength-based community organizing models.

5 List the steps for a generalized model for community organizing/building.

6 Explain what is meant by community building.

7 Explain the difference between health education and health promotion.

8 State and summarize the steps involved in creating a health promotion program.

9 Define the term *needs assessment.*

10 Briefly explain the six steps used in assessing needs.

11 Explain the difference between goals and objectives.

12 List the different types of intervention strategies.

13 Explain the differences among best practices, best experiences, and best processes.

14 Explain the purposes of pilot testing in program development.

15 State the difference between formative and summative evaluation.

SCENARIO

It was becoming obvious to many that the suburb of Kenzington now had a drug problem, but few wanted to admit it. The community's residents liked their quiet neighborhoods, and most never thought that drugs would be a problem. In fact, the problem really sneaked up on everyone. The town had only one bar, and although occasionally someone drank too much, the bar's patrons usually controlled their drinking and didn't bother anyone. Occasionally, two or three high school seniors would be caught drinking beer purchased at a store in a nearby town. Yet these isolated incidents gave no indication of Kenzington's impending drug problem.

Within the past year, the climate of the town had changed considerably. Incidents of teenagers being arrested for possession of alcohol or even other drugs, such as marijuana, were being reported more regularly in the newspaper. There seemed to be more reports of burglaries, too. There had even been a robbery and two assaults reported within the last month. The population of young adults in the community seemed to be increasing, and many of these seemed to be driving impressive cars, using the hottest new digital devices, and wearing the latest clothes. All of these signs were obvious to a group of concerned citizens in Kenzington and suggested the possibility of a drug problem. So the concerned citizens decided to take their concern to the city council.

INTRODUCTION

To deal with the health issues that face many communities, community health professionals must possess specific knowledge and skills. They need to be able to identify problems, develop a plan to attack each problem, gather the resources necessary to carry out that plan, implement that plan, and then evaluate the results to determine the degree of progress that has been achieved. In the previous two chapters, we described epidemiological methods as essential tools of the community health professional. In this chapter, we present two other important tools that each successful community health worker must master: the skills to organize/build a community and to plan a health promotion program. Prior to presenting information about community organizing/building and health promotion programming, we need to introduce the concept of *social ecological approach*.

Inherent in the community organizing/building and health promotion programming processes is behavior change. That is, for community organizing/building and health promotion programming efforts to be successful people must change their behavior. Some of the behaviors that need to change as part of these processes are health-related and others are not. The underlying foundation of the social ecological approach is that behavior has multiple levels of influences. This approach "emphasizes the interaction between, and the interdependence of factors within and across all levels of a health problem"[1] That is to say, seldom does behavior change based on influence from a single level. People "live in social, political, and economic systems that shape behaviors and access to the resources they need to maintain good health."[2] Scholars who study and write about the levels of influence have used various labels to describe them. However, commonly used labels include intrapersonal, interpersonal, institutional or organizational, community, and public policy.[3] These five levels are presented in a hierarchical order with the first level, intrapersonal, affecting a single person, with successive levels affecting greater numbers, and the highest level—public policy—affecting the most. For example, to get a person to participate in a community coalition it may take someone to talk with the person (e.g., intrapersonal-level influence) about the importance of the work of the coalition, but it might also take the organization with which the person is affiliated to include the work of the coalition in its mission statement (i.e., organizational-level influence). Or, to get a person to stop smoking it may take a conversation with his/her physician (i.e., intrapersonal-level influence), a company policy (i.e., institutional- or organizational-level), and also a county ordinance prohibiting smoking in public places (i.e., community-level influence). Thus, a central conclusion of the social ecological approach "is that it usually takes the combination of both individual-level and environmental/policy-level interventions to achieve substantial changes in health behavior."[4]

As you read the rest of this chapter, consider the impact of the social ecological approach on both community/organizing and health promotion programming.

COMMUNITY ORGANIZING/BUILDING

Community health problems can range from small and simple to large and complex. Small, simple problems that are local and involve few people can be solved with the effort of a small group of people and a minimal amount of organization. Large, complex problems that involve whole communities require significant skills and resources for their solution. For these larger problems, a considerable effort must be expended to organize the citizens of the community to work together to implement a lasting solution to their problem. For example, a trained smoking cessation facilitator could help a single person or a small group of people to stop smoking. But to reduce the smoking rates community-wide, community collaboration is needed. The same smoking cessation facilitators are needed to work with individuals, but others are also needed. Schools are needed to provide appropriate tobacco education programs to youth, organizations (e.g., worksites) and institutions (e.g., religious communities) are needed to create smoking policies, government agencies are needed to enforce the laws associated with the sale of tobacco, and cities, counties, and states are needed to create clean indoor air ordinances or laws. This more comprehensive approach to reducing smoking rates needs to bring together, in an organized and coordinated effort, the people and groups interested in the issue and the resources necessary for change. In other words, a community organization effort is needed.

community organizing process through which communities are helped to identify common problems or goals, mobilize resources, and in other ways develop and implement strategies for reaching their goals they have collectively set

"The term *community organization* was coined by American social workers in the late 1880s to describe their efforts to coordinate services for newly arrived immigrants and the poor."[5] More recently, *community organization* has been used by a variety of professionals, including community health workers, and refers to various methods of interventions to deal with social problems. More formally, **community organizing** has been defined as a "process through which communities are helped to identify common problems or goals, mobilize resources, and in other ways develop and implement strategies for reaching their goals they have collectively set."[5] Community organizing is not a science but an art of consensus building within a democratic process.[6] (See Table 5.1 for terms associated with community organizing/building).

Table 5.1
Terms Associated with Community Organizing/Building

Community capacity	"The characteristics of communities that affect their ability to identify, mobilize, and address social and public health problems"[7]
Empowerment	"Social action process for people to gain mastery over their lives and the lives of their communities"[8]
Participation and relevance	"Community organizing that starts where the people are and engages community members as equals"[5]
Social capital	"Relationships and structures within a community that promote cooperation for mutual benefit"[5]

Need for Organizing Communities

In recent years, the need to organize communities seems to have increased. Advances in electronics (e.g., handheld digital devices) and communications (e.g., multifunction cell phones and the Internet), household upgrades (e.g., energy efficiency), and increased mobility (i.e., frequency of moving and ease of worldwide travel) have resulted in a loss of a sense of community. Individuals are much more independent than ever before. The days when people knew everyone on their block are past. Today, it is not uncommon for people to never meet their neighbors (see Figure 5.1). In other cases, people see or talk to their neighbors only once or twice each year. Because of these changes in community social structure, it now takes specific skills to organize a community to act together for the collective good. Note that the usefulness of community organizing skills extends beyond community health.

Assumptions of Community Organizing

According to Ross,[6] those who organize communities do so while making certain assumptions. The assumptions Ross outlines can be summarized as follows:

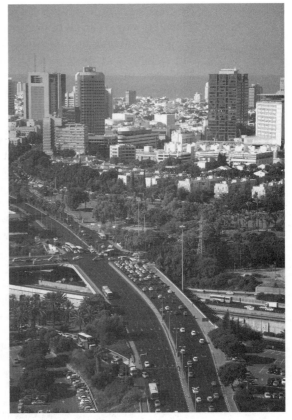

FIGURE 5.1
In today's complex communities, it is not uncommon for people never to meet their neighbors.

1. Communities of people can develop the capacity to deal with their own problems.
2. People want to change and can change.
3. People should participate in making, adjusting, or controlling the major changes taking place within their communities.
4. Changes in community living that are self-imposed or self-developed have a meaning and permanence that imposed changes do not have.
5. A "holistic approach" can successfully address problems with which a "fragmented approach" cannot cope.
6. Democracy requires cooperative participation and action in the affairs of the community, and people must learn the skills that make this possible.
7. Frequently, communities of people need help in organizing to deal with their needs, just as many individuals require help in coping with their individual problems.

Community Organizing Methods

There is no single, preferred method for organizing a community. In fact, a careful review reveals that several different approaches have been successful, which led Rothman and Tropman to state, "We would speak of community organization methods rather than the community organization method."[9]

The early approaches to community organization used by social workers emphasized the use of consensus and cooperation to deal with community problems.[10] However, Rothman created a typology of three primary methods of community organization.[11] Included were locality development, social planning, and social action.[9] *Locality development* is based on the concept of broad self-help participation from the local community. It is "heavily process oriented, stressing consensus and cooperation aimed at building group identity and a sense of community."[5]

Social planning is heavily task oriented, stressing rational-empirical problem solving and involves various levels of participation from many people and outside planners.[5]

The third method, *social action,* is "both task and process oriented"[5] and has been useful in helping to organize disadvantaged segments of the population. It often involves trying to redistribute power or resources, which enables institutional or community change. This method is not used as much as it once was, but it was useful during the civil rights and gay rights movements and in other settings where people have been oppressed.

Though locality development, social planning, and social action methods have been the primary means by which communities have organized over the years, they do have their limitations. Maybe the greatest limitation is that they are primarily "problem-based and organizer-centered, rather than strength-based and community-centered."[12] Thus, some of the newer models are based more on collaborative empowerment and community building. However, all models—old or new—revolve around a common theme: The work and resources of many have a much better chance of solving a problem than the work and resources of a few.

Minkler and Wallerstein have done a nice job of summarizing the models, old and new, by presenting a typology that incorporates both needs- and strength-based approaches (see Figure 5.2).[5] Their typology is divided into four quadrants, with strength-based and needs-based on the vertical axis and consensus and conflict on the horizontal axis. Though this typology separates and categorizes the various methods of community organizing and building, Minkler and Wallerstein point out that

> Community organizing and community building are fluid endeavors. While some organizing efforts primarily have focused in one quadrant, most incorporate multiple tendencies, possibly starting from a specific need or crisis and moving to a strength-based community capacity

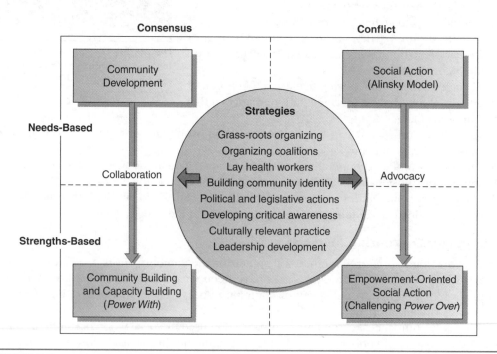

FIGURE 5.2

Community organization and community building typology.

Source: Minkler, M., and N. Wallerstein (2005). "Improving Health through Community Organization and Community Building." In M. Minkler, ed., *Community Organizing and Community Building for Health,* 2nd ed. Rutgers University Press, 32. Reprinted with permission.

approach. Different organizing models, such as coalitions, lay health worker programs, political action groups, leadership development or grassroots organizing may incorporate needs- or strength-based approaches at different times, depending on the starting place and the ever changing social dynamic. It is important, however, that organizing efforts clarify their assumptions and make decisions about primary strategies based on skills of group members, history of the group, willingness to take risks, or comfort level with different approaches.[5]

No matter what community organizing/community building approach is used, they all incorporate some fundamental principles. These include "the principle of relevance, or starting where the people are; the principle of participation; and the importance of creating environments in which individuals and communities can become empowered as they increase their community problem-solving ability."[5]

THE PROCESS OF COMMUNITY ORGANIZING/BUILDING

It is beyond the scope of this textbook to explain all the approaches to community organizing and building in detail. Instead, we will present a generic approach (see Figure 5.3) created by McKenzie, Neiger, and Thackeray that draws upon many of these other approaches.[13] The 10 steps of this generic approach are briefly reviewed in the sections that follow.

Recognizing the Issue

The process of community organizing/building begins when someone recognizes that a problem exists in a community and decides to do something about it. This person (or persons) is referred to as the initial organizer. This individual may not be the primary organizer throughout the community organizing/building process. He or she is the one who gets things started. For the purposes of this discussion, let us assume the problem is violence. People in most communities would like to have a violence-free community, but it would be most unusual to live in a community that was without at least some level of violence. How much violence is too much? At what point is a community willing to organize to deal with the problem? In a small-town community, an acceptable level of violence would be very low, while in a large city, an acceptable level would be much higher.

The people, or organizers, who first recognize a problem in the community and decide to act can be members of the community or individuals from outside the community. If those who initiate community organization are members of the community, then the movement is

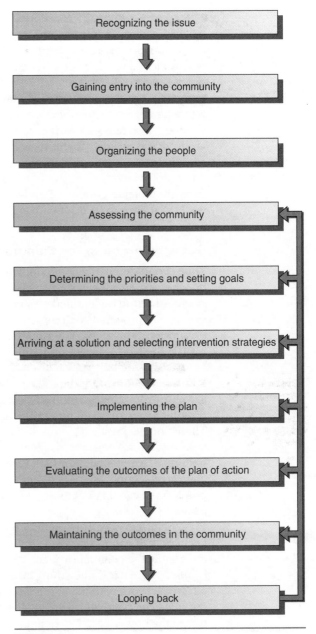

FIGURE 5.3

A summary of steps in community organizing and building.

Source: McKenzie, J. F., B. L. Neiger, and R. Thackeray (2009). *Planning, Implementing, and Evaluating Health Promotion Programs: A Primer,* 5th ed. San Francisco, CA: Benjamin Cummings. Reprinted with permission from Pearson Education, Inc.

grass-roots
a process that begins with those who are affected by the problem/concern

referred to as being **grass-roots**, *citizen initiated,* or organized from the *bottom up.* "In *grassroots organizing,* community groups are built from scratch, and leadership is developed where none existed before."[14] Community members who might recognize that violence is a problem could include teachers, police officers, or other concerned citizens. When community organization is initiated by individuals from outside of the community, the problem is said to be organized from the *top down* or *outside in.* Individuals from outside the community who might initiate organization could include a judge who presides over cases involving violence, a state social worker who handles cases of family violence, or a politically active group that is against violent behavior wherever it happens. In cases where the person who recognizes the community problem is not a community member, great care must be taken when notifying those in the community that a problem exists. "It is difficult for someone from the outside coming in and telling community members that they have problems or issues that have to be dealt with and they need to organize to take care of them."[13]

Gaining Entry into the Community

This second step in the community organizing process may or may not be needed, depending on whether the issue in step 1 was identified by someone from within the community or outside. If the issue is identified by someone outside the community, this step becomes a critical step in the process.[13] Gaining entry may seem like a relatively easy matter, but an error by organizers at this step could ruin the chances of successfully organizing the community. This may be the most crucial step in the whole process.

gatekeepers
those who control, both formally and informally, the political climate of the community

Braithwaite and colleagues have stressed the importance of tactfully negotiating entry into a community with the individuals who control, both formally and informally, the "political climate" of the community.[15] These people are referred to as the **gatekeepers**. Thus the term indicates that you must pass through this "gate" to get to your priority population.[16] These "power brokers" know their community, how it functions, and how to accomplish tasks within it. Long-time residents are usually able to identify the gatekeepers of their community. A gatekeeper can be a representative of an intermediary organization—such as a church or school—that has direct contact with your priority population.[16] Examples include politicians, leaders of activist groups, business and education leaders, and clergy, to name a few.

Organizers must approach such figures on the gatekeepers' own terms and play the gatekeepers' ball game. However, before approaching these important individuals, organizers must study the community well. They must be *culturally sensitive* and work toward *cultural competence.* That is, they must be aware of the cultural differences within a community and effectively work with the cultural context of the community. Tervalon and Garcia have stated the need for *cultural humility*—openness to others' culture.[17] Organizers need to know where the power lies, the community power dynamics, what type of politics must be used to solve a problem, and whether the particular problem they wish to solve has ever been dealt with before in the community.[18] In the violence example, organizers need to know (1) who is causing the violence and why, (2) how the problem has been addressed in the past, (3) who supports and who opposes the idea of addressing the problem, and (4) who could provide more insight into the problem. This is a critical step in the community organization process because failure to study the community carefully in the beginning may lead to a delay in organizing it later, a subsequent waste of time and resources, and possibly the inability to organize at all.

Once the organizers have a good understanding of the community, they are then ready to approach the gatekeepers. In keeping with the violence example, the gatekeepers would probably include the police department, elected officials, school board members, social service personnel, members of the judicial system, and possibly some of those who are creating the violence.

When the top-down approach is being used, organizers might find it advantageous to enter the community through a well-respected organization or institution that is already established in the community, such as a church, a service group, or another successful local group. If those who make up such an organization/institution can be convinced that the problem exists and needs to be solved, it can help smooth the way for gaining entry and achieving the remaining steps in the process.

Organizing the People

Obtaining the support of community members to deal with the problem is the next step in the process. It is best to begin by organizing those who are already interested in seeing that the problem is solved. This core group of community members, sometimes referred to as "executive participants,"[19] will become the backbone of the workforce and will end up doing the majority of the work. For our example of community violence, the core group could include law enforcement personnel, former victims of violence and their families (or victims' support groups), parent-teacher organizations, and public health officials. It is also important to recruit people from the subpopulation that is most directly affected by the problem. For example, if most of the violence in a community is directed toward teenagers, teenagers need to be included in the core group. If elderly persons are affected, they need to be included.

"From among the core group, a leader or coordinator must be identified. If at all possible, the leader should be someone with leadership skills, good knowledge of the concern and the community, and most of all, someone from within the community. One of the early tasks of the leader will be to help build group cohesion."[13]

Although the formation of the core group is essential, this group is usually not large enough to do all the work itself. Therefore, one of the core group's tasks is to recruit more members of the community to the cause. This step can take place via a *networking process*, which is when organizers make personal contacts with others who might be interested. Or, the organizers can call an organizing meeting at a local school, community center, or religious organization. By broadening the constituency, the core group can spread out the workload and generate additional resources to deal with the problem. However, recruiting additional workers can often be difficult. Over the last 30 years, the number of people in many communities interested in volunteering their time has decreased. Today, if you ask someone to volunteer, you may hear the reply, "I'm already too busy." There are two primary reasons for this response. First, there are many families in which both husband and wife work outside the home. And second, there are more single-parent households.

task force
a temporary group that is brought together for dealing with a specific problem

Therefore, when organizers are expanding their constituencies, they should be sure to (1) identify people who are affected by the problem that they are trying to solve, (2) provide "perks" for or otherwise reward volunteers, (3) keep volunteer time short, (4) match volunteer assignments with the abilities and expertise of the volunteers, and (5) consider providing appropriate training to make sure volunteers are comfortable with their tasks. For example, if the organizers need someone to talk with law enforcement groups, it would probably be a good idea to solicit the help of someone who feels comfortable around such groups and who is respected by them, such as another law enforcement person.

coalition
formal alliance of organizations that come together to work for a common goal

When the core group has been expanded to include these other volunteers, the larger group is sometimes referred to as a task force. A **task force** has been defined as "a self-contained group of 'doers' that is not ongoing, but rather brought together due to a strong interest in an issue and for a specific purpose."[14] There may even be an occasion where a coalition is formed. A **coalition** is "a formal alliance of organizations that come together to

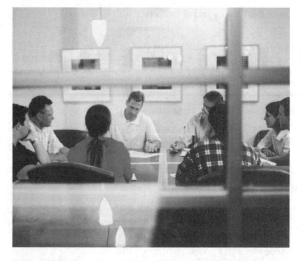

FIGURE 5.4
Coalition building is often an important step in successful community organization.

work for a common goal"[14]—often, to compensate for deficits in power, resources, and expertise. A larger group with more resources, people, and energy has a greater chance of solving a community problem than a smaller, less powerful group (see Figure 5.4). "Building and maintaining effective coalitions have increasingly been recognized as vital components of much effective community organizing and community building."[20]

Assessing the Community

Earlier in this chapter we referred to Rothman and Tropman's typology for organizing a community—locality development, social planning, and social action.[9] Each of these community organizing strategies operates "from the assumption that problems in society can be addressed by the community becoming better or differently 'organized,' with each strategy perceiving the problems and how or whom to organize in order to address them somewhat differently."[15] In contrast to these strategies is community building. **Community building** "is an orientation to community that is strength-based rather than need-based and stresses the identification, nurturing, and celebration of community assets."[21] Thus, one of the major differences between community organizing and community building is the type of assessment that is used to determine where to focus the community's efforts. In the community organizing approach, the assessment is focused on the needs of the community, while in community building, the assessment focuses on the assets and capabilities of the community. It is assumed that a clearer picture of the community will be revealed and a stronger base will be developed for change if the assessment includes the identification of both needs and assets/capacities and involves those who live in the community. It is from these capacities and assets that communities are built.[22]

community building
an orientation to community that is strength-based rather than need-based and stresses the identification, nurturing, and celebration of community assets

To determine the needs and assets/capacities of a community, an assessment must be completed. There are two reasons for completing an effective and comprehensive assessment: "Information is needed for change, and it is also needed for empowerment."[23] This could include a traditional *needs assessment* and/or a newer technique called *mapping community capacity*. A needs assessment is a process by which data about the issues of concern are collected and analyzed. From the analyzed data, concerns or problems emerge and are prioritized so that strategies can be created to tackle them.

Traditional forms of data collection for needs assessments have included techniques such as completing written questionnaires or interviewing people in the community. Because of the importance of getting participation from community members and "starting where the people are,"[24] some organizers have used *participatory data collection* processes. Such processes get those from whom the data are to be collected to help with data collection. One newer technique for doing this is call *photovoice*.[25,26] With this technique community members are provided with cameras and skills training, and then they use the cameras to convey their own images of community problems and strengths.[5] "Participants then work together to select the pictures that best capture their collective wisdom and use these both to tell their stories and to stimulate change through local organizing and institutional—and policy-level action."[8] (*Note:* Needs assessment is discussed in greater length in the second half of this chapter, with regard to program planning.)

Mapping community capacity, on the other hand, is a process of identifying community assets, not concerns or problems. It is a process by which organizers literally use a map to identify the different assets of a community. McKnight and Kretzmann[22] have categorized assets into three different groups based on their availability to the community and refer to them as building blocks. *Primary building blocks* are the most accessible assets. They are located in the neighborhood and are controlled by those who live in the neighborhood. Primary building blocks can be organized into the assets of individuals (e.g., skills and talents) and those of organizations or associations (e.g., religious and citizen organizations). The next most accessible building blocks are secondary building blocks. *Secondary building blocks* are assets located in the neighborhood but largely controlled by people outside (e.g., social service agencies, schools, hospitals, and housing structures). The least accessible assets are referred to as potential building blocks. *Potential building blocks* are resources originating outside the neighborhood and controlled by people outside (e.g., welfare expenditures and public information). By knowing both the needs and assets of the community, organizers can work to identify the true concerns or problems of the community and use the assets of the community as a foundation for dealing with the concerns or problems.

Determining the Priorities and Setting Goals

An analysis of the community assessment data should result in the identification of the problems to be addressed. However, more often than not, the resources needed to solve all identified problems are not available. Therefore, the problems that have been identified must be prioritized. This prioritization is best achieved through general agreement or consensus of those who have been organized so that "ownership" can take hold. It is critical that all those working with the process feel that they "own" the problem and want to see it solved. Without this sense of ownership, they will be unwilling to give of their time and energy to solve it. For example, if a few highly vocal participants intimidate people into voting for certain activities to be the top priorities before a consensus is actually reached, it is unlikely that those who disagreed on this assignment of priorities will work enthusiastically to help solve the problem. They may even drop out of the process because they feel they have no ownership in the decision-making process.

Miller (as cited in Minkler and Wallenstein[5]) has identified five criteria that community organizers need to consider when selecting a priority issue or problem. The issue or problem (1) must be winnable, ensuring that working on it does not simply reinforce fatalistic attitudes and beliefs that things cannot be improved; (2) must be simple and specific, so that any member of the organizing group can explain it clearly in a sentence or two; (3) must unite members of the organizing group and must involve them in a meaningful way in achieving resolution of the issue or problem; (4) should affect many people and build up the community; and (5) should be a part of a larger plan or strategy to enhance the community.[27]

Once the problems have been prioritized, goals need to be identified and written that will serve as guides for problem solving. The practice of consensus building should again be employed during the setting of goals. These goals, which will become the foundation for all the work that follows, can be thought of as the "hoped-for end result." In other words, once community action has occurred, what will have changed? In the community where violence is a problem, the goal may be to reduce the number of violent crimes or eliminate them altogether. Sometimes at this point in the process, some members of the larger group drop out because they do not see their priorities or goals included on consensus lists. Unable to feel ownership, they are unwilling to expend their resources on this process. Because there is strength in numbers, efforts should be made to keep them in. One strategy for doing so is to keep the goal list as long as possible.

Arriving at a Solution and Selecting Intervention Strategies

There are alternative solutions for every community problem. The group should examine the alternatives in terms of probable outcomes, acceptability to the community, probable long- and short-term effects on the community, and the cost of resources to solve the problem.[28] A solution involves selecting one or more intervention strategies (see Table 5.2). Each type of intervention strategy has advantages and disadvantages. The group must try to agree on the best strategy and then select the most advantageous intervention activity or activities. Again, the group must work toward consensus through compromise. If the educators in the group were asked to provide a recommended strategy, they might suggest offering more preventive-education programs; law enforcement personnel might recommend more enforceable laws; judges might want more space in the jails and prisons. The protectionism of the subgroups within the larger group is often referred to as *turfism*. It is not uncommon to have turf struggles when trying to build consensus.

The Final Steps in the Community Organizing/Building Process: Implementing, Evaluating, Maintaining, and Looping Back

The last four steps in this generalized approach to organizing/building a community include implementing the intervention strategy and activities that were selected in the previous step, evaluating the outcomes of the plans of action, maintaining the outcomes over time, and if necessary, going back to a previous step in the process—"looping back"—to modify or restructure the work plan to organize the community.

Implementation of the intervention strategy includes identifying and collecting the necessary resources for implementation and creating the appropriate time line for implementation. Often the resources can be found within a community, and thus horizontal relationships, the interaction of local units with one another, are needed.[29] Other times the resources

---

Table 5.2
Intervention Strategies and Example Activities

1. *Health communication strategies:* Mass media, billboards, booklets, bulletin boards, flyers, direct mail, newsletters, pamphlets, posters, and video and audio materials
2. *Health education strategies:* Educational methods (such as lecture, discussion, and group work) as well as audiovisual materials, computerized instruction, laboratory exercises, and written materials (books and periodicals)
3. *Health policy/enforcement strategies:* Executive orders, laws, ordinances, policies, position statements, regulations, and formal and informal rules
4. *Environmental change strategies:* Those that are designed to change the structure of services or systems of care to improve health promotion services, such as safety belts and air bags in cars, speed bumps in parking lots, or environmental cues such as No Smoking signs
5. *Health-related community services:* The use of health risk appraisals (HRAs), community screening for health problems, and immunization clinics
6. Other strategies
   a. *Behavior modification activities:* Modifying behavior to stop smoking, start to exercise, manage stress, and regulate diet
   b. *Community advocacy activities:* Mass mobilization, social action, community planning, community service development, community education, and community advocacy (such as a letter-writing campaign)
   c. *Organizational culture activities:* Activities that work to change norms and traditions
   d. *Incentives and disincentives:* Items that can either encourage or discourage people to behave a certain way, which may include money and other material items or fines
   e. *Social intervention activities:* Support groups, social activities, and social networks
   f. *Technology-delivered activities:* Educating or informing people by using technology (e.g., computers and telephones)

Source: Adapted from McKenzie, J. F., B. L. Neiger, and R. Thackeray (2009). *Planning, Implementing, and Evaluating Health Promotion Programs: A Primer,* 5th ed. San Francisco, CA: Benjamin Cummings, 201–225.

must be obtained from units located outside the community; in this case, vertical relationships, those where local units interact with extracommunity systems, are needed.[29] An example of this latter relationship is the interaction "between a local nonprofit organization and a state agency with which it has contact."[21]

Evaluation of the process often involves comparing the long-term health and social outcomes of the process to the goals that were set in an earlier step. Some scholars[8] have indicated that such traditional evaluations of community organizing efforts are not easy to carry out and have some limitations. There are times when evaluations are not well planned or funded. As such they "may fail to capture the shorter-term, system-level effects with which community organizing is heavily concerned, such as improvements in organizational collaboration, community involvement, capacity, and healthier public policies or environments."

Maintaining or sustaining the outcomes may be one of the most difficult steps in the entire process. It is at this point that organizers need to seriously consider the need for a long-term capacity for problem solving. Finally, through the steps of implementation, evaluation, and maintenance of the outcomes, organizers may see the need to "loop back" to a previous step in the process to rethink or rework before proceeding onward in their plan.

A Special Note about Community Organizing/Building

Before we leave the processes of community organizing/building, it should be noted that no matter what approach is used in organizing/building a community—locality development, social planning, social action, or the generalized approach outlined here—not all problems can be solved. In other cases, repeated attempts may be necessary before a solution is reached. In addition, it is important to remember that if a problem exists in a community, there are probably some people who benefit from its existence and who may work toward preventing a successful solution to the problem. Whether or not the problem is solved, the final decision facing the organized group is whether to disband the group or to reorganize in order to take on a new problem or attack the first problem from a different direction.

HEALTH PROMOTION PROGRAMMING

In Chapters 2 through 4, we discuss how communities describe, analyze, and intervene to solve existing health problems such as disease outbreaks or other community problems. However, the 1979 Surgeon General's report on health promotion and disease prevention, *Healthy People* (see Figure 5.5), charted a new course for community health—away from curing diseases and toward preventing diseases and promoting health. Health promotion programming has now become an important tool of community health professionals. The second half of this chapter presents the process of health promotion programming.

Basic Understanding of Program Planning

Prior to discussing the process of program planning, two relationships must be presented. These are the relationships between health education and health promotion, and program planning and community organizing/building.

Health education and *health promotion* are terms that are sometimes used interchangeably. This is incorrect because health

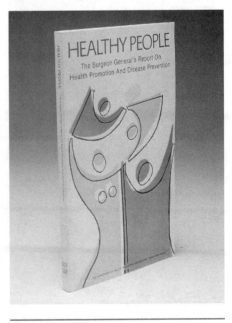

FIGURE 5.5

Healthy People, the 1979 Surgeon General's report on health promotion and disease prevention, charted a new course for community health.

health education
any combination of planned learning experiences based on sound theories that provide individuals, groups, and communities the opportunity to acquire information and the skills to make quality health decisions

health promotion
any planned combination of educational, political, environmental, regulatory, or organizational mechanisms that support actions and conditions of living conducive to the health of individuals, groups, and communities

program planning
a process by which an intervention is planned to help meet the needs of a priority population

education is only a part of health promotion. The Joint Committee on Health Education and Promotion Terminology defined the process of **health education** as "any combination of planned learning experiences based on sound theories that provide individuals, groups, and communities the opportunity to acquire information and the skills to make quality health decisions."[30] The committee defined **health promotion** as "any planned combination of educational, political, environmental, regulatory, or organizational mechanisms that support actions and conditions of living conducive to the health of individuals, groups, and communities."[30] From these definitions, it is obvious that the terms are not the same and that *health promotion* is a much more encompassing term than *health education*. Figure 5.6 provides a graphic representation of the relationship between the terms.

The first half of this chapter described the process of community organizing/building—the process by which individuals, groups, and organizations engage in planned action to influence social problems. Program planning may or may not be associated with community organizing/building. **Program planning** is a process in which an intervention is planned to help meet the needs of a specific group of people. It may take a community organizing/building effort to be able to plan such an intervention. The antiviolence campaign used earlier in the chapter is such an example, where many resources of the community were brought together to create interventions (programs) to deal with the violence problem. However, program planning need not be connected to community organizing/building. For example, a community organizing/building effort is not needed before a company offers a smoking cessation program for its employees or a religious organization offers a stress management class for its members. In such cases, only the steps of the program planning process need to be carried out. These steps are described in the following section.

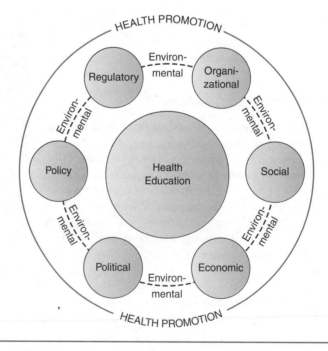

FIGURE 5.6
The relationship of health education and health promotion.

Source: McKenzie, J. F., B. L. Neiger, and R. Thackeray (2009). *Planning, Implementing, and Evaluating Health Promotion Programs: A Primer*, 5th ed. San Francisco, CA: Benjamin Cummings. Reprinted with permission from Pearson Education, Inc.

CREATING A HEALTH PROMOTION PROGRAM

The process of developing a health promotion program, like the process of community organizing/building, involves a series of steps. Success depends on many factors, including the assistance of a professional experienced in program planning.

Experienced program planners use models to guide their work. Planning models are the means by which structure and organization are given to the planning process. Many different planning models exist, some of which are used more often than others. Some of the more frequently used models include the PRECEDE/PROCEED model,[31] probably the best known and most often used; the Multilevel Approach to Community Health (MATCH),[32] Intervention Mapping,[33] and the more recently developed consumer-based planning models that are based on health communication and social marketing such as CDCynergy[34] and Social Marketing Assessment and Response Tool (SMART).[35] Each of these planning models has its strengths and weaknesses, and each has distinctive components that make it unique. In addition, each of the models has been used to plan health promotion programs in a variety of settings, with many successes.

It is not absolutely necessary that the student studying community health for the first time have a thorough understanding of the models mentioned here, but it is important to know the basic steps in the planning process. Therefore, we present a generalized program development model[13] that draws on the major components of these other models. The steps of this generalized model are presented in Figure 5.7 and explained in the following paragraphs.

Prior to undertaking the first step in the generalized model it is important to understand the community and engage the **priority population (audience)**, those whom the health promotion program is intended to serve. Understanding the community means finding out as much as possible about the priority population and the environment in which it exists. Engaging the priority population means getting those in the population involved in the early stages of the health promotion program planning process. If the priority population was composed of the employees of a corporation, the planners would want to read all the material they could find about the company, spend time talking with various individuals and subgroups in the company (e.g., new employees, employees who had been with the company for a long time, management, clerical staff, labor representatives) to find out what they wanted from a health promotion program, and review old documents of the company (e.g., health insurance records, labor agreements, written history of the company). Also, the planners should consider forming a program planning committee with representation from the various subgroups of the workforce (i.e., management, labor, and clerical staff). The planning committee can help ensure that all segments of the priority population will be engaged in the planning process.

priority population (audience)
those whom a program is intended to serve

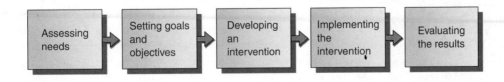

FIGURE 5.7
A generalized model for program planning.

Source: McKenzie, J. F., B. L. Neiger, and R. Thackeray (2009). *Planning, Implementing, and Evaluating Health Promotion Programs: A Primer*, 5th ed. San Francisco, CA: Benjamin Cummings. Reprinted with permission from Pearson Education, Inc.

Assessing the Needs of the Priority Population

needs assessment
the process of collecting and analyzing information, to develop an understanding of the issues, resources, and constraints of the priority population, as related to the development of the health promotion program

To create a useful and effective program for the priority population, planners, with the assistance of the planning committee, must determine the needs and wants of the priority population. This procedural step is referred to as a *needs assessment*. A **needs assessment** is the process of collecting and analyzing information to develop an understanding of the issues, resources, and constraints of the priority population, as related to the development of the health promotion program.[36] The assessment's purpose is to determine whether the needs of the people are being met.

For those interested in a detailed explanation of the process of conducting a needs assessment, extensive accounts are available.[37,38] The following is a simplified six-step approach.[13]

Step 1: Determining the Purpose and Scope of the Needs Assessment

The first step in the needs assessment process is to determine the purpose and the scope of the needs assessment. That is, what is the goal of the needs assessment? What does the planning committee hope to gain from the needs assessment? How extensive will the assessment be? What kind of resources will be available to conduct the needs assessment? Once these questions are answered, the planners are ready to begin gathering data.

Step 2: Gathering Data

The second step in the process is gathering the data that will help to identify the true needs of the priority population. Such data are categorized into two groups—primary and secondary. Primary data are those that are collected specifically for use in this process. An example is having those in the priority population complete a needs assessment questionnaire about their health behavior. The completion of the questionnaire may be in a traditional paper–pencil format, as an online survey, or via face-to-face or telephone interviews (see Figure 5.8). Secondary data are data that have already been collected for some other purpose, such as health insurance claims records or Behavioral Risk Factor Surveillance System (BRFSS) data. Using both primary and secondary data usually presents the clearest picture of the priority population's needs.

Step 3: Analyzing the Data

Collected data can be analyzed in one of two ways—formally or informally. Formal analysis consists of some type of statistical analysis, assuming that the appropriate statistical criteria have been met. However, a more common means of analysis is an informal technique referred to as "eyeballing the data." With this technique, program planners look for the obvious differences between the health status or conditions of the priority population and the programs and services available to close the gap between what is and what ought to be. Regardless of the method used, data analysis should yield a list of the problems that exist, with a description of the nature and extent of each.

The final part of this step is prioritizing the list of problems. Prioritization must take place because though all needs are important, seldom are there enough resources (money and time) available to deal with all the problems identified. When prioritizing, planners should consider (1) the importance of the need, (2) how changeable the need is, and (3) whether adequate resources are available to deal with the problem.

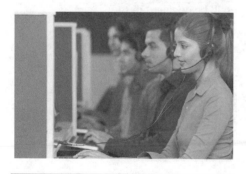

FIGURE 5.8
A telephone survey is a common form of data collection for a health needs assessment.

Step 4: Identifying the Factors Linked to the Health Problem

In this step of the process, planners need to identify and prioritize the risk factors that are associated with the health problem. Thus, if the prioritized health problem identified in step 3 is heart disease, planners must analyze the health behaviors and environment of the priority population for known risk factors of heart disease. For example, higher than expected smoking behavior may be present in the priority population in addition to a community that lacks recreational areas for exercise. Once these risk factors are identified, they also need to be prioritized.

Step 5: Identifying the Program Focus

With risk factors identified and prioritized, planners need to identify those *predisposing*, *enabling*, and *reinforcing* factors that seem to have a direct impact on the targeted risk factors. In the heart disease example, those in the priority population may not (1) have the knowledge to begin an exercise program (predisposing factor), (2) have access to recreational facilities (enabling factor), or (3) have people around them who value the benefits of exercise (reinforcing factor). Once the predisposing, enabling, and reinforcing factors have been identified, they too need to be prioritized. As in step 2 earlier, planners can prioritize these factors according to their importance and changeability.[31] The resulting prioritized list provides the program focus.

Step 6: Validating the Prioritized Need

The final step in this process is to double-check or to confirm that the identified need and resulting program focus indeed need to be addressed in the priority population. For example, a limited amount of data may indicate the primary need of the priority group to be one thing—knowledge about heart disease, for example. However, more extensive data or more comprehensive networking may identify another problem such as lack of free or inexpensive recreational facilities. Before step 6 is completed, planners must make sure they have indeed identified a true need. In short, all work should be double-checked.

At the conclusion of a needs assessment, planners should be able to answer the following questions:[38]

1. Who is the priority population?
2. What are the needs of the priority population?
3. Which subgroups within the priority population have the greatest need?
4. Where are the subgroups located geographically?
5. What is currently being done to resolve identified needs?
6. How well have the identified needs been addressed in the past?

Setting Appropriate Goals and Objectives

Once the problem has been well defined and the needs prioritized, the planners can set goals and develop objectives for the program. The goals and objectives should be thought of as the foundation of the program and for the evaluation. The remaining portions of the programming process—intervention development, implementation, and evaluation—will be designed to achieve the goals by meeting the objectives.

The words *goals* and *objectives* are often used interchangeably, but there is really a significant difference between the two. "A goal is a future event toward which a committed endeavor is directed; objectives are the steps taken in pursuit of a goal."[39] To further distinguish between goals and objectives, McKenzie and colleagues[13] have stated that goals (1) are much more encompassing and global than objectives, (2) are written to cover all aspects of a program, (3) provide overall program direction, (4) are more general in nature, (5) usually take longer to complete, (6) do not have a deadline, (7) are usually not observed but inferred,[40] and (8) often not measured in exact terms. Goals are easy to write and include two basic components—who will be affected and what will change because of the program. Here are some examples of program goals:

1. To help employees learn how to manage their stress
2. To reduce the number of teenage pregnancies in the community
3. To help cardiac patients and their families deal with the lifestyle changes that occur after a heart attack

Objectives are more precise and, as noted earlier, can be considered the steps to achieve the program goals. Because some program goals are more complex than others, the number and type of objectives will vary from program to program. For example, the process of getting a group of people to exercise is a more complex activity than trying to get a group to learn the four food groups. The more complex a program, the greater the number of objectives needed. To deal with these different types of programs, McKenzie and colleagues[13] adapted a hierarchy of program objectives first developed by Deeds[41] and later updated by Cleary and Neiger.[42] Table 5.3 presents the hierarchy and an example of an objective at each of the levels within the hierarchy.

From the examples presented in Table 5.3, it should be obvious that the hierarchy goes from less complex to more complex levels. Thus, it takes less energy and fewer resources to increase awareness in the priority population than to improve its health status. Close examination of the example objectives reveals that the objectives are written in specific terms. They are composed of four parts (who, what, when, and how much) and outline changes

Table 5.3
Hierarchy of Objectives and Examples of Each

Type of Objective	Program Outcomes	Possible Evaluation Measures	Type of Evaluation	Example Objective
Process objectives	Activities presented and tasks completed	Number of sessions held, exposure, attendance, participation, staff performance, appropriate materials, adequacy of resources, tasks on schedule	Process (form of formative)	On June 12, 2011, a breast cancer brochure will be distributed to all female customers over the age of 18 at the Ross grocery store.
Impact objectives				
Learning objectives	Change in awareness, knowledge, attitudes, and skills	Increase in awareness, knowledge, attitudes, and skill development/acquisition	Impact (form of summative)	When asked in class, 50% of the students will be able to list the four principles of cardiovascular conditioning.
Action/behavioral objectives	Change in behavior	Current behavior modified or discontinued, or new behavior adopted	Impact (form of summative)	During a telephone interview, 35% of the residents will report having had their blood cholesterol checked in the last 6 months.
Environmental objectives	Change in the environment	Measures associated with economic, service, physical, social, psychological, or political environments, e.g., protection added to, or hazards or barriers removed from, the environment	Impact (form of summative)	By the end of the year, all senior citizens who requested transportation to the congregate meals will have received it.
Outcome objectives	Change in quality of life (QOL), health status, or risk, and social benefits	QOL measures, morbidity data, mortality data, measures of risk (e.g., HRA)	Outcome (form of summative)	By the year 2015, infant mortality rates will be reduced to no more than 7 per 1,000 in Franklin County.

Source: Adapted from Deeds, S. G. (1992). *The Health Education Specialist: Self-Study for Professional Competence.* Los Alamitos, CA: Loose Cannon; Cleary, M. J., and B. L. Neiger (1998). *The Certified Health Education Specialist: A Self-Study Guide for Professional Competence,* 3rd ed. Allentown, PA: National Commission for Health Education Credentialing; and McKenzie, J. F., B. L. Neiger, and R. Thackeray (2009). *Planning, Implementing, and Evaluating Health Promotion Programs: A Primer,* 5th ed. San Francisco, CA: Benjamin Cummings.

| BOX 5.1 | HEALTHY PEOPLE 2020: OBJECTIVES |

Educational and Community-Based Programs

Goal: Increase the quality, availability, and effectiveness of educational and community-based programs designed to prevent disease and injury, improve health, and enhance quality of life.

Objective: ECBP-10 Increase the number of community-based organizations (including local health departments, tribal health services, nongovernmental organizations, and state agencies) providing population-based primary prevention services in the following areas:

ECBP 10.8 Nutrition

Target: 94.7 percent.

Baseline: 86.4 percent of community-based organizations (including local health departments, tribal health services, nongovernmental organizations, and state agencies) provided population-based primary prevention services in nutrition in 2008.

Target setting method: 10 percent improvement.

Data source: National Profile of Local Health Departments, National Association of County and City Health Officials (NACCHO)

ECBP 10.9 Physical Activity

Target: 88.5 percent.

Baseline: 80.5 percent of community-based organizations (including local health departments, tribal health services, nongovernmental organizations, and State agencies) provided population-based primary prevention services in physical activity in 2008.

Target setting method: 10 percent improvement.

Data source: National Profile of Local Health Departments, National Association of County and City Health Officials (NACCHO).

Note: Other areas covered by this objective include: 10.1 Injury, 10.2 Violence, 10.3 Mental Illness, 10.4 Tobacco Use, 10.5 Substance Abuse, and 10.6 Unintended Pregnancy, and 10.7 Chronic Diseases Programs.

For Further Thought

If you had the opportunity to write one more objective dealing with the implementation of health promotion programs for use in *Healthy People 2020*, what would it be? What is your rationale for selecting such an objective?

Source: U.S. Department of Health and Human Services, Office of Disease Prevention and Health Promotion (2010). *Healthy People 2020*. Available at http://www.healthypeople.gov/2020/default.aspx. Accessed January 4, 2011.

that should result from the implementation of the program.[43] As such, the objectives are written so that the level of their attainment is observable and measurable.

One final note about objectives: In Chapter 1, *Healthy People 2020,* the national health goals and objectives of the nation, was discussed. Selected objectives from this publication are presented in boxes throughout this text (see Box 5.1). These goals and objectives provide a good model for developing goals and objectives for a new program. In fact, these goals and objectives can be adapted for use in most community health promotion programs.

Creating an Intervention That Considers the Peculiarities of the Setting

The next step in the program planning process is to design activities that will help the priority population meet the objectives and, in the process, achieve the program goals. These activities are collectively referred to as an **intervention**, or treatment. This intervention or treatment constitutes the program that the priority population will experience.

intervention
an activity or activities designed to create change in people

The number of activities in an intervention may be many or only a few. Although no minimum number has been established, it has been shown that multiple activities are often more effective than a single activity. For example, if the planners wanted to change the attitudes of community members toward a new landfill, they would have a greater chance of doing so by distributing pamphlets door to door, writing articles for the local newspaper, and speaking to local service groups, than by performing any one of these activities by itself. In other words, the size and amount of intervention are important in health promotion programming. Few people change their behavior based on a single exposure; instead, multiple exposures are generally needed to change most behaviors. It stands to reason that "hitting" the priority population from several angles or through multiple channels should increase the chances of making an impact.[13]

Two terms that relate to the size and amount of an intervention are *multiplicity* and *dose*. **Multiplicity** refers to the number of activities that make up the intervention, while **dose** refers to the number of program units delivered. Thus, if an intervention has two activities—say, an educational workshop and a public service announcement for radio—they define multiplicity, while the number of times each of the activities is presented defines the dose.[13]

The actual creation of the intervention should begin by asking and answering a series of questions.[13] The first is, what needs to change? The answer to this question comes from the needs assessment and the resulting goals and objectives. The second question is, at what level of prevention (i.e., primary, secondary, or tertiary) will the program be aimed? The approach taken to a primary prevention need, that is, preventing a problem before it begins, would be different from a tertiary prevention need of managing a problem after it has existed for a while. The third question asks, at what level of influence will the intervention be focused? The various levels of influence (i.e., intrapersonal, interpersonal, institutional or organizational, community, and public policy) that were presented at the beginning of the chapter as part of the social ecological approach need to be considered. These levels provide the planners with a framework from which to think about how they will "attack" the needs of the priority population. For example, if the goal of a program is to reduce the prevalence of smoking in a community, the intervention could attack the problem by focusing the intervention on individuals through one-on-one counseling, via groups by offering smoking cessation classes, by trying to change policy by enacting a state law prohibiting smoking in public places, or by attacking the problem using more than one of these strategies.

The fourth question asks, has an effective intervention strategy to deal with the focus of the problem already been created? Three sources of guidance for selecting intervention strategies (see Table 5.2 for a list of strategies)—*best practices, best experiences,* and *best processes*.[31] **Best practices** refers to "recommendations for an intervention, based on critical review of multiple research and evaluation studies that substantiate the efficacy of the intervention in the populations and circumstances in which the studies were done, if not its effectiveness in other populations and situations where it might be implemented."[31] Examples of best practices related to health promotion programs are provided in *The Community Guide: What Works to Promote Health*[44] (see Community Health on the Web at the end of this chapter).

When best practice recommendations are not available for use, planners need to look for information on best experiences. **Best experience** intervention strategies are those of prior or existing programs that have not gone through the critical research and evaluation studies and thus fall short of best practice criteria but nonetheless show promise in being effective. Best experiences can often be found by networking with others professionals and by reviewing the literature.

If neither best practices nor best experiences are available to planners, then the third source of guidance for selecting an intervention strategy is using best processes. **Best processes** intervention strategies are original interventions that the planners create based on

---

multiplicity
the number of activities that make up the intervention

dose
the number of program units as part of the intervention

best practices
recommendations for interventions based on critical review of multiple research and evaluation studies that substantiate the efficacy of the intervention

best experience
intervention strategies used in prior or existing programs that have not gone through the critical research and evaluation studies and thus fall short of best practice criteria

best processes
original intervention strategies that the planners create based on their knowledge and skills of good planning processes including the involvement of those in the priority population and the use of theories and models

their knowledge and skills of good planning processes including the involvement of those in the priority population and the theories and models used to change behaviors such as social cognitive theory[45] or the transtheoretical model.[46]

The fifth question asks, is the intervention an appropriate fit for the priority population? In other words, does the planned intervention meet the specific characteristics of the priority population such as the educational level, developmental stages, or the specific cultural characteristics of the people being served?

The sixth, and/final, question that needs to be asked is, are the resources available to implement the intervention selected? Planners need to evaluate the amount of money, time, personnel, and/or space that is needed to carry out the various interventions and make a determination if such resources are available to implement the intervention.

Once all of these questions have been asked and answered the planners can then decide which intervention would be best for the priority population with whom they are working. The general intervention strategies presented in Table 5.2 associated with community organizing/building are the same ones that planners can use with health promotion interventions.

Implementing the Intervention

The moment of truth is when the intervention is implemented. **Implementation** is the actual carrying out or putting into practice the activity or activities that make up the intervention. More formally, implementation has been defined as "the act of converting planning, goals, and objectives into action through administrative structure, management activities, policies, procedures, regulations, and organizational actions of new programs."[47] It is at this point that the planners will learn whether the product (intervention) they developed will be useful in producing the measurable changes as outlined in the objectives.

> **implementation**
> putting a planned program into action

To ensure a smooth-flowing implementation of the intervention, it is wise to pilot test it at least once and sometimes more. A **pilot test** is a trial run. It is when the intervention is presented to just a few individuals who are either from the intended priority population or from a very similar population. For example, if the intervention is being developed for fifth graders in a particular school, it might be pilot tested on fifth graders with similar educational backgrounds and demographic characteristics but from a different school.

> **pilot test**
> a trial run of an intervention

The purpose of pilot testing an intervention is to determine whether there are any problems with it. Some of the more common problems that pop up are those dealing with the design or delivery of the intervention; however, any part of it could be flawed. For example, it could be determined during pilot testing that there is a lack of resources to carry out the intervention as planned or that those implementing the intervention need more training. When minor flaws are detected and corrected easily, the intervention is then ready for full implementation. However, if a major problem surfaces—one that requires much time and many resources to correct—it is recommended that the intervention be pilot tested again with the improvements in place before implementation.

An integral part of the piloting process is collecting feedback from those in the pilot group. By surveying the pilot group, planners can identify popular and unpopular aspects of the intervention, how the intervention might be changed or improved, and whether the program activities were effective. This information can be useful in fine-tuning this intervention or in developing future programs.

Once the intervention has been pilot tested and corrected as necessary, it is ready to be disseminated and implemented. If the planned program is being implemented with a large priority population and there is a lot at stake with the implementation, it is advisable that the intervention be implemented gradually rather than all at once. One way of doing so is by phasing in the intervention. **Phasing in** refers to a step-by-step implementation in which the

> **phasing in**
> implementation of an intervention with a series of small groups instead of the entire population

intervention is introduced first to smaller groups instead of the entire priority population. Common criteria used for selecting participating groups for phasing in include participant ability, number of participants, program offerings, and program location.[13]

The following is an example of phasing in by location. Assume that a local health department wants to provide smoking cessation programs for all the smokers in the community (priority population). Instead of initiating one big intervention for all, planners could divide the priority population by residence location. Facilitators would begin implementation by offering the smoking cessation classes on the south side of town during the first month. During the second month, they would continue the classes on the south side and begin implementation on the west side of town. They would continue to implement this intervention until all sections of the town were included.

Evaluating the Results

The final step in the generalized planning model is the evaluation. Although evaluation is the last step in this model, it really takes place in all steps of program planning. It is very important that planning for evaluation occur during the first stages of program development, not just at the end.

Evaluation is the process in which planners determine the value or worth of the object of interest by comparing it against a **standard of acceptability**.[48] Common standards of acceptability include, but are not limited to, mandates (policies, statutes, and laws), values, norms, and comparison/control groups.

Evaluation can be categorized further into summative and formative evaluation. **Formative evaluation** is done during the planning and implementing processes to improve or refine the program. For example, validating the needs assessment and pilot testing are both forms of formative evaluation. **Summative evaluation** begins with the development of goals and objectives and is conducted after implementation to determine the program's effect on the priority population. Often, the summative evaluation is broken down into two categories—*impact* and *outcome evaluation*. **Impact evaluation** focuses on immediate observable effects of a program such as changes in awareness, knowledge, attitudes, skills, environmental surroundings, and behavior of those in the priority population, whereas **outcome evaluation** focuses on the end result of the program and is generally measured by improvements in morbidity, mortality, or vital measures of symptoms, signs, or physiologic indicators.[48]

Like other steps in the planning model, the evaluation step can be broken down into smaller steps. The mini-steps of evaluation include planning the evaluation, collecting the necessary evaluative data, analyzing the data, and reporting and applying the results.

Planning the Evaluation

As noted earlier, planning for summative evaluation begins with the development of the goals and objectives of the program. These statements put into writing what should happen as a result of the program. Also in this planning mini-step, it should be determined who will evaluate the program—an *internal evaluator* (one who already is involved in the program) or an *external evaluator* (one from outside the program). In addition, this portion of the evaluation process should identify an evaluation design and a time line for carrying out the evaluation.

Collecting the Data

Data collection includes deciding how to collect the data (e.g., with an online survey, from existing records, by observation), determining who will collect them, pilot testing the procedures, and performing the actual data collection.

---

evaluation
determining the value or worth of an object of interest

standard of acceptability
a comparative mandate, value, norm, or group

formative evaluation
the evaluation that is conducted during the planning and implementing processes to improve or refine the program

summative evaluation
the evaluation that determines the effect of a program on the priority population

impact evaluation
focuses on immediate observable effects of a program

outcome evaluation
focuses on the end result of the program

Analyzing the Data

Once the data are in hand, they must be analyzed and interpreted. Also, it must be decided who will analyze the data and when the analysis is to be completed.

Reporting the Results

Next the evaluation report should be written. Decisions must be made (if they have not been made already) regarding who should write the report, who should receive the report, in what form, and when.

Applying the Results

With the findings in hand, it then must be decided how they will be used. When time, resources, and effort are spent on an evaluation, it is important that the results be useful for reaching a constructive end and for deciding whether to continue or discontinue the program or to alter it in some way.

CHAPTER SUMMARY

- A knowledge of community organizing and program planning is essential for community health workers whose job it is to promote and protect the health of the community.

- Community organizing is a process through which communities are helped to identify common problems or goals, mobilize resources, and in other ways develop and implement strategies for reaching their goals that they have collectively set.

- Community building is an orientation to community that is strength-based rather than need-based and stresses the identification, nurturing, and celebration of community assets.

- The steps of the general model for community organizing/building include recognizing the issue, gaining entry into the community, organizing the people, assessing the community, determining the priorities and setting goals, arriving at a solution and selecting the intervention strategies, implementing the plan, evaluating the outcomes of the plan of action, maintaining the outcomes in the community, and, if necessary, looping back.

- Program planning is a process in which an intervention is planned to help meet the needs of a priority population (audience).

- The steps in the program planning process include assessing the needs of the priority population, setting

SCENARIO: ANALYSIS AND RESPONSE

The town of Kenzington sounds like a good candidate for a community organizing/building effort. Assume that Kenzington is the town in which you now live and you belong to the group that has taken the issue to the city council. Based on what you know about the problem in the scenario and what you know about your town, answer the following questions.

1. What is the real problem?
2. Who do you think the gatekeepers are in the community?
3. What groups of people in the community might be most interested in solving this problem?
4. What groups might have a vested interest in seeing the problem remain unsolved?
5. What interventions would be useful in dealing with the problem?
6. How would you evaluate your efforts to solve the problem?
7. What strategies might you recommend to make the solution lasting?
8. If you were to look for help on the Internet to deal with this problem, what key words would you use to search the Web for help?

appropriate goals and objectives, creating an intervention that considers the peculiarities of the setting, implementing the intervention, and evaluating the results.

REVIEW QUESTIONS

1. What is community organizing?

2. What are the assumptions (identified by Ross) under which organizers work when bringing a community together to solve a problem?

3. What is the difference between top-down and grassroots community organizing?

4. What is meant by the term *gatekeepers*? Who would they be in your home community?

5. Identify the steps in the generalized approach to community organizing/building presented in this chapter.

6. What is meant by community building?

7. What is a needs assessment? Why is it important in the health promotion programming process?

8. What are the five major steps in program development?

9. What are the differences between goals and objectives?

10. What are intervention strategies? Provide five examples.

11. What are *best practices, best experiences*, and *best processes*? How are they different?

12. What is meant by the term *pilot testing*? How is it useful when developing an intervention?

13. What is the difference between formative and summative evaluation? What are impact and outcome evaluation?

14. Name and briefly describe the five major components of program evaluation.

ACTIVITIES

1. From your knowledge of the community in which you live (or from the yellow pages of the telephone book), generate a list of 7 to 10 agencies that might be interested in creating a coalition to deal with community drug problems. Provide a one-sentence rationale for each why it might want to be involved.

2. Ask your instructor if he or she is aware of any community organizing/building efforts in a local community. If you are able to identify such an effort, make an appointment—either by yourself or with some of your classmates—to meet with the person who is leading the effort and ask the following questions:

   What is the problem that faces the community?

   What is the goal of the group?

What steps have been taken so far to organize/build the community, and what steps are yet to be taken?

Who is active in the core group?

Did the group conduct a community assessment?

What intervention will be/has been used?

Is it anticipated that the problem will be solved?

3. Using a smoking cessation program, write one program goal and an objective for each of the levels presented in Table 5.3.

4. Visit a voluntary health agency in your community, either by yourself or with classmates. Ask employees if you may review any of the standard health promotion programs the agency offers to the community. Examine the program materials, locating the five major components of a program development discussed in this chapter. Then, in a two-page paper, summarize your findings.

COMMUNITY HEALTH ON THE WEB

The Internet contains a wealth of information about community and public health. Increase your knowledge of some of the topics presented in this chapter by accessing the Jones & Bartlett Learning Web site at **http://health .jbpub.com/book/communityhealth/7e** and follow the links to complete the following Web activities.

- MAPP
- CDC's Healthy Communities Program
- The Guide to Community Preventive Services

REFERENCES

1. Rimer, B. K., and K. Glanz (2005). *Theory at a Glance: A Guide for Health Promotion Practice*, 2nd ed. [NIH Pub. No. 05-3896]. Washington, DC: National Cancer Institute.

2. Pellmar, T. C., E. N. Brandt, Jr., and M. Baird (2002). "Health and Behavior: The Interplay of Biological, Behavioral, and Social Influences: Summary of an Institute of Medicine Report." *American Journal of Health Promotion*, 16(4): 206-219.

3. McLeroy, K. R., D. Bibeau, A. Steckler, and K. Glanz (1988). "An Ecological Perspective for Health Promotion Programs." *Health Education Quarterly*, 15(4): 351-378.

4. Sallis, J. F., N. Owen, and E. B. Fisher (2008). "Ecological Models of Health Behavior." In K. Glanz, B. K. Rimer, and K. Viswanath, eds., *Health Behavior and Health Education Practice: Theory, Research, and Practice*, 4th ed. San Francisco, CA: Jossey-Bass, 465-485.

5. Minkler, M., and N. Wallerstein (2005). "Improving Health through Community Organization and Community Building: A Health Education Perspective." In M. Minkler, ed., *Community Organizing and Community Building for Health*, 2nd ed. New Brunswick, NJ: Rutgers University Press, 26-50.

6. Ross, M. G. (1967). *Community Organization: Theory, Principles, and Practice*. New York: Harper and Row, 86-92.

7. Goodman, R. M., M. A. Speers, K. McLeroy, S. Fawcett, M. Kegler, E. Parker, S. R. Smith, T. D. Sterling, and N. Wallerstein (1999). "Identifying and Defining the Dimensions of Community Capacity to Provide a Basis for Measurement." *Health Education and Behavior*, 25(3): 258-278.

8. Minkler, M., N. Wallerstein, and N. Wilson (2008). "Improving Health through Community Organizing and Community Building." In K. Glanz, B. K. Rimer, and K. Viswanath, eds., *Health Behavior and Health Education Practice: Theory, Research, and Practice*, 4th ed. San Francisco, CA: Jossey-Bass, 287-312.

9. Rothman, J., and J. E. Tropman (1987). "Models of Community Organization and Macro Practice Perspectives: Their Mixing and Phasing." In F. M. Cox, J. L. Erlich, J. Rothman, and J. E. Tropman, eds., *Strategies of Community Organization: Macro Practice*. Itasca, IL: Peacock, 3-26.

10. Garvin, C. D., and F. M. Cox (2001). "A History of Community Organizing Since the Civil War with Special Reference to Oppressed Communities." In J. Rothman, J. L. Erlich, and J. E. Tropman, eds., *Strategies of Community Intervention*, 5th ed. Itasca, IL: Peacock, 65-100.

11. Rothman, J. (2001). "Approaches to Community Intervention." In J. Rothman, J. L. Erlich, and J. E. Tropman, eds., *Strategies of Community Intervention*, 6th ed. Itasca, IL: Peacock.

12. Checkoway, B. (1989). "Community Participation for Health Promotion: Prescription for Public Policy." *Wellness Perspectives: Research, Theory, and Practice*, 6(1): 18-26.

13. McKenzie, J. F., B. L. Neiger, and R. Thackeray (2009). *Planning, Implementing, and Evaluating Health Promotion Programs: A Primer*, 5th ed. San Francisco, CA: Benjamin Cummings.

14. Butterfoss, F. D. (2007). *Coalitions and Partnerships in Community Health*. San Francisco, CA: Jossey-Bass.

15. Braithwaite, R. L., F. Murphy, N. Lythcott, and D. S. Blumenthal (1989). "Community Organization and Development for Health Promotion within an Urban Black Community: A Conceptual Model." *Health Education*, 20(5): 56-60.

16. Wright, P. A. (1994). *A Key Step in Developing Prevention Materials Is to Obtain Expert and Gatekeepers' Reviews* (Technical Assistance Bulletin). Bethesda, MD: Center for Substance Abuse Prevention (CASP) Communications Team, 1-6.

17. Tervalon, M., and J. Garcia (1998). "Cultural Humility versus Cultural Competence: A Critical Distinction in Defining Physician Training Outcomes in Multicultural Education." *Journal of Health Care for the Poor and Underserved*, 9(2): 117-125.

18. Perlman, J. (1978). "Grassroots Participation from Neighborhood to Nation." In S. Langton, ed., *Citizen Participation in America*. Lexington, MA: Lexington Books, 65-79.

19. Brager, G., H. Specht, and J. L. Torczyner (1987). *Community Organizing*. New York: Columbia University Press, 55.

20. Minkler, M. (2005). "Introduction to Community Organizing and Community Building." In M. Minkler, ed., *Community Organizing and Community Building for Health*, 2nd ed. New Brunswick, NJ: Rutgers University Press, 1-21.

21. Walter, C. L. (2005). "Community Building Practice: A Conceptual Framework." In M. Minkler, ed., *Community Organizing and Community Building for Health*, 2nd ed. New Brunswick, NJ: Rutgers University Press, 66-78.

22. McKnight, J. L., and J. P. Kretzmann (2005). "Mapping Community Capacity." In M. Minkler, ed., *Community Organizing and Community Building for Health*, 2nd ed. New Brunswick, NJ: Rutgers University Press, 158-172.

23. Hancock, T., and M. Minkler (2005). "Community Health Assessment or Healthy Community Assessment." In M. Minkler, ed., *Community Organizing and Community Building for Health*, 2nd ed. New Brunswick, NJ: Rutgers University Press, 138-157.

24. Nyswander, D. B. (1956). "Education for Health: Some Principles and Their Application." *Health Education Monographs*, 14: 65-70.

25. Wang, C. C., and M. A. Burris (1994). "Empowerment through Photovoice: Portraits of Participation." *Health Education Quarterly*, 21(2): 171-186.

26. Wang, C. C., and M. A. Burris (1997). "Photovoice: Concept, Methodology, and Use for Participatory Needs Assessment." *Health Education and Behavior*, 24(3): 369-387.

27. Miller, M. (1986). "Turning Problems into Actionable Issues." Unpublished paper. San Francisco, CA: Organize Training Center.

28. Archer, S. E., and R. P. Fleshman (1985). *Community Health Nursing*. Monterey, CA: Wadsworth Health Sciences.

29. Warren, R. L. (1963). *The Community in America*. Chicago: Rand-McNally.

30. Joint Committee on Health Education and Promotion Terminology (2001). "Report of the 2000 Joint Committee on Health Education and Promotion Terminology." *American Journal of Health Education*, 32(2): 89-103.

31. Green, L. W., and M. W. Kreuter (2005). *Health Program Planning: An Educational and Ecological Approach*, 4th ed. Boston: McGraw-Hill.

32. Simons-Morton, D. G., W. H. Greene, and N. H. Gottlieb (1995). *Introduction to Health Education and Health Promotion*, 2nd ed. Prospect Heights, IL: Waveland Press.

33. Bartholomew, L. K., G. S. Parcel, G. Kok, and N. H. Gottlieb (2006). *Planning Health Promotion Programs: An Intervention Mapping Approach*, 2nd ed. San Francisco, CA: Jossey-Bass.

34. Centers for Disease Control and Prevention, U.S. Department of Health and Human Services (2003). *CDCynergy 3.0: Your Guide to Effective Health Communication* [CD-ROM Version 3.0]. Atlanta, GA: Author.

35. Neiger, B. L., and R. Thackeray (1998). *Social Marketing: Making Public Health Sense*. Paper presented at the annual meeting of the Utah Public Health Association, Provo, UT.

36. Anspaugh, D. J., M. B. Dignan, and S. L. Anspaugh (2000). *Developing Health Promotion Programs*. Boston: McGraw-Hill Higher Education.

37. Gilmore, G. D., and M. D. Campbell (2005). *Needs and Capacity Assessment Strategies for Health Education and Health Promotion*, 3rd ed. Sudbury, MA: Jones & Bartlett.

38. Peterson, D. J., and G. R. Alexander (2001). *Needs Assessment in Public Health: A Practical Guide for Students and Professionals*. New York, NY: Kluwer Academic/Plenum Publishers.

39. Ross, H. S., and P. R. Mico (1980). *Theory and Practice in Health Education*. Palo Alto, CA: Mayfield, 219.

40. Jacobsen, D., P. Eggen, and D. Kauchak (1989). *Methods for Teaching: A Skills Approach*, 3rd ed. Columbus, OH: Merrill.

41. Deeds, S. G. (1992). *The Health Education Specialist: Self-Study for Professional Competence*. Los Alamitos, CA: Loose Cannon Publications.

42. Cleary, M. J., and B. L. Neiger (1998). *The Certified Health Education Specialist: A Self-Study Guide for Professional Competence*, 3rd ed. Allentown, PA: National Commission for Health Education Credentialing.

43. McKenzie, J. F. (2005). "Planning and Evaluating Interventions." In J. Kerr, R. Weitkunat, and M. Moretti, eds., *ABC of Behavior Change: A Guide to Successful Disease Prevention and Health Promotion*. Oxford, England: Elsevier, 41-54.

44. Centers for Disease Control and Prevention (2010). *Guide to Community Preventive Services—The Community Guide: What Works to Promote Health*. Available at http://www.thecommunityguide.org/index.html.

45. McAlister, A. L., C. L. Perry, and G. S. Parcel (2008). How Individuals, Environments, and Health Behaviors Interact: Social Cognitive Theory. In K. Glanz, B. K. Rimer, and K. Viswanath, eds., *Health Behavior and Health Education: Theory, Research, and Practice*, 4th ed. San Francisco, CA: Jossey-Bass, 167-188.

46. Prochaska, J. O., C. A. Redding, and K. E. Evers (2008). The Transtheoretical Model and Stages of Change. In K. Glanz, B. K. Rimer, and K. Viswanath, eds., *Health Behavior and Health Education: Theory, Research, and Practice*, 4th ed. San Francisco, CA: Jossey-Bass, 97–121.

47. Timmreck, T. C. (1997). *Health Services Cyclopedic Dictionary*, 3rd ed. Sudbury, MA: Jones & Bartlett.

48. Green, L. W., and F. M. Lewis (1986). *Measurement and Evaluation in Health Education and Health Promotion*. Palo Alto, CA: Mayfield.

Chapter 6

The School Health Program: A Component of Community Health

Chapter Objectives

After studying this chapter, you will be able to:

1 Define *coordinated school health program*.

2 List the ideal members of a school health council.

3 Explain why a school health program is important.

4 Identify the major foundations of a coordinated school health program.

5 Define written school health policies and explain their importance to the school health program.

6 Explain processes for developing and implementing school health policies.

7 List the eight components of a coordinated school health program.

8 Describe the role of the school health coordinator.

9 Identify those services offered as part of school health services and explain why schools are logical places to offer such services.

10 Explain what is meant by a healthy school environment and discuss the two major environments.

11 Define *school health education*.

12 Identify the eight National Health Education Standards.

13 Explain how a health education specialist could locate credible health education curricula.

14 Identify and briefly explain four issues that are faced by school health advocates.

SCENARIO

Seldom does an elementary school teacher have a typical day. Each day seems to bring a variety of new experiences. Take, for example, the day Ms. Graff experienced last Wednesday. Even before the first bell at 8:30 A.M. she was summoned to the hallway, where one of her second-graders became ill and threw up. Remembering her teachers' in-service workshop on universal precautions, Ms. Graff put into action her new knowledge for handling blood and body fluids.

After that incident, her day seemed to be going along well until two of Ms. Graff's students began fighting in the lunch room. They were arguing over who had the healthier lunch. It seemed that Billy thought his school lunch was healthier than Tommy's cheese sandwich and bag of potato chips. Ms. Graff was skillful in helping to settle the dispute.

After lunch, Ms. Graff began her lesson on drug education. She wasn't 10 minutes into her lesson when the school nurse stuck her head in the door and asked if Ms. Graff could send five students for their annual vision screening. Reluctantly, Ms. Graff excused five of her students.

During the last half-hour of the school day, students were engaged in success time—focused instruction in preparation for standardized testing. Just before the last bell was to ring, Annie came up to Ms. Graff's desk and told her that the girl sitting in front of her kept rubbing her eye and it seemed really red. Annie said, "I think she has pinkeye."

Just another "typical day" for Ms. Graff.

INTRODUCTION

coordinated school health program (CSHP)
an organized set of policies, procedures, and activities designed to protect, promote, and improve the health and well-being of students and staff, thus improving a student's ability to learn. It includes, but is not limited to, comprehensive school health education; school health services; a healthy school environment; school counseling; psychological and social services; physical education; school nutrition services; family and community involvement in school health; and school-site health promotion for staff

The school health program is an important component of community health. Though the primary responsibility for the health of school-aged children lies with their parents/guardians, the schools have immeasurable potential for affecting the health of children, their families, and the health of the community. As former U.S. Surgeon General David Satcher states, "The school setting is a great equalizer, providing all students and families—regardless of ethnicity, socio-economic status or level of education—with the same access to good nutrition and physical activity. Because children also teach their parents, important lessons learned at school can help the entire family,"[1] thus improving the health of the entire community. Full-service community schools provide a good example of the link between school health and community health. These schools, using an integrated approach, offer a variety of educational, counseling, social, and health services to families in one location, resulting in improved educational outcomes. Such schools focus on the well-being of the child and family, and some of their services are available on a 24-hour basis. These school buildings serve as neighborhood hubs and institutions that are safe, attentive, and comfortable.[2,3]

In this chapter, we define *coordinated school health program*, explain who is involved in school health programs, explore the reasons why school health is important, discuss the components of school health, and present some of the issues facing school health programs today.

Coordinated School Health Program Defined

A **coordinated school health program (CSHP)** has been defined as

an organized set of policies, procedures, and activities designed to protect, promote, and improve the health and well-being of students and staff, thus improving a student's ability to learn. It includes, but is not limited to comprehensive school health education; school health services; a healthy school environment; school counseling; psychological and social services; physical education; school nutrition services; family and community involvement in school health; and school-site health promotion for staff.[4]

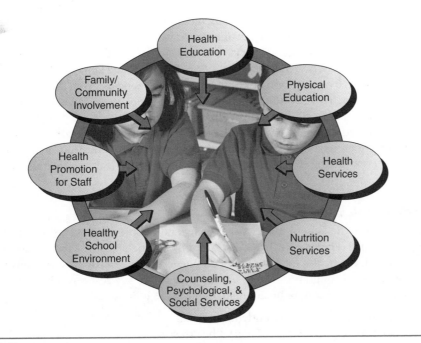

FIGURE 6.1

The coordinated school health program.

Source: Division of Adolescent and School Health, Centers for Disease Control and Prevention (2008). *Coordinated School Health Program.* Available at http://www.cdc.gov/healthyyouth/CSHP. Accessed November 29, 2010.

This definition is based on the work of Allensworth and Kolbe[5] and is represented in Figure 6.1.

The school health program has great potential for affecting the health of many. An estimated 56 million school-aged children attend more than 125,000 schools, and there are more than 7.2 million instructional and noninstructional employees in the United States.[6] This represents about one-fifth of the entire U.S. population. "The knowledge, attitudes, behavior, and skills developed as a result of effective school health programs enable individuals to make informed choices about behavior that will affect their own health throughout their lives, as well as the health of the families for which they are responsible, and the health of the communities in which they live."[7] However, in practice the quality and quantity of CSHPs in school districts throughout the United States vary greatly. Most likely, every school has some elements of a coordinated school health program. Significant improvements would be seen if energy and resources were dedicated to coordinating these services.[8,9] For example, it is not unusual for a health teacher to talk about the importance of aerobic exercise but to never tell the physical education teacher. Similarly, a science teacher may teach about pathogens and the prevention of communicable diseases, but yet the restrooms in a school are not properly equipped for adequate hand washing. Additionally, there is little coordination between school districts and community health agencies to improve the health of the school-aged child.

The School Health Council

For CSHPs to fulfill their potential, a great deal of time and effort must be expended by those involved in the program's various components. When these individuals work together to plan and implement a school health program, they are referred to as the **school health council**, sometimes called a school health advisory council. The primary role of this council is to provide coordination of the various components of CSHP to help students reach and maintain

school health council individuals from a school or school district and its community who work together to provide advice on aspects of the school health program

high-quality health. An ideal council would include representation from administrators, food service workers, counseling personnel, maintenance workers, medical personnel (especially a school nurse and school physician), social workers, parents and other caregivers, students, teachers (especially those who teach health, physical education, and family and consumer science classes), and personnel from appropriate community health agencies. From this group must come a leader or coordinator. This coordinator should have an educational background that includes training in school health. In addition, the coordinator should "be able to plan, implement, and evaluate a coordinated school health program; be familiar with existing community resources; and have connections to local, state, and national health and education organizations."[10,11] Most often the coordinator of the school health council is a health education specialist or school nurse.

The School Nurse

As previously noted, the school nurse is one of several people who is positioned to provide leadership for a CSHP (Figure 6.2). The nurse not only has medical knowledge, but should also have formal training in health education and an understanding of the health needs of all children in kindergarten through the twelfth grade. Some of the key responsibilities of the school nurse as a member of the school health team include the following:[12]

1. Providing direct health care to students and staff
2. Providing leadership for the provision of health services
3. Providing screening and referral for health conditions
4. Promoting a healthy school environment
5. Promoting health
6. Serving in a leadership role for health policies and programs
7. Serving as a liaison between school personnel, family, community, and health care providers

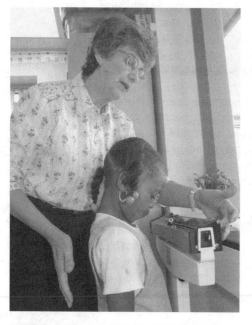

FIGURE 6.2

The school nurse is in a good position to guide the school health program.

Note that even though school nurses are in a good position to provide leadership to the school health council, many school districts do not have the resources to hire a full-time school nurse. It is not uncommon for a school district to contract with an outside health agency such as a local health department or hospital for nursing services. When this scenario occurs, it is normal for the contracted nurse to complete only the nursing tasks required by state law and not to take on the leadership responsibilities for the school health council. This task may then be fulfilled by a school health education specialist. In fact, the health educator may even be responsible when a full-time nurse is present.

The Teacher's Role

Though the school nurse might provide the leadership for a CSHP, the classroom teachers carry a heavy responsibility in seeing that the program works (see Figure 6.3). On the average school day, teachers spend more waking hours with school-aged children than do the parents of many children. A teacher may spend 6 to 8 hours a day with any given child, while the parents spend an hour with that child before school and maybe 4 to 5 hours with the child after school and before bedtime. Teachers are also in a position to make observations on the "normal and abnormal" behaviors and conditions of children because they are able to compare the students in their classroom each day. Furthermore, many health teachers are receiving leadership training regarding CSHPs in their undergraduate or postgraduate coursework, thus making them ideal individuals to lead the coordination. Table 6.1 presents a suggested list of competencies for teachers who expect to be involved in school health education and leadership of a CSHP.

THE NEED FOR SCHOOL HEALTH

The primary role of schools is to educate. However, an unhealthy child has a difficult time learning. Consider, for example, a student who arrives at school without having breakfast, with poor hygiene, and without adequate sleep. This student will be unable to concentrate on schoolwork and may distract others. As a reader, you know how difficult it is to study for a test or even to read this textbook when you do not feel well or are depressed or hungry (see Box 6.1). See Chapters 7 and 8 for specific information related to the health behaviors of school-aged children and adolescents.

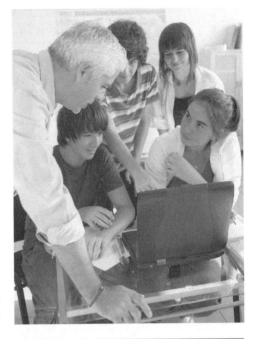

FIGURE 6.3

The classroom teacher's participation is essential for a successful school health program.

"Health and success in school are interrelated. Schools cannot achieve their primary mission of education if students and staff are not healthy and fit physically, mentally, and socially."[13] More specifically, a "student who is not healthy, who suffers from an undetected vision or hearing defect, or who is hungry, or who is impaired by drugs or alcohol, is not a student who will profit from the educational process. Likewise, an individual who has not been provided assistance in the shaping of healthy attitudes, beliefs, and habits early in life, will be more likely to suffer the consequences of reduced productivity in later years."[14] A CSHP provides the integration of education and health.

The importance of the school health program is also evident by its inclusion in the national health objectives for the year 2020. Of all the objectives listed in the publication *Healthy People 2020: Understanding and Improving Health,* a significant number can either be directly attained by schools or their attainment can be influenced in important ways by schools (see Box 6.2).

Nevertheless, a CSHP is not a cure-all. There are no quick and easy solutions to improving the overall health of a community. However, a CSHP provides a strong base on which to build.

FOUNDATIONS OF THE SCHOOL HEALTH PROGRAM

The true foundations of any school health program are (1) a school administration that supports such an effort; (2) a well-organized school health council that is genuinely interested in providing a coordinated program for the students, families, and staff; and (3) written school health policies. A highly supportive administration is a must for a quality CSHP. In almost all organizations—and schools are no different—the administration controls resources. Without leadership and support from top school administrators, it will be an ongoing struggle to provide a quality program. Furthermore, every effort should be made to employ personnel who are appropriately trained to carry out their responsibilities as members of the school health council. For example, the National Association of School Nurses has taken the position that "every school-aged child deserves a school nurse who is a graduate of a baccalaureate degree program from an accredited college or university and licensed by that state as a registered nurse,"[15] yet many school nurses without college degrees and training in health education are

Table 6.1
Health Education Standards for School Health Educators

Standard I: Demonstrate the knowledge and skills of a health literate educator
   A. Describe the theoretical foundations of health behavior and principles of learning.
   B. Describe the National Health Education Standards.
   C. Describe practices that promote health or safety.
   D. Describe behaviors that might compromise health or safety.
   E. Describe disease etiology and prevention practices.
   F. Demonstrate the health literacy skills of an informed consumer of health products and services.

Standard II: Assess needs to determine priorities for school health education
   A. Access a variety of reliable data sources related to health.
   B. Collect health-related data
   C. Infer needs for health education from data obtained.

Standard III: Plan effective comprehensive school health education curricula and programs
   A. Design strategies for involving key individuals and organizations in program planning for School Health Education.
   B. Design a logical scope and sequence of learning experiences that accommodate all students.
   C. Create appropriate and measurable learner objectives that align with assessments and scoring rubrics.
   D. Select developmentally appropriate strategies to meet learning objectives.
   E. Align health education curricula with needs assessment data and the National Health Education Standards.
   F. Analyze the feasibility of implementing selected strategies.

Standard IV: Implement health education instruction
   A. Demonstrate multiple strategies that reflect effective pedagogy, and health education theories and models that facilitate learning for all students.
   B. Utilize technology and resources that provide instruction in challenging, clear, and compelling ways and engage diverse learners.
   C. Exhibit competence in classroom management.
   D. Reflect on their implementation practices, adjusting objectives, instructional strategies and assessments as necessary to enhance student learning.

Standard V: Assess student learning
   A. Develop assessment plans.
   B. Analyze available assessment instruments.
   C. Develop instruments to assess student learning.
   D. Implement plans to assess student learning.
   E. Utilize assessment results to guide future instruction.

Standard VI: Plan and coordinate a school health education program.
   A. Develop a plan for comprehensive school health education within a coordinated school health program.
   B. Explain how a health education program fits the culture of a school and contributes to the school's mission.
   C. Design a plan to collaborate with others such as school personnel, community health educators, and students' families in planning and implementing health education programs.

Standard VII: Serve as a resource person in health education
   A. Use health information resources.
   B. Respond to requests for health information.
   C. Select educational resource materials for dissemination.
   D. Describe ways to establish effective consultative relationships with others involved in Coordinated School Health Programs.

Standard VIII: Communicate and advocate for health and school health education
   A. Analyze and respond to factors that impact current and future needs in comprehensive school health education.
   B. Apply a variety of communication methods and techniques.
   C. Advocate for school health education.
   D. Demonstrate professionalism.

Source: American Association for Health Education (2008). "2008 NCATE Health Education Teacher Preparation Standards." Available at http://www.ncate.org/institutions/programStandards.asp?ch=4. Accessed October 15, 2010.

BOX
6.1

IT IS HARDER TO LEARN IF YOU ARE NOT HEALTHY! A LOOK AT THE IMPACT OF CHILDHOOD OBESITY

It stands to reason that if children are not healthy, it is harder for them to concentrate and in turn to have a meaningful learning experience. One such example that is significantly affecting students and schools is the obesity epidemic. Childhood obesity has more than tripled in the past 30 years, with the prevalence affecting nearly 20% of children and adolescents. Experts have determined that body mass index (BMI) is the most practical tool available to define obesity and screen for it.

Childhood obesity is often accompanied by numerous other health conditions, such as increased rates of type 2 diabetes, cardiovascular problems, sleep apnea, and bone and joint problems. The reasons for the obesity epidemic are varied but are slowly becoming understood. Increased soft drink consumption is one such reason: Consumption of soft drinks increased 41% in the first 5 years of the 1990s. The impact of soft drink consumption is not just felt by those who consume the drinks, but also by those who benefit from the consumption—schools. In 2006, the School Health Policies and Practices Study (SHPPS) found that nearly 65% received a percentage of the sales receipts from soft drinks and one-third received incentives such as cash awards or donations of equipment once receipts totaled a specified amount. Couple this with schools failing to provide the recommended daily physical education and providing poor nutritional offerings, and it is no wonder that the obesity problem is affecting schools. Researchers are beginning to determine some of the social, psychological, and educational consequences of obesity. A review of the literature determined that overweight and obese children are more likely to have low self-esteem, higher rates of anxiety disorders, and depression. Severely obese kids report many more missed days of school than the general student population. What is yet to be understood is why these kids miss more school—are they embarrassed to participate in physical activity? Are health conditions keeping them from school? Are they experiencing bullying or teasing? Although there is no known reason, the consequences are significant.

One way schools are addressing concerns about overweight children is by establishing policies related to improved nutritional offerings in the cafeteria, school parties and events, and vending machines, as well as increasing nutrition education and physical activity. The Child Nutrition and WIC Reauthorization Act of 2004 (Public Law 108-265) required all schools participating in the federally funded school feeding programs to establish a local wellness policy by the first day of the 2006–2007 school year. This law helped many districts begin the process of improving the school environment, not just to improve the obesity problem, but to make school a healthier place for all.

Most recently the issue of obesity has become a priority in the White House with First Lady Michelle Obama's *Let's Move!* campaign. The *Let's Move!* campaign "has an ambitious national goal of solving the challenge of childhood obesity within a generation so that children born today will reach adulthood at a healthy weight." The campaign includes a comprehensive approach that will provide schools, families, and communities simple tools to help kids be more active, eat better, and get healthy. As part of this campaign, chefs across the country are getting involved in the fight against obesity by adopting a school in their community and working with teachers, parents, school nutritionists, and administrators to help educate kids about food and nutrition. Further, President Obama has established the first ever Task Force on Childhood Obesity with the charge of "conducting a review of every single program and policy relating to child nutrition and physical activity and develop a national action plan to maximize federal resources and set concrete benchmarks toward the First Lady's national goal." What are you doing in the fight against obesity? The time to take action is now!

Sources: Division of Adolescent and School Health, Centers for Disease Control and Prevention (2010). School Health Policies and Practices Study. Available at http://www.cdc.gov/healthyyouth/shpps/index.htm; Taras, H., and W. Potts-Datema (2005). "Obesity and Student Performance at School." *Journal of School Health*, 75(8): 291–295; Division of Adolescent and School Health, Centers for Disease Control and Prevention (2010). "Childhood Obesity." Available at http://www.cdc.gov/healthyyouth/obesity/index.htm; and The White House (2010). "Let's Move." Available at http://www.letsmove.gov/. Accessed January 4, 2011.

BOX
6.2

HEALTHY PEOPLE 2020: OBJECTIVES

Educational and Community-Based Programs

Goal: Increase the quality, availability, and effectiveness of educational and community-based programs designed to prevent disease and injury, improve health, and enhance quality of life.

Objective: ECBP-2. Increase the proportion of elementary, middle, and senior high schools that provide comprehensive school health education to prevent health problems in the following areas: unintentional injury; violence; suicide; tobacco use and addiction; alcohol or other drug use; unintended pregnancy, HIV/AIDS, and STD infection; unhealthy dietary patterns; and inadequate physical activity.

ECBP 2.2 Unintentional Injury

Target: 89.9 percent.

Baseline: 81.7 percent of elementary, middle, and senior high schools provided comprehensive school health education to prevent unintentional injury in 2006.

Target setting method: 10 percent improvement.

Data source: School Health Policies and Programs Study (SHPPS), CDC, NCCDPHP.

ECBP 2.6 Alcohol and Other Drug Use

Target: 90.0 percent.

Baseline: 81.8 percent of elementary, middle, and senior high schools provided comprehensive school health education to prevent alcohol and other drug use in 2006.

Target setting method: 10 percent improvement.

Data source: School Health Policies and Programs Study (SHPPS), CDC, NCCDPHP.

ECBP 2.8 Unhealthy Dietary Patterns

Target: 92.7 percent.

Baseline: 84.3 percent of elementary, middle, and senior high schools provided comprehensive school health education to prevent unhealthy dietary patterns in 2006.

Target setting method: 10 percent improvement.

Data source: School Health Policies and Programs Study (SHPPS), CDC, NCCDPHP.

Note: Other areas covered by this objective include: 2.1 All Priority Areas, 2.3 Violence, 2.4 Suicide, 2.5 Tobacco Use and Addition, 2.7 Unintended Pregnancy, HIV/AIDS, and STD Infection, and 2.9 Inadequate Physical Activity.

For Further Thought

Assuming money is available, why doesn't every school district in the nation have a coordinated school health program?

Source: U.S. Department of Health and Human Services, Office of Disease Prevention and Health Promotion (2010). *Healthy People 2020.* Available at http://www.healthypeople.gov/2020/default.aspx. Accessed January 4, 2011.

---

asked to provide health education. Conversely, certified teachers who lack preparation in school health are required to teach health to secure a job.[16] Qualified personnel are a must.

school health policies
written statements that describe the nature and procedures of a school health program

SCHOOL HEALTH POLICIES

School health policies, which "include laws, mandates, regulations, standards, resolutions, and guidelines, provide a foundation for school district practices and procedures."[17] The written policy also describes the nature of the program and the procedure for its implementation to those outside the program.[18] Well-written school health policies provide a sense of direction and a means of accountability and credibility, and strengthen the possibility that a school health program will become "an institutionalized part of the school culture."[19] Steps for creating local health-related policies include the following:[20,21]

1. Identify the policy development team.
2. Assess the district's needs.
3. Prioritize needs and develop an action plan.
4. Draft a policy.
5. Build awareness and support.
6. Adopt and implement the policy.
7. Maintain, measure, and evaluate.

Policy Development

The development of a set of written policies is not an easy task. This challenging and time-consuming task should be executed by the school health council because the council includes those most knowledgeable about the school health program in addition to representing many different constituencies in the school community.

The policies should cover all facets of the school health program. Table 6.2 provides a checklist that can be used for developing policies. Also, several professional associations that have an interest in school health programs have written a number of policy statements relating to school health issues. A few such associations are the American Academy of Pediatrics (information available at www.aap.org), the American School Health Association (information available at www.ashaweb.org), the American Association for Health Education (information available at www.aahperd.org/aahe), and the Association for Supervision and Curriculum Development (information available at www.ascd.org).

Once the policies have been written, it is important that they receive approval from key stakeholders. Although the school board is the final authority that adopts policies, approval from school administrators, school-based committees, parents, and other key stakeholders can aid in the implementation process.[22] The approval process provides credibility to the policies as well as legal protection for those who must implement the policies.[18]

Policy Implementation

The development of written policies is an important step in building a solid base for a CSHP. However, if the policies are never implemented, the school district will be no better off than before their development.

Implementation begins with the distribution of the policies to those who will be affected by them—faculty, staff, students, and parents. Some ideas for carrying out this process include (1) distributing the policies with a memorandum of explanation, (2) placing the policies in both faculty/staff and student handbooks, (3) presenting them at a gathering of the different groups (e.g., at staff or parent-teacher organization [PTO] meetings, or an open house), (4) holding a special meeting for the specific purpose of explaining the policies, and (5) placing them in the school district newsletter. News releases might even be considered if the policies include major changes. Each school district must decide the best way to disseminate its school health policies.

Policy Development Resources

Because of the requirements of the Child Nutrition and WIC Reauthorization Act of 2004 to implement a school wellness policy by districts,[23] numerous resources have become available to help schools develop policies. Action for Healthy Kids (AFHK) is one such organization that is advocating and providing support for making changes in schools to address childhood obesity and undernourishment by working with schools to improve nutrition and physical activity.

Table 6.2
A Checklist for Developing Written Policies

	PIP	PN	NA
I. Administration and Organization			
A. Duties and Responsibilities of the Coordinator of the School Health Program			
B. Duties and Responsibilities of the School Health Council			
C. Responsibilities of School Health Personnel			
D. School Health Records			
E. General School Health Policies			
1. Use of prescribed medication in the school including self-administration of asthmas medications			
2. Report of child abuse and neglect			
3. Substance use/abuse			
4. Student health insurance			
5. Health policies for after-school activities (including emergency care)			
6. Sending ill/injured students home			
7. Relationships with community health agencies/organizations			
8. In-service health programs for teachers			
II. School Health Services			
A. Emergency Care for Illness/Injury			
B. Students with Special Needs			
C. Health Appraisal			
1. Medical examinations			
2. Screening programs			
3. Dental examinations			
4. Social and psychological evaluations			
5. Policy for health referrals to parents			
D. Communicable Disease Control			
III. Healthy School Environment			
A. Safety Program			
B. Safety Patrol and Bus Safety			
C. Emergency Drills (fire, tornado, etc.)			
D. Drug-Free Schools			
E. Safe/Violence-Free Schools Including Bullying and Electronic Aggression			
F. Student Discipline			
G. Universal Precautions			
H. Hazardous Materials			
IV. School Health Education			
A. Procedures for Curriculum Development and Revision			
B. Individual Education Programs for Special Needs Students			
V. School Food Service			
VI. School Counseling, Psychological, and Social Services			
VII. School Physical Education			
VIII. School-Site Health Promotion for Faculty and Staff			
IX. Integrated School, Family, and Community Health Promotion Efforts			

Code: PIP = Policy in place. PN = Policy needed. NA = Not applicable to our district.

Source: Adapted from McKenzie, J. F. (1983). "Written Policies: Developing a Solid Foundation for a Comprehensive School Health Program." *Future Focus: Ohio Journal of Health, Physical Education, Recreation and Dance*, 4(3): 9–11.

AFHK has created a partner network of more than 65 national organizations and associations representing leaders in health, education, nutrition, fitness, business, government agencies, and other organizations that serve and care about youth.[24] Sample wellness policies and a clearinghouse of related resources, including policy development guides, are available at the AFHK Web site (www.actionforhealthykids.org). Tools to assist schools in conducting needs assessments related to the CSHP include the School Health Index, available free from the Centers for Disease Control and Prevention (CDC) (www.cdc.gov/healthyyouth/shi/index.htm) and Creating a Healthy School Using the Healthy School Report Card: An ASCD Action Tool, available for purchase from the Association for Supervision and Curriculum Development (ASCD) (http://shop.ascd.org).

Monitoring the Status of School Health Policy in the United States

Because school health policy is an important foundation for CSHPs, the Division of Adolescent Health at the CDC conducts a national survey to assess school health policies and practices at the state, district, school, and classroom levels. The survey, which is titled the School Health Policies and Practices Study (SHPPS), has been conducted every 6 years since 1994. Specifically, SHPPS is used to do the following:[25]

- Describe characteristics of each component of school health at various levels and across elementary, middle, and high schools.
- Describe the professional background of the personnel who deliver each component of the school health program.
- Describe collaboration among components of school health programs.
- Describe how key policies and practices have changed over time.

Results of these national surveys are available at the Division of Adolescent and School Health's Web site.

COMPONENTS OF A COORDINATED SCHOOL HEALTH PROGRAM

If implemented appropriately, a coordinated approach to school health can have a significant positive impact on the overall health status of students, staff, and the community, which, in turn, can be linked to higher academic achievement for students. To do so, all eight components illustrated in Figure 6.1 need to be provided in a coordinated fashion. Because of the limitation of space, we discuss the importance of the administration and organization of the eight components, provide an overview of the three traditional components of the school health program—(1) school health services, (2) healthy school environment, and (3) health education—and provide a brief explanation of the five additional components.

Administration and Organization

Effective administration and organization of the school health program ensure that the people and activities that constitute the program work in a coordinated manner to meet the program's goals. As previously noted, the responsibility for coordinating the program in each school district should be delegated to a properly trained and knowledgeable individual. Logical choices for this position of **school health coordinator** would be a trained school nurse or a health education specialist.[8] Whereas nearly two-thirds of school districts in the United States employ school health coordinators, there are only a few states that require such a person.[25,26]

The American Cancer Society has taken a leadership role in training leaders for school health programs. In 1999, the American Cancer Society conducted the first National School Health Coordinator Leadership Institute, the beginning of a 3-year training program for school health coordinators around the United States. As a result of the success of the institute, a number of replications have been implemented around the country, some as state replication programs and others with specific school districts, such as urban school districts.[27] The following are responsibilities common to school health coordinators:[28,29]

school health coordinator
a professional at the district (or school) level responsible for management and coordination of all school health policies, activities, and resources

- Ensuring that the instruction and services provided through various components of the school health program are mutually reinforcing and present consistent messages
- Facilitating collaboration among school health program personnel and between them and other school staff
- Assisting the superintendent/school principal and other administrative staff with the integration, management, and supervision of the school health program
- Providing or arranging for necessary technical assistance
- Identifying necessary resources
- Facilitating collaboration between the district/school and other agencies and organizations in the community who have an interest in the health and well-being of children and their families
- Conducting evaluation activities that assess the implementation and results of the school health program, as well as assisting with reporting evaluation results

School Health Services

school health services
health services provided by school health workers to appraise, protect, and promote the health of students

School health services are those health "services provided for students to appraise, protect, and promote health."[30] Specifically, those services offered by schools include health appraisals (screenings and examinations), emergency care for injury and sudden illness, management of chronic disease, prevention and control of communicable disease, provisions for special needs students, health counseling, and remediation of detected health problems within the limits of state laws through referral and follow-up by the school nurse and teachers (see Figure 6.4). Originally, the intent of school health services was to supplement rather than to supplant the family's responsibility for meeting the health care needs of its children. However, because of the poorer health status of youth, the involvement of youth in high-risk behaviors (such as smoking, drinking, substance abuse, and unprotected sexual intercourse), and such barriers to health care as inadequate health insurance and lack of providers, there has been a broadening of the role of schools in providing health care.

Because school attendance is required throughout the United States, schools represent our best opportunity to reach many of those children in need of proper health care. More than 95% of all youths aged 5 to 17 years are enrolled in schools.[31]"The school's ability to reach children and youth slipping through the cracks of the health care system and at highest risk for poor health and potentially health-threatening behaviors is unmatched."[32] The advantages of having school health services include the following:[33]

- *Equitability.* School health services provide a point of entry into the health care system for all children in school.
- *Breadth of coverage.* Many preventive services are provided that are not covered in a majority of health insurance policies.
- *Confidentiality.*
- *User friendliness.* The school is an environment with which students are familiar and in which they feel comfortable.
- *Convenience.* Services are accessible to all students.

Each school district is unique, from the demographics of its students to the availability of its health resources. The American Academy of Pediatrics (AAP) recommends that at minimum schools should provide the following three types of services: (1) state-mandated services, including health screenings, verification of immunization status, and infectious disease reporting; (2) assessment of minor health complaints, medication administration, and care for students with special needs; and (3) management of emergencies and other urgent situations.[33] When resources permit, more comprehensive services may be offered, such as administration of immunizations, case management, wellness promotion, and patient education.[34]

Expanded services are increasingly being offered through school-based, mobile, and school-linked programs. School-based health centers (SBHCs) have been defined as "a health center located in a school or on school grounds that provides, at a minimum, on-site primary and preventive health care, mental health counseling, health promotion, referral and follow-up services for young people enrolled."[35] Mobile programs are those "without a fixed site that rotate a health care team through a number of schools."[36] School-linked health centers (SLHCs) are typically coordinated at the school but delivered off campus through collaborations with community clinics, hospitals, or other health care professionals and agencies.[37] A number of health care professionals are employed on a full-time basis for these programs to function successfully. The idea of young people receiving more comprehensive health care within the context of the school setting is gaining momentum throughout the country and is discussed in greater detail later in this chapter.

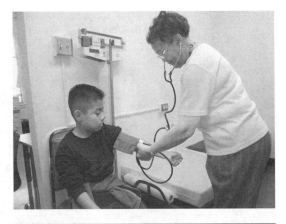

FIGURE 6.4
Health screenings are important components of school health services.

Healthy School Environment

The term *healthy school environment* designates the part of a CSHP that provides for a safe—both physically and emotionally—learning environment (see Figure 6.5). If children are not placed in a safe environment, learning becomes difficult at best. The most comprehensive definition of **healthy school environment** was provided by the 1972–1973 Joint Committee on Health Education Terminology. They stated that providing a healthy school environment includes "the promotion, maintenance, and utilization of safe and wholesome surroundings, organization of day-by-day experiences and planned learning procedures to influence favorable emotional, physical and social health."[38] The CDC, while brief, expands the definition to include school culture, defining the healthy school environment as "the physical and aesthetic surroundings and the psychosocial climate and culture of the school."[30]

By law, school districts are required to provide a safe school environment. However, the responsibility for maintaining this safe environment should rest with all who use it. Everyone, including those on the board of education, administrators, teachers, custodial staff, and students, must contribute to make a school a safer place through their daily actions. An unsafe school environment can exist only if those responsible for it and those who use it allow it to exist.

healthy school environment the promotion, maintenance, and utilization of safe and wholesome surroundings in a school

The Physical Environment

The physical environment of a school can be divided into two major categories. The first is the actual physical plant—the buildings and surrounding areas and all that come with them. The second is the behaviors of those using the buildings. The factors that must be considered when looking at the physical plant include (1) where the school is located, (2) the age of the buildings, (3) the traffic patterns in and around the school, (4) indoor air quality, (5) pest management, (6) temperature control, (7) lighting, (8) acoustics, (9) water supply/quality, (10) sanitation, (11) food service, (12) playgrounds, (13) school bus safety, and, more recently

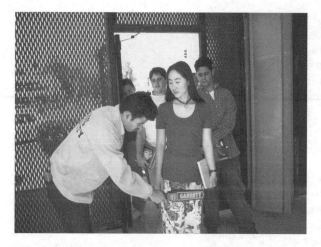

FIGURE 6.5
The school should be a safe and healthy place to learn.

(14) green building design, among other items. Each school district should have an appropriate protocol for dealing with and maintaining these aspects of the physical environment.[39]

The behavior of both the school personnel and students in the school environment also affects the safety of the environment. Each year a significant number of students throughout the country are injured on their way to, at, or on their way home from school. Some of these injuries occur from an unsafe physical plant that is in need of repair, but many occur from inappropriate behavior. Unsafe behavior that is observed too frequently in schools includes acts of violence between students and lack of proper supervision by school employees. However, most do not worry about a safe environment until they are faced with a problem. Every school building in the United States could become a safer environment if greater attention were given to prevention than to a cure.

The Psychosocial Environment

Although a safe physical environment is important, a safe psychosocial environment is equally important. This portion of the school environment "encompasses the attitudes, feelings, and values of students and staff."[40] Students who are fearful of responding to a teacher's question because the teacher might make fun of them if they answer incorrectly or students who avoid being in the halls during passing time because of fear of being bullied are not learning in a healthy psychosocial environment. For many, learning does not come easily, and anxiety-producing factors such as these can only make it more difficult.

The ways in which school personnel and students treat each other can also add much to the teaching/learning process (see Figure 6.6). All individuals within the school should be treated with respect. People should be polite and courteous to each other. This does not mean that high academic standards should be abandoned and that everyone should agree with all that others do, but students and teachers should not be afraid to express themselves in a cooperative, respectful way. For example, think back to your middle school and high school days. Think about the teachers you liked best. Did you like them because they were great teachers and knew their subject well? Or did you like them because of the way they treated and respected you? The psychosocial environment can have a significant impact on the school environment!

Implementing a school crisis plan can assist with addressing situations that affect both the physical and social environments. A clear, written plan that includes procedures for handling various emergencies (e.g., fire, tornado, death of a student or staff member, mass illness, terrorism, suicide attempt), communication procedures, staff training, practice drills, coordination with local public safety agencies, among other procedures, can help ensure, when threats occur, that safe practices are implemented.[25,39]

school health education
the development, delivery, and evaluation of a planned curriculum, kindergarten through grade 12

School Health Education

School health education provides students with a "planned, sequential, K–12 curriculum that addresses the physical, mental, emotional and social dimensions of health. The curriculum is designed to motivate and assist students to maintain and improve their health, prevent disease, and reduce health-related risk behaviors."[30] If designed properly, school health education could be one of the most effective means to reduce serious health problems in the

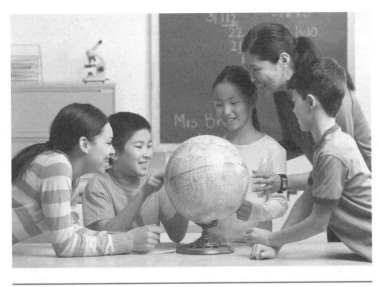

FIGURE 6.6
A healthy social environment, conducive to learning, is an important component
of good school health.

United States, including cardiovascular disease, cancer, motor vehicle crashes, homicide, and
suicide.[41] Such a curriculum should focus on promoting the following priority health
content:[42]

- Alcohol and other drugs
- Healthy eating
- Mental and emotional health
- Personal health and wellness
- Physical activity
- Safety/unintentional injury prevention
- Sexual health (abstinence and risk avoidance)
- Tobacco
- Violence prevention

School health education includes all health education in the school. It includes health
education that takes place in the classroom as well as any other activities designed to positively influence the health knowledge and skills of students, parents, and school staff. For
example, health education can take place when the school nurse gives a vision screening test
to a student or when coaches talk with their teams about the abuse of drugs.

For health education to be effective, it should be well conceived and carefully planned.
The written plan for school health education is referred to as the health **curriculum**. The
curriculum not only outlines the **scope** (what will be taught) and the **sequence** (when it
will be taught) but also provides (1) learning objectives, (2) standards (see Box 6.3),
(3) learning activities, (4) possible instructional resources, and (5) methods for assessment to
determine the extent to which the objectives and standards are met. If health instruction is to
be effective, the health curriculum should include lessons of appropriate scope and sequence
for all grades from kindergarten through the twelfth grade.

curriculum
a written plan for
instruction

scope
part of the curriculum
that outlines what will
be taught

sequence
part of the curriculum
that states in what
order the content will
be taught

BOX
6.3

NATIONAL HEALTH EDUCATION STANDARDS

1. Students will comprehend concepts related to health promotion and disease prevention to enhance health.
2. Students will analyze the influence of family, peers, culture, media, technology, and other factors on health behaviors.
3. Students will demonstrate the ability to access valid information and products and services to enhance health.
4. Students will demonstrate the ability to use interpersonal communication skills to enhance health and avoid or reduce health risks.
5. Students will demonstrate the ability to use decision-making skills to enhance health.

6. Students will demonstrate the ability to use goal setting to enhance health.
7. Students will demonstrate the ability to practice health-enhancing behaviors to avoid or reduce health risks.
8. Students will demonstrate the ability to advocate for personal, family, and community health.

Source: Reprinted with permission, from the American Cancer Society. *National Health Education Standards: Achieving Excellence*, 2nd ed. (Atlanta, GA: American Cancer Society), 8. Available at cancer.org/bookstore. Accessed November 29, 2010.

As with the CSHP, results from CDC's School Health Policies and Practices Study (SHPPS) show that good school health instruction is not widespread. To enhance the state of health instruction in schools National Health Education Standards have been developed. The National Health Education Standards delineate the essential knowledge and skills that every student should know and be able to do following the completion of quality school health education. The standards are not a federal mandate or national curriculum, but rather provide a foundation for curriculum development, instructional delivery, and assessment of student knowledge and skills for students in grades pre-K–12.[43] There are eight standards (see Box 6.3), and each standard has grade-level performance indicators set for grades pre-K–2, 3–5, 6–8, and 9–12. "The standards evolved from the health education profession's current thinking about what constitutes grade-appropriate and challenging content and performance expectations for students."[44] Currently, 72% of states mandating standards-based health education have used the National Health Education Standards as their basis for requirements and recommendations.[25]

Development of and Sources of Health Education Curricula

Each year, many school districts throughout the United States are faced with the task of developing a curriculum to guide health education. Such a task can be completed in one of several ways. First, a school district could obtain a prepackaged curriculum that has been developed by nationally recognized specialists. Some of these are prepared and sold by for-profit organizations, and others are available free of charge from nonprofit agencies (i.e., voluntary health agencies). A second means is to use the approved curriculum of either the state departments of education or health. A third method is to adopt a new health textbook series and consider the series as a district's curricular guide. And fourth, some districts may even develop their own in-house curriculum. Each of these approaches has its strengths and weaknesses, and school districts have to decide which approach best suits their particular situation.

Determining what is and what is not a good curriculum can be a difficult process. Some very poor curricula, packaged in a slick way, can convince administrators that they have purchased a very fine product. Conversely, some educationally sound programs may not be well packaged. Fortunately, resources are available to help reduce the guesswork for those who must select curricula. See Box 6.4 for a summary of characteristics of effective health education curricula, which can serve as a guide when evaluating and selecting materials.

BOX
6.4

CHARACTERISTICS OF EFFECTIVE HEALTH EDUCATION CURRICULA

- Focuses on clear health goals and related behavioral outcomes
- Is research-based and theory-driven
- Addresses individual values and group norms that support health-enhancing behaviors
- Focuses on increasing the personal perception of risk and harmfulness of engaging in specific health risk behaviors and reinforcing protective factors
- Addresses social pressures and influences
- Builds personal competence, social competence, and self-efficacy by addressing skills
- Provides functional health knowledge that is basic, accurate, and directly contributes to health-promoting decisions and behaviors
- Uses strategies designed to personalize information and engage students
- Provides age-appropriate and developmentally appropriate information, learning strategies, teaching methods, and materials

- Incorporates learning strategies, teaching methods, and materials that are culturally inclusive
- Provides adequate time for instruction and learning
- Provides opportunities to reinforce skills and positive health behaviors
- Provides opportunities to make positive connections with influential others (e.g., peers, parents or other caregivers, families, and other positive adult role models)
- Includes teacher information and plans for professional development and training that enhances the effectiveness of instruction and student learning

Source: Centers for Disease Control and Prevention (2007). *Health Education Curriculum Assessment Tool.* Atlanta, GA: Author, 5–6.

A number of federal agencies have created processes for reviewing, approving, and recommending health education programs that are effective. The CDC maintains a list of registries sponsored by federal agencies that include programs effective in reducing youth risk behaviors.[45] Most of these registries allow curriculum developers to nominate their curricula for review. The review process typically involves peer review by three or more professionals with expertise in the specific area. Programs deemed worthy of recommendation based on the expert review process can be found on the various registries identified on the CDC Web site.[45] Additionally, the CDC has developed the Health Education Curriculum Analysis Tool (HECAT), a resource school districts, schools, and others involved in the curriculum process can use to conduct their own analysis of health curricula. The HECAT, which is based on the National Health Education Standards and CDC's Characteristics of Effective Health Education Curriculum, can help in the selection or development of appropriate and effective health education curricula and improve the delivery of health education.[42]

In addition to using programs described on the various registries or evaluating curriculum yourself, a number of other sources are available for obtaining health curricula. Some of them may be comprehensive (include a variety of topics and for every grade level, K–12), and others may be topic and/or grade-level specific. These other sources include the following:

- *State departments of education or health.* A number of states have either recommended or required a particular curriculum. Some states do not have comprehensive curricula but require instruction in some of the more controversial health topics, such as substance use and abuse and sexuality education.

- *Health agencies and associations.* Many of the voluntary health agencies (e.g., American Cancer Society, American Heart Association, and American Lung Association) and other health-related organizations (e.g., National Dairy Council, Hazelden Foundation [cyber bullying], and Indiana Organ Procurement Organization) have developed curricula for grades K–12. Most of these are not comprehensive, but they are usually well done, supported by audiovisuals and handouts, and available either at very low or no cost.

- *Commercially produced curricula.* These curricula have been developed by private corporations for schools.

Counseling, Psychological, and Social Services

Counseling, psychological, and social services are services provided to improve students' mental, emotional, and social health. These services can include individual and group assessments, interventions, and referrals. Professionals such as certified school counselors, psychologists, and social workers provide these services.[30]

Physical Education

Physical education is defined as a "planned, sequential K–12 curriculum that provides cognitive content and learning experiences in a variety of activity areas."[30] Emphasis is placed on physical fitness and skill development that lead to lifelong physical activity. Physical education should be taught by qualified teachers.[30]

School Nutrition Services

School nutrition services should provide access to a variety of nutritious and appealing meals that accommodate the health and nutrition needs of all students in a school district. Additionally, the school nutrition services program should offer students a learning laboratory for classroom nutrition and health education. The program should also serve as a resource for links with nutrition-related community services.[30]

Family/Community Involvement for School Health

Family/community involvement allows for an "integrated school, parent, and community approach for enhancing the health and well-being of students."[30] The school is an agency within a community that cannot function in isolation. Schools that actively engage parents and community resources in their school health councils, curriculum committees, and other health-related programming respond more effectively to the health-related needs of students.[30]

School-Site Health Promotion for Staff

School-site health promotion for staff includes "opportunities for school staff to improve their health status" through health-related assessments and activities.[30] These opportunities encourage staff to engage in healthy behaviors, resulting in improved health status, improved morale, positive health role modeling, reduced health insurance costs, and decreased absenteeism.[30]

ISSUES AND CONCERNS FACING THE SCHOOL HEALTH PROGRAM

Like most other community health programs, the school health program is not without its issues and concerns. "In the 1940s, the three leading school discipline problems were talking, chewing gum, and making noise."[46] Today, many of the leading school discipline problems are related to health, such as the distribution of prescription medications, violence, obesity, and the consequences of low self-esteem. In the remainder of this chapter, we summarize a few of the challenges that still lie ahead for those who work in school health.

Lack of Support for Coordinated School Health Programs

"Schools offer the most systematic and efficient means available to improve the health of youth and enable young people to avoid health risks,"[47] yet, ironically, school health advocates have had limited success in getting a CSHP implemented in school districts across the country.

We have already pointed out that healthy children are better learners and that a CSHP can contribute to the health of children. A CSHP "can provide a safe haven for teaching and learning by addressing the immediate needs of the whole child. In the long term, it can have a significant effect on youth development and academic achievement."[10]

Although many Americans support the idea that everyone is entitled to good health, we have not supported through legislation the notion that everyone is entitled to a CSHP. Obviously, getting legislation passed is a complicated process and is dependent on a number of different circumstances, including, but not limited to, economics, social action, and politics. Additionally, limited resources, lack of buy-in and investment, the inability of schools to demonstrate competence and effectiveness to stakeholders, lack of organizational capacity, leadership support, and continued emphasis on high-stakes testing have made it difficult for school districts to make a CSHP a priority.[48,49] This difficult task should not deter those who feel coordinated school health is vital. It is becoming clearer that many of the answers to current and future health problems lie with the resources found in the school—the one institution of society through which all of us must pass. The following are a few examples of the impact coordinated school health can have:

- At the present time, the key to dealing with the AIDS problem is education.
- The biggest stride in improving the health of the country will not come from new technology but from the health behavior in which we engage.
- Many of the primary health care services needed by the children of this country are not available because of the barriers of the health care system.[50]
- Effective school-based prevention programs have been estimated to save society $18 per $1 invested. "If effective prevention programs were implemented nationwide, substance abuse initiation would decline for 1.5 million youth and be delayed for 2 years on average."[51]

The need for coordinated school health should be obvious to all. We have taken the liberty to rephrase a quote from a group of school health experts who say it best: Society should not be as concerned with what happens when we implement a CSHP as about what is likely to happen if we do not.[52] Although garnering support for CSHPs has been an uphill battle, we are moving in the right direction. As mentioned earlier in the chapter, with the passing of the Child Nutrition and WIC Reauthorization Act of 2004,[23] school districts are required to institute local wellness policies promoting better nutrition, physical activity, and wellness. Some states have taken this one step further by passing state legislation requiring districts to institute coordinated school health advisory councils.[53] The inclusion of "coordinated school health" in the title of these councils encourages many districts to begin talking about, developing, and/or implementing a CSHP.

School Health Curriculum Challenges

Controversy

The words *sexual intercourse*, *suicide*, *substance use and abuse*, *sexually transmitted diseases*, *dating violence*, *contraception*, *death and dying*, and even *abstinence* get attention. The very nature of the topics covered in a school health education curriculum today continue

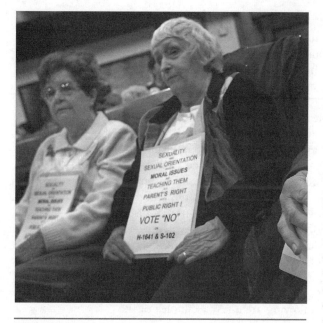

FIGURE 6.7

There are still many controversial issues that surround health coordinated school health programs.

to create controversy in some districts and in different parts of the country. Yet, controversy is not new to school health education; it has followed health education ever since it first attempted to deal with the many issues that face youth (see Figure 6.7).

Controversy continues to be a challenge for health education for a number of reasons. Part of it deals with the pressure that has been applied to schools by conservative groups. These groups are interested in discouraging health instruction that includes values-clarification activities and open-ended decision-making processes.[54] Others believe that controversy exists because of the differences in family value systems and religious beliefs. Questions such as (1) Do students really need to learn in school how to use a condom? (2) Doesn't talk of suicide lead some students to think that it might be the best alternative for them? (3) Aren't chiropractors just health quacks? and (4) Why do students need to know about funeral preplanning in high school? create legitimate concerns, but they are also issues that today's adolescents face. Lack of awareness, knowledge, and skills is not an excuse for undesirable health behavior. If the students do not get this information at school, where will they get it? Studies have shown that the institutions of church and family have taught little about the controversial topics included in health curricula.

Improper Implementation

Improper implementation of the curriculum is another challenge to school health (see Box 6.5). Because health is not considered a "core" subject in most school districts, it has received little attention and support. In many school districts throughout the United States, the low priority given to health has meant that much of the health education is provided by individuals other than health education specialists. These people are not incapable of teaching health, but they have not been educated to do so. Reliance on a textbook as the curriculum, lack of awareness/implementation of state or national standards, an emphasis on content rather than skills, and limited, if any, coverage of topics that cause discomfort are some of the outcomes of improperly prepared teachers in the health classroom. The long-term result is young people do not learn the skills necessary to live a healthy lifestyle.

School districts can help reduce controversy and improve the quality of health instruction provided by (1) implementing age-appropriate curricula, (2) using acceptable teaching methods, (3) gaining parent/guardian approval of curricula and teaching methods, (4) developing a school policy that enables parents/guardians to review the curricula and to withdraw their children from lessons that go against family or religious beliefs, (5) implementing a school policy that provides for the handling of concern by parents/guardians,[50] and (6) making sure qualified and interested teachers teach health.

School-Based Health Centers or School-Linked Health Centers

Earlier in the chapter, we mentioned that a number of school districts across the country are opening school-based, mobile, or linked health centers to help meet the health needs of their students. Yet, the concept of offering comprehensive health care services through school-based or school-linked health centers is still a relatively new one. In 1970, only one U.S. school

---

BOX
6.5

BARRIERS TO SCHOOL HEALTH EDUCATION

Although the importance of school health education is being recognized more and more, there are several barriers to its implementation. Research by various authors has informed health education specialists of barriers to establishing effective health instruction. Those barriers include the following:

1. Lack of local administrative commitment
2. Lack of adequately prepared teachers
3. Lack of time in the school day/year
4. Lack of money/funds
5. Health education's lack of credibility as an academic subject
6. Lack of community/parental support for controversial topics
7. Policy constraints
8. Teacher priorities
9. Pressure to focus on subjects included in high-stakes tests
10. General lack of reinforcement by state and local education policymakers

The top three barriers tend to be seen as the most significant. Recommendations to address them include the following:

1. Inviting administrators to workshops and conferences dealing with current health issues
2. Conducting quality in-service programs
3. Advocacy to school administrators and professors of education

Sources: Bender, S. J., J. J. Neutens, S. Skonie-Hardin, and W. D. Sorochan (1997). *Teaching Health Science: Elementary and Middle School*, 4th ed. Sudbury, MA: Jones & Bartlett, 32; Butler, S. C. (1993). "Chief State School Officers Rank Barriers to Implementing Comprehensive School Health Education." *Journal of School Health*, 63(3): 130–132; Telljohann, S. K., C. W. Symons, and B. Pateman (2009). *Health Education: Elementary and Middle School Applications*, 6th ed. New York, NY: McGraw-Hill; Thackeray, R., B. L. Neiger, H. Bartle, S. C. Hill, and M. D. Barnes (2002). "Elementary School Teachers' Perspectives on Health Instruction: Implications for Health Education." *American Journal of Health Education*, 33(2): 77–82; and Sy, A., and K. Glanz (2008). "Factors Influencing Teachers' Implementation of an Innovative Tobacco Prevention Curriculum for Multiethnic Youth: Project SPLASH." *Journal of School Health*, 78(5): 264–273.

---

had a SBHC/SLHC.[55] By 1984, that number had jumped to 31; by 1989 it had increased to 150.[56] In 2009, there were 1,906 school-based, mobile, and linked health centers in 48 states.[36] The majority (96%) of SBHCs are located in the school building. Most (56%) of the SBHCs operating today are found in urban areas. Of the SBHCs currently operating, 33% are found in high schools, 7.8% in middle schools, and 9.6% in elementary schools. The other 50% are located in alternative, K–8, 6–12, or K–12 schools.[36]

Although there is no single model for SBHCs, they share some common features:[57]

- They are located in schools or on school grounds.
- They work cooperatively within the school to become an integral part of the school.
- They provide a comprehensive range of services that meet the specific physical and behavioral health needs of young people in the community.
- They employ a multidisciplinary team of providers to care for students: nurse practitioners, registered nurses, physician assistants, social workers, physicians, alcohol and drug counselors, and other health professionals.
- They provide clinical services through a qualified health provider such as a hospital, health department, or medical practice.
- They require parents to sign written consents for their children to receive the full scope of services provided by the SBHC.
- They have an advisory board of community representatives, parents, youth, and family organizations participate in planning and oversight.

As mentioned earlier in the chapter, there are a number of sound reasons why health centers should be based in schools—the primary reason being the ability to reach, in a cost-effective manner, a large segment of the population that is otherwise without primary health care. "School-based health centers are the best model of health care in this country for at-risk populations. . . . SBHCs increase access to health care, eliminate barriers and improve health outcomes for essentially every patient enrolled."[58] Yet, SBHCs have not experienced the level of implementation that might be expected of a program that could make such a positive impact on the health of young people. Early on, SBHCs were frequent targets of intense criticism at the local and national levels by political and religious groups.[59-61] Much of the controversy surrounding SBHCs centered around cultural wars and partisan politics.[62] The issue of cultural wars revolved around the views of conservatives versus liberals, and how and where people should receive their health care. Whereas some people who support SBHCs would want their child treated as quickly and effectively as possible for a health problem, others who oppose the centers can see nothing but the "image of a condom on a cafeteria tray."[62] The key to working through the "cultural wars" problem is compromise. That is, each area of the country is different and what are reasonable health services provided in an SBHC in one area are unacceptable in another. Thus, advocates of the centers say that the services provided by SBHCs are so badly needed that a single issue such as reproductive health care should not keep an SBHC from existing.[62]

Since their inception, funding for SBHCs has always been an issue. They do not have the sophisticated computers to bill for services, and they are typically not open 24 hours a day to qualify, at least in the eyes of insurance companies, as primary care health centers.[60] Also, the SBHCs' means of operation really do not match well with the concept of managed care (see Chapter 13). Therefore, most of the SBHCs receive funding from a variety of revenue sources including state government (76%), sponsor organizations (49%), and school or school district (46%). Thirty-nine percent of SBHCs receive funding from the federal government.[36]

Another one of the challenges facing SBHCs is the pressure for schools and school-related programs to be accountable for demonstrating their impact on improving the learning environment and academic outcomes.[63] Research studies have explored the link between SBHCs and health outcomes, resulting in positive findings. For example, there is a correlation between asthma and lower student attendance. For those students with asthma attending a school with an SBHC, there were fewer hospitalization days and school absences when compared with children at control schools without an SBHC.[64] In this current climate of accountability within the educational system, indirect links do not provide enough evidence that SBHCs positively affect academic outcomes. Research demonstrating the correlation between SBHCs and health and academic outcomes is needed for SBHCs to gain greater implementation.[63]

Violence in Schools

Over the years, schools have been viewed as safe havens for teaching and learning.[65] But more recently, there have been a number of high-profile incidents of violence in schools (e.g., Paducah, Kentucky; Pearl, Missouri; Moses Lake, Washington; Springfield, Oregon; Littleton, Colorado; and San Diego, California) that have made the general public more aware of the violence in schools. "Any instance of crime or violence at school not only affects the individuals involved, but also may disrupt the educational process and affect bystanders, the school itself, and the surrounding community."[65] The difference between violence in the schools today and years past is the means by which disagreements are settled. "Today the possibility that a disagreement among students will be settled with some type of weapon rather than an old-fashioned fist fight has significantly increased."[66] CDC Youth Risk Behavior data indicate that 1 of 20 U.S. high school students had missed at least one day of school in the preceding month because that student felt unsafe either being at school or going to and from school; 1

of 13 students had been threatened or injured with a weapon on school property during the preceding year; and 1 of 9 had been in a physical fight on school property.[67]

We know that males are involved in more violent acts than are females.[67] We also know that certain racial and ethnic groups participate and are victims of violence at school more often than other students are.[67] Yet, it is close to impossible to predict who will be next to commit a violent act in a school. (See Chapter 8 for a more detailed description of adolescent risk behaviors.)

Another form of violence that has received significant attention recently is bullying. *Bullying* can be defined as "aggressive behavior that is intentional and that involves an imbalance of power or strength."[68] Bullying can take many forms, such as physical (hitting); verbal (teasing or name calling); emotional (gestures or social exclusion); and cyber (sending insulting messages or pictures by mobile phone or using the Internet).[68] Research indicates that between 15% and 25% of students are bullied with some frequency, and 15% to 20% report that they engage in bullying behavior. Being bullied can affect academic achievement and self-esteem. Bullying can also affect bystanders by creating a climate of fear and disrespect in schools. Furthermore, bullying behavior can be a sign of other serious antisocial or violent behavior by those who bully their peers.[68]

With the technologic advances of late, concern has increased about the connection between electronic media and youth violence. *Electronic aggression*, which has been defined as "any kind of aggression perpetrated through technology—any type of harassment or bullying that occurs through email, a chat room, instant messaging, a Web site (including blogs), or text messaging,"[69] is a recent phenomenon among youth. Because electronic aggression is fairly new, limited information is available. However, 9% to 35% of young people say they have been a victim of electronic aggression. Some evidence suggests that electronic aggression may peak around the end of middle school/beginning of high school.[69] Instant messaging appears to be the most common way electronic aggression is perpetrated, and it is most often experienced between a victim and perpetrator who know each other. Whether electronic aggression occurs at home or at school, it has implications for school. "Young people who were harassed on-line were more likely to get a detention or be suspended, to skip school, and to experience emotional distress than those who were not harassed."[69] This behavior also influences students' sense of safety at school.[69]

Like most other health problems, risk factors need to be identified and steps taken to reduce the risk of violent acts occurring in the schools. Many schools have taken steps to try to reduce the chances for violence, yet many more have stated that violence is not a problem at "our school." These are the schools that are most vulnerable to such a problem. The CDC makes the following recommendations for educators and educational policymakers for improving the school climate as it relates to violence, bullying, and electronic aggression:[69]

- *Explore current bullying prevention policies.* Determine if they need to be modified to reflect electronic aggression.
- *Work collaboratively to develop policies.* States, school districts, and boards of education must work in conjunction with other stakeholders to meet the needs of the state or district and those it serves. The CDC School Health Guidelines provide a general outline of steps to follow.[70]
- *Explore current programs to prevent bullying and youth violence.* A number of evidence-based programs exist.
- *Offer training on electronic aggression for educators and administrators.*
- *Talk to teens.* Provide opportunities for students to discuss their concerns.

- *Work with technology staff.* Ensure that all involved are aware and working on strategies for minimizing risk.
- *Create a positive school atmosphere.* Students who feel connected to their school are less likely to perpetrate any type of violence or aggression.
- *Have a plan in place for what should happen if an incident is brought to the attention of school officials.*

With the new phenomenon of electronic aggression, it becomes clear that violence is not a problem that will go away soon. Many school personnel do not believe it is a problem in their schools. As life has shown us, it can happen anywhere. Violence is an issue that all schools need to face and something for which they need to plan to reduce the risks to school children and personnel. "We send our children out into the world every day to explore and learn, and we hope that they will approach a trusted adult if they encounter a challenge; now, we need to apply this message to the virtual world."[69]

CHAPTER SUMMARY

- The potential impact of a coordinated school health program on the health of children, their families, and the community is great because the school is the one institution through which we all must pass.
- To date, the full potential of school health has not been reached because of lack of support and interest.
- If implemented properly, coordinated school health programs can improve access to health services, educate students about pressing health issues, and provide a safe and healthy environment in which students can learn and grow.
- The foundations of the school health program include (1) a school administration that supports such an effort, (2) a well-organized school health council that is genuinely interested in providing a coordinated program for the students, and (3) written school health policies.
- School health policies are critical for ensuring accountability, credibility, and the institutionalization of programs and efforts to make schools a healthy learning environment.
- The components of a coordinated school health program include (1) school health services; (2) a healthy school environment; (3) school health education; (4) counseling, psychological, and social services; (5) physical education; (6) school nutrition services; (7) family/community involvement for school health; and (8) school-site health promotion for staff.
- The eight National Health Education Standards emphasize a skills-based curriculum focusing on the following: (1) core concepts; (2) analyzing influences; (3) accessing valid health information, products, and services; (4) demonstrating interpersonal communication

skills; (5) utilizing decision-making skills; (6) utilizing goal-setting skills; (7) practicing health-enhancing behaviors; and (8) advocating for personal, family, and community health.
- A number of resources exist to assist health education specialists in locating and assessing available curricula.
- A number of issues face school health advocates, including a lack of support for coordinated school health, health curriculum challenges, the implementation of school-based health centers, and violence in schools.

REVIEW QUESTIONS

1. What is meant by the term *coordinated school health program*?
2. Which individuals (name by position) should be considered for inclusion on the school health council?
3. What foundations are needed to ensure a coordinated school health program? Why?
4. Why are written school health policies needed?
5. Who should approve written school health policies?
6. What are the eight components of a coordinated school health program?
7. The American Academy of Pediatrics recommends that at minimum schools should provide three types of services. What are the three types of services?
8. Explain the importance of using a standards-based health curriculum.
9. How would a health education specialists go about locating credible health education curricula?
10. State four issues facing school health advocates and explain why they are issues.

SCENARIO: ANALYSIS AND RESPONSE

It was obvious that Ms. Graff had a very full day, which included several issues related to a coordinated school health program. Based on what you read in this chapter and other knowledge you have about school health, respond to the following questions:

1. Identify five school health concerns with which Ms. Graff had to deal.
2. For each of the concerns you identified in question 1, state how written policies may have helped or hindered Ms. Graff with her responsibilities.

3. How important do you think is the role of the classroom teacher in making a coordinated school health program work? Why do you feel this way?
4. Say the school district in which Ms. Graff works was interested in opening up a school-based health center, but the superintendent needed more data to help "sell" the idea to the school board. Using a search engine on the Internet (e.g., Google), enter "school-based health centers." Could you recommend some Web sites to the superintendent that would be useful?

ACTIVITIES

1. Make arrangements to observe an elementary classroom in your town for a half day. While observing, keep a chart of all the activities that take place in the classroom that relate to a coordinated school health program. Select one activity from your list and write a one-page paper describing the activity, why it was health related, how the teacher handled it, and what could have been done differently to improve the situation.

2. Visit a voluntary health agency in your community and ask the employees to describe the organization's philosophy on health education and inquire if their health education materials are available for use in a school health program. Summarize your visit with a one-page reaction paper.

3. Make an appointment to interview either a school nurse or a school health coordinator. During your interview, ask the person to provide an overview of what his or her school offers in the way of a coordinated school health program. Ask specifically about the eight components of the school health program and the issues of controversy presented in this chapter. Summarize your visit with a two-page written paper.

4. Make arrangements to interview a school administrator or school board member in a district where a school-based, mobile, or linked center exists. Ask the person to describe the process that the school district went through to start the center, what resistance the district met in doing so, and what the district would do differently if it had to implement it again or start another center.

COMMUNITY HEALTH ON THE WEB

The Internet contains a wealth of information about community and public health. Increase your knowledge of some of the topics presented in this chapter by accessing the Jones & Bartlett Learning Web site at **http://health .jbpub.com/book/communityhealth/7e** and follow the links to complete the following Web activities:

- American School Health Association
- Action for Healthy Kids
- Division of Adolescent and School Health

REFERENCES

1. Satcher, D. (2005). "Healthy and Ready to Learn." *Educational Leadership*, 63(1): 26–30.

2. Office of Planning, Evaluation and Policy Development (2010). *ESEA Blueprint for Reform*. Washington, DC: U.S. Department of Education.

3. Dryfoos, J. (2008). "Centers of Hope." *Educational Leadership*, 65(7): 38–43.

4. Joint Committee on Health Education and Promotion Terminology (2001). "Report of the 2000 Joint Committee on Health Education and Promotion Terminology." *American Journal of Health Education*, 32(2): 89–103.

5. Allensworth, D. D., and L. J. Kolbe (1987). "The Comprehensive School Health Program: Exploring an Expanded Concept." *Journal of School Health*, 57(10): 409–412.

6. U.S. Census Bureau (2010). "Back to School: 2010–2011." In *U.S. Census Bureau News: Facts for Features*. Washington, DC: U.S. Department of Commerce.

7. McGinnis, J. M., and C. DeGraw (1991). "Healthy Schools 2000: Creating Partnerships for the Decade." *Journal of School Health*, 61(7): 292–296.

8. American Cancer Society (2000). *School Health Programs Elements of Excellence: Helping Children to Grow Up Healthy and*

Able to Learn. Available at http://www.cancer.org/Healthy/
MoreWaysACSHelpsYouStayWell/SchoolHealth/WhatsSchoolHealthAll
About/index.

9. Fetro, J. V., C. Givens, and K. Carroll (2010). "Coordinated School
Health: Getting It All Together." *Educational Leadership*, 67(4): 32–37.

10. Fetro, J. V. (1998). "Implementing Coordinated School Health
Programs in Local Schools." In E. Marx, S. F. Wooley, and D. Northrop,
eds., *Health Is Academic: A Guide to Coordinated School Health
Programs*. New York, NY: Teachers College Press, 15–42.

11. Ottoson, J., G. Streib, J. Thomas, M. Rivera, and B. Stevenson
(2004). "Evaluation of the National School Health Coordinator
Leadership Institute." *Journal of School Health*, 74(5): 170–176.

12. National Association of School Nurses (2002). "Issue Brief: Role of
the School Nurse." Available at http://www.nasn.org/Default.aspx?
tabid=279.

13. National Association of State Boards of Education (2000). *Fit,
Healthy, and Ready to Learn: Part 1: Physical Activity, Healthy
Eating, and Tobacco-Use Prevention*. Alexandria, VA: Author.

14. McGinnis, J. M. (1981). "Health Problems of Children and Youth: A
Challenge for Schools." *Health Education Quarterly*, 8(1): 11–14.

15. National Association of School Nurses. (2002). "Position Statement:
Education, Licensure, and Certification of School Nurses." Available at
http://www.nasn.org/default.aspx?tabid=219.

16. Kann, L., S. Telljohann, and S. Wooley (2007). "Health Education:
Results from the School Health Policies and Programs Study 2006."
Journal of School Health, 77(8): 408–434.

17. Centers for Disease Control and Prevention (2010). School Health
Policy. Available at http://www.cdc.gov/healthyyouth/policy/index
.htm.

18. McKenzie, J. F. (1983). "Written Policies: Developing a Solid
Foundation for a Comprehensive School Health Program." *Future
Focus: Ohio Journal of Health, Physical Education, Recreation, and
Dance*, 4(3): 9–11.

19. Grebow, P. M., B. Z. Greene, J. Harvey, and C. J. Head (2000).
"Shaping Health Policies." *Educational Leadership*, 57(6): 63–66.

20. Bureau of Health and Nutrition Services and Child/Family/School
Partnerships (2009). *Action Guide for School Nutrition and Physical
Activity Policies*. Middletown: Connecticut State Department of
Education.

21. U.S. Department of Agriculture, Food and Nutrition Service (2010).
"The Local Process: How to Create and Implement a Local Wellness
Policy." Available at http://www.fns.usda.gov/tn/Healthy/wellnesspolicy_
steps.html.

22. Action for Healthy Kids. (2009). "Wellness Policy Tool." Available at
http://www.actionforhealthykids.org/school-programs/our-programs/
wellness-policy-tool/.

23. Child Nutrition and WIC Reauthorization Act of 2004, Pub. L. No.
108-265, § 204 (2004). Available at http://www.fns.usda.gov/TN/
Healthy/108-265.pdf.

24. Action for Healthy Kids (2009). "About Us." Available at http://
www.actionforhealthykids.org/about-us.

25. Division of Adolescent and School Health, Centers for Disease
Control and Prevention (2010). "School Health Policies and Practices
Study." Available at http://www.cdc.gov/healthyyouth/shpps/index.htm.

26. National Association of State Boards of Education (2010). "State-by-
State School Health Program Coordinators." Available at http://
nasbe.org/healthy_schools/hs/bytopics.php.

27. Winnail, S., S. Dorman, and B. Stevenson (2004). "Training Leaders
for School Health Programs: The National School Coordinator
Leadership Institute." *Journal of School Health*, 74(3): 79–84.

28. American Cancer Society (2010). "The Role of the School Health
Coordinator." Available at http://www.cancer.org/Healthy/MoreWays
ACSHelpsYouStayWell/SchoolHealth/WhatsSchoolHealthAllAbout/index.

29. National Association of School Board Education (2010). "Health
and Safety Coordinator for School, for District." Available at http://
www.nasbe.org/healthy_schools/hs/natstandbytopics.php#School
HealthProgramCoordinators.

30. Division of Adolescent and School Health, Centers for Disease
Control and Prevention (2008). "Coordinated School Health Program."
Available at http://www.cdc.gov/healthyyouth/CSHP/.

31. U.S. Department of Commerce, Census Bureau (2009). "Digest of
Education Statistics: 2009." Available at http://nces.ed.gov/programs/
digest/d09.

32. Schlitt, J. J. (June 1991). "Issue Brief—Bringing Health to School:
Policy Implications for Southern States." Washington, DC: Southern
Center on Adolescent Pregnancy Prevention and Southern Regional
Project on Infant Mortality. Printed in *Journal of School Health*, 62(2):
60a–60h.

33. Klein, J. D., and L. S. Sadowski (1990). "Personal Health Services as
a Component of Comprehensive Health Programs." *Journal of School
Health*, 60(4): 164–169.

34. American Academy of Pediatrics (2004). *School Health: Policy and
Practice*. Elk Grove Village, IL: Author.

35. National Health and Education Consortium (1995). *Starting
Young: School-Based Health Centers at the Elementary Level*.
Washington, DC: Author.

36. Strozer, J., L. Juszczak, and A. Ammerman (2010). *2007–2008
National School-Based Health Care Census*. Washington, DC: National
Assembly on School-Based Health Care.

37. Committee on School Health (2001). "School Health Centers and
Other Integrated School Health Services." *Pediatrics*, 107(1).

38. Joint Committee on Health Education Terminology (1974). "New
Definitions: Report of the 1972–73 Joint Committee on Health
Education Terminology." *Journal of School Health*, 44(1): 33–37.

39. Centers for Disease Control and Prevention (2005). *School Health
Index: A Self-Assessment and Planning Guide*. Atlanta, GA: Author.
Available at http://www.cdc.gov/healthyyouth/shi.

40. Henderson, A., and D. E. Rowe. (1998). "A Healthy School
Environment." In E. Marx, S. F. Wooley, and D. Northrop, eds., *Health
Is Academic: A Guide to Coordinated School Health Programs*. New
York, NY: Teachers College Press, 96–115.

41. Institute of Medicine (1997). *Schools and Health: Our Nation's
Investment*. Washington, DC: National Academies Press.

42. Centers for Disease Control and Prevention (2009). "Health
Education Curriculum Assessment Tool." Atlanta, GA: Author. Available
at http://www.cdc.gov/healthyyouth/HECAT/index.htm.

43. Joint Committee on National Health Education Standards (2007).
National Health Education Standards (2nd ed.). Atlanta, GA: Author.

44. Joint Committee on National Health Education Standards (1995).
National Health Education Standards. Atlanta, GA: American Cancer
Society.

45. Division of Adolescent and School Health, Centers for Disease
Control and Prevention (2009). "Adolescent Health: Registries of
Programs Effective in Reducing Youth Risk Behaviors." Available at
http://www.cdc.gov/healthyyouth/AdolescentHealth/registries.htm.

46. U.S. Department of Health and Human Services, Office for
Substance Abuse Prevention (1989). *Drug-Free Committees: Turning
Awareness into Action* (DHHS pub. no. ADM 89-1562). Washington,
DC: U.S. Government Printing Office.

47. "*Healthy People 2000*: National Health Promotion and Disease
Prevention Objectives and Health Schools." (1991). *Journal of School
Health*, 61(7): 298–299.

48. Rosas, S., J. Case, and L. Tholstrup (2009). "A Retrospective
Examination of the Relationship Between Implementation Quality of
the Coordinated School Health Program Model and School-Level
Academic Indicators Over Time." *Journal of School Health*, 79(3):
108–115.

49. Weiler, R., R. M. Pigg, and R. McDermott (2003). "Evaluation of the
Florida Coordinated School Health Program Pilot Project." *Journal of
School Health*, 73(1): 3–8.

50. Centers for Disease Control and Prevention, Division of Adolescent
and School Health (1997). "Is School Health Education Cost-Effective?
An Exploratory Analysis of Selected Exemplary Components." As
quoted in F. D. McKenzie and J. B. Richmond (1998). "Linking Health

and Learning: An Overview of Coordinated School Health Programs." In E. Marx, S. F. Wooley, and D. Northrop, eds., *Health Is Academic: A Guide to Coordinated School Health Programs*. New York, NY: Teachers College Press, 1–14.

51. Miller, T. and D. Hendrie (2009). *Substance Abuse Prevention Dollars and Cents: A Cost-Benefit Analysis*. (DHHS pub. no. [SMA] 07-4298). Rockville, MD: Center for Substance Abuse Prevention, Substance Abuse and Mental Health Services Administration.

52. Gold, R. S., G. S. Parcel, H. J. Walberg, R. V. Luepker, B. Portnoy, and E. J. Stone (1991). "Summary and Conclusions of the THTM Evaluation: The Expert Work Group Perspective." *Journal of School Health*, 61(1): 39–42.

53. Student Nutrition and Physical Activity. S. Enrolled Act No. 111, 114th Gen. Assem., 2d Reg. Sess. (Ind. 2006). Available at http://www.in.gov/legislative/bills/2006/SE/SE0111.1.html.

54. Cleary, M. J. (1991). "School Health Education and a National Curriculum: One Disconcerting Scenario." *Journal of School Health*, 61(8): 355–358.

55. Council on Scientific Affairs, American Medical Association (1990). "Providing Medical Services through School-Based Health Programs." *Journal of School Health*, 60(3): 87–91.

56. Lear, J. G., L. L. Montgomery, J. J. Schlitt, and K. D. Rickett (1996). "Key Issues Affecting School-Based Health Centers and Medicaid." *Journal of School Health*, 66(3): 83–88.

57. National Assembly on School-Based Health Care (2010). "About School-Based Health Care." Available at http://www.nasbhc.org/site/c.jsJPKWPFJrH/b.2561553/k.843D/about_sbhcs.htm.

58. Ammerman, A. (2010). "School Based Healthcare: Why It Is Common Sense." *SEEN Magazine*. Charlotte, NC: Knight Communications. Available at http://www.seenmagazine.us/Sections/ArticleDetail/tabid/79/ArticleID/582/smid/403/reftab/317/Default.aspx.

59. Pacheco, M., W. Powell, C. Cole, N. Kalishman, R. Benon, and A. Kaufmann (1991). "School-Based Clinics: The Politics of Change." *Journal of School Health*, 61(2): 92–94.

60. Rienzo, B. A., and J. W. Button (1993). "The Politics of School-Based Clinics: A Community-Level Analysis." *Journal of School Health*, 63(6): 266–272.

61. The School-Based Adolescent Health Care Program (1993). *The Answer Is at School: Bringing Health Care to Our Students*. Washington, DC: Author.

62. Morone, J. A., E. H. Kilbreth, and K. M. Langwell (2001). "Back to School: A Health Care Strategy for Youth." *Health Affairs*, 20(1): 122–136.

63. Strolin-Goltzman, J. (2010). "The Relationship between School-Based Health Centers and the Learning Environment." *Journal of School Health*, 80(3): 153–159.

64. Webber, M., K. Carpiniello, T. Oruwariye, Y. Lo, W. Burton, and D. Appel. (2003). "Burden of Asthma in Inner-City Elementary School Children: Do School-Based Health Centers Make a Difference?" *Archives of Pediatrics and Adolescent Medicine*, 157: 125–129.

65. National Center for Education Statistics (2009). "Indicators of School Crime and Safety: 2009." Available at http://nces.ed.gov/programs/crimeindicators/crimeindicators2009/.

66. Anspaugh, D. J., and G. Ezell (2001). *Teaching Today's Health*, 6th ed. Boston: Allyn and Bacon.

67. Centers for Disease Control and Prevention (2010). "Youth Risk Behavior Surveillance—United States, 2009." *MMWR Surveillance Summaries*, 59(SS-5).

68. Health Resources and Services Administration (2010). "What Do We Know About Bullying." Available at http://www.stopbullyingnow.hrsa.gov/adults.

69. Hertz, M. F. and C. David-Ferdon (2008). *Electronic Media and Youth Violence: A CDC Issue Brief for Educators and Caregivers*. Atlanta, GA: Centers for Disease Control and Prevention.

70. Centers for Disease Control and Prevention (2001). "School Health Guidelines to Prevent Unintentional Injuries and Violence." *Morbidity and Mortality Weekly Report*, 50(RR-22): 1–75.

UNIT
TWO

THE NATION'S HEALTH AND HEALTH CARE DELIVERY

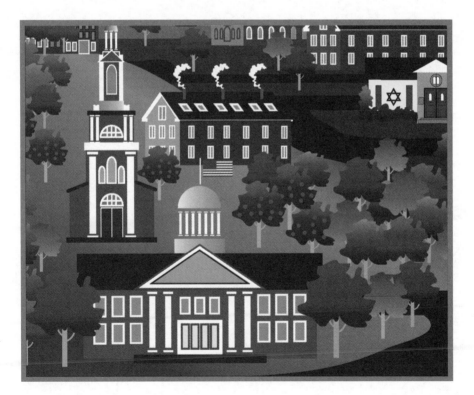

Chapter 7

Maternal, Infant, and Child Health

Chapter Objectives

After studying this chapter, you will be able to:

1 Define *maternal, infant,* and *child health.*

2 Explain the importance of maternal, infant, and child health as indicators of a society's health.

3 Define *family planning* and explain why it is important.

4 Identify consequences of teenage pregnancies.

5 Define *legalized abortion* and discuss *Roe v. Wade* and the pro-life and pro-choice movements.

6 Define *maternal mortality rate.*

7 Define *prenatal care* and the influence this has on pregnancy outcome.

8 List the major factors that contribute to infant health and mortality.

9 Explain the differences among infant mortality, neonatal mortality, and postneonatal mortality.

10 Identify the leading causes of childhood morbidity and mortality.

11 List the immunizations required for a 2-year-old child to be considered fully immunized.

12 Explain how health insurance and health care services affect childhood health.

13 Identify important governmental programs developed to improve maternal and child health.

14 Briefly explain what WIC programs are and who they serve.

15 Identify the major groups that are recognized as advocates for children.

SCENARIO

Joan is 18 years old and a recent high school graduate. She lives in a small town of about 2,700 people. Most of the town's residents rely on a larger city nearby for shopping, recreation, and health care. Joan had dated Dave the past 2 years, but there was never any talk of marriage. Just before graduation she learned that she was pregnant. At Thanksgiving, just as she was completing her seventh month of pregnancy, she went into premature labor. An ambulance rushed her to the emergency room of the hospital in the nearby city for what became a premature birth of her baby. While Joan was in recovery, doctors determined that her baby was not only premature, it also appeared to have other "developmental abnormalities." When asked whether she had received any prenatal care, Joan replied, "No, I couldn't afford it; besides, I didn't know where to go to get help."

INTRODUCTION

Creating a health profile of Americans requires a clear understanding of the health-related problems and opportunities of all Americans. In Chapter 3 we dicussed the role of descriptive epidemiology in understanding the health of populations. In describing the personal characteristics of a population, age is the first and perhaps the most important population characteristic to consider when describing the occurrence of disease, injury, and/or death in a population. Almost every health-related event or state has greater differences with age than any other population characteristic. For this reason, community health professionals use age-specific rates when comparing the amount of disease between populations. When they analyze data by age, they use groups that are narrow enough to detect any age-related patterns, which may be present as a result of either the natural life cycle or behavioral patterns. Viewing age-group profiles in this manner enables community health workers to identify risk factors for specific age groups within the population and to develop and propose interventions aimed at reducing these risk factors. Health promotion and disease prevention programs successful at reducing exposure of specific age groups to such risk factors can improve the health status of the entire population.

In this chapter, we present a health profile of mothers, infants (those younger than 1 year), and children (ages 1–14 years). In the following two chapters, the health profiles will be presented of adolescents and young adults (15–24), adults (25–64), and older adults or seniors (65 and older). These same age subgroupings are used by the *Healthy People 2020* report and many other documents produced by the National Center for Health Statistics (NCHS) to describe and measure the health status of Americans.

maternal, infant, and child health the health of women of childbearing age from pre-pregnancy, through pregnancy, labor, and delivery, and the postpartum period and the health of the child prior to birth through adolescence.[1] In this chapter, we define and discuss commonly used indicators for measuring maternal, infant, and child health; examine the risk factors associated with maternal, infant, and child morbidity and mortality; and review selected community programs aimed at improving the health of women of childbearing age, infants, and children in the United States.

Maternal, infant, and child health is important to a community for several reasons. First, maternal, infant, and child health statistics are regarded as important indicators of the effectiveness of the disease prevention and health promotion services in a community. It is known

maternal, infant, and child health the health of women of childbearing age and that of the child through adolescence that unintended pregnancies, lack of prenatal care, poor maternal and child nutrition, maternal drug use, low immunization rates, poverty, limited education, and insufficient child care—combined with a lack of access to health care services in a community—are precursors to high rates of maternal, infant, and childhood morbidity and mortality. Second, we now know that many of the risk factors specified can be reduced or prevented with the early intervention of educational programs and preventive medical services for women, infants, and children. These early community efforts provide a positive environment that supports the physical and emotional needs of the woman, infant, and family and reduce the need for more costly medical or social assistance to these same members of society later in their lives (see Figure 7.1).

During the past several decades the United States has made important progress in reducing infant and maternal mortality. However, despite these declines in mortality rates, challenges remain. Possibly the most important concern is that infant and maternal mortality data for the United States are characterized by a continual and substantial disparity between mortality rates for whites and blacks. The mortality rate among non-Hispanic black infants (13.8 per 1,000 live births) was about two and one-half times the rate among white, non-Hispanic and Hispanic infants (5.6 and 5.5 per 1,000 live births) in 2006 (see Figure 7.2). The mortality rate among black women (34.8 per 100,000 births) was about four times the

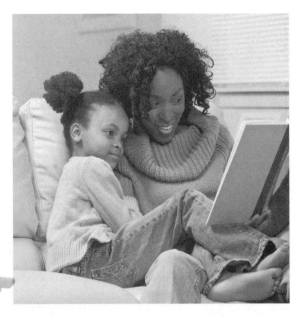

FIGURE 7.1

The health of a nation is often judged by the health of its mothers and children.

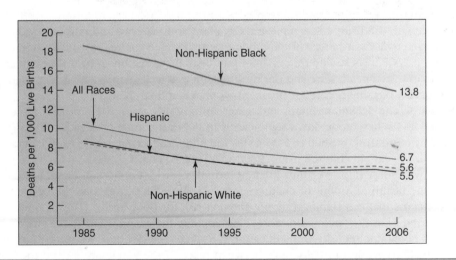

FIGURE 7.2

U.S. mortality rates among infants younger than 1 year, by maternal race/ethnicity, 1985–2006.

Source: U.S. Department of Health and Human Services, Health Resources and Services Administration, Maternal and Child Health Bureau. *Child Health USA 2008–2009.* Rockville, Maryland: U.S. Department of Health and Human Services, 2009

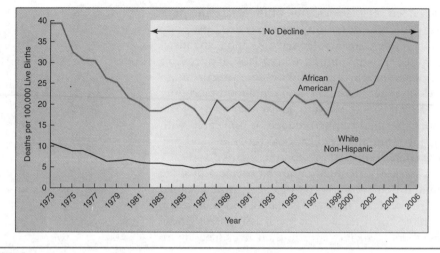

FIGURE 7.3

African American and white women who died of pregnancy-related complications: United States, 1973–2006 (annual number of deaths during pregnancy or within 42 days after delivery, per 100,000 live births).

˙The apparent increase in the number of maternal deaths between 1998 and 1999 is the result of changes in how maternal deaths are classified and coded.

Source: U.S. Department of Health and Human Services, Health Resources and Services Administration, Maternal and Child Health Bureau. *Child Health USA 2008–2009.* Rockville, Maryland: U.S. Department of Health and Human Services, 2009

rate among white women (9.1 per 100,000 live births) in 2006 (see Figure 7.3). These disparities are not directly attributable to race or ethnicity, although certain diseases occur more often in certain races or ethnicities. Rather, the disparity can be traced to differences in the socioeconomic status between segments of the American population. For example, research indicates that low income and limited education correlate very highly with poor health status.[2] Second, the United States has higher infant and maternal mortality rates than other industrialized nations; it ranked 30th in infant mortality (see Figure 7.4) and 20th in maternal mortality in 2005.[2] These differences among industrialized nations mirror differences in the health status of women before and during pregnancy as well as the ease of access and quantity and quality of primary care for pregnant women and their infants.

Similar to the decline in infant and maternal mortality rates, the mortality rates of *children* (ages 1–14) have gone down significantly in the past couple of decades. The death rate declined by more than one-half in 1- to 4-year-old children (see Figure 7.5) and by nearly one-half in 5- to 14-year-old children from 1980 to 2006 (see Figure 7.6).[2]

Even with these improvements in child mortality rates, there is still much to be done to improve the health of American children. First, we must recognize that children today face other concerns that can significantly put them at risk for poor health. These concerns have been referred to as the "new morbidities" and include their family and social environments, behaviors, economic security, and education (see Box 7.1).[2] Second, we must be concerned about the difference in mortality rates between races. If the young are indeed the hope for the future, the United States must continue to work hard to ensure the health of each infant and child, regardless of race or socioeconomic status.

Whereas numerous factors affect the health of both infant and child, many reflect or are related to the health status of the mother and her immediate environment. One of the first

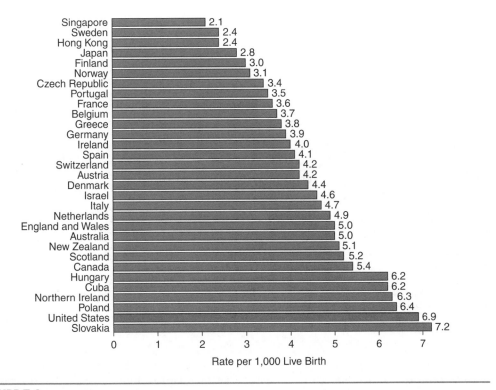

FIGURE 7.4

Comparison of national infant mortality rates, 2005.

Source: National Center for Health Statistics. *Health, United States, 2008 With Special Feature on the Health of Young Adults.* Hyattsville, MD: 2009.

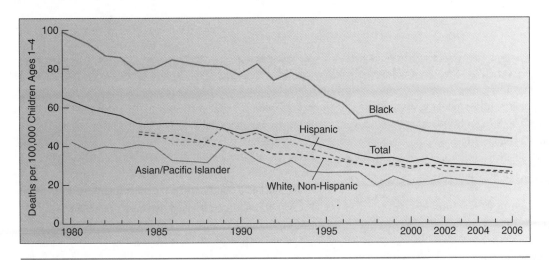

FIGURE 7.5

Death rates among children ages 1–4 by race and Hispanic origin, 1980–2006.

Note: Death rates for American Indians/Alaska Natives are included in the total but are not shown separately because the numbers of deaths were too small to calculate reliable rates.

Source: Data from *Infant, Child, and Teen Death Rates (per 100,000) for Selected Years, 1980–2007.* Child Trends DataBank.

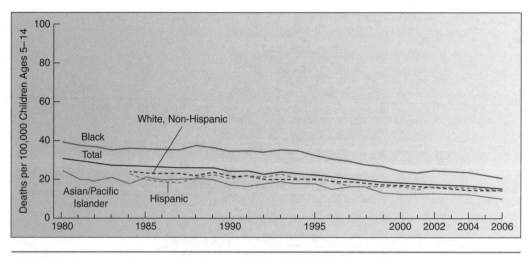

FIGURE 7.6

Death rates among children ages 5 to 14 by race and Hispanic origin, 1980–2006.

Note: Death rates for American Indians/Alaska Natives are included in the total but are not shown separately because the numbers of deaths were too small to calculate reliable rates.

Source: Data from *Infant, Child, and Teen Death Rates (per 100,000) for Selected Years, 1980–2007.* Child Trends DataBank.

steps to ensure healthy children is to ensure that pregnant women have access to prenatal care early in a pregnancy and that they receive proper care throughout it. There is nothing more dependent than a fetus in a mother's uterus relying on her to eat nutritiously and to avoid drugs or a newborn that is reliant on an adult to survive and develop into a healthy child. Therefore, we begin by looking at the health status of mothers and the family structure.

BOX
7.1

MOMENTS IN AMERICA FOR <u>ALL</u> CHILDREN

Every second a public school student is suspended.*

Every 11 seconds a high school student drops out.*

Every 19 seconds a child is arrested.

Every 19 seconds a baby is born to an unmarried mother.

Every 20 seconds a public school student is corporally punished.*

Every 32 seconds a baby is born into poverty.

Every 41 seconds a child is confirmed as abused or neglected.

Every 42 seconds a baby is born without health insurance.

Every minute a baby is born to a teen mother.

Every minute a baby is born at low birth weight.

Every 4 minutes a child is arrested for a drug offense.

Every 7 minutes a child is arrested for a violent crime.

Every 18 minutes a baby dies before his or her first birthday.

Every 45 minutes a child or teen dies from an accident.

Every 3 hours a child or teen is killed by a firearm.

Every 5 hours a child or teen commits suicide.

Every 6 hours a child is killed by abuse or neglect.

Every 15 hours a mother dies from complications of childbirth or pregnancy.

*Based on calculations per school day (180 days of 7 hours each).

Source: Children's Defense Fund (2010). *The State of America's Children 2010.* Reprinted with permission. Available at http://www.childrensdefense.org/child-research-data-publications/data/state-of-americas-children-2010-report.html. Accessed December 21, 2010.

FAMILY AND REPRODUCTIVE HEALTH

The family is one of society's most treasured foundations. It represents a primary social group that influences and is influenced by other people and establishments. Moreover, families are the primary unit in which infants and children are nurtured and supported regarding their healthy development.[1] The U.S. Census Bureau defines a family as "a group of two people or more (one of whom is the householder) related by birth, marriage, or adoption and residing together; all such people (including related subfamily members) are considered as members of one family."[3] This definition does not include a variety of cultural styles and optional family structures that exist in our society today. Friedman broadens the definition of family to include "two or more persons who are joined together by bonds of sharing and emotional closeness and who identify themselves as being part of the family."[4] These definitions not only provide a basis for delineating a family, but are important to consider because most people, at some point in their life, will consider becoming a parent.

From a community health perspective, a marriage, or having two parents, serves as an important family characteristic in relation to a child's well-being. Research indicates there are increased health risks for infants and children who are raised in single-parent families, including adverse birth outcomes, low birth weight, and infant mortality, and that these children are more likely to live in poverty than children of married mothers.[5,6] Additionally, unmarried mothers generally have lower education, lower incomes, and greater dependence on welfare assistance than do married mothers. In 2007, the percentage of births to unmarried women was 40%, or more than double that of the 18.4% of live births to unmarried women that occurred in 1980.[6] Teenage women who give birth are substantially more likely than women age 20 and older to have that birth outside of marriage. In fact, between 1980 and 2007 the proportion of births to unmarried women rose from 62% to 93% for ages 15–17 and from 40% to 82% for ages 18–19 (see Figure 7.7).[7]

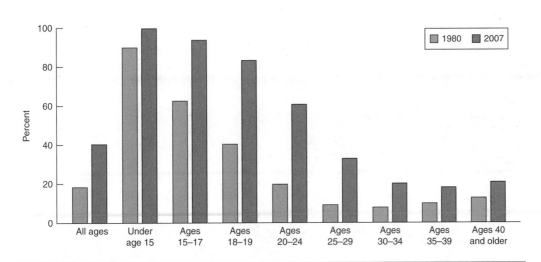

FIGURE 7.7

Percentage of all births that were to unmarried women, by age, 1980–2007.

Note: Data for 2007 are preliminary.

Source: National Center for Health Statistics (2010). *Health, United States, 2009 with Special Feature on Medical Technology.* (DHHS pub. No. 2010-1232), Hyattsville, MD. Available at http://www.cdc.gov/nchs/hus.htm. Accessed October 1, 2010.

Teenage Births

Teenage childbearing represents a significant social and financial burden on both the family and the community. Teenagers who become pregnant and have a child are more likely than their peers who are not mothers to (1) drop out of school, (2) not get married or to have a marriage end in divorce, (3) rely on public assistance, and (4) live in poverty.[5,8] Teenage pregnancy and childbearing also have substantial economic consequences for society in the form of increased welfare costs. Each year teenage childbearing costs taxpayers at least $9 billion in direct costs associated with health care, foster care, criminal justice, and public assistance, as well as lost tax revenues.[9] Furthermore, teenage pregnancy and childbearing have considerable long-term consequences for teenage parents and their children. For instance, teenagers who give birth are less likely to graduate from high school and more likely to have a larger number of children in poverty than are nonparenting teenagers. Also, children born to teenage mothers may experience lower educational attainment and higher rates of teenage childbearing themselves when compared with children born to older mothers.

Teenage pregnancies also result in serious health consequences for these women and their babies. Teenage mothers are much less likely than women older than the age of 20 to receive early prenatal care and are more likely to smoke during pregnancy and have a preterm birth and low-birth-weight baby (see Figure 7.8).[8] As a consequence of these and other factors, babies born to teenagers are more likely to die during the first year of life and more likely to suffer certain serious health problems than a baby born to a mother in her twenties and thirties. A teenage mother is at greater risk than a woman older than the age of 20 for pregnancy complications (such as premature labor, anemia, and high blood pressure).[8] Therefore, teenage pregnancies are a significant community health concern in the United States.

In large part as a result of effective community and public health campaigns aimed at reducing teenage pregnancies, teen pregnancy and birth rates have declined steadily in recent years. Between 1991 and 2008, the teenage birth rate in the United States declined by one-third to 41.5 births per 1,000 teenage girls in 2008.[6] Despite the recently declining rates,

FIGURE 7.8

Selected characteristics for teenage mothers and mothers aged 20 years and older: United States, 1999.

Note: Smoking data exclude information for California and South Dakota.

Source: Ventura, S. J., T. J. Mathew, and B. E. Hamilton (2001). "Births to Teenagers in the United States, 1940–2000." *National Vital Statistics Reports,* 49(10).

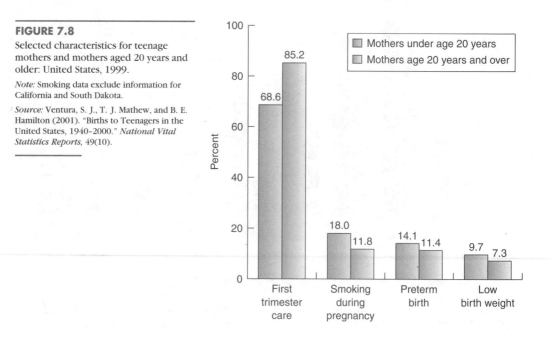

one-third of teenage girls get pregnant at least once before they reach age 20, resulting in approximately 750,000 teen pregnancies a year.[6] In fact, the United States still leads the industrialized world in teen pregnancy and birth rates by a large margin. U.S. rates are at least double those of other Western countries, which places the United States at a significant competitive disadvantage in the global economy.[10]

As stated in the introduction, the future of our nation depends on our children. The extent to which we actually believe this can be measured by the degree to which we plan, provide for, educate, and protect our children. Yet, every day in America, 4,498 babies are born to unmarried mothers; 2,692 babies are born into poverty; 2,222 are born to mothers who are not high school graduates; 2,175 are confirmed abused or neglected; 2,062 babies are born without health insurance; 1,200 babies are born to teenage mothers; 964 babies are at low birth weight; and 78 babies die before their first birthday.[11] The need to plan a pregnancy and thereby place children first in families and in communities must be reemphasized. Unwanted and unplanned childbearing has long been linked with adverse consequences for mothers, couples, and families, as well as for the children themselves.[12]

The choice to become a parent is a critical decision that affects the individual and the community. People who become parents acquire the major responsibility for another human being. They must provide an environment conducive to child development—one that protects and promotes health. However, the broader community also contributes to this growth and development.[12] This is best illustrated by an African proverb "it takes an entire village to educate and raise a child."[13] Therefore, the community must also make provisions for a child's care, nurture, and socialization.

Family Planning

Planning for the birth of a child can be one of life's splendid experiences. The first step is making a conscious decision on whether or not to become a parent. This determination will perhaps be one of the most important and consequential decisions couples will make during their lifetime. Parenthood requires enormous amounts of time, energy, and financial commitment, but most notably it requires the willingness to take full responsibility for a child's growth and development. In general, it is considered important that a pregnancy be planned to ensure the best health for the mother and fetus during the pregnancy. Unfortunately, approximately one-half of pregnancies in the United States are unintended, and 40% of those end in abortion.[14] The United States has set a national goal of increasing intended pregnancies to 56% by 2020.[12]

An unintended pregnancy is a pregnancy that is either mistimed (the woman did not want to be pregnant until later) or unwanted (the woman did not want to be pregnant at any time) at the time of conception. Unintended pregnancy is associated with a range of behaviors that can adversely affect the health of mothers and their babies. These risky behaviors include delayed entry into prenatal care, inadequate weight gain, cigarette smoking, and the use of alcohol and other drugs.[15] Women of all ages may have unintended pregnancies, but some groups are at a higher risk, including teenagers, those living in poverty, and those with limited education.[15,16]

The National Family Growth Study collects information to better understand unintended pregnancy. Using a 10-point scale, with 1 being "very unhappy to be pregnant" and 10 being "very happy to be pregnant," women were asked to report their feelings of pregnancy. The average mean rating was 9.2 for intended pregnancies and 4.2 for unintended pregnancies.[17] These indicators reemphasize the importance of community health education programs regarding family planning.

family planning
determining the preferred number and spacing of children and choosing the appropriate means to accomplish it

Therefore, an important approach to reducing unwanted pregnancies and their adverse consequences is effective family planning by the community.[12] **Family planning** is defined as the process of determining the preferred number and spacing of children in one's family and choosing the appropriate means to achieve this preference. Although many maternal, infant, and child morbidity and mortality outcomes cannot be completely prevented by effective family planning, the frequency of occurrence can be reduced. Thus, preconception education and good gynecological, maternal, and child health care are required for effective family planning.[12]

Title X
a portion of the Public Health Service Act of 1970 that provides funds for family planning services for low-income people

Community involvement in family planning and care programs has historically included both governmental and nongovernmental health organizations in the United States (see Box 7.2). The federal and state governments provide funding assistance through a myriad of family planning services, including Title X of the Public Health Service Act, Medicaid, state funds, the Maternal and Child Health Bureau, and Social Service block grants. Of these, Title X, or the Family Planning Act, is the only federal program dedicated solely to funding family planning and related reproductive health care services through the National Family Planning Program (PL 91-572).[18] **Title X** of the Public Health Service Act was signed into law by President Nixon in 1970 to provide family planning services and help to all who wanted them but could not afford them. For more than three decades, Title X has been this nation's major program to reduce unintended pregnancy by providing contraceptive and other reproductive health care services to low-income women. Currently, it provides funding support to approximately 61% of the 4,000-plus family planning clinics nationwide. Every year more than 5 mil-

---

BOX 7.2 | **TEN GREAT PUBLIC HEALTH ACHIEVEMENTS, 1900–1999: FAMILY PLANNING**

Changes in Family Planning

In 1900, the average life span was 47 years, and 10% of infants died during their first year of life. The average woman had 3.5 children, and 6 to 9 women per 1,000 died in childbirth. Distribution of information regarding contraception and contraceptive devices was generally illegal under federal and state Comstock laws, which had been enacted in the late 1800s. In 1900, the most common methods of contraception included withdrawal before ejaculation, rhythm, contraceptive douches, and vaginal pessaries (diaphragms, for example).

Milestones in Family Planning, United States, 1900–1999

1914	Margaret Sanger arrested for distributing information regarding birth control
1916	First birth control clinic, Brooklyn, New York; closed after 10 days by the New York City Vice Squad
1917	Federal registration of birth certificates
1928	Timing of ovulation during the menstrual cycle established
1955	First national fertility survey
1960	First licensure of birth control pills
1960	Modern intrauterine device licensed
1965	*Griswold v. Connecticut;* Supreme Court legalizes contraception
1970	Title X created
1972	Medicaid funding for family planning services authorized
1972	*Roe v. Wade;* Supreme Court legalizes abortion
1973	First National Survey of Family Growth taken
1990	Norplant licensed
1992	Depo-Provera licensed
1993	Female condom licensed

Source: Centers for Disease Control and Prevention. (1999). "Ten Great Public Health Achievements-United States, 1900-1999." *Morbidity and Mortality Weekly Report,* 48(12): 241–242. Available at www.cdc.gov/mmwr/PDF/wk/mm4812.pdf. Accessed October 26, 2010.

lion women receive health care services at family planning clinics funded by Title X.[19,20] Those served are predominantly young, poor, uninsured, and have never had a child.[21]

These family planning clinics are located in every state and in 85% of all counties. The administration of all Title X grants is through state health departments or regional agencies that subcontract with local agencies and clinics. Currently, slightly more than half of the grants are administered by state and local health departments, one-fifth by Planned Parenthood affiliates, and the remaining one-fourth by regional or local family planning councils located in community organizations and hospitals.[21]

For clinics to receive funding under the Title X program, they must offer a broad range of acceptable family planning methods (oral contraceptives, condoms, sterilization, and abstinence); they must encourage family participation; they must give priority to low-income families, and they must not use abortion as a method of family planning.[18] In addition to family planning methods, clinics also provide a comprehensive group of other health services critical to their clients' sexual and reproductive health (see Figure 7.9).

In 1981, family planning clinics that received federal funds were required to provide counseling on all options open to a pregnant woman, including abortion, as outlined in Title X. However, these facilities were not allowed to perform abortions. In 1984, the "**gag rule**" regulations were enacted. These regulations barred physicians and nurses in clinics receiving federal funds from counseling clients about abortions. Family planning providers challenged this legislation on the grounds that it denied women their rights to information that was needed to make an informed decision. Many health care providers felt that the gag rule restricted their rights to counsel a client even when childbirth could be detrimental to her health.[18] Supporters of the gag rule regulation felt that Title X was created to help prevent unwanted pregnancy by providing education and contraception services and was not intended to provide services related to pregnancy options.

In 1992, congressional action loosened the gag rule and allowed for abortion options to be discussed between a client and her physician at Title X facilities. Although this may appear to be a reasonable compromise, in reality most women who visit family planning clinics are served by

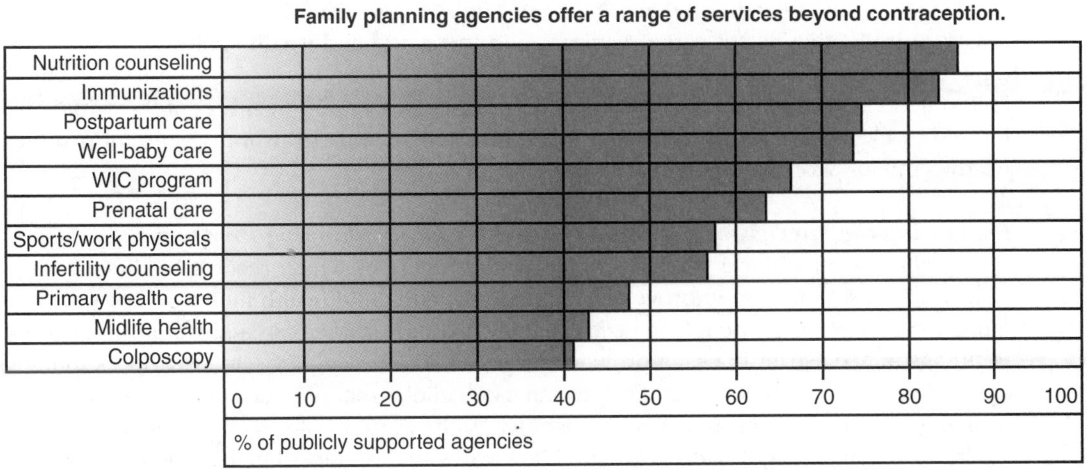

gag rule regulations that barred physicians and nurses in clinics receiving federal funds from counseling clients about abortions

Family planning agencies offer a range of services beyond contraception.

FIGURE 7.9

A significant proportion of women rely on family planning clinics for their reproductive health care.

Source: Alan Guttmacher Institute (AGI). *Fulfilling the Promise: Public Policy and U.S. Family Planning Clinics.* New York: AGI, 2000, p. 18.

a nurse or nurse-practitioner and never see a physician; therefore, this change in the gag rule still did not permit the free exchange of information between clients and all professionals in the clinic. In 1993, President William Clinton signed a presidential memorandum to reverse the gag rule regulations. This change enabled Title X facilities to discuss abortion as an option to pregnancy. In 2003, President George W. Bush reimposed the gag rule to cover State Department family-planning grants. In 2009, President Obama rescinded the gag rule. This tug-of-war over the gag rule is expected to continue.

Controversy regarding acceptable family planning methods is not new in our country. In the early 1900s, a maternity nurse by the name of Margaret Sanger delivered babies in the homes of poor, mostly immigrant women. She described her experiences by writing: "Tales were poured into my ears, a baby born dead, great relief, the death of an older child, sorrow but again relief of a sort, . . . the story told a thousand times of death and abortion and children going into institutions. I shuddered with horror as I listened to the details and studied the reasons in back of them—destitution with excessive childbearing. The waste of life seemed utterly senseless."[22]

The women Sanger cared for knew nothing of how to prevent pregnancy and because of the "Comstock Laws" they could get no information from their doctors. Sanger further explained her experiences by writing "I came to a sudden realization that my work as a nurse and my activities in social service were entirely palliative and consequently futile and useless to relieve the misery I saw all about me."[22] So, disheartened by her ability to care for them, she decided to try to prevent these unwanted conditions in the first place.

In 1914, Margaret Sanger, with the help of funds from numerous supporters worldwide, founded the National Birth Control League. The establishment of this organization is credited with starting the birth control movement in the United States. The purpose of this organization was to win greater public support for birth control by demonstrating the association between a woman's ability to limit her fertility and the improvement of both her health and the health of children. In addition, Sanger also challenged the morality of the times by declaring that women had the right to experience sexual pleasure and that freeing them from the fear of pregnancy would assist women in achieving this. In 1942, the National Birth Control League joined with hundreds of family planning clinics nationwide and formed the Planned Parenthood Federation of America.

Today, Planned Parenthood Federation of America, Inc., has grown to be the largest voluntary reproductive health care organization in the world and is still dedicated to the principle that every woman has the fundamental right to choose when or whether to have children.[23] Currently, Planned Parenthood operates nearly 900 health centers, which are located in every state and the District of Columbia. This not-for-profit organization serves nearly 5 million women and men each year.[23]

Evaluating the Success of Community Health Family Planning Programs

The establishment of local family planning clinics, many of which receive funding through Title X, has resulted in an improvement in maternal and child health indicators for the communities served.[21] Many people in need of family planning services are uninsured, and private health insurance usually does not provide coverage for contraceptive services. Title X funding enables for the support network of more than 4,000 clinics that provide comprehensive family planning services to more than 9 million women each year, 85% of whom are low income and a third of whom are adolescents. By providing access to contraceptive materials and instructions on how to use these materials effectively and counseling about reproductive health matters, community family planning clinics are able to show large reductions in unintended pregnancies, abortions, and births. Each year, publicly subsidized family planning services help prevent 1.9 million unplanned pregnancies, which would otherwise result in 860,000 unintended births, 810,000 abortions, and 270,000 miscarriages.[21]

Publicly funded family planning services are vital to enabling low-income women to avoid unintended pregnancy. From an economic perspective, each public health dollar spent by federal and state governments to provide family planning services saves $4 in Medicaid costs for pregnancy-related and newborn care.[24] The total annual savings is estimated at nearly $5 billion, which represents money currently being spent on welfare, medical, and nutritional services as required by law. A 2010 report showed that more women are in need of publicly funded family services.[25] This is due in large part to the increase in the number of poor women needing publicly funded contraceptive services and supplies.

Abortion

One of the most important outcomes of community family planning programs is preventing abortions. Abortion has been legal throughout the United States since 1973 when the Supreme Court ruled in the **Roe v. Wade** case that women, in consultation with their physician, have a constitutionally protected right to have an abortion in the early stages of pregnancy free from government interference.[26] Since the early 1970s, the Centers for Disease Control and Prevention (CDC) has been documenting the number and characteristics of women obtaining legal induced abortions to monitor unintended pregnancy and to assist with efforts to identify and reduce preventable causes of morbidity and mortality associated with abortions.[27] As a result of the *Roe v. Wade* decision, the number of women dying from illegal abortions has diminished sharply during the last three decades in the United States. However, doubters remain, largely among those whose main strategy for reducing abortion is to outlaw it. However, although it may seem paradoxical, the legal status of abortion appears to have relatively little connection to its overall pervasiveness.

Starting in 1973, the number, ratio, and rate of legal abortions in the United States increased steadily until 1979 and remained stable in the 1980s and early 1990s; it has declined in most years thereafter (see Figure 7.10). In 2006, 846,181 legal induced abortions were reported.[27] According to the CDC, the overwhelming majority of all abortions were performed on unmarried mothers (83.5%), of whom 55% were white and approximately half (52%) were younger than age 25 (see Figure 7.11).

Roe v. Wade
a 1973 Supreme Court decision that made it unconstitutional for state laws to prohibit abortions

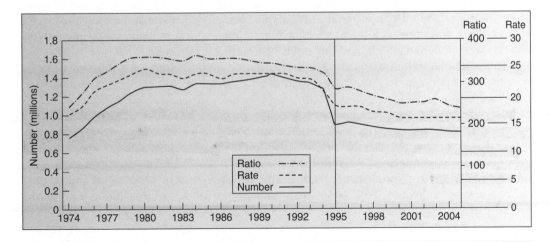

FIGURE 7.10

Number, ratio, and rate of legal abortions performed, by year: United States, 1974–2005.

Note: Ratio is calculated as number of abortions per 1,000 live births; rate is calculated as number of abortions per 1,000 women aged 15 to 44 years. For 1995–2005, data are from 46 reporting areas.

Source: Gamble, S. B., L. T. Strauss, W. Y. Parker, D. A. Cook, S. B. Zane, and S. Hamdan (2008). "Abortion Surveillance—United States, 2005." *Morbidity and Mortality Weekly Report*, 57(SS 13): 1–32.

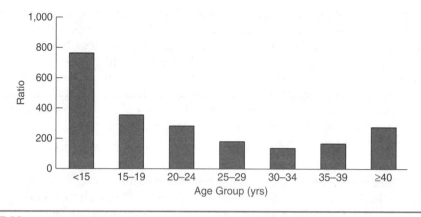

FIGURE 7.11

Abortion ratio, by age group of women who obtained a legal abortion in selected states: United States, 2005.

Note: Ratio is calculated as number of abortions per 1,000 live births. Data are from 46 states, the District of Columbia, and New York City.

Source: Gamble, S. B., L. T. Strauss, W. Y. Parker, D. A. Cook, S. B. Zane, and S. Hamdan (2008). "Abortion Surveillance—United States, 2005." *Morbidity and Mortality Weekly Report,* 57(SS 13): 1-32.

The fate of legalized abortion itself is as unclear as the right of a client to discuss abortion options in federally funded clinics. The Hyde Amendment of 1976 made it illegal to use federal funds to perform an abortion except in cases where the woman's life was in danger. In 1992, the Supreme Court was asked to rule on the constitutionality of the landmark court decision of *Roe v. Wade.* The *Roe v. Wade* Supreme Court ruling made it unconstitutional for state laws to prohibit abortions. In effect, this decision concluded that an unborn child is not a person and therefore has no rights under the law. The decision of whether to have an abortion or not was left up to the woman until she was 12 weeks' pregnant. After the twelfth week, an abortion was permissible only when the health of the mother was in question. In 1989, the Supreme Court appeared to reverse this decision. It ruled that the individual states could place restrictions on a woman's right to obtain an abortion. Some states now have a 24-hour waiting period after counseling before permitting an abortion.

The issue of abortion has become a hotly debated topic. Political appointments can be won or lost depending on a candidate's stance as "pro-life" or "pro-choice" on the abortion issue (see Figure 7.12).

pro-life
a medical/ethical position that holds that performing an abortion is an act of murder

Pro-life groups argue that performing an abortion is an act of murder. Generally, they believe that life begins at conception and that an embryo is a person. The **pro-choice** position is that women have a right to reproductive freedom. Pro-choice advocates feel that the government should not be allowed to force a woman to carry to term and give birth to an unwanted child. They support this argument by raising issues of child abuse and neglect against unwanted children. To counter this argument, pro-life advocates support adoption as an alternative. Clearly, there is no easy solution to the question of abortion. The question of when life begins can only be decided by each individual based on his or her own values and beliefs.[23]

pro-choice
a medical/ethical position that holds that women have a right to reproductive freedom

Maternal Health

Maternal health encompasses the health of women in the childbearing years, including those in the pre-pregnancy period, those who are pregnant, and those who are caring for young children (see Figure 7.13). The effect of pregnancy and childbirth on women is an important indi-

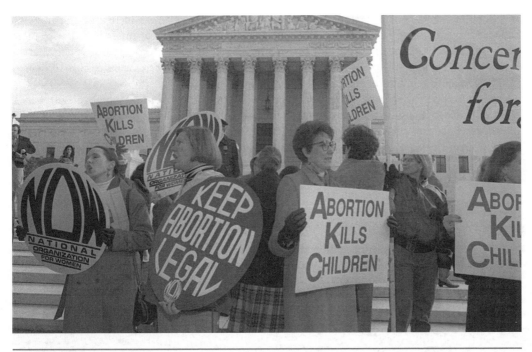

FIGURE 7.12
Political appointments and elections can be won or lost on the issue of abortion.

cator of their health. Pregnancy and delivery can lead to serious health problems. Maternal mortality rates are the most severe measure of ill health for pregnant women.

The Tenth Revision of the *International Classification of Diseases* (ICD 10) defines a *maternal death* (maternal mortality) as "the death of a woman while pregnant or within 42 days of termination of pregnancy, irrespective of the duration and site of the pregnancy, from any cause related to or aggravated by the pregnancy or its management but not from accidental or incidental causes."[28] The *maternal mortality rate* is the number of mothers dying per 100,000 live births in a given year. The number of live births is used in the denominator because the total number of pregnant women is unknown.

In the United States, two to three women die of pregnancy-related complications every day. Between 1970 and 1982, maternal mortality decreased from 21.5 deaths per 100,000 live births to 9.1 deaths per 100,000 live births, more than a 50% decline (see Figure 7.3). However, since 1982 the risk of dying has remained relatively stable, and there has been no marked decrease since that time. This is disturbing because many studies indicate that as many as half of all maternal deaths could be prevented if women had better

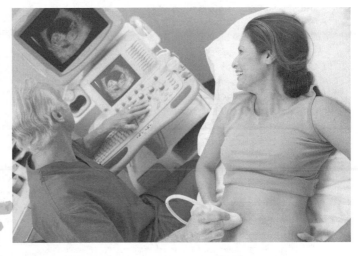

FIGURE 7.13
Maternal health encompasses the health of women in the childbearing years.

access to health care and better quality of care, and made changes in health and lifestyle habits. Causes of maternal death are classified as direct, indirect, or unspecified. The most common direct causes include complications related to the puerperium (period after delivery), eclampsia and preeclampsia, and hemorrhage. Indirect causes comprise deaths from preexisting conditions complicated by pregnancy.

Additionally, the gap between rates for black and white women remains, with black women being four times more likely than white women to die from pregnancy and its complications. Ensuring early initiation of prenatal care during maternity greatly contributes to reductions in perinatal illness, disability, and death for both the mother and the infant.[29] In addition, a number of underlying causes of high maternal morbidity and mortality rates include poverty, the sociocultural factor, and a limited education.

Prenatal Health Care

prenatal health care
medical care provided to a pregnant woman from the time of conception until the birth process occurs

High-quality **prenatal health care** is one of the fundamentals of a safe motherhood program and includes three major components—risk assessment, treatment for medical conditions or risk reduction, and education.[12,29] Prenatal health care should begin before pregnancy when a couple is considering having a child, and it should continue throughout pregnancy (see Box 7.3). The goals of prenatal care include providing the best care for the pregnant woman

---

BOX 7.3 — OPPORTUNITIES TO REDUCE MATERNAL AND INFANT MORTALITY

Prevention measures that reduce maternal and infant mortality and promote the health of all childbearing women and their newborns should start before conception and continue through the postpartum period. Some of these prevention measures include the following.

Before Conception

- Screen women for health risks and preexisting chronic conditions such as diabetes, hypertension, and sexually transmitted diseases.
- Counsel women about contraception and provide access to effective family planning services (to prevent unintended pregnancies and unnecessary abortions).
- Counsel women about the benefits of good nutrition; encourage women especially to consume adequate amounts of folic acid supplements (to prevent neural tube defects) and iron.
- Advise women to avoid alcohol, tobacco, and illicit drugs.
- Advise women about the value of regular physical exercise.

During Pregnancy

- Provide women with early access to high-quality care throughout the phases of pregnancy, labor, and delivery. Such care includes risk-appropriate care, treatment for complications, and use of antenatal corticosteroids when appropriate.
- Monitor and, when appropriate, treat preexisting chronic conditions.
- Screen for and, when appropriate, treat reproductive tract infections, including bacterial vaginosis, group B streptococcus, and human immunodeficiency virus.
- Vaccinate women against influenza, if appropriate.
- Continue counseling against use of alcohol, tobacco, and illicit drugs.
- Continue counseling about nutrition and physical exercise.
- Educate women about the early signs of pregnancy-related problems.

During Postpartum Period

- Vaccinate newborns at age-appropriate times.
- Provide information about well-baby care and the benefits of breastfeeding.
- Warn parents about exposing infants to secondhand smoke.
- Counsel parents about placing infants to sleep on their backs.
- Educate parents about how to protect their infants from exposure to infectious diseases and harmful substances.

Source: Centers for Disease Control and Prevention. (1999). "Ten Great Public Health Achievements-United States, 1900–1999." *Morbidity and Mortality Weekly Report*, 48(12): 241–242. Available at www.cdc.gov/mmwr/PDF/wk/mm4812.pdf. Accessed October 26, 2010.

and the unborn child, as well as preparing the mother-to-be for the delivery of a healthy baby. During prenatal visits, tests are performed on both the mother and fetus to assess any potential risks, to treat any maternal or fetal complications, and to monitor the growth and development of the fetus. In addition, counseling and guidance are provided regarding the various aspects of pregnancy, including weight gain, exercise, nutrition, and overall health.

Prenatal care is crucial to maternal and infant health. Women who receive early and continuous prenatal health care have better pregnancy outcomes than women who do not. A pregnant woman who receives no prenatal care is three times as likely to give birth to a **low-birth-weight infant** (one that weighs less than 5.5 pounds or 2,500 grams) as one who receives the appropriate care, and she is four times as likely to have her baby die in infancy. Getting pregnant women into prenatal care early (during the first three months of pregnancy) is the main policy goal of most publicly funded programs designed to reduce the incidence of low birth weight and infant mortality in the United States. The percentage of women receiving prenatal care during the first trimester was 70.8% in 2007. The target goal for 2010 is 77.9%. Non-Hispanic black, Hispanic, and American Indian/Alaska Native women were 2.5 to 3.5 times more likely to begin care late or to receive no prenatal care at all in 2006 (see Figure 7.14). Black, Native American, Hispanic, poorly educated women, and those most likely to be poor and without health insurance are significantly less likely to receive early and comprehensive prenatal care.[29]

low-birth-weight infant
one that weighs less than 2,500 grams, or 5.5 pounds, at birth

INFANT HEALTH

An infant's health depends on many factors, which include the mother's health and her health behavior prior to and during pregnancy, her level of prenatal care, the quality of her delivery, and the infant's environment after birth. The infant's environment includes not only the home and family environment, but also the availability of essential medical services such as a post-

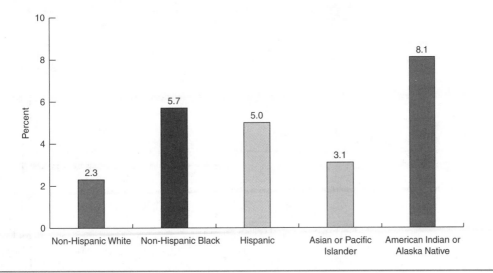

FIGURE 7.14

Percentage of mothers receiving late or no prenatal care by race and hispanic origin, 2006.

Note: Data include those jurisdictions (32 states, the District of Columbia, and New York City) using the 1989 revision of the birth certificates.

Source: National Center for Health Statistics, National Vital Statistics System, *VitalStats*. Available at http://205.207.175.93/VitalStats/TableViewer/tableView.aspx?Reportid=15101. Accessed November 30, 2010.

natal physical examination by a *neonatologist* (a medical doctor who specializes in the care of newborn children up to 2 months of age), regular visits to a physician, and the appropriate immunizations. The infant's health also depends on proper nutrition and other nurturing care in the home environment. Shortcomings in these areas can result in illness, developmental problems, and even the death of the child.

Infant Mortality

Infant death is an important measure of a nation's health because it is associated with a variety of factors, such as maternal health, quality of access to medical care, socioeconomic conditions, and public health practices.[12] An *infant death* (infant mortality) is the death of a child younger than 1 year (see Figure 7.15). The *infant mortality rate* is expressed as the number of deaths of children younger than 1 year per 1,000 live births.

   The infant mortality rate gradually declined from 1980 to 2000 (see Figure 7.2). Decreases in the infant mortality rate during this period have been attributed to improved disease surveillance, advanced clinical care, improved access to health care, better nutrition, the recommendation that infants be placed on their backs when sleeping, and increased educational levels.[12] Since 2000, the infant mortality rate in the United States has shown no further significant decline, maintaining a rate of between 6.7 and 7.0 deaths per 1,000 live births (see Figure 7.2).[30] This is unfortunate because many of the causes of infant deaths could be eliminated by modifying the behaviors, lifestyles, and conditions that affect birth outcomes, such as smoking, substance abuse, poor nutrition, lack of prenatal care, medical problems, and chronic illness.

   The leading causes of infant death include congenital abnormalities, preterm/low birth weight, sudden infant death syndrome (SIDS), problems related to complications of pregnancy, and respiratory distress syndrome.[30]

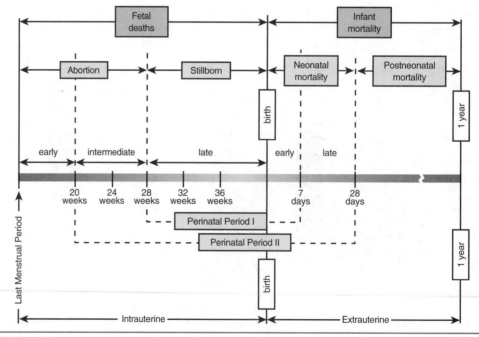

FIGURE 7.15
Important early-life mortality time periods.

Infant deaths, or infant mortality, can be further divided into neonatal mortality and post-neonatal mortality (see Figure 7.15). *Neonatal mortality* is deaths that occur during the first 28 days after birth. Approximately two-thirds of all infant deaths take place during this period. The most common causes of neonatal death are disorders related to short gestation (premature births) and low birth weight, and congenital birth defects. These causes currently account for approximately one-half of all neonatal deaths. *Postneonatal mortality* is deaths that occur between 28 days and 365 days after birth. The most common causes of post-neonatal deaths are sudden infant death syndrome and congenital birth defects.

Improving Infant Health

In part because of medical research and public health and social services supported by both public and private organizations, infant mortality has declined considerably during the past couple of decades. However, there are many opportunities for decreasing infant deaths and improving infant health even further through reducing risk factors associated with these conditions.

Premature Births

Premature (or preterm) babies are born prior to 37 weeks of gestation. The average length of gestation is 40 weeks, and normal is considered 38 to 42 weeks. The number of babies born prematurely in the United States has risen steadily since 1980, and only recently leveled off to 12.3% of all births in 2008.[31,32] Disorders related to short gestation and low birth weight are the leading causes of neonatal death in the United States. Since premature babies usually have less developed organs than full-term babies, they are more likely to face serious multiple health problems following delivery. Premature babies often require neonatal intensive care, which utilizes specialized medical personnel and equipment. In 2005, the economic burden of preterm births was $26.2 billion, or $51,600 per infant. The majority of the expense was for medical care provided in infancy. Other factors that contribute to the economic burden are maternal care services, early intervention services, special education for preterm infants with learning difficulties, and lost labor productivity.[31,32]

Approximately half of all premature births have no known cause. Known major risk factors associated with preterm labor and birth include a woman's past history of preterm delivery, multiple fetuses, late or no prenatal care, cigarette smoking, drinking alcohol, using illegal drugs, exposure to domestic violence, lack of social support, low income, diabetes, anemia, high blood pressure, obesity, and women younger than 17 or older than 35.[31]

Therefore, although a number of causes of premature birth may have eluded researchers and are currently beyond our control, prenatal care and lifestyle changes can help women reduce their risk of having a premature delivery. Consequently, there is a lot that community health programs can do to assist a woman in reducing her risk of having a premature baby—specifically, educating parents about premature labor and what can be done to prevent it and expanding access to health care coverage so that more women can get prenatal care.

Low Birth Weight

Today, it is widely accepted that low birth weight (LBW) is the single most important factor in neonatal death, as well as being a significant predictor of postneonatal mortality and infant and later childhood morbidity. Most infants weigh 3,400 grams (7 pounds) at birth. LBW infants are those that weigh 2,500 grams, or about 5.5 pounds. LBW infants are 40 times more likely to die in their first year of life than normal-weight babies. LBW babies often require extensive medical attention early in life and subsequently may suffer from a variety of physical, emotional, and intellectual problems. LBW babies have a higher incidence of cerebral palsy, deafness, blindness, epilepsy, chronic lung disease, learning disabilities, and attention deficit disorder.[33]

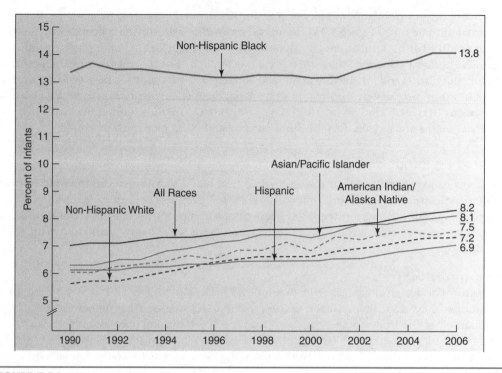

FIGURE 7.16

Percentage of infants born at low birth weight by race/ethnicity, 1990–2007.

*Persons of Hispanic origin may be of any race.

Note: Data for 2007 are preliminary.

Source: U.S. Department of Health and Human Services, Health Resources and Services Administration, Maternal and Child Health Bureau. *Child Health USA 2008–2009.* Rockville, Maryland: U.S. Department of Health and Human Services, 2009.

The percentage of U.S. infants born at LBW has remained relatively stable (between 7.0% and 8.3%) in the last two decades (see Figure 7.16). LBW must continually be aggressively targeted, especially among various racial/ethnic groups, because significant differences exist among these groups (see Chapter 10).

The two factors that are generally recognized to govern infant birth weight are the duration of gestation (premature births) and intrauterine growth rate. Approximately two-thirds of LBW infants are born premature. Therefore, reduction in premature births holds the most potential for overall reduction in LBW. Research on the causes of intrauterine growth retardation (IUGR) leading to LBW babies finds that maternal cigarette smoking during pregnancy is by far the most important risk factor. Other maternal characteristics that are risk factors connected with IUGR include maternal LBW, prior LBW history, low pre-pregnancy weight, drinking alcohol, multiple births, and low pregnancy weight gain.[12] Therefore, all pregnant women should (1) get early, regular prenatal care; (2) eat a balanced diet, including adequate amounts of folic acid; (3) gain enough weight; and (4) avoid smoking and drinking alcohol.[34]

Cigarette Smoking

Research has shown that maternal cigarette smoking during pregnancy is the leading modifiable cause of LBW in the United States, therefore making it an ideal target for intervention. Researchers estimate that smoking during pregnancy is linked to 20% to 30% of LBW infants and 10% of infant deaths.[35] The incidence of LBW infants among mothers who smoke is more than twice that of nonsmokers. The good news is that the percentage of births to women who

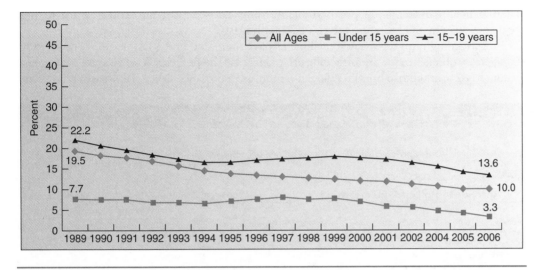

FIGURE 7.17

Percentage of mothers who smoked during pregnancy, by age: 1989–2006.

Source: National Center for Health Statistics, 2008. Table 11. Mothers Who Smoked Cigarettes During Pregnancy, by Selected Characteristics: United States, Selected Years 1990–2000 and Selected States, 2005–2006. *Health, United States, 2008 With Special Feature on the Health of Young Adults.* Hyattsville, MD: 2009. Author. Available at http://ftp.cdc.gov/pub/Health_Statistics/ NCHS/Publications/Health_US/hus99/Excel/table011.xls. Accessed November 30, 2010.

smoked during pregnancy has been dropping, from 19.5% in 1989 to 10% in 2006 (see Figure 7.17). This would seem to indicate that the United States is definitely progressing in the right direction when it comes to reaching its goal of 98.6% of females abstaining from smoking cigarettes during pregnancy by 2020.[12]

Alcohol and Other Drugs

Prenatal exposure to alcohol can cause a range of disorders, known as fetal alcohol spectrum disorders (FASDs). FASD refers to conditions such as **fetal alcohol syndrome (FAS)**, fetal alcohol effects (FAE), alcohol-related neurodevelopmental disorder (ARND), and alcohol-related birth defects (ARBD) (see Chapter 12). A safe level of alcohol consumption during pregnancy has not been determined, but adverse effects are associated with heavy consumption during the first few months of pregnancy.[35] In general, no alcohol during pregnancy is strongly recommended.

Other drug use can also result in a number of deleterious effects on the developing fetus, including impaired fetal growth, that can lead to congenital defects. Crack cocaine use during pregnancy can result in genital and urinary tract malformations in the baby. Marijuana use has also been associated with an increased risk of birth defects. A study showed that infants born to women using marijuana and/or cocaine were significantly smaller than infants of nonusers. Marijuana's effect of increasing maternal heart rate, blood pressure, and carbon monoxide levels may be responsible for impairing the growth of the fetus. Maternal use of cocaine results in lower fetal oxygen levels by inducing uterine contractions.[35]

fetal alcohol syndrome (FAS) a group of abnormalities that may include growth retardation, abnormal appearance of face and head, and deficits of central nervous system function, including mental retardation, in babies born to mothers who have consumed heavy amounts of alcohol during their pregnancies

Breastfeeding

The American Academy of Pediatrics recommends that babies be breast-fed for the first year of life. Breast milk is the ideal food for babies, newborn through 4 to 6 months. Breastfeeding has many advantages for both baby and mother. Breast milk contains substances that help babies resist infections and other diseases. Breastfed babies have fewer ear infections and colds, less diarrhea, and vomit less often. In addition, breastfeeding has been shown to improve maternal health by reducing postpartum bleeding, allowing for an earlier return to pre-pregnancy weight and reducing the risk of osteoporosis.[12]

Breastfeeding rates for women of all races have increased in the last decade. The *Healthy People 2020* objectives for breastfeeding are to increase the percentage of women ever breast-feeding to 82%, and those breastfeeding at 6 months to 60% (see Box 7.4). Breastfeeding rates

---

BOX 7.4

HEALTHY PEOPLE 2010: OBJECTIVES

Objective MICH-21:   Increase the proportion of infants who are breastfed.

Target and baseline:

Objective	Increase in Mothers Who Breastfeed	2005–2007 Status	2020 Target
		Percent	
21.1	Ever breastfed	74	82
21.2	At 6 months	43	61
21.3	At 1 year	23	34
21.5	Exclusively through 6 months	12	24

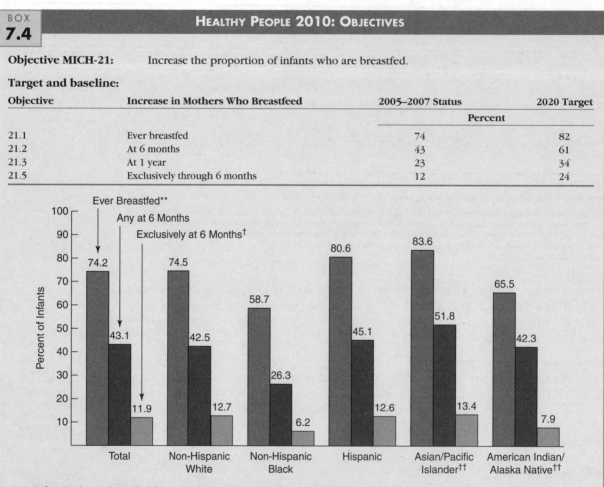

Infants* who are breastfed, by race/ethncity and duration, 2005–2007.

Source: Centers for Disease Control and Prevention, National Immunization Survey.

*Includes only infants born in 2005: data are provisional. **Reported that child was ever breastfed or fed human breastmilk. †Exclusive breastfeeding is defined as only human breastmilk—no solids, water, or other liquids. ††Includes Hispanics.

Source: U.S. Department of Health and Human Services, Health Resources and Services Administration, Maternal and Child Health Bureau (2009). *Women's Health USA 2009.* Rockville, Maryland: U.S. Department of Health and Human Services.

For Further Thought

An important public health goal is to increase the number of mothers who breastfeed. Human milk is acknowledged by the American Academy of Pediatrics as the most complete form of nutrition for infants, with a broad realm of benefits for infants' growth and development. What types of programs would you recommend to educate new mothers and their partners and to educate health care providers?

Source: U.S. Department of Health and Human Services, Office of Disease Prevention and Health Promotion (2010). *Healthy People 2020.* Available at http://www.healthypeople.gov/2020/default.aspx. Accessed December 2, 2010.

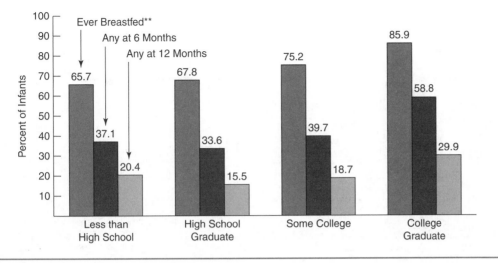

FIGURE 7.18

Infants who are breastfed, by maternal education and duration, 2005–2007.

*Includes only infants born in 2005; data are provisional. **Reported that child was ever breastfed or fed human breastmilk.

Source: U.S. Department of Health and Human Services, Health Resources and Services Administration, Maternal and Child Health Bureau (2009). *Women's Health USA 2009.* Rockville, Maryland: U.S. Department of Health and Human Services.

are highest among those who are college educated (see Figure 7.18), among women 35 years and older, and women participating in the Women, Infants, and Children (WIC) dietary supplemental program. Women least likely to breastfeed were those younger than 20 years of age, those not employed, those with a low income, and those who were black.[12] Two voluntary community groups, the La Leche League and the Nursing Mother's Council, are good sources for breastfeeding information, advice, and support.

Sudden Infant Death Syndrome

Sudden infant death syndrome (SIDS) strikes approximately 2,500 babies each year in the United States. SIDS is defined as the sudden unanticipated death of an infant in whom, after examination, there is no recognizable cause of death. Because most cases of SIDS occur when a baby is sleeping in a crib, SIDS has been referred to as *crib death*. SIDS is the third leading cause of infant death. Moreover, after the first month of life, it is the leading cause of infant death (postneonatal mortality), accounting for one-third of deaths during the period.[12,36]

There is currently no way of predicting which infants will die because of SIDS. However, research has shown that sleeping on the side or back rather than the stomach greatly decreases the risk of SIDS among healthy full-term infants.[37] In response to this research, the federal government initiated a national "Back to Sleep" campaign in 1992 to educate parents and health professionals with the message that placing babies on their backs or sides to sleep can reduce the risk of SIDS. Since the dissemination of the recommendation, more infants have been put to bed on their backs and sides, and the rate of SIDS has fallen by more than 50% (see Figure 7.19).

sudden infant death syndrome (SIDS)
sudden unanticipated death of an infant in whom, after examination, there is no recognized cause of death

CHILD HEALTH

Good health during the childhood years (ages 1–14) is essential to each child's optimal development and America's future. America cannot hope for every child to become a productive member of society if children in this country are allowed to grow up with poverty or live in a violent environment, with mediocre child care, or with no health insurance. Failure to provide

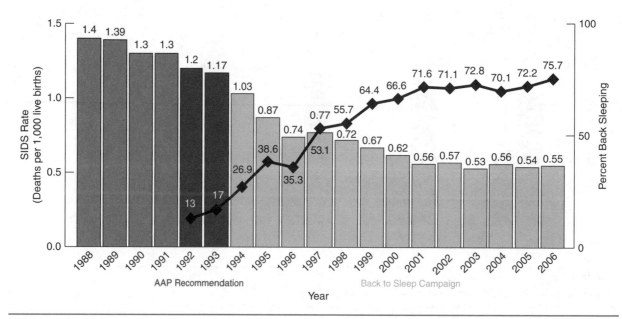

FIGURE 7.19

Rate of sudden infant death syndrome and sleep position: 1988–2006.

Source: National Institutes of Heath, Eunice Kennedy Shriver National Institute of Child Health and Human Development, Sleep Position Data: NICHD, National Infant Sleep Position Study. Available at www.nichd.nih.gov/SIDS/upload/SIDS_rate_back_sleep_2006.pdf. Accessed November 30, 2010.

timely and remedial care leads to unnecessary illness, disability, and death—events that are associated with much greater costs than the timely care itself. The previous example of the cost of not providing prenatal care given earlier in this chapter presents a vivid example. For those who believe that access to basic care is a standard of justness and fairness in any socialized society, America lingers sadly behind many other nations in the health of her children (see Box 7.5).[38]

Childhood Mortality

Childhood mortality rates are the most severe measure of health in children. The death of a child is an enormous tragedy for family and friends, as well as a loss to the community. As

---

BOX 7.5

HOW AMERICA RANKS AMONG INDUSTRIALIZED COUNTRIES IN INVESTING IIN AND PROTECTING CHILDREN

1st in gross domestic product
1st in number of billionaires
1st in number of persons incarcerated
1st in health expenditures
1st in military technology
1st in defense expenditures
1st in military weapons exports
21st in 15-year-olds' science scores
21st in low-birth-weight rates
25th in 15-year-olds' math scores

28th in infant mortality rates
Last in relative child poverty
Last in the gap between the rich and the poor
Last in adolescent birth rates (ages 15 to 19)
Last in protecting our children against gun violence

Source: Children's Defense Fund (2010). *The State of America's Children 2010.* Reprinted with permission. Available at http://www.childrensdefense.org/child-research-data-publications/data/state-of-americas-children-2010-report.html. Accessed December 21, 2010.

mentioned in the introduction of this chapter, the mortality rates of children have generally declined over the past couple of decades (see Figures 7.5 and 7.6). Unintentional injuries are the leading cause of mortality in children (see Figure 7.20). In fact, unintentional injuries kill more children than all diseases combined. The overwhelming majority of unintentional injury deaths in children are the result of to motor vehicle crashes. Moreover, the majority of children were not wearing a seat belt or other restraint.[38] All 50 states have primary child restraint laws. They allow law enforcement officers to stop a driver if a child is not restrained according to the state law. However, the provisions of these laws vary from state to state.

Childhood Morbidity

Although childhood for many children represents a time of relatively good overall health, it is a time when far too many suffer from acute illness, chronic disease, and disabilities. Morbidity statistics on children are more difficult to calculate because they consist of a variety of perspectives. These include unintentional injuries, child maltreatment, and infectious diseases.

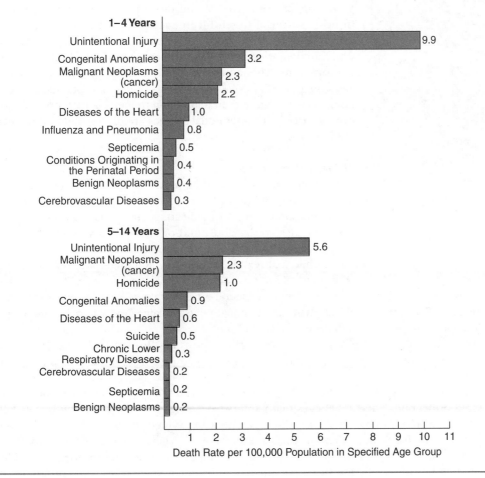

FIGURE 7.20

Leading causes of death in children aged 1 to 14: 2006.

Source: U.S. Department of Health and Human Services, Health Resources and Services Administration, Maternal and Child Health Bureau. *Child Health USA 2008–2009.* Rockville, Maryland: U.S. Department of Health and Human Services, 2009.

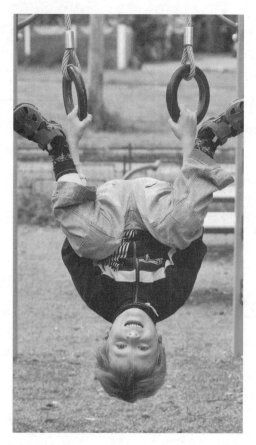

FIGURE 7.21

Unintentional injuries are the leading cause of childhood morbidity and mortality.

Unintentional Injuries

The United States needs to do a better job of protecting its children from unintentional injuries. Even though unintentional injuries are the leading cause of death among children, deaths are a rare event. However, injury-related morbidity is much more prevalent among children (see Figure 7.21). For each childhood death by injury, there are approximately 40 hospitalizations and 1,000 emergency department visits.[39] Every year about one-fourth of all children sustain an injury severe enough to require medical attention, missed school, or bed rest. Moreover, injuries are the leading cause of disability in children, with approximately 100,000 children becoming permanently disabled annually.[39]

In addition to the physical and emotional effects on children and their families, these injuries have enormous financial costs. Injuries requiring medical attention or resulting in restricted activity cost $17 billion annually for medical treatment.[40] Estimates are that 90% of the more than 4,000 unintentional injuries suffered by children each day in a manner seriously enough to require medical treatment could be prevented. Childhood injuries can deprive the country of the child's potential contributions. The injuries incurred in 2000 by children aged 14 and younger will have lasting effects, including total lifetime economic costs of more than $50 billion in medical expenses and lost productivity.[40] (Unintentional injuries are discussed in more detail in Chapter 15.)

Child Maltreatment

Child maltreatment is another source of injury to children. Child maltreatment includes physical abuse, neglect (physical, educational, emotional, and/or medical), sexual abuse, emotional abuse (psychological/verbal abuse and/or mental injury), and other types of maltreatment such as abandonment, exploitation, and/or threats to harm the child. The causes of child maltreatment are not well understood. Child abuse or neglect is often associated with physical injuries and delayed physical growth. However child abuse and neglect is also associated with psychological problems such as aggression and depression. The rate of children maltreated annually has remained between 10 and 15 per 1,000 children over the past decade (see Table 7.1).[41]

The oldest federal agency for children, the Children's Bureau (CB), located in the Administration for Children and Families, has worked to lead the public in taking a more informed and active part in child abuse prevention. The CB has been instrumental in defining the scope of the problem of child maltreatment and in promoting community responsibility for child protection. The CB believes that parents have a right to raise their children as long as they are willing to protect them. When parents cannot meet their children's needs and keep them from harm, the community has a responsibility to act on behalf of the child. If one suspects a child is being abused or neglected, it is important to call the proper authorities. Any action into the family life should be guided by federal and state laws. According to the CB, the community's responsibility for child protection is based on the following:[42]

- Communities should develop and implement programs to strengthen families and prevent the likelihood of child abuse and neglect.

Table 7.1 Child Maltreatment: Rate of Substantiated Maltreatment Reports of Children Ages 0–17 by Selected Characteristics, 1998–2007

(Substantiated maltreatment reports per 1,000 children ages 0–17)

Characteristic	1998	1999	2000	2001	2002	2003	2004	2005	2006	2007[a]
Total	12.9	11.8	12.2	12.5	12.3	12.2	12.0	12.1	12.1	10.6
Gender										
Male	—	—	11.4	11.7	11.5	11.5	11.3	11.3	11.4	10.0
Female	—	—	12.9	13.2	13.0	12.9	12.7	12.7	12.7	11.2
Race and Hispanic Origin[b]										
White, non-Hispanic	—	—	10.7	10.9	10.9	11.0	10.9	10.8	10.7	9.1
Black, non-Hispanic	—	—	21.5	21.8	20.8	20.7	20.1	19.5	19.8	16.7
Asian	—	—	2.0	3.7	3.2	3.0	2.9	2.5	2.5	2.4
Native Hawaiian or Other Pacific Islander	—	—	21.7	20.7	18.6	18.6	18.0	16.1	14.3	14.1
American Indian or Alaska Native	—	—	20.5	26.5	21.8	21.5	16.5	16.5	15.9	13.6
Multiple races	—	—	12.3	11.1	13.0	12.9	14.5	15.0	15.4	14.0
Hispanic	—	—	10.2	10.3	8.2	10.2	10.1	10.7	10.8	10.3
Age										
Ages 0–3	—	—	15.7	16.1	16.1	16.1	16.0	16.5	16.8	15.0
Age <1	—	—	—	—	21.6	21.7	22.0	23.4	23.9	22.0
Ages 1–3	—	—	—	—	14.2	14.2	13.9	14.1	14.2	12.6
Ages 4–7	—	—	13.4	13.8	13.6	13.7	13.5	13.5	13.5	11.6
Ages 8–11	—	—	11.8	12.2	11.9	11.6	11.1	10.9	10.8	9.4
Ages 12–15	—	—	10.4	10.8	10.7	10.6	10.3	10.2	10.2	8.7
Ages 16–17	—	—	5.8	6.0	6.0	6.0	6.1	6.2	6.3	5.4

— Not available.

[a]Data since 2007 are not directly comparable with prior years as differences may be partially attributed to changes in one state's procedures for determination of maltreatment. Other reasons include the increase in children who received an "other" disposition, the decrease in the percentage of children who received a substantiated or indicated disposition, and the decrease in the number of children who received an investigation or assessment.

[b]The revised 1997 OMB standards were used for Race and Hispanic origin, where respondents could choose one or more of five racial groups: White, Black or African American, Asian, Native Hawaiian or Other Pacific Islander, or American Indian or Alaska Native. Those reporting more than one race were classified as "Two or more races." In addition, data on race and Hispanic origin are collected separately, but are combined for reporting. Persons of Hispanic origin may be of any race.

Note: The count of child victims is based on the number of investigations by Child Protective Services that found the child to be a victim of one or more types of maltreatment. The count of victims is, therefore, a report-based count and is a "duplicated count," because an individual child may have been maltreated more than once. Substantiated maltreatment includes the dispositions of substantiated, indicated, or alternative response-victim. Rates are based on the number of states submitting data to the National Child Abuse and Neglect Data System (NCANDS) each year: states include the District of Columbia and Puerto Rico. The overall rate of maltreatment is based on the following number of states for each year: 51 in 1998, 50 in 1999, 50 in 2000, 51 in 2001, 51 in 2002, 51 in 2003, 50 in 2004, 52 in 2005, 51 in 2006, 50 in 2007, and 51 in 2008. The number of states reporting on sex for each year from 2000 to the present was 50 in 2000, 51 in 2001, 51 in 2002, 51 in 2003, 50 in 2004, 51 in 2005, 51 in 2006, 50 in 2007, and 51 in 2008. The number of states reporting on race and Hispanic origin for each year from 2000 to the present was 48 in 2000, 49 in 2001, 50 in 2002, 50 in 2003, 49 in 2004, 50 in 2005, 49 in 2006, 46 in 2007, and 47 in 2008. The number of states reporting on age for each year from 2000 to the present was 50 in 2000, 51 in 2001, 51 in 2002, 51 in 2003, 50 in 2004, 51 in 2005, 51 in 2006, 50 in 2007, and 51 in 2008. Rates from 1998 to1999 are based on aggregated data submitted by states; rates from 2000 to 2008 are based on case-level data submitted by the states. The reporting year changed in 2003 from the calendar year to the Federal fiscal year. Additional technical notes are available in the annual reports entitled Child Maltreatment. These reports are available on the Internet at http://www.acf.hhs.gov/programs/cb/stats_research/index.htm#can.

Source: Federal Interagency Forum on Child and Family Statistics. National Child Abuse and Neglect Data System. Available at www.childstats.gov/americaschildren/tables.asp. Accessed November 30, 2010.

- Child maltreatment is a community problem; no single agency or individual has the necessary knowledge, skills, resources, or societal mandate to provide the assistance to abused and neglected children and their families.
- Intervention must be sensitive to culture, values, religion, and other differences.
- Professionals must recognize that most parents do not intend to harm their children. Rather, abuse and neglect may be the result of a combination of psychological, social, situational, and societal factors.
- Service providers should recognize that many maltreating adults have the capacity to change their abusive/neglectful behavior, when given sufficient help and resources to do so.
- To help families protect their children and meet their basic needs, the community's response should be nonpunitive, noncritical, and conducted in the least intrusive manner possible.
- Growing up in their own family is optimal for children, as long as the children's safety can be assured.
- When parents cannot or will not meet their child's needs, removal from the home may be necessary. All efforts to develop a permanent plan for a child should be made as quickly as possible.[42]

See Chapter 15 for more detailed information on child abuse and neglect.

Infectious Diseases

In the past, infectious diseases were the leading health concern among children, but increased public health action has resulted in a substantial reduction in both morbidity and mortality rates. Infectious disease control resulted from improvements in sanitation and hygiene and the implementation of universal vaccination programs. Because many vaccine-preventable diseases are more common and more deadly among infants and children, the CDC recommends vaccinating children against most vaccine-preventable diseases early in life. The 2010 recommended immunization schedule is shown in Figure 7.22.

The CDC's immunization schedule for very young children recommends four doses of the diphtheria, tetanus, and pertussis (DTP) vaccine, three or more doses of polio vaccine, one or more doses of measles-mumps-rubella (MMR) vaccine, three or more doses of

Vaccine ▼ Age ▶	Birth	1 month	2 months	4 months	6 months	12 months	15 months	18 months	19–23 months	2–3 years	4–6 years
Hepatitis B	HepB	HepB			HepB						
Rotavirus			RV	RV	RV						
Diphtheria, Tetanus, Pertussis			DTaP	DTaP	DTaP		DTaP				DTaP
Haemophilus influenzae type b			Hib	Hib	Hib	Hib					
Pneumococcal			PCV	PCV	PCV	PCV			PPSV		
Inactivated Poliovirus			IPV	IPV		IPV					IPV
Influenza						Influenza (Yearly)					
Measles, Mumps, Rubella						MMR					MMR
Varicella						Varicella					Varicella
Hepatitis A						HepA (2 doses)				HepA Series	
Meningococcal										MCV	

Range of recommended ages for all children except certain high-risk groups

Range of recommended ages for certain high-risk groups

FIGURE 7.22

Recommended 2010 immunization schedule for ages 0–6 years: United States, 2010.

Source: Centers for Disease Control and Prevention. Recommended Immunization Schedules for Persons Aged 0 Through 18 Years—United States, 2010. *Morbidity and Mortality Weekly Report,* 58(51&52):1–4.

Haemophilus influenzae type b (Hib) vaccine, the hepatitis B vaccine, and the varicella (chickenpox) vaccine. The combined immunization series is referred to as the 4:3:1:3 series. Immunization rates are considered an important indicator of the adequacy of health care for children and of the level of protection a community values related to preventable infectious diseases. The proportion of children aged 19 months to 35 months receiving the recommended combined series has increased from 69% in 1994 to 80% in 2008 (see Figure 7.23).

All children should be immunized at regular health care visits, beginning at birth and continuing to age 6.[43] By immunizing, the community safeguards its children against the potentially devastating effects of vaccine-preventable diseases. No child should ever have to endure the effects of these diseases simply because he or she was not vaccinated on time.

Although progress in improving immunization rates has been substantial, about 1 million children in the United States under 2 years of age have not been fully vaccinated with the most critical vaccines. In addition, the National Immunization Survey data showed considerable variation between states and urban areas, indicating that children are not equally well protected in all parts of the United States. This large number of unvaccinated children has been attributed to cost, lack of access to medical care, uneducated parents, and confusion on when to vaccinate children. The U.S. government's Childhood Immunization Initiative includes five strategies: (1) improving immunization services for needy families, especially in public health clinics; (2) reducing vaccine costs for lower-income and uninsured families, especially for vaccines provided in private physicians' offices; (3) building community networks to reach out to families and ensure that young children are vaccinated as needed; (4) improving systems for monitoring diseases and vaccinations; and (5) improving vaccines and vaccine use.[43]

More stringent measures by the medical community are needed to ensure that all children are immunized. Opportunities to vaccinate are frequently missed by health care practitioners in primary care settings that do not routinely inquire about the immunization status of the child. Parents and health practitioners need to work together to ensure that youth are protected from communicable diseases. Timely immunization of children must be accepted as a national obligation because America cannot afford the waste that results from unnecessary illness, disability, and death.[43]

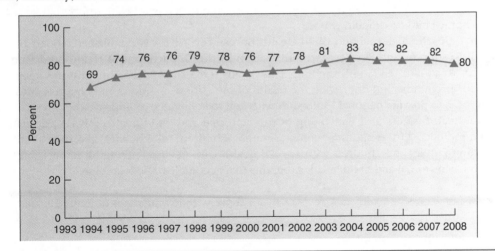

FIGURE 7.23

Percentage of children aged 19 to 35 months receiving the combined series vaccination (4:3:1:3), 1994–2008.

Sources: Data for 1994: Eberhardt, M. S., D. D. Ingram, D. M. Makuc, et al. (2001). *Urban and Rural Health Chartbook: Health, United States, 2001.* Hyattsville, MD: National Center for Health Statistics. Data for 1995–2001: National Center for Health Statistics (2003). *Health, United States 2003 with Chartbook on Trends in the Health of Americans.* Hyattsville, MD: Author. Data for 2002: National Immunization Program (2003). *Immunization Coverage in the U.S.* Results from National Immunization Survey, Centers for Disease Control and Prevention. Data for 2003: National Immunizaton Program (2004). Immunization Coverage.

Community Programs for Women, Infants, and Children

In the preceding pages, many problems associated with maternal, infant, and child health have been identified. Solutions to many of these problems have been proposed, and in many cases programs are already in place. Some of these programs are aimed at preventing or reducing the levels of maternal and infant morbidity and mortality, whereas others are aimed at the prevention or reduction of childhood morbidity and mortality.

The federal government has more than 35 health programs in 16 different agencies to serve the needs of our nation's children. The majority of these programs are well respected and help meet the needs of many children. However, others are **categorical programs**, meaning they are only available to people who can be categorized into a specific group based on disease, age, family means, geography, financial need, or other variables. This means that too many children fall through the cracks and are not served. Some children require services from multiple programs, which complicates the eligibility determination of each child. At times, this can lead to an inefficient system of child health care. Nonetheless, federal programs have contributed to a monumental improvement in maternal, infant, and child health. We discuss some of the more consequential government programs and their past successes and future objectives in the following text.

categorical programs programs available only to people who can be categorized into a group based on specific variables

Maternal and Child Health Bureau

In 1935, Congress enacted Title V of the Social Security Act. Title V is the only federal legislation dedicated to promoting and improving the health of our nation's mothers and children. Since its enactment, Title V–sponsored projects have been incorporated into the ongoing health care system for children and families. Although Title V has been frequently modified over the last couple of decades, the fundamental goal has remained constant: continued progress in the health, safety, and well-being of mothers and children. The most notable landmark achievements of Title V are projects that have produced "guidelines for child health supervision from infancy through adolescence; influenced the nature of nutrition care during pregnancy and lactation; recommended standards for prenatal care; identified successful strategies for the prevention of childhood injuries; and developed health safety standards for out-of-home child care facilities."[44]

In 1990, the Maternal and Child Health Bureau (MCHB) was established as part of the Health Resources and Services Administration in the Department of Health and Human Services to administer Title V funding. This means the MCHB is charged with the responsibility for promoting and improving the health of our nation's mothers and children. MCHB's mission "is to provide national leadership with key stakeholders, to improve the physical and mental health, safety and well-being of the maternal and child health (MCH) population which includes all the nation's women, infants, children, adolescents, and their families, including fathers and children with special health care needs."[45] To fulfill its mission, the MCHB has maternal and child health programs that accomplish the following:[45]

- Ensure access to quality care, especially for those with low incomes or limited availability of care
- Reduce infant mortality
- Provide and ensure access to comprehensive prenatal and postnatal care, especially for low-income and at-risk women
- Increase the number of children receiving health assessments and follow-up diagnostic and treatment services
- Provide and ensure access to preventive and child care services, as well as rehabilitative services for certain children

- Implement family-centered, community-based systems of coordinated care for children with special health care needs
- Provide assistance in applying for services to pregnant women with infants and children who are eligible for Medicaid

The MCHB works on accomplishing its goals through the administration of four core public health services: (1) infrastructure-building services, (2) population-based services, (3) enabling services, and (4) direct health care (gap-filling) services. MCHB uses the construct of a pyramid to provide a useful framework for understanding programmatic directions and resource allocation by the bureau and its partners (see Figure 7.24). MCHB continues to strive for a "society that recognizes and fully supports the important role that public health

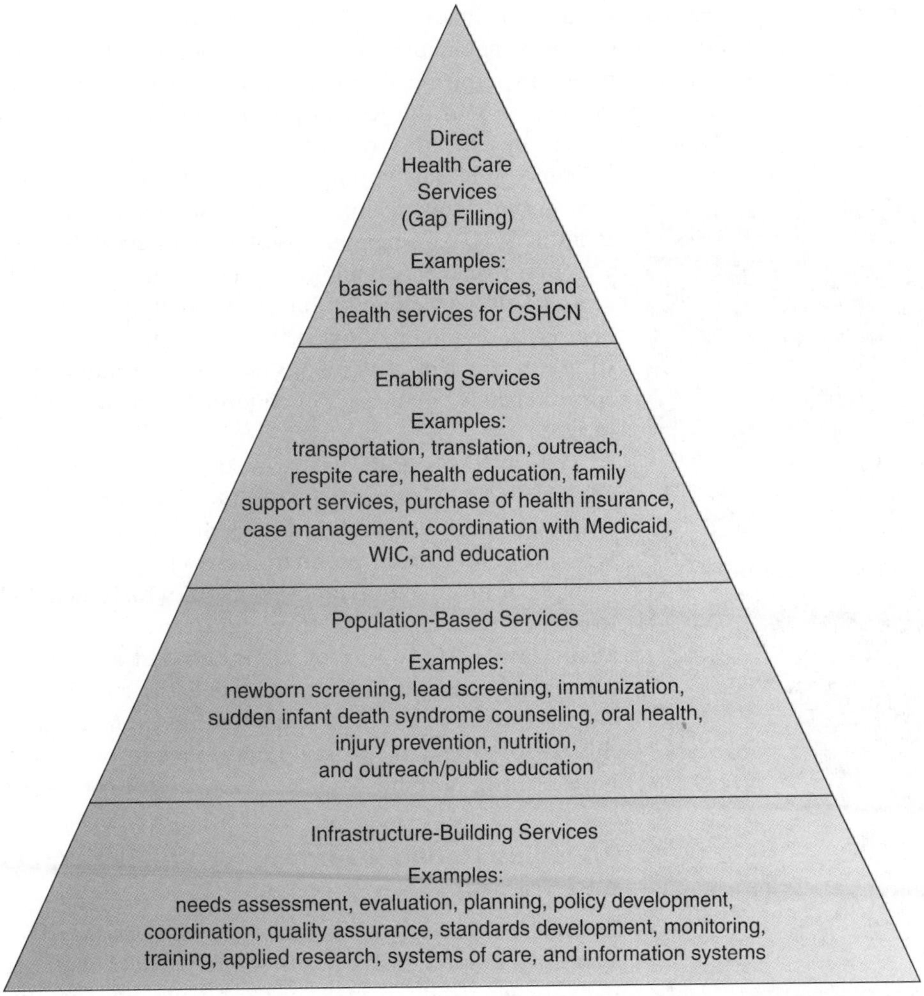

Direct
Health Care
Services
(Gap Filling)

Examples:
basic health services, and
health services for CSHCN

Enabling Services

Examples:
transportation, translation, outreach,
respite care, health education, family
support services, purchase of health insurance,
case management, coordination with Medicaid,
WIC, and education

Population-Based Services

Examples:
newborn screening, lead screening, immunization,
sudden infant death syndrome counseling, oral health,
injury prevention, nutrition,
and outreach/public education

Infrastructure-Building Services

Examples:
needs assessment, evaluation, planning, policy development,
coordination, quality assurance, standards development, monitoring,
training, applied research, systems of care, and information systems

FIGURE 7.24

MCH pyramid of health services. The conceptual framework for the services of Title V Maternal and Child Health is envisioned as a pyramid with four tiers of services and levels of funding that provide comprehensive services for mothers and children.

Source: U.S. Department of Health and Human Services (2003). *Understanding Title V of the Social Security Act.* Washington, DC: Health Resources and Service Administration, Maternal and Child Health Bureau.

plays in promoting the health of the MCH population, including building, strengthening and assuring MCH health services and infrastructure at all levels."[45]

Women, Infants, and Children Program

The Women, Infants, and Children (**WIC**) program is a clinic-based program designed to provide a variety of nutritional and health-related goods and services to pregnant, postpartum, and breastfeeding women, infants, and children under the age of 5. The WIC program began as a pilot in 1972 and received permanent federal funding in 1974, in response to growing evidence linking nutritional inadequacies to mental and physical health defects. Congress intended that WIC, unlike other food programs, would serve as "an adjunct to good health care, during critical times of growth and development, to prevent the occurrence of health problems."[46]

> **WIC**
> a special supplemental food program for women, infants, and children, sponsored by the USDA

The U.S. Department of Agriculture (USDA) administers WIC. The USDA administers grants to the states, where the WIC programs are most often offered through local health departments or state health and welfare agencies (see Figure 7.25). Pregnant or postpartum women, infants, and children up to age 5 are eligible if they meet the following three criteria: (1) residency in the state in which they are applying, (2) income requirements (applicant must have a household income at or below 185% of the federal poverty income guidelines), (3) determination to be at "nutritional risk" by a health professional.

Since WIC's inception as a national nutrition program, it has grown dramatically. In 1974, the average number of monthly WIC participants was 88,000; in 2008 that number was more than 9.5 million women, infants, and children. Among WIC participants, children make up half, infants one-quarter, and women one-quarter (see Figure 7.26). This constitutes nearly half of all infants born in the United States and approximately one-quarter of children between 1 and 5 years of age.

The WIC program has proved to be one of the most effective ways to improve the health of mothers, infants, and young children. Research indicates that participation in the WIC program during pregnancy provides women with a number of positive outcomes, some of which include birth to babies with higher birth weights and fewer fetal and infant deaths. The WIC program is also cost effective. USDA research has shown that for every dollar spent on WIC, the taxpayer saves $4 in future expenditures on Medicaid.[47] For this reason, the WIC program continues to possess strong bipartisan support in Congress.

Providing Health Insurance for Women, Infants, and Children

All children deserve to start life on the right track and to have access to comprehensive health services that provide preventive care when they are well and treatment when they are ill or injured. Health insurance provides access to critical preventive medical services as well as acute medical care in the case of illness or injury (see Chapter 13). When compared with children who are privately insured or have governmental insurance, children without health insurance are much more likely

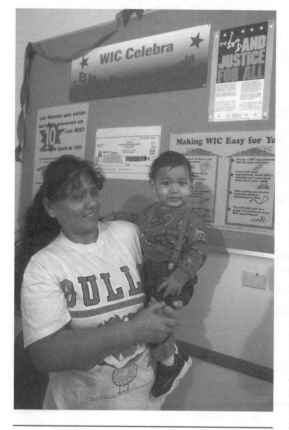

FIGURE 7.25

The WIC program has proven to be extremely effective in improving the health of women, infants, and children in America.

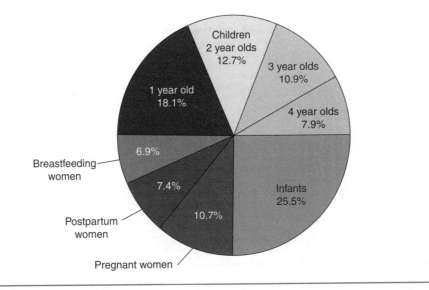

FIGURE 7.26

Distribution of individuals enrolled in the WIC program.

Note: Percentages may not add to 100.0% due to rounding.

Source: Conner, P., S. Bartlett, M. Mendelson, K. Condon, and J. Sutcliffe (January 2010). *WIC Participant and Program Characteristics, 2008* (WIC-08-PC). Alexandria, VA: U.S. Department of Agriculture, Food and Nutrition Service, Office of Research and

to have necessary care delayed or receive no care for health problems, putting them at greater risk for hospitalization.[48] Therefore, providing health insurance to low-income children is a critical health care safety net.

The government has two principal programs aimed at providing health care coverage to low-income children: the Medicaid program and the State Children's Health Insurance Program (formerly called SCHIP, now called CHIP). Medicaid, created in 1965, provides medical assistance for certain low-income individuals and families, mostly women and children (see Chapter 13). Children represent slightly more than half of all Medicaid beneficiaries, yet account for only 17% of program spending. A major reason that Medicaid is working well for American children is the multiphase program for preventive health called the Early and Periodic Screening, Diagnostic, and Treatment (EPSDT) for individuals younger than the age of 21. The Medicaid EPSDT provisions entitle poor children to a comprehensive package of preventive health care and medically necessary diagnosis and treatment.

Although the Medicaid program is a critical health care program for low-income children, being poor does not automatically qualify a child for Medicaid. Medicaid eligibility is determined by each state based on various age and income requirements. As a result, Medicaid coverage varies across the states and leaves a significant number of poor children uninsured. To broaden coverage to low-income children, Congress created CHIP under provisions in the Balanced Budget Act of 1997 (see Chapter 13). The program targets uninsured children younger than 19 with family incomes below 200% of poverty who are not eligible for Medicaid or covered by private insurance. Government-funded health insurance is an important source of coverage for children, and its significance has been growing. Medicaid coverage for children increased from 20% of all children in 2000 to 30% in 2008 (see Figure 7.27). During the same time period, the percentage of children with private health insurance coverage decreased from 71% in 2000 to 63% in 2008 (see Figure 7.27). The success in increasing the number of children with coverage is attributable not just to Medicaid but to the combined effects of Medicaid and CHIP. However, despite these programs, approximately

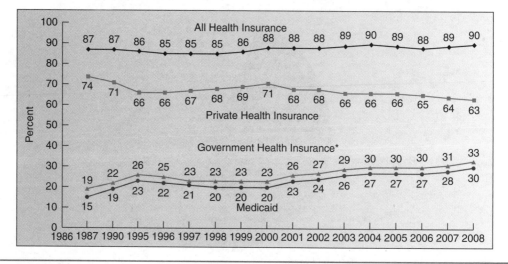

FIGURE 7.27

Percentage of children covered by health insurance, by type of insurance, selected years, 1987–2008.

*Government health insurance consists primarily of Medicaid, but also includes such coverage as Medicare, State Children's Health Insurance Programs (SCHIP), and Medical Care Program of the Uniformed Services (CHAMPUS/Tricare).

Source: U.S. Census Bureau (2009). *Income, Poverty, and Health Insurance Coverage in the United States, 2008. Current Population Reports, Consumer Income* (P60-236).Washington, DC: U.S. Government Printing Office.

10% of youth younger than the age of 19 were uninsured in 2008. Advocates have encouraged state and community decision makers to continue the expansion of Medicaid and CHIP programs to cover as many uninsured children as possible.

Providing Child Care

Experiences during the first years of childhood significantly influence the health of a child. Research shows that early investments in the nurturing of children provides major advantages for families and society later. Whereas parents should accept the primary responsibility for raising their children, the government can assist families who need help making important investments. Two important investments to the health and welfare of America's children are parenting during the first months of life and the accompanying need for secure relationships with a small number of adults in safe settings as they develop during the first few years of life.

To support new parents, the **Family and Medical Leave Act (FMLA)** was signed into law in 1993. The FMLA grants 12 weeks of unpaid job-protected leave to men or women after the birth of a child, an adoption, or in the event of illness in the immediate family.[49] This legislation has provided employed parents with the time to nurture their children and develop their parenting skills. However, the FMLA only affects businesses with 50 or more employees. Those employees covered by the law include those who have worked 1,250 hours for an employer over a 12-month period (an average of 25 hours per week). This excludes about 40% of American employees who work in small businesses that do not fall under the law's guidelines. Also, employers covered by the FMLA can exempt key salaried employees who are among their highest paid 10%, if they are needed to prevent "substantial and grievous" economic harm to the employer. Some experts feel the law divides the people by class, helping those who can afford the 3 months without pay, and bypassing those who cannot. Experts have recommended a 6- to 12-month family care leave program with partial pay for at least 3 months. America is the only industrialized nation that has not enacted a paid infant-care leave.

Today more families are in need of child care than ever before. Estimates are that as many as 13 million children younger than age 6 are in child care every day. The need for increased

Family and Medical Leave Act (FMLA)
federal law that provides up to a 12-week unpaid leave to men and women after the birth of a child, an adoption, or an event of illness in the immediate family

use of professional child care has come about as women increasingly are working outside the home and as more children grow up in single-parent households. However, for many families, especially those with low and moderate incomes, high-quality, affordable child care is simply not available. According to a recent study, much of the care we offer children is inadequate, yet a full day of child care costs an average of $4,000 to $10,000 annually per child.[11] These costs are beyond the reach of many working parents, half of whom earn $35,000 or less a year. The lack of high-quality child care prevents children from entering school ready to learn, hinders their success in school, and limits the ability of their parents to be productive workers. Furthermore, after-school care is crucial because juvenile crime peaks between the hours of 3 P.M. and 7 P.M., and school-aged children may be at greater risk of engaging in activities that lead to problems such as violence and teen pregnancy.

In 1988, Congress passed the Family Support Act, which provided funding for child care assistance to welfare parents who are employed or participating in an approved training program. Unfortunately, states must match federal funds for this program, which makes meeting the needs of eligible participants difficult for poor states.

In 1990, Congress passed the Child Care and Development Block Grant (CCDBG), which provides child care subsidies for low-income children and funding to improve the quality of child care services. The "At Risk" Child Care Program, also passed in 1990, provides additional funding to support child care assistance to low-income families at risk of going on welfare. With the initiation of the "At Risk" Child Care Program and the CCDBG, states were able to provide additional assistance to many more low-income families. However, according to state-reported statistics, of the 15 million children eligible for federal support, only 12% are receiving federal help because of limited federal funding.[50] This means that only 1 of 10 children who are eligible for child care assistance under federal law receive any help. Not one state is currently serving all eligible families. This means that too many parents are unable to obtain necessary child care assistance.

Other Advocates for Children

Numerous groups advocate for children's health and welfare. Among them are the Children's Defense Fund, UNICEF, and the American Academy of Pediatrics.

Children's Defense Fund

Since 1973, the Children's Defense Fund (CDF) has been working to create a nation in which the network of family, community, private-sector, and government supports for children is so tightly intertwined that no child can slip through the cracks. The CDF is a private, nonprofit organization headquartered in Washington, D.C., and it is dedicated to providing a voice for the children of America. It has never accepted government funds and supports its programs through donations from foundations, corporate grants, and individuals. The CDF focuses on the needs of poor, minority, and handicapped children and their families. The aim of the CDF is to educate the nation about the needs of children and to encourage preventive investment in children before they get sick or suffer. It provides information and technical assistance to state and local child advocates.

United Nations Children's Fund

Founded in 1946, the United Nations Children's Fund (UNICEF) is the only organization of the United Nations assigned exclusively to children. This organization works with other United Nations' members, governments, and nongovernmental organizations to improve child conditions through community-based services in primary health care, basic education, and safe water and sanitation in more than 140 developing countries. UNICEF gathers data on the health of children throughout the world. UNICEF has assisted in mass vaccinations and has been involved in other international health efforts to protect children.

American Academy of Pediatrics

The American Academy of Pediatrics (AAP) was founded in 1930 by 35 pediatricians who felt the need for an independent pediatric forum to address children's needs. When the Academy was established, the idea that children have special developmental and health needs was a new one. Preventive health practices now associated with child care, including immunizations and regular health exams, were only just beginning to change the custom of treating children as "miniature adults." The Academy is committed to the attainment of optimal physical, mental, and social health and well-being for all infants, children, adolescents, and young adults. The activities and efforts of the AAP include research, advocacy for children and youth, and public and professional education.

An example of a program that the AAP coordinates is the Healthy Child Care America (HCCA) program. HCCA is partly funded by the Child Care Bureau (CCB), Office of Family Assistance (OFA), Administration for Children and Families (ACF), the Maternal and Child Health Bureau, HRSA, and the U.S. Department of Health and Human Services. The specific goals of the HCCA program are the following:

- To promote the healthy development and school readiness of children in early education and child care by strengthening partnerships between health and child care professionals
- To provide information and support necessary to strengthen children's access to health services
- To promote the cognitive, social, and physical development of children in early education and child care
- To provide technical assistance regarding health and safety for health professionals and the early childhood community
- To enhance the quality of early education and child care with health and safety resources
- To support the needs of health professionals interested in promoting healthy and safe early education and child care programs

Since the Healthy Child Care America program was launched in 1995, many communities around the country have been promoting collaborative partnerships between health and child care professionals to ensure that children receive the best and the highest-quality care possible. By expanding and creating partnerships between families, child care providers, and government, the best care for millions of children continues to occur.

CHAPTER SUMMARY

- Maternal, infant, and child health are important indicators of a community's overall health. Maternal health encompasses the health of women of childbearing age from pre-pregnancy through pregnancy, labor, and delivery, and in the postpartum period. Infant and child health refers to individuals through 14 years of age.

- Families are the primary unit in which infants and children are nurtured and supported regarding healthy development. Significant increases in births to unmarried women in the last two decades, especially among teenagers, are among the many changes in American society that have affected family structure and the economic security of children. Teenage childbearing represents a significant social and financial burden on both the family and the community.

- The establishment of local Family Planning Clinics with Title X funding has resulted in an improvement in maternal and child health indicators for the communities served.

- High-quality prenatal care is one of the fundamentals of a safe motherhood program. Ensuring early initiation of prenatal care during pregnancy greatly contributes to reductions in perinatal illness, disability, and death for the mother and the infant.

SCENARIO: ANALYSIS AND RESPONSE

- Good health during the childhood years (ages 1–14) is essential for each child's optimal development and America's future. America cannot hope for every child to become a productive member of society if children in this country are allowed to grow up with poor or mediocre child care, have no health insurance, live in poverty, or live in a violent environment.

- The federal government has more than 35 health programs within 16 different agencies helping states to serve the needs of our nation's children. The majority of these programs are well respected and help meet the needs of many children.

We have learned that a lack of prenatal care increases the risk of premature delivery and possible health problems for the infant.

1. If Joan had received prenatal care, how could it have helped in the normal development of the infant? How could the doctor have counseled Joan?

2. How could Joan have found out about opportunities for affordable prenatal care?

3. The cost of treating Joan's infant could run into the hundreds of thousands of dollars, and there is no guarantee that the child will survive. Do you think it would be more cost effective to ensure prenatal care to all women or to continue under the system that is in place now? How would you suggest the United States approach this problem?

4. What programs mentioned in this chapter could have helped Joan?

5. Visit the Web site of the USDA (www.usda.gov) and read about WIC. After reading about WIC, do you think this is something that could help Joan with the raising of her child? Why or why not?

REVIEW QUESTIONS

1. What has been the trend in infant mortality rates in the United States in the last 30 years? What is the current rate? How does this rate compare with that of other industrial countries?

2. What has been the trend in maternal mortality rates in the United States in the last 30 years? What factors have influenced this trend?

3. Why is prenatal care so important for mothers and infants? What types of services are included?

4. What are the consequences of teen pregnancy to the mother? To the infant? To the community?

5. What is included in family planning? Why is family planning important?

6. Discuss the pro-life and pro-choice positions on the abortion issue.

7. Why was the *Roe v. Wade* court decision so important?

8. What are the leading causes of death in children ages 1 to 4 and ages 5 to 14 years?

9. Why are childhood immunizations so important?

10. What is the WIC program?

11. Why is health insurance important for women, infants, and children?

12. Name three groups that are advocates for the health of children and what they have done to show their support.

ACTIVITIES

Write a two-page paper summarizing the results and/or information you gain from one of the following activities.

1. Survey 10 classmates and friends and ask them what leads to teen pregnancy. What prompts adolescents to risk pregnancy when they have adequate knowledge of contraception? Ask if they know anyone who became pregnant as an adolescent. Are the reasons given the same as your own? Divide your list into categories of personal beliefs, barriers to action, and social pressure. For example, a comment that might fit under beliefs is "they don't think they can get pregnant the first time"; under barriers, "they are too embarrassed to buy contraception"; and under social pressure, "all the messages in society promoting sex." Which of the three categories had the most responses?

Does this surprise you? What implications does this have for programs trying to reduce the incidence of teen pregnancy?

2. Call your local health department and ask for information about the local WIC program. Ask permission to visit and talk to a representative about the program and clientele.

3. Visit, call, or get on the Web site of your state health department and obtain information concerning the number of childhood communicable diseases reported in your state. What are your state laws concerning immunization of children? Does your state provide immunizations free of charge? What qualifications must a person meet to receive free immunizations?

4. Call a local obstetrician's office and ask if he or she accepts Medicaid reimbursement. What is the normal fee for prenatal care and delivery? If he or she does not take Medicaid, ask the obstetrician to whom he or she would refer a pregnant woman with no private insurance.

5. Create a record of your own (or a family member's) immunizations. Find out when and where you were immunized for each of the immunizations listed in Figure 7.22. Are there any immunizations that are still needed? When are you scheduled to get your next tetanus/toxoid immunization?

COMMUNITY HEALTH ON THE WEB

The Internet contains a wealth of information about community and public health. Increase your knowledge of some of the topics presented in this chapter by accessing the Jones & Bartlett Learning Web site at **http://health .jbpub.com/book/communityhealth/7e** and follow the links to complete the following Web activities.

* Maternal and Child Health Bureau
* Women, Infants, and Children Program
* Insure Kids Now!

REFERENCES

1. Pillitteri, A. (2010). *Maternal and Child Health Nursing: Care of the Childbearing and Childrearing Family*, 6th ed. Philadelphia: J. B. Lippincott.

2. U.S. Department of Health and Human Services (2009). *Child Health—USA 2009*. Washington, DC: U.S. Government Printing Office.

3. U.S. Census Bureau, Population Division, Fertility and Family Statistics Branch (2010). *Current Population Survey (CPS), Definitions and Explanations*. Available at http://www.census.gov/population/www/cps/cpsdef.html.

4. Friedman, M. (2003). *Family Nursing: Research, Theory and Practice*, 5th ed. Stamford, CT: Appleton & Lange.

5. Terry-Humen, E., J. Manlove, and K. A. Moore (2001). "Births Outside of Marriage: Perceptions vs. Reality." In *Child Trends Research Brief*. Washington, DC: Child Trends.

6. Martin, J. A., B. E. Hamilton, P. D. Sutton, S. J. Ventura, F. Menacker, and S. Kirmeyer (2006). "Births: Final Data for 2004." *National Vital Statistics Reports*, 55(1): 1–31.

7. Hamilton, B. E., J. A. Martin, and S. J. Ventura (2009). "Births: Preliminary Data for 2007." *National Vital Statistics Reports*, 54(2): 1–30.

8. Ventura, S. J., T. J. Mathew, and B. E. Hamilton (2001). "Births to Teenagers in the United States, 1940–2000." *National Vital Statistics Reports*, 57(12): 1–24.

9. National Campaign to Prevent Teen and Unplanned Pregnancy (2010). "The Public Costs of Teen Childbearing." Available at http://www.thenationalcampaign.org/costs/pdf/resources/key_data.pdf.

10. United Nations (2010). *Demographic Yearbook, 2006*. New York, NY: Author. Available at http://unstats.un.org/unsd/demographic/sconcerns/natality/default.htm.

11. Children's Defense Fund (2010). *The State of America's Children 2010*. Washington, DC: Author.

12. U.S. Department of Health and Human Services, Office of Disease Prevention and Health Promotion (2010). *Healthy People 2020*. Available at http://www.healthypeople.gov/2020/default.aspx.

13. Jackson, S. (1993). "Opening Session Comments: Laying the Groundwork for Working Together for the Future." *Journal of School Health*, 63(1): 11.

14. Finer, L. B., and S. K. Henshaw (2006). "Disparities in Rates of Unintended Pregnancy in the United States, 1994 and 2001." *Perspectives on Sexual and Reproductive Health*, 38(2): 90–96.

15. Sonfield, A., C. Alrich, and R. B. Gold (2008). "Public Funding for Family Planning, Sterilization, and Abortion Services, FY 1980–2006, Occasional Report." New York, NY: Guttmacher Institute, No. 38.

16. Sonfield, A. (2003). "Preventing Unintended Pregnancy: The Need and the Means." *Guttmacher Report on Public Policy*, 6(5): 7–11.

17. Chandra, A., G. M. Martinez, W. D. Mosher, J. C. Abma, and J. Jones (2005). "Fertility, Family Planning and Women's Health: Data from the 2002 National Survey of Family Growth." *Vital Health Statistics*, 23(25).

18. "Title X Pregnancy Counseling Act." (1991). *Congressional Digest*, 70(8,9): 195–224.

19. Frost, J. J., L. Frohwirth, and A. Purcell (2004). "The Availability and Use of Publicly Funded Family Planning Clinics: U.S. Trends, 1994–2001." *Perspectives on Sexual and Reproductive Health*, 36(5): 206–215.

20. Alan Guttmacher Institute (2005). *Family Planning Annual Report: 2004 Summary*. Submitted to the Office of Population Affairs, Department of Health and Human Services. Available at http://www.hhs.gov/opa/familyplanning/toolsdocs/2004-fpar-part1.pdf.

21. R. B. Gold, A. Sonfield, C. L. Richards, and J. J. Frost (2009). *Next Steps for America's Family Planning Program: Leveraging the Potential of Medicaid and Title X in an Evolving Health Care System*. New York, NY: Guttmacher Institute. Available at http://www.guttmacher.org/pubs/summaries/NextStepsExec.pdf.

22. Hyde, J., and J. DeLamater (2003). *Understanding Human Sexuality*, 8th ed. Boston: McGraw-Hill.

23. Planned Parenthood Federation of America (2009). *2007–2008 Annual Report*. New York, NY: Author. Available at http://www.plannedparenthood.org/about-us/annual-report-4661.htm.

24. Frost J., S. Henshaw, and A. Sonfield (2010). *Contraceptive Needs and Services: National and State Data, 2008 Update*. New York, NY: Guttmacher Institute.

25. Frost, J. J., A. Sonfield, and R. B. Gold (2006). *Estimating the Impact of Expanding Medicaid Eligibility for Family Planning Services* (Occasional Report no. 28). New York, NY: Guttmacher Institute.

26. "Court Reaffirms Roe but Upholds Restrictions." (1992). *Family Planning Perspectives*, 24: 174-185.

27. Pazol, K., S. Gamble, W. Parker, D. Cook, S. Zane, and S. Hamdan (2009). "Abortion Surveillance—United States, 2006." *Morbidity and Mortality Weekly Report*, 58(SS 08): 1-35.

28. World Health Organization (1992). *International Statistical Classification of Diseases and Related Health Problems*, 10th Revision. Geneva, Switzerland: Author.

29. Centers for Disease Control and Prevention (2000). "Entry into Prenatal Care—United States, 1989-1997." *Morbidity and Mortality Weekly Report*, 49(18): 393-398.

30. Xu, J., K. Kochanek, S. Murphy, and B. Fejada-Vera (2010). "Deaths: Final Data for 2007." *National Vital Statistics Reports*, 58(19): 1-31.

31. Behrman, R. E., and A. Stith Buter, eds. (2006). *Preterm Birth: Causes, Consequences, and Prevention*. Washington, DC: National Academies Press.

32. Martin, J., J. K. Michelle, M. H. S. Osterman, and P. D. Sutton (2010). "Are Preterm Births on the Decline in the United States? Recent Data from the National Vital Statistics System." Available at http://www.cdc.gov/nchs/data/databriefs/db39.pdf.

33. S. Nigel Paneth (1995). "The Problem of Low Birth Weight." *Future of Children*, 5(1): 35-56.

34. Chomitz, O. R., L. W. Cheung, and E. Lieberman (1995). "The Role of Lifestyle in Preventing Low Birthweight." *Future of Children*, 5(1): 162-175.

35. Centers for Disease Control and Prevention (1998). "Trends in Infant Mortality Attributable to Birth Defects—United States, 1980-1995." *Morbidity and Mortality Weekly Report*, 47(37): 773-778.

36. Centers for Disease Control and Prevention (2010). "Sudden Infant Death Syndrome (SIDS)." Available at http://www.cdc.gov/SIDS/.

37. Willinger, M., M. J. Hoffman, K. T. Wu, J. R. Hou, R. C. Kessler, S. L. Ward, T. G. Keens, and M. J. Corwin (1998). "Factors Associated with the Transition to Non-prone Sleep Positions of Infants in the United States. The National Infant Sleep Position Study." *Journal of the American Medical Association*, 280: 329-335.

38. National Highway Traffic Safety Administration (2009). *Traffic Safety Facts 2008: Occupant Protection*. Washington, DC: U.S. Department of Transportation.

39. National Center for Injury Prevention and Control (2010). *Childhood Injury Fact Sheet*. Available at http://www.cdc.gov/ncipc/factsheets/childh.htm.

40. Finkelstein, E. A., P. S. Corso, and T. R. Miller (2006). *Incidence and Economic Burden of Injuries in the United States*. New York, NY: Oxford University Press.

41. U.S. Department of Health and Human Services, Administration for Children and Families (2009). *Child Maltreatment 2007*. Washington, DC: U.S. Government Printing Office.

42. U.S. Department of Health and Human Services, Administration for Children and Families (2004). "Community Responsibility for Child Protection." Available at http://nccanch.acf.hhs.gov/pubs/otherpubs/commresp.cfm.

43. Centers for Disease Control and Prevention (2000). *Immunization 2000: A History of Achievement, a Future of Promise*. Atlanta, GA: Author.

44. U.S. Department of Health and Human Services, Health Resources and Services Administration (2003). *Understanding Title V of the Social Security Act*. Rockville, MD: Author.

45. U.S. Department of Health and Human Services, Health Resources and Services Administration (2010). "Maternal and Child Health Bureau Mission." Available at http://mchb.hrsa.gov/about/default.htm.

46. Special Supplemental Nutrition Program for Women, Infants, and Children (7CFR246) (January 1, 2002). Available at http://frwebgate.access.gpo.gov/cgi-bin/multidb.cgi.

47. U.S. Department of Agriculture, Food and Nutrition Service (2010). "About WIC." Available at http://www.fns.usda.gov/wic/aboutwic/.

48. Institute of Medicine (2002). *Health Insurance Is a Family Matter*. Washington, DC: National Academies Press. Available at http://nap.edu/books/0309085187/html/.

49. Ruhm, C. J. (1997). "The Family and Medical Leave Act." *Journal of Economic Perspectives*, 3: 10-14.

50. U.S. Department of Health and Human Services (2000). "National Study of Child Care for Low-Income Families, State, and Community Substudy." Available at http://acf.dhhs.gov/news/ccstudy.htm.

Chapter 8

Adolescents, Young Adults, and Adults

Chapter Objectives

After studying this chapter, you will be able to:

1 Explain why it is important for community health
workers to be aware of the different health concerns of the various age groups in the United
States.

2 Define by age the groups of adolescents and young
adults and adults.

3 Briefly describe key demographic characteristics of
adolescents and young adults.

4 Explain what the Youth Risk Behavior Surveillance
System (YRBSS) and the Behavioral Risk Factor
Surveillance System (BRFSS) are and what type of
data they generate.

5 Provide a brief behavioral risk profile for adolescents, college students, and adults.

6 Outline the health profiles for the various age
groups—adolescents and young adults, and
adults—listing the major causes of mortality, morbidity, and risk factors for each group.

7 Give examples of community health strategies for
improving the health status of adolescents, young
adults, and adults.

SCENARIO

Annie and Latasha are about halfway through their sophomore year at Garber University. Though they came from very different environments—Annie came from a small rural community with a population of about 1,500, and Latasha grew up in a large metropolitan area—they have become good friends. This year, as chance would have it, they have similar class schedules and have ended up in the dining hall each morning at about the same time for breakfast.

One morning, while reading the school newspaper over breakfast, Annie came across an article that described an automobile crash involving some university students. Four university students riding in one car collided with a second car driven by a local middle-aged businessman. Annie asked Latasha if she knew any of the students. Latasha asked who they were, and Annie read their names. Latasha did not know them.

Annie said it looked like the students were in big trouble because they had all been drinking alcohol, and no one was 21 years old. When the police tested the driver, her blood alcohol concentration was 0.14%. So, not only was she being charged with underage drinking, but also with driving while intoxicated. Luckily, none of the students was injured, but the local businessman was in serious condition in the hospital. The newspaper article indicated that the students were wearing their safety belts, but the businessman was not. Annie told Latasha that she knew of only one similar incident like this back home. She added, "Why would anyone drink and drive?" Latasha replied, "Don't worry about this Annie. It's no big deal. It happens all the time in the city; in fact it is so common this type of news seldom makes the papers."

INTRODUCTION

In this chapter, we present a profile of the health of Americans in two different groups—adolescents and young adults (15 to 24 years of age) and adults (25 to 64 years of age). Just like the age groups of Americans presented in Chapter 7, each of these groups has its own sets of health risks and problems. Viewing these age group profiles enables public health workers to detect the sources of diseases, injury, and death for specific priority populations and to propose programs to reduce those sources. Effective programs aimed at specific population age groups can reduce the risk factors that contribute to disease, injury, and death for the entire population. We hope that you, the student, will become knowledgeable about the specific health problems of each age group and also become mindful of the subpopulations within these groups that are at special risk.

The years of life between the ages of 15 and 64 are some of the most productive, if not the most productive, of people's lives. Consider all that takes place during these years. Most people complete their formal education, meet and commit to their lifelong partners, become parents and raise a family, find and develop their vocation, become owners (or at least mortgage holders) of property, earn their greatest amount of wealth, actively engage in the development of their community, travel more than during any other time in their lives, become aunts or uncles and grandparents, become valued employees, serve as role models and mentors, and plan and save for retirement. It is also a time when they enjoy some of the best health of their lives as well as shape their health (through their lifestyle and health behavior) for their later years.

ADOLESCENTS AND YOUNG ADULTS

adolescents and young adults are considered to be those people who fall into the 15- to 24-year-old age range. The individuals in this age group are considered very important by our society because they represent the future of our nation. If the United States is going to maintain its standard of living and preeminent position among the countries of the world that it enjoys today, it will depend in large part on these young people.[1]

This period of development of adolescence and young adulthood, often combined when reporting data about young people, can be further split into two subgroups. "Adolescence is generally regarded as the period of life from puberty to maturity."[2] This is not an easy stage of life for most because it is a period of transition from childhood to adulthood. Adolescence "is a time when children psychologically move from areas of relative comfort and emotional security to places and situations that are far more complex and often much more challenging."[3] In addition to the psychological changes, this population of teenagers is also experiencing "hormonal changes, physical maturation, and frequently, opportunities to engage in risk behaviors."[2]

Young adults also face many physical, emotional, and educational changes. For example, young adults complete their physical growth and maturity, leave home, marry and start families, attend postsecondary education, enlist in the military, or begin careers. Couple the demands of these personal changes with the demands of a fast-paced, ever-changing society and it is easy to see why this stage in life is considered one of the most difficult.[1]

The combined period of adolescence and young adulthood is a critical one healthwise. It is during this period in one's life that many health-related beliefs, attitudes, and behaviors are adopted and consolidated.[2,4,5] During this stage of life, young people have increased freedom and access to health-compromising substances and experiences—such as alcohol, tobacco, other drugs, and sexual risk taking—as well as opportunities for health-enhancing experiences such as regularly scheduled exercise and healthful diets.[2,4,5] It is also during this stage that certain lifestyle decisions are made that will have long-term influences on health in later years of life.

adolescents and young adults
those people who fall into the 15- to 24-year-old age range

Demography

Several demographic variables affect the health of this age group, but the three variables that are most important to community health are the number of young people, their living arrangements, and their employment status.

Number of Adolescents and Young Adults

The number of adolescents and young adults peaked in 1979, when the baby boomers swelled their ranks to about 21% of the total population. Since 1979, the proportion of 15- to 24-year-olds has declined. Thus, in 2010 they are estimated to make up 14% of the population, roughly the same proportion they made up in 1960.[6-8]

As we look to the future, the proportion of adolescents and young adults in the general population will continue to increase, and at the same time the racial and ethnic makeup will become increasingly more diverse (see Figure 8.1). In 2008, approximately 60% of the adolescents were non-Hispanic white. It is estimated that in 2050, this percentage will decrease to 44%.[2,8,9]

Living Arrangements

The percentage of children younger than the age of 18 living in a single-parent family has been on the rise ever since 1965. In fact, the percentage increased sharply in the 1970s and continued to rise slowly through the 1990s. The sharp rise in the 1970s can be attributed to the great increase in the divorce rate.[1] In 2008, almost one-third (32%)[10] of all children lived in

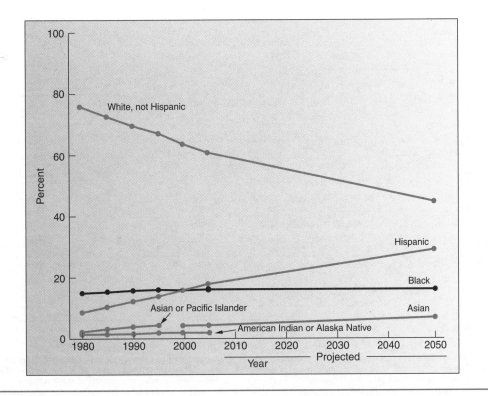

FIGURE 8.1

Race and Hispanic origin of adolescents 10–19 years of age: United States, 1980–2050.

Notes: Data for 1980–1995 are for Asian or Pacific Islander persons; data for 2000–2050 are for Asian person only. Population projections are not available for American Indian or Alaska Native persons. Persons of Hispanic origin may be of any race. See data table for data points and additional notes.

Source: MacKay, A. P., and C. Duran (2007). *Adolescent Health in the United States*. Hyattsville, MD: National Center for Health Statistics, 9.

single-parent families versus approximately one-tenth (11%) in 1970.[7] Additionally, more black children (59%) lived in a single-parent home than did white children (25%) or Hispanic children (30%).[8]

Family household statistics on single-parent families are only a snapshot of children's living status during a single year. Unfortunately, many children are affected over their lifetimes by growing up in single-parent families. Though the psychological and emotional consequences of single-parent families are not clear, the economic consequences are indeed. Children living in single-parent families are more likely to experience severe economic disadvantages.[1] These economic disadvantages adversely affect health.

Employment Status

Since the years of 1960 and the early 1980s, when there were significant increases in the participation of young women in the labor force, the proportion of all adolescents and young adults in the labor force has remained relatively constant (see Figure 8.2). However, this age group is beginning to see some significant permanent changes in its labor-force participation, particularly 16- to 19-year-old males, mainly because of increased school attendance and enrollment in high school, college, and summer school over the past decade.[11] The youth labor force, composed of 16- to 24-year-olds, makes up approximately 14% of the overall labor force.[12] When the unemployment rates of this age group are separated by race and ethnicity,

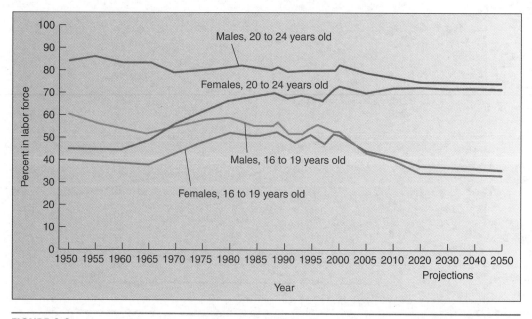

FIGURE 8.2

Labor force participation rate of young adults by sex and age, 1950–2050.

Sources: U.S. Department of Labor, Bureau of Labor Statistics, *Employment and Earnings* (January issues); *Handbook of Labor Statistics,* Bulletin 2217. U.S. Department of Commerce, Bureau of the Census, *Statistical Abstract of the United States, 1956, 1987, and 1999;* and *Current Population Reports,* Series P-50, nos. 31 and 72; and unpublished data. Council of Economic Advisers, *Economic Report of the President,* 1987. Tossi, M. (2006). "A New Look at Long-Term Labor Force Projections to 2050." *Monthly Labor Review Online,* 129(11).

differences appear. Regardless of sex, black adolescents and young adults are more likely to be unemployed than are whites or Hispanics. White adolescents and young adults have the lowest proportion of unemployment.[13] These proportions, like so many others already discussed, are disproportionate by race/ethnicity. These figures are important to community health because most health insurance, and thus access to health care, is connected to employment status.

A Health Profile

With regard to the health profile of this age group, three major areas stand out—mortality, morbidity from specific infectious diseases, and health behavior and lifestyle choices.

Mortality

Although, on average, Americans live longer than ever before, adolescents and young adults suffer their share of life-threatening problems.[1] As it has been with most other age groups, the death rate for adolescents and young adults has significantly declined. Between 1950 and 2006, the death rate of adolescents and young adults declined by 36%, from 128.1 to 82.2 per 100,000.[14] This decline in death rates for adolescents and young adults, like that for children, can be attributed to advances in medicine and injury and disease prevention.[1,14]

Regardless of race or ethnicity, men have higher mortality rates than women.[14] Mortality rates for men and women were highest among blacks and American Indians/Alaska Natives. The lowest mortality rates of both men and women belong to Asian/Pacific Islanders.[14]

Much of the physical threat to adolescents and young adults stems from their behavior rather than from disease.[1] For young people overall, approximately three-fourths of all mortality can be attributed to three causes—unintentional injuries (mainly motor vehicle crashes)

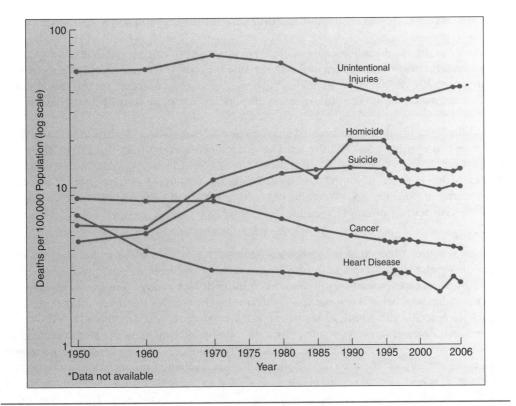

FIGURE 8.3

Death rates for leading causes of death for ages 15 to 24, 1950–2006.

Sources: Fried, V. M., K. Prager, A. P. MacKay, and H. Xia (2003). *Health, United States, 2003, with Chartbook on Trends in Health of Americans.* Hyattsville, MD: National Center for Health Statistics, 50; National Center for Health Statistics (2006). *Health, United States, 2006, with Chartbook on Trends in the Health of Americans.* Hyattsville, MD: Author; and National Center for Health Statistics (2010). *Health, United States, 2009, with Special Feature on Medical Technology.* Hyattsville, MD: Author.

(46.5%), homicide (16%), and suicide (12%).[14] Mortality from unintentional injuries in this age group declined during the last half of the twentieth century. Even so, unintentional injury deaths remain the leading cause of death in adolescents and young adults, accounting for almost half of all deaths in this age group (see Figure 8.3).

Deaths from motor vehicle–related injuries account for one-quarter of all deaths for young people in this age group, and in more than half of all the fatal crashes, alcohol was a contributing factor, which is down from 72% in 1982.[15] Unlike other mortality data in this age group, white males have a higher rate of death in motor vehicles than do black males. Motor vehicle–related death rates of Hispanic and Native American males are the highest for this age group. The mortality rates for white and black women combined are lower than those for males of either race. Overall, the rate of motor vehicle deaths for 15- to 24-year-olds is lower now than it was in 1950.[14]

The most alarming mortality trend in this age group is the growing number of homicides and suicides. Over the last 50 years, homicide and suicides rates increased between 200% and 300%.[14] Homicide is the second leading cause of death in the 15- to 24-year age group, and it is the leading cause of death among black Americans.[16] It is not race, per se, that is a risk factor for violent death, but rather socioeconomic status and environment. Differences in homicide rates between races are significantly reduced when socioeconomic factors are taken into account. However, alcohol and drugs are involved in a majority of homicides and legal interventions.[17]

Suicide is the third leading cause of death in adolescents and young adults, and it is the second leading cause of death of white males in this age group. The rate among black males is just under two-thirds that of white males.[14] The suicide rate in females is significantly lower than that for males, although young women attempt suicide more frequently than do young men.[14,18]

Although the number of completed suicides by adolescents and young adults is alarming, it represents only a fraction of all the suicides contemplated. Data from the 2009 Centers for Disease Control and Prevention's Youth Risk Behavior Surveillance System (YRBSS) indicate that nearly one in seven ninth to twelfth graders in the United States have thought seriously about attempting suicide (13.8%), while 10.9% have made a specific plan to attempt suicide, and 6.3% have actually attempted suicide.[18]

Morbidity

Although a higher proportion of adolescents and young adults survive to age 24 than ever before, this group still suffers significantly from a number of different communicable diseases. One of these diseases, measles (rubeola), once thought to be only a childhood disease and close to eradication, made a resurgence in the late 1980s. Measles is a much more severe disease for adolescents and young adults than it is for children. It was first thought that a single vaccination for measles (taken concurrently with mumps and rubella, as the MMR vaccination, at 15 months of age) would confer lifelong immunity against the disease. However, measles is much more communicable than once believed so that a second immunization at the time of first entering school is now recommended. As shown in Table 8.1, this change in the immunization schedule has significantly reduced the number of measles cases. The recommendations for measles and other vaccinations are presented in Chapter 7.

The other diseases that cause considerable morbidity in adolescents and young adults are sexually transmitted diseases (STDs) (see Table 8.1). "Compared to older adults, sexually-active adolescents 15 to 19 years of age and young adults 20 to 24 years of age are at higher risk for acquiring STDs for a combination of behavioral, biological, and cultural reasons."[19] Whereas many STDs are completely curable with antibiotics, some viral infections, such as hepatitis, human immunodeficiency virus (HIV), or human papillomavirus (HPV), can be treated but never cured.[20] The effects of some STDs can last a lifetime. For example, some forms of HPV are the precursor to cervical cancer, and the effects of chlamydia, if untreated, can lead to infertility. As in the case of HIV, the precursor to AIDS, the result may even be death.[20] Chlamydia and gonorrhea are the most common curable STDs among this age group,[19] and more than half of all new HIV infections occurring in the United States are found in people under the age of 29.[21] "Estimates suggest that while representing 25% of the sexually experienced population, 15- to 24-year-olds acquire nearly half of all new STDs."[19]

Health Behaviors and Lifestyle Choices of High School Students

Whereas many behavioral patterns begin during the childhood years (ages 1–14), others begin in adolescence and young adulthood. During this period of experimentation, young people are susceptible to developing deleterious behaviors such as the abuse of alcohol and/or tobacco and other drugs, fighting, and weapon carrying.

In 1990, the Centers for Disease Control and Prevention (CDC) initiated the Youth Risk Behavior Surveillance System (YRBSS) to better track selected health behaviors among young people (see Chapter 3 for more information on the YRBSS). The YRBSS includes a national school-based survey, as well as state, territorial, tribal, and district surveys. In the spring of 1991, CDC conducted for the first time the national school-based Youth Risk Behavior Survey. This survey continues to be conducted biennially during odd-numbered years among

Table 8.1
Number of Reported Cases (and Incidence Rates) of Selected Communicable Diseases among 15- to 24-Year-Olds, 1981 to 2008

Disease and Age	1981#	1990#	2000	2008
AIDS	—	1,715	1,567 (4.16)	11,321 (47.34)
Chlamydia	—	—	508,736 (1,349.42)	856,189 (3,580.47)
Gonorrhea*	617,994	384,490	212,679 (564.13)	205,816 (860.70)
Measles	594	5,646	17 (0.05)	16 (0.07)
Syphilis*	12,965	16,408	1,338 (3.55)	3,300 (13.80)
Tuberculosis	2,198	1,867	1,623 (4.31)	1,440 (3.39)

Note: # = rates not available. — = data not collected. * = civilian cases only, primary and secondary. Incidence rates per 100,000 population.

Sources: Centers for Disease Control and Prevention. *Morbidity and Mortality Weekly Report*: Annual Summaries, various years; "Summary of Notifiable Diseases—United States, 2000." *Morbidity and Mortality Weekly Report*, 49(53): 23; and "Summary of Notifiable Diseases—United States, 2008." *Morbidity and Mortality Weekly Report*, 57(54): 32–33.

national probability samples of ninth- through twelfth-grade students from private and public schools. Results of the 2009 survey are included in the following sections. In 1990, CDC began offering to each state and to selected local education departments the YRBSS questionnaire and fiscal and technical assistance to conduct the Youth Risk Behavior Survey. During 2009, 47 states, 4 territories, 2 tribal governments, and 23 local surveys were conducted.[18] In the time the YRBSS has been in operation, it has proved to be very helpful at both the state and local levels. A number of states and local communities have put into place programs and policies to reduce risk behaviors in youth. For example, "in Wyoming, YRBS data on alcohol use were used to help keep the minimum legal drinking age at 21 and are being used to support an amendment to a bill addressing underage use and possession of alcohol."[18] Continued support of YRBSS will help monitor and ensure the success of many public health and school health programs.

Behaviors That Contribute to Unintentional Injuries
Five different behaviors of high school students that relate to unintentional injuries are monitored as part of the YRBSS: seat belt use, bicycle helmet use, motorcycle helmet use, riding with a driver who has been drinking alcohol, and driving after drinking alcohol. Since 1991, the numbers of students engaging in these risk behaviors have declined. Yet in 2009, more than one-fourth of students nationwide had, in the 30 days preceding the survey, ridden with a driver who had been drinking alcohol and 9.7% had driven a vehicle after drinking alcohol.[18]

Behaviors That Contribute to Violence
Behaviors that contribute to violence-related injuries of high school students include carrying a weapon (e.g., gun, knife, or club), engaging in a physical fight, engaging in dating violence, having been forced to have sexual intercourse, engaging in school-related violence including bullying, suicide ideation, and suicide attempts. Nationwide more than one-sixth (17.5%) of high school students reported having carried a weapon during the 30 days prior to the survey, and about one-third (31.5%) of all high school students reported having been in a fight in the past 12 months. Additionally, one in five students (19.9%) had been bullied on school property in the past 12 months before the survey. It is no wonder that many school districts around the country are taking steps to reduce violent behavior in school. Males are more likely than females are to get in a fight or carry a weapon. However, females are more likely than males to have been forced to have sexual intercourse and to report sadness, suicide ideation, and suicide attempts.[18] (See Chapter 15 for more on violence.)

Tobacco Use

The use of tobacco products represents one of the most widespread, high-risk health behaviors for this group. In 2009, approximately one-fifth of high school students (19.5%) nationwide were current smokers—that is, smoked on at least one day in the past 30 days—which is a significant decrease from 1997, when 36.4% of students were current smokers. Similarly, a significant decrease has been seen among current frequent smokers—those who had smoked on 20 or more days in the past 30 days (2009, 7.3%; 1999, 16.8%). Overall, white students (22.5%) were significantly more likely to report current cigarette use than were Hispanic (18.0%) and black (9.5%) students, as well as more frequent use of cigarettes (9.5%, 4.2%, and 2.1%, respectively).[18] The vast majority of people who become dependent on nicotine develop that dependency between the ages of 15 and 24, and most before they reach the age of 18.[22] (See Figure 8.4.)

In addition to cigarette smoking, the use of **smokeless tobacco** or *spit tobacco* (snuff and chewing tobacco) and cigars is a threat to the health of teenagers. In 2009, the overall prevalence of current smokeless tobacco use was 8.9% in high school students, which is a significant decrease from 1995 (11.4%). The prevalence was higher in males (15.0%) than in females (2.2%), and higher in whites (11.9%) than in Hispanics (5.1%) or blacks (3.3%). White males reported the highest rates of smokeless tobacco use (20.1%). Although the number of students using cigars has significantly decreased since 1997 (22%), approximately one-sixth (14.0%) of students reported current cigar use.[18]

> **smokeless tobacco, or spit tobacco,** includes oral snuff, loose leaf chewing tobacco, plug chewing tobacco, and nasal snuff

Because use of tobacco that begins during adolescence can lead to a lifetime of nicotine dependence and a variety of negative health consequences, the federal government has exerted considerable effort to keep tobacco out of the hands of adolescents. Many believed, and data from the YRBSS verified, that most adolescents have had easy access to tobacco products. During his term of office, President Clinton was proactive in trying to restrict the distribution of tobacco to youth. One piece of legislation that was approved during President Clinton's term included a requirement that retailers must verify the age of persons who purchase cigarettes or smokeless tobacco products.[23] That guideline stated that anyone who appears to be 27 years of age or younger must be "carded" by retailers.

The most sweeping changes related to the sale of cigarettes came in 1998 when 46 state attorneys general agreed to a settlement with tobacco companies. (Florida, Minnesota, Mississippi, and Texas were not included in the settlement because they had already settled individually with the tobacco companies.) The settlement called for the companies to make payments of $206 billion to the states over 25 years beginning in 2000 and to finance antismoking programs in exchange for the states dropping their health care lawsuits for smokers who were treated with Medicaid funds. In addition to paying the states, the tobacco companies agreed to spend $1.7 billion to study youth smoking and to finance antismoking advertising and accept restrictions on marketing practices that appeal to children, such as the use of cartoon characters (e.g., Joe Camel).[23] The Congress and President Obama have continued to positively affect the number of children who begin smoking. In 2009, an increase in federal tobacco

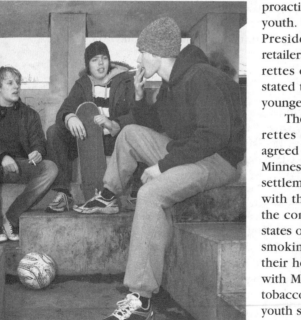

FIGURE 8.4
An estimated 1,100 young people become new smokers each day.

taxes, including a 62-cent increase in the cigarette tax, was passed, which will help fund the Children's Health Insurance Program (CHIP).[24]

Alcohol and Other Drugs

Although, for some, the first use of alcohol or other drugs begins during the childhood years, for most experimentation with these substances occurs between the ages of 15 and 24 years. YRBSS data from 2009 indicate that 41.8% of all high school students reported drinking during the previous month. Further, the data indicate that 24.2% have experienced episodic heavy drinking, and 20.8% have used marijuana at least once in the preceding month.[18]

Although one-fifth of all high school students have used marijuana during the preceding month, alcohol use and abuse continue to be major problems for adolescents, particularly among high school dropouts. As was reported earlier in this chapter, alcohol contributes significantly to motor vehicle crashes and violence in this age group.[14]

In addition to the use of marijuana, high school students are reporting the use of other illicit drugs. The 2009 YRBSS data indicated 6.4% of students had used some form of cocaine, 11.7% had used an inhalant, 6.7% had used Ecstasy, 4.1% had used methamphetamines, 3.3% had used steroids without a doctor's prescription, and 8.0% had used hallucinogenic drugs on one or more occasions during their life.[18] (Chapter 12 presents a more detailed examination of the problems of alcohol and other drug misuse and abuse.)

Sexual Behaviors That Contribute to Unintended Pregnancy and Sexually Transmitted Diseases

Since the early 1980s, adolescents in the United States have experienced high rates of unintended pregnancies and STDs, including HIV infection.[25,26] YRBSS data from 2009 show that almost half (46.0%) of all high school students have engaged in sexual intercourse sometime in their lifetime. The prevalence of sexual intercourse ranged between 29.3% for ninth-grade girls to 59.6% for high school senior boys. Furthermore, it was much more likely for black (65.2%) and Hispanic (49.1%) students to have engaged in sexual intercourse than for whites (42.0%).[18] Table 8.2 shows the trends of selected sexual risk behaviors for high school students since 1991.

As you learned in Chapter 7, each year nearly 750,000 women in the United States between the ages of 15 and 19 become pregnant.[27] In 2005, the U.S. teenage pregnancy rate reached its lowest point in more than 30 years, down 41% since its peak in 1990. However, in 2006, the rate increased by 3%, which is the first increase in more than a decade.[27] More than 80% of these pregnancies are unintended.[28] The teenage pregnancy rate in the United States is substantially higher than in England, France, Canada, and Sweden.[29] In addition to the health risks associated with teenage pregnancies for both mother and child, there are educational, economic, and psychosocial risks as well. Teenage mothers are less likely to get or stay

---

Table 8.2
Percentage of High School Students Who Reported Selected Sexual Risk Behaviors, by Year— Youth Risk Behavior Survey, United States, 1991, 1999, and 2009

Behavior	1991	1999	2009
Ever had sexual intercourse	54.1	49.9	46.0
Ever had sexual intercourse with four or more partners	18.7	16.2	13.8
Had sexual intercourse during the three months preceding the survey	37.5	36.3	34.2
Used alcohol or drugs before last sexual intercourse	21.6	24.8	21.6
Used or partner used birth control pills or Depo-Provera before last sexual intercourse	NA	19.5	29.9
Used or partner used condom at last sexual intercourse	46.2	58.0	61.1

Note: NA indicates data not available.

Source: Centers for Disease Control and Prevention (2010). "National Youth Risk Behavior Survey: 1991–2009—Trends in the Prevalence of Sexual Behaviors." Available at http://www.cdc.gov/healthyyouth/yrbs/index.htm. Accessed November 30, 2010.

married, less likely to complete high school or college, and more likely to require public assistance and to live in poverty than their peers who are not mothers.[30]

Physical Activity

Lack of physical activity by young people has increasingly become a concern. In 2009, nearly two-thirds (63%) of students had not been physically active for at least 60 minutes per day on 5 or more days during the 7 days prior to the survey. Males (45.6%) were more likely than females (27.7%) to engage in sufficient physical activity. The prevalence of lack of participation in a sufficient amount of physical activity was highest among black students. Nationally, 23.1% of students had not participated in 60 minutes of any kind of physical activity that increased their heart rate or made them breathe hard some of the time on at least 1 day during the 7 days preceding the survey.[18]

Overweight and Weight Control

Much like the concern for insufficient physical activity, the concern regarding students becoming overweight has received significant attention recently (see Figure 8.5). In 2009, approximately one-quarter of students were obese (12.0%) or overweight (15.8%), while 27.7% described themselves as slightly or very overweight. Almost one-half of students were trying to lose weight (44.4%). Eating less food, fewer calories, or foods low in fat (39.5%) and exercising (61.5%) were commonly documented behaviors for losing weight or avoiding weight gain. The prevalence for engaging in weight loss behaviors was higher among females (59.3%) than males (30.5%). Nationally, 10.6% of students had gone without eating for 24 hours or more to lose weight or to keep from gaining weight during the 30 days preceding the survey.[18]

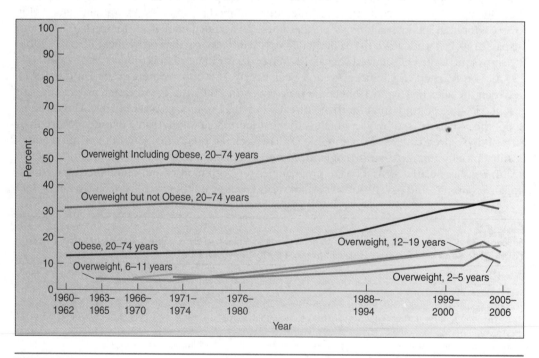

FIGURE 8.5

Overweight and obesity by age: United States, 1960–2006.

Source: National Center for Health Statistics (2010). *Health, United States, 2009, with Special Feature on Medical Technology.* Hyattsville, MD: Author.

Health Behaviors and Lifestyle Choices of College Students

Two currently available data sources regarding the health behaviors of college students are the National College Health Assessment (NCHA)[31] and Monitoring the Future.[32] The NCHA, first implemented in spring 2000, is a national, nonprofit research effort organized by the American College Health Association.[31] Monitoring the Future is conducted at the University of Michigan's Institute for Social Research and, since its inception in 1975, has been funded by the National Institute on Drug Abuse. Monitoring the Future specifically examines drug behaviors and related attitudes of a broad participant age range: eighth, tenth, and twelfth graders to adults through age 40,[32] whereas the NCHA examines a wide range of health behaviors in college students. These data sources, among others, can be helpful to those responsible for delivering health promotion education and services to many of the 18.2 million students enrolled in the nation's 4,200-plus colleges and universities.[33]

Behaviors That Contribute to Unintentional Injuries

Motor vehicle crashes, operating motor vehicles after consuming alcohol, riding with a driver who has consumed alcohol, swimming or boating while using alcohol, and not wearing seat belts are common incidences causing unintentional injuries to college-aged students.[18] Unintentional injuries have been the leading cause of death for young adults throughout the past 50 years (see Figure 8.3 presented earlier).[14]

Behaviors That Contribute to Violence

College campuses are communities just like small towns or neighborhoods in large cities. Thus, they have their share of violence. Knowing this, most colleges and universities have programs in place to address this issue. Though weapon carrying, fighting, and suicide ideation and attempts are important public health issues, sexual assault seems to be particularly prevalent among college students. Collectively, approximately one-fourth of female college students reported experiencing some form of sexual abuse/assault in the past school year—sexual touching (7.2%), verbal threats (17.4%), attempted penetration (3.1%), or sexual penetration (2.0%). Additionally, 11.2% of females and 7.1% of males reported being involved in an emotionally abusive relationship in the past school year.[31] Though not all the reasons for these sexual assaults are clear, alcohol is a contributing factor in many of these episodes.

Tobacco Use

Statistics indicate that the more education a person has, the less likely he or she is to use tobacco. In 2008, the prevalence of daily smoking for college students was 9% versus 25% for age-mates not enrolled full-time in college.[32] As shown in Figure 8.6a and 8.6b, the use of tobacco by college students had been steadily declining until the early 1990s, was inconsistent during the 1990s, and had an obvious decline again in the 2000s. The reason for the inconsistencies in prevalence over the past 20 years is unknown.[32]

Alcohol and Other Drug Use

College and university campuses have long been thought of as places where alcohol and other drugs have been abused. Table 8.3 shows that alcohol is the drug of choice on college campuses, with 69.0% of the students reporting that they had consumed alcohol in the previous 30 days. Table 8.3 also shows that illicit drug use continues to rise, but it is still considerably lower than it was in 1980.[32] Figure 8.7a presents the 28-year trend for alcohol use on college campuses. The figure shows that the number of individuals consuming one or more drinks over the past 30-day period has remained fairly stable for the past 10 years, with approximately 85.3% of college students having tried alcohol.[32] Although the number of individuals consuming alcohol has decreased over the past 25 years, Figure 8.7b demonstrates the need for concern regarding the number of college students participating in binge drinking, which is commonly defined as consuming five or more drinks in a row. According to the National

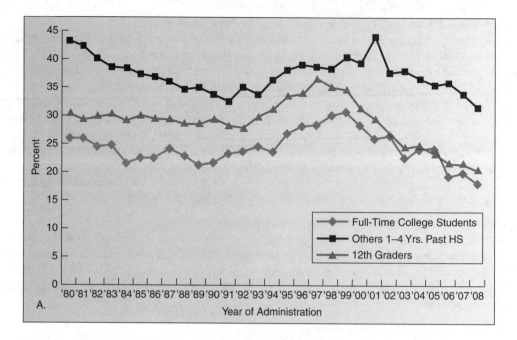

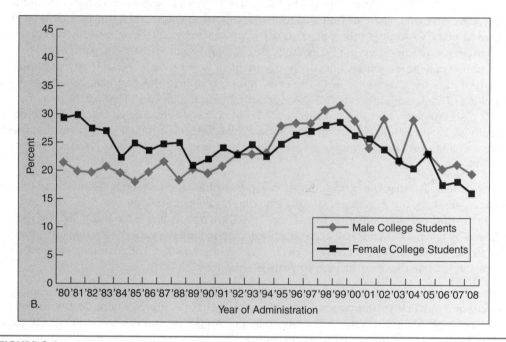

FIGURE 8.6

A. Cigarettes: trends in 30-day prevalence among college students vs. others 1 to 4 years beyond high school;
B. Cigarettes: trends in 30-day prevalence among male vs. female college students.

Source: Johnston, L. D., P. M. O'Malley, and J. G. Bachman (2010). *Monitoring the Future National Survey Results on Drug Use, 1975–2009. Vol. II: College Students and Adults Ages 19–50.* Bethesda, MD: National Institute on Drug Abuse.

Table 8.3
Trends in 30-Day Prevalence of Various Types of Drugs among College Students 1 to 4 Years Beyond High School

	Percentage Who Used in Past 30 Days			
	1980	**1990**	**2000**	**2008**
Any illicit drug[a]	38.4	15.2	21.5	18.9
Any illicit drug other than marijuana	20.7	4.4	6.9	7.3
Marijuana	34.0	14.0	20.0	17.0
Inhalants[b]	1.5	1.0	0.9	0.4
Hallucinogens[c]	2.7	1.4	1.4	1.7
LSD	1.4	1.1	0.9	0.8
MDMA (Ecstasy)[d]	NA	0.6	2.5	0.6
Cocaine	6.9	1.2	1.4	1.2
Heroin	0.3	0.0	0.2	*
Other narcotics[e,f]	1.8	0.5	1.7	2.3
Amphetamines, adj.[c,g]	NA	1.4	2.9	2.8
Barbiturates[e]	0.9	0.2	1.1	1.4
Tranquilizers[e,f]	2.0	0.5	2.0	1.6
Alcohol	81.8	74.5	67.4	69.0
Cigarettes	25.8	21.5	28.2	17.9

Notes: NA indicates data not available.

*indicates a prevalence rate of less than 0.05%.

[a]"Any illicit drug" includes use of marijuana, hallucinogens, cocaine, or heroin, or other narcotics, amphetamines, sedatives (barbiturates), methaqualone (until 1990), or tranquilizers not under a doctor's orders.

[b]This drug was asked about in four of the five questionnaire forms in 1980–1989 and in three of the six forms in 1999–2005. Total *N* in 2005 (for college students) is 680.

[c]In 2001, the question text was changed on half the questionnaire forms. "Other psychedelics" was changed to "other hallucinogens," and "shrooms" was added to the list of examples. For tranquilizers, "Miltown" was replaced with "Xanax" in the list of examples. Beginning in 2002, the remaining forms were changed to the new wording.

[d]This drug was asked about in two of the five questionnaire forms in 1989, in two of the six questionnaire forms in 1990–2001, and in three of the six questionnaire forms in 2002–2005. Total *N* in 2005 (for college students) is approximately 680.

[e]Only drug use that was not under a doctor's orders is included here.

[f]In 2002 the question text was changed on half of the questionnaire forms. The list of examples of narcotics other than heroin was updated: Talwin, laudanum, and paregoric—all of which had negligible rates of use by 2001—were replaced by Vicodin, OxyContin, and Percocet. In 2003, the remaining forms were changed to the new wording. The data are based on all forms in 2003 and beyond.

[g]Based on the data from the revised question, which attempts to exclude inappropriate reporting of nonprescription amphetamines.

Source: Johnston, L. D., P. M. O'Malley, J. G. Bachman, and J. E. Schulenberg (2010). *Monitoring the Future National Survey Results on Drug Use, 1975–2009. Vol. II: College Students and Adults Ages 19–50*. Bethesda, MD: National Institute on Drug Abuse.

College Health Association, 36.4% of males and 25.9% of females binge drank on at least one occasion during the 2 weeks prior to survey administration.[31] Excessive alcohol intake is associated with a number of adverse consequences, including fatal and nonfatal injuries, alcohol poisoning, academic failure, STDs and unintended pregnancy, and various forms of violence.[34]

Sexual Behaviors That Contribute to Unintended Pregnancy and Sexually Transmitted Diseases

Like adolescents, many college students put themselves at risk for unintended pregnancies and infections with STDs through the practice of unprotected sexual activity. Approximately 60%

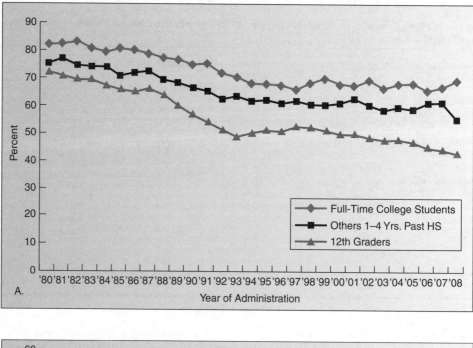

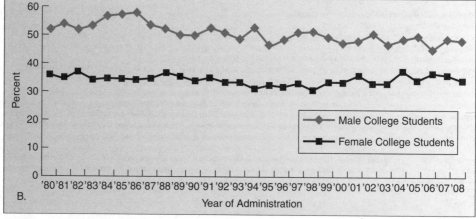

FIGURE 8.7

A. Alcohol: trends in 30-day prevalence among college students vs. others 1 to 4 years beyond high school;
B. Alcohol: trends in 2-week prevalence of 5 or more drinks in a row among male vs. female college students.

Source: Johnston, L. D., P. M. O'Malley, and J. G. Bachman (2010). *Monitoring the Future National Survey Results on Drug Use, 1975–2009. Vol. II: College Students and Adults Ages 19–50.* Bethesda, MD: National Institute on Drug Abuse.

of all gonorrhea cases and nearly three-fourths of all chlamydia cases occur among persons under 25 years of age (see Box 8.1).[35] Only approximately one-half (51.6%) of college students always or mostly used a condom when having vaginal intercourse in the 30 days prior to being surveyed, and 26.1% relied on the withdrawal method for pregnancy prevention.[31]

**BOX
8.1**

HEALTHY PEOPLE 2020: OBJECTIVES

Sexually Transmitted Diseases

Goal: Promote healthy sexual behaviors, strengthen community capacity, and increase access to quality services to prevent STDs and their complications.

Objective: STD-1 Reduce the proportion of adolescents and young adults with *Chlamydia trachomatis* infections.

STD 1.1 Among females aged 15 to 24 years attending family planning clinics:

Target: 6.7 percent.

Baseline: 7.4 percent of females aged 15 to 24 years who attended family planning clinics in the past 12 months tested positive for *Chlamydia trachomatis* infections in 2008.

Target setting method: 10 percent improvement.

Data source: STD Surveillance System (STDSS), CDC, NCHHSTP.

For Further Thought

If you were given the responsibility of lowering the incidence of chlamydia in the United States, what community health activities would you recommend?

Source: U.S. Department of Health and Human Services, Office of Disease Prevention and Health Promotion (2010). *Healthy People 2020.* Available at http://www.healthypeople.gov/2020/default.aspx. Accessed December 2, 2010.

Community Health Strategies for Improving the Health of Adolescents and Young Adults

There are no easy, simple, or immediate solutions to reducing or eliminating the health problems of adolescents and young adults. As noted in Chapter 1, community health is affected by four major factors—physical factors, community organizing, individual behavior, and social and cultural factors. Of these four, the two that need special attention when dealing with the health problems of adolescents and young adults are social and cultural factors and community organizing. Many health problems originate from the social and cultural environments in which people have been raised and live, and the culture and social norms that have been with us in some cases for many years. Take, for example, the use of alcohol. It is safe to say that the biggest health problem facing adolescents and young adults in the United States today is the use of alcohol. Alcohol contributes to all the leading causes of mortality and morbidity in these age groups. If the norm of a community is to turn its back on adolescents consuming alcohol or young adults (of legal age) abusing alcohol, efforts need to be made to change the culture. However, in most communities, culture and social norms do not change quickly. Efforts to turn these health problems around will need to be community-wide in nature and sustained over a long period of time. By "community-wide," we mean the involvement of all the stakeholders in a community, not just those who are associated with health-related professions—in other words, a community organizing effort is needed. By "sustained over a long period," we mean institutionalizing the change in the culture. For examples of programs that have been effective in preventing or reducing substance abuse and other related high-risk behaviors in communities and schools, including college campus communities, visit the SAMHSA (Substance Abuse and Mental Health Services Administration) National Registry of Evidence-Based Programs and Practices (NREPP) Web site at http://nrepp.samhsa.gov, which includes a searchable online registry of mental health and substance abuse interventions that have been reviewed and rated by independent reviewers.[36]

To change the culture as it relates to adolescents' use of alcohol, research has shown that alcohol prevention efforts need to be a part of a comprehensive school health education effort and should include components outside the classroom. Thus, prevention programs need to include components that focus on changing norms, interaction among peers, social skills training, and developmental and cultural appropriateness.[37-39]

Many colleges and universities are trying to change the culture on campus as it relates to the use of alcohol. In fact, some schools have signed up for national programs to change campus culture to reduce drinking. Some schools are increasing the number of Friday classes to try to reduce the amount of Thursday-night partying. Others have banned alcohol from campus and toughened penalties for those caught drinking, while still others have restricted tailgating and stadium sales.[40] Research strongly supports an integrated approach to programming that targets: (1) individuals, including at-risk or alcohol-dependent drinkers; (2) the student population as a whole; and (3) the college and the surrounding community. Strategies such as cognitive-behavioral skills training, norms or values clarification, strengthening of students' intrinsic desire to change behavior, and challenging alcohol expectations have proved effective in changing the culture with college students.[40]

ADULTS

The adult age group (those 25 to 64 years old) represents slightly more than half of the U.S. population. The size of this segment of the overall population is expected to remain stable over the next couple of decades, but in proportion to the rest of the population this segment will become smaller. Therefore, provisions to deal with the health concerns of this age group will need to be maintained.

A Health Profile

The health profile of this age group of adults is characterized primarily by mortality from chronic diseases stemming from poor health behavior and poor lifestyle choices made during the earlier years of life.

Mortality

With life expectancy at birth between 75 and 80 years,[14] most Americans can expect to live beyond their 65th birthday. However, many do not. During the 1950s and 1960s, it was revealed that many of the leading causes of death in this age group resulted from preventable conditions associated with unhealthy behaviors and lifestyles. As such, many adults have quit smoking, and more Americans than ever before are exercising regularly and eating healthier diets. These lifestyle improvements, along with successes in public health and advances in medicine, have resulted in a significant decline in the death rate for adults.

In the past, leading causes of death for adults were reported only for the 25- to 64-year-old age group. More recently, the adult years have been subdivided into two groups: 25 to 44 years and 45 to 64 years, with some data being reported in 10-year age spans. In 2007, the death rate for all adults aged 25 to 34 years was 104.9 per 100,000, and for ages 35 to 44 years it was 184.4 per 100,000.[41] The leading causes of death for those in this age group in 2007 were unintentional injuries, malignant neoplasms (cancer), heart disease, suicide, homicide, and HIV. With the exception of HIV, the current leading causes of death were also at the top of the list in 1980.[14] When these mortality data were broken down in 2006 by age, sex, and ethnicity, some differences appear. For 25- to 34-year-olds, with the exception of diabetes mellitus for whites and HIV among blacks and Hispanics, the six leading causes of death are the same, but differ in rank order by race and ethnic group. For 35- to 44-year-olds, diabetes mellitus is among the six leading causes for whites replacing homicide, liver disease and cirrhosis replaces suicide among Hispanics, whereas among blacks, the six leading causes include cerebrovascular disease (stroke) rather than suicide (see Table 8.4).[42]

Table 8.4
2006 Death Rates, Adults, Ages 25–34 and 35–44 (Rate per 100,000 Population)

Cause	Non-Hispanic White		Non-Hispanic Black		Hispanic	
	25–34 (102.1)	35–44 (184.8)	25–34 (185.7)	35–44 (325.2)	25–34 (81.5)	35–44 (134.4)
Unintentional injuries	41.8	43.6	35.6	42.4	29.7	31.6
Cancer	9.2	32.4	11.9	45.8	7.2	21.6
Heart disease	7.4	27.6	19.1	55.8	4.6	14.0
Suicide	15.3	19.1	8.7	7.5	7.1	6.6
Homicide	3.9	3.6	49.3	24.5	12.3	8.1
HIV	0.9	4.1	14.3	39.7	2.4	8.8
Liver disease and cirrhosis	0.7	5.9	—	4.6	1.1	6.7
Diabetes mellitus	1.4	4.4	4.4	10.6	0.9	2.8
Stroke	1.0	3.8	2.8	12.7	1.2	4.6

Source: Heron, M. (2010). "Deaths: Leading causes for 2006." *National Vital Statistics Reports*, 58(14). Hyattsville, MD: National Center for Health Statistics.

In 2007, the death rate for 45- to 54-year-olds was 420.9 per 100,000, more than twice that of the 35 to 44 age group. The death rate for 55- to 64-year-olds was 877.7 per 100,000, more than two times greater than the 45 to 54 age group.[41] The majority of these deaths were the result of noncommunicable health problems. They include cancer, heart disease, unintentional injuries, diabetes, stroke, and chronic lower respiratory disease, which includes emphysema, asthma, and bronchitis. Like with the 25- to 44-year-olds, there are racial and ethnic disparities. Though cancer and heart disease are the first and second causes of death for all three groups presented in Table 8.5, chronic lower respiratory disease appears in the list of the six leading causes for whites, HIV appears in the list for blacks, and liver disease and cirrhosis appears in the Hispanic list.[42]

Cancer
Since 1983, the number 1 cause of death in the adult age group has been cancer (malignant neoplasms). (For a review of malignant neoplasms, see Chapter 4.) Age-adjusted cancer death rates have remained relatively steady since 1950 (193.9 per 100,000 in 1950 compared to 180.7 per 100,000 in 2006). However, the crude death rates have jumped from 139.8 per 100,000 to 187.0 per 100,000 during that same time, reflecting an aging American population.[14]

Four types of cancers account for these large numbers—prostate, lung, and colorectal for men; and breast, lung, and colorectal for women. The leading cause of cancer deaths and the most preventable type of cancer for both men and women is lung cancer. This trend is expected to continue as large numbers of smokers continue to age. Of all lung cancer deaths, upward of 87% can be attributed to smoking.[43] The second leading cause of death resulting from cancer is colorectal cancer. Risk factors for this type of cancer include personal or family history, obesity, lack of physical activity, alcohol consumption, a diet high in red or processed meats, and possibly smoking and inadequate intake of fruits and vegetables.[43]

Breast cancer is the other cancer of much concern. Until it was surpassed by lung cancer in the mid-1980s, it was the leading cause of cancer deaths in women. Although it is less deadly than is lung cancer, the number of cases of breast cancer is nearly twice that of lung cancer in women.[43] Because of increased community awareness and the availability of diagnostic screening for breast cancer, survival rates are much higher than for lung cancer. However, breast cancer rates could be reduced even further if a higher percentage of women older than 39 years of age complied with the screening recommendations.[43]

Table 8.5
2006 Death Rates, Adults, Ages 45–54 and 55–64 (Rate per 100,000 Population)

Cause	Non-Hispanic White		Non-Hispanic Black		Hispanic	
	45–54 (406.6)	55–64 (861.2)	45–54 (738.5)	55–64 (1,472.4)	45–54 (310.7)	55–64 (657.6)
Cancer	115.8	325.1	174.0	450.1	74.7	198.6
Heart disease	83.1	196.8	170.1	382.6	51.7	142.2
Unintentional injuries	46.5	35.4	56.2	49.5	35.6	33.2
Diabetes mellitus	11.0	30.3	28.0	79.3	13.2	42.6
Stroke	11.1	29.8	37.9	83.0	14.4	34.2
Chronic lower respiratory disease	9.9	43.7	12.3	38.1	2.6	12.0
Liver disease and cirrhosis	17.6	22.1	15.8	22.4	23.7	34.2
Suicide	21.0	17.1	6.0	—	6.5	6.0
Kidney disease	3.5	10.3	16.7	42.7	4.9	14.4
Septicemia	4.2	11.0	13.4	31.6	4.0	9.9

Source: Heron, M. (2010). "Deaths: Leading causes for 2006." *National Vital Statistics Reports*, 58(14). Hyattsville, MD: National Center for Health Statistics.

Cardiovascular Diseases

Some of the greatest changes in cause-specific mortality rates in adults are those for the cardiovascular diseases. Age-adjusted mortality rates from diseases of the heart dropped from 588.8 per 100,000 in 1950 to 200.2 per 100,000 in 2006, while deaths from strokes dropped from 180.7 per 100,000 to 43.6 per 100,000 during the same period of time.[14] These figures represent drops of about 65% and 75%, respectively. These changes are primarily the result of public health efforts that have encouraged people to stop smoking, increase their physical activity, and eat more nutritionally. The reduction or postponement of deaths from heart disease has resulted in cancer becoming the leading cause of deaths in adults 45 to 64 years of age.

Health Behaviors and Lifestyle Choices

Many of the risk factors associated with the leading causes of morbidity and mortality in American adults are associated with health behavior and lifestyle choices. Adults have a unique opportunity to take personal action to substantially decrease their risk of ill health, and in recent years, many have taken such action. Today, more than ever before, adults are watching what they eat, wearing their seat belts, controlling their blood pressure, and exercising with regularity. The prevalence of smoking among adults has declined, as has the incidence of drinking and driving. Although these are encouraging signs, still much more can be done.

As with the other age groups discussed in this chapter, the National Center for Heath Statistics (NCHS) collects self-reported behavior risk data on adults. These data are collected via the Behavioral Risk Factor Surveillance System (BRFSS). (See Chapter 3 for a discussion of the BRFSS.) One limitation of the data from this system is that they are collected, and usually reported, on all adults older than 18 years of age; the data are not broken down by the specific age groups (18–24, 25–44, and 45–64) discussed in this chapter. More detailed information about the health behaviors and lifestyle choices of adults in the United States is presented next.

Risk Factors for Chronic Disease

The best single behavioral change Americans can make to reduce morbidity and mortality is to stop smoking. Smoking is responsible for 30% of deaths in the United States.[44] It is an important risk factor for cancer, heart disease, and stroke. In 2008, approximately one-fifth (21%) of those aged 18 years and older smoked. This amounts to about 46 million Americans.[43] The proportion of Americans who smoke has dropped considerably since 1965, when 40% of all

Americans smoked. Whereas more men than women (22% versus 17.5%) smoke,[14] the gap between the genders is decreasing. In general, smoking rates are higher among American Indians and Alaska Natives, people with fewer years of education, and those with lower incomes.[14,29]

Three other interrelated risk factors that contribute to disease and death in this age group are lack of exercise, failure to maintain an appropriate body weight, and alcohol consumption. Though American adults are exercising more than ever before, few are exercising on a regular basis. Less than 10% of U.S. adults are getting the recommended amount of moderate-vigorous physical activity each day.[45] Although it was once thought that **intensity** had to be high for cardiovascular benefits from exercise to accrue, it is believed that even light-to-moderate physical activity can have significant health benefits if done regularly and long term. Such activities include walking, gardening, housework, and dancing.

Being overweight increases one's chances of encountering a number of health problems, including heart disease, some cancers, hypertension, elevated blood cholesterol, diabetes, stroke, gallbladder disease, and osteoarthritis. Results from the 2007–2008 National Health and Nutrition Examination Surveys (NHANES) indicate that 73% of 20- to 74-year-olds were overweight (including obese and extremely obese), with nearly 34% being obese and almost 6% being extremely obese as defined by **body mass index (BMI)**.[46] Obesity in the United States is truly an epidemic (see Figure 8.8).[47] Although significant increases in the prevalence

Intensity
cardiovascular workload measured by heart rate

body mass index (BMI)
the ratio of weight (in kilograms) to height (in meters, squared)

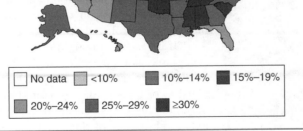

FIGURE 8.8

Obesity trends among U.S. adults, 1990, 1999, and 2008.

Note: Obesity is defined as a BMI > 30, or about 30 pounds overweight for a five-foot, four-inch person.

Source: Source: Centers for Disease Control and Prevention. *Obesity Trends Among U.S. Adults, BRFSS, 1990, 1999, 2008.* Behavioral Risk Factor Surveillance System.

of obesity were observed between the mid-1970s and 2000, the prevalence does not appear to be continuing at the same rate over the past 10 years, particularly for women.[48] The trend of weight gain increases with age. The key to maintaining an appropriate weight throughout life is a combination of diet and exercise; total reliance on either factor alone makes it a difficult process.[49]

As with other age groups, alcohol consumption often places adults at greater health risk. Approximately 65% of adult Americans consume alcohol.[50] Although most do so in moderation, a relatively small percentage develop serious problems with their alcohol use. In 2009, 15.5% of adults reported binge drinking (males having five or more drinks on one occasion, females having four or more drinks on one occasion) in the previous month.[47] Men are twice as likely to report binge drinking than are women.[47] It has been estimated that the 5% who consume the greatest amount of alcohol consume about 36% of all the alcohol consumed in the United States.[51] These people are at greatest risk for developing a dependence on alcohol and for developing such alcohol-related health problems as cirrhosis, alcoholism, and alcohol psychosis.

One does not have to become dependent on alcohol to have a drinking problem. Alcohol contributes to society's problems in a great many other ways. As noted in other chapters of this text, alcohol increases the rates of homicide, suicide, family violence, and unintentional injuries such as those from motor vehicle crashes, boating incidents, and falls. The use of alcohol by pregnant women can cause fetal alcohol spectrum disorder, one of the most common causes of mental retardation in children.[52] Clearly, alcohol consumption adversely affects the health and well-being of Americans.

Risk Factors for Personal Injury

hypertension
systolic pressure equal to or greater than 140 mm of mercury (Hg) and/or diastolic pressure equal to or greater than 90 mm Hg for extended periods of time

Like individuals in the other age groups, adults also put themselves at risk for personal injury by the way they behave. Two such areas of concerns are both related to the operation of motor vehicles—the use of seat belts and the operation of a motor vehicle after drinking alcohol. Most Americans (84%) report wearing seat belts when driving or riding in a motor vehicle, which is an improvement from 15 years ago, when approximately 60% of the population reported wearing a seat belt when in a motor vehicle.[53] Among drivers 21 years or older, an estimated 15% drive under the influence of alcohol annually.[54] The data on both of these behaviors are interesting because both behaviors are regulated by public health laws. This suggests that a society can be controlled by regulations only to the extent that it wants to be.

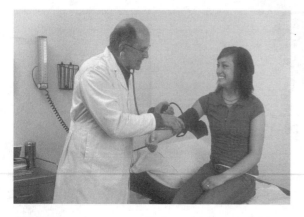

FIGURE 8.9
Hypertension is a highly modifiable risk factor.

Awareness and Screening of Certain Medical Conditions

A number of regular, noninvasive or minimally invasive health screenings are recommended for adults to participate in, such as screenings for hypertension, diabetes, high blood cholesterol, and cancer.

There is no "ideal" blood pressure. Instead, the acceptable blood pressure falls within a range considered healthy. **Hypertension** exists when systolic pressure is equal to or greater than 140 mm of mercury (Hg) and/or diastolic pressure is equal to or greater than 90 mm Hg for extended periods of time. Statistics show that hypertension is found in about one in three adults in the United States, with one-third of those unaware they have it, making it the most prevalent risk factor for cardiovascular disease in the United States.[55] Fortunately, once detected hypertension is a risk factor that is highly modifiable (see

Figure 8.9). The most desirable means of controlling hypertension is through a combination of diet modification, appropriate physical exercise, and weight management. In cases in which these measures prove ineffective, hypertension can usually still be controlled with medication. The keys to reducing morbidity and mortality resulting from hypertension are mass screenings that result in early detection of previously unidentified cases and their appropriate treatment.

Diabetes results from failure of the pancreas to make or use a sufficient amount of insulin. Without insulin, food cannot be properly used by the body. Diabetes cannot be cured, but it can be controlled through a combination of diet, exercise, medications, and insulin injections. It has already been reported earlier in the chapter that with the exception of 15- to 24-year-olds, diabetes is one of the leading causes of death for all adults. The death rates are highest in American Indians/Alaska Natives and black Americans.[14] However, many deaths resulting from diabetes could be postponed if diabetes was detected and treated appropriately. Approximately 20 million Americans have diabetes, with almost 1.6 million new cases diagnosed in people aged 20 years or older in 2007.[56] The percentage of adults with diagnosed diabetes has increased significantly over the past 20 years (see Figure 8.10).[47] Furthermore, many individuals with diabetes are unaware they have the disease.[56]

Cholesterol is a soft, fatlike substance that is necessary to build cell membranes. About 75% of cholesterol is produced by the liver and other cells in the body, with the other 25% coming from the foods we eat, specifically animal products. Elevated cholesterol levels in blood can put people at greater risk for heart disease and stroke. The higher the cholesterol level, the greater the risk.[57] A person's cholesterol level is affected by age, heredity, and diet. There is nothing we can do about heredity and age, but diet is something we can modify.[57]

Dietary factors are associated with 4 of the 10 leading causes of death in this age group. Many dietary components are involved in the diet–health relationship, but chief among them is the disproportionate consumption of foods high in fat, often at the expense of foods high in complex carbohydrates and dietary fiber. Total dietary fat (saturated and unsaturated) accounts for too many total calories consumed in the United States. A diet that contains between 20% and 35% fat, with less than 10% of calories from saturated fats, is recommended.[58] Currently, the largest source of fat in diets comes from cheeses and oils. Diets high

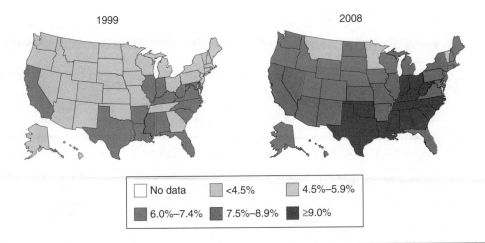

FIGURE 8.10

Age-adjusted percentage of U.S. adults who had diagnosed diabetes, 1999 and 2008.

Source: Centers for Disease Control and Prevention, Division of Diabetes Translation. National Diabetes Surveillance System. Available at http://www.cdc.gov/diabetes/statistics. Accessed November 30, 2010.

in fat and cholesterol are part of the reason why an estimated 50% of American adults have blood cholesterol levels of 200 mg/dL (milligrams per deciliter) and higher, and why about 20% have levels of 240 mg/dL or above.[59] Based on several studies, blood cholesterol levels less than 200 mg/dL in middle-aged adults seem to indicate a relatively low risk of coronary heart disease. In contrast, people with a blood cholesterol level of 240 mg/dL have twice the risk of having a coronary heart attack as do people who have a cholesterol level of 200 mg/dL.[59] **Hypercholesterolemia** is the term used for high levels of cholesterol in the blood. Like diabetes, the key to controlling hypercholesterolemia is screening and treatment.

> **hypercholesterolemia** high levels of cholesterol in the blood

The other prevalent medical condition in this age group that should be screened for on a regular basis is cancer. As noted earlier, malignant neoplasms are the leading cause of death in 45- to 64-year-olds. The American Cancer Society recommends a number of screenings for various age groups (see Table 8.6). However, many more adults in the United States could be getting screened. The earlier that cancer is detected, the greater the chance for successful treatment.

Community Health Strategies for Improving the Health of Adults

As noted in the previous pages, adults in the United States face a number of health issues. Even so, for most individuals the years between 25 and 64 are some of the healthiest of their lifetime. A key for keeping these people healthy is to reemphasize the importance of individual responsibility for health. That is, individuals must engage in behaviors that are health enhancing. From a community health perspective, this means that community health workers must continue to offer primary, secondary, and tertiary prevention programs that are aimed at the needs of this age group. For example, primary prevention programs could include exercise and nutrition programs that help reduce the risks of cancer and cardiovascular disease. Secondary prevention programs that emphasize self or clinical screenings to identify and control disease processes in their early stages, such as mammography, self-testicular exams, and cholesterol screenings, are also appropriate for this age group. In addition, tertiary prevention programs such as medication compliance to prevent disability by restoring individuals to their optimal level of functioning after the onset of disease or injury could also be useful.

SCENARIO: ANALYSIS AND RESPONSE

1. What primary prevention measures would have been helpful for the four university students? What primary prevention measures would have helped the businessman?

2. Why do you think that adolescents and young adults and adults engage in high-risk behaviors such as those presented in the scenario? If you were a community health worker in this community, what kind of programs would you recommend to lower the health risks of these individuals?

3. Comment on the attitudes of Annie and Latasha toward drunk driving and the automobile crash. Do you agree with one or the other? Why or why not?

4. Do colleges and universities have an obligation to develop prevention programs to keep students out of situations like the one described in the scenario? Why or why not?

5. Say you were friends with Annie. She got so concerned with the problem of alcohol abuse on campus that she wanted to take action. She thought that maybe she should look into starting a chapter of the BACCHUS Network (formerly called Boost Alcohol Consciousness Concerning the Health of University Students [BACCHUS]). She wanted to see what was on the Web about the BACCHUS Network, but because of a busy afternoon of classes she knew she wouldn't have time to check it, so she asked you if you would do it for her. Go to the Web and use a search engine (e.g., Google) and enter "BACCHUS." What did you find that might be of help to Annie?

Table 8.6
Summary of American Cancer Society Recommendations for the Early Detection of Cancer in Asymptomatic People

Cancer Site	Population	Test or Procedure	Frequency
Breast	Women, age 20+	Breast self-examination	Beginning in their early 20s, women should be told about the benefits and limitations of breast self-examination (BSE). The importance of prompt reporting of any new breast symptoms to a health professional should be emphasized. Women who choose to do BSE should receive instruction and have their technique reviewed on the occasion of a periodic health examination. It is acceptable for women to choose not to do BSE or to do BSE irregularly.
		Clinical breast examination	For women in their 20s and 30s, it is recommended that clinical breast examination (CBE) be part of a periodic health examination, preferably at least every three years. Asymptomatic women aged 40 and over should continue to receive a clinical breast examination as part of a periodic health examination, preferably annually.
		Mammography	Begin annual mammography at age 40.*
Colorectal†	Men and women, age 50+	*Tests that find polyps and cancer:*	
		Flexible sigmoidoscopy,‡ or	Every five years, starting at age 50
		Colonoscopy, or	Every 10 years, starting at age 50
		Double-contrast barium enema (DCBE),‡ or	Every five years, starting at age 50
		CT colonography (virtual colonoscopy)‡	Every five years, starting at age 50
		Tests that mainly find cancer:	
		Fecal occult blood test (FOBT) with at least 50% test sensitivity for cancer, or fecal immunochemical test (FIT) with at least 50% test sensitivity for cancer‡§ or	Annual, starting at age 50
		Stool DNA test (sDNA)‡	Interval uncertain, starting at age 50

(continued)

Table 8.6
Summary of American Cancer Society Recommendations for the Early Detection of Cancer in Asymptomatic People (continued)

Prostate	Men, age 50+	Prostate-specific antigen test (PSA) with or without digital rectal exam (DRE)	Asymptomatic men who have at least a 10-year life expectancy should have an opportunity to make an informed decision with their health care provider about screening for prostate cancer after receiving information about the uncertainties, risks, and potential benefits associated with screening. Men at average risk should receive this information beginning at age 50. Men at higher risk, including African American men and men with a first degree relative (father or brother) diagnosed with prostate cancer before age 65, should receive this information beginning at age 45. Men at appreciably higher risk (multiple family members diagnosed with prostate cancer before age 65) should receive this information beginning at age 40.
Cervix	Women, age 18+	Pap test	Cervical cancer screening should begin approximately three years after a woman begins having vaginal intercourse, but no later than 21 years of age. Screening should be done every year with conventional Pap tests or every two years using liquid-based Pap tests. At or after age 30, women who have had three normal test results in a row may get screened every two to three years with cervical cytology (either conventional or liquid-based Pap test) alone, or every three years with an HPV DNA test plus cervical cytology. Women 70 years of age and older who have had three or more normal Pap tests and no abnormal Pap tests in the past 10 years and women who have had a total hysterectomy may choose to stop cervical cancer screening.
Endometrial	Women, at menopause		At the time of menopause, women at average risk should be informed about risks and symptoms of endometrial cancer and strongly encouraged to report any unexpected bleeding or spotting to their physicians.
Cancer-related checkup	Men and women, age 20+		On the occasion of a periodic health examination, the cancer-related checkup should include examination for cancers of the thyroid, testicles, ovaries, lymph nodes, oral cavity, and skin, as well as health counseling about tobacco, sun exposure, diet and nutrition, risk factors, sexual practices, and environmental and occupational exposures.

*Beginning at age 40, annual clinical breast examination should be performed prior to mammography.

†Individuals with a personal or family history of colorectal cancer or adenomas, inflammatory bowel disease, or high-risk genetic syndromes should continue to follow the most recent recommendations for individuals at increased or high risk.

‡Colonoscopy should be done if test results are positive.

§For FOBT or FIT used as a screening test, the take-home multiple sample method should be used. A FOBT or FIT done during a digital rectal exam in the doctor's office is not adequate for screening.

Source: Reprinted from American Cancer Society. *Cancer Facts and Figures 2010.* Atlanta: American Cancer Society, Inc. Available at www.cancer.org. Accessed October 15, 2010.

CHAPTER SUMMARY

- Adolescence and young adulthood (15 to 24 years old) and adulthood (25 to 64 years old) are the most productive periods of people's lives. Although most people enjoy good health during these years, there is substantial room for improvement.

- The overall health status of these age groups could be improved by reducing the prevalence of high-risk behaviors (e.g., cigarette smoking, excessive alcohol consumption, and physical inactivity) and by increasing participation in health screenings and institutionalizing preventive health care in our society.

- Approximately 75% of adolescent and young adult mortality can be attributed to motor vehicle crashes, other unintentional injuries, homicide and legal intervention, and suicide.

- Adolescents and young adults remain at considerable risk for STD morbidity.

- College students put themselves at considerable risk through unprotected sexual activity and the use of alcohol, tobacco, and other drugs.

- Mortality rates for older adults (45 to 64 years old) have declined in recent years, but cancer is still the overall leading cause of death, followed by cardiovascular disease.

- Reductions in deaths from cardiovascular diseases in adults have been substantial, but health problems resulting from unhealthy behaviors—such as smoking, poor diet, and physical inactivity—can be reduced further if adults are willing to modify their behavior.

- No matter how the health of adolescents and young adults and adults in the United States is broken down and described, it can be summarized by saying that the health of Americans in these age groups has come a long way in the past 50 years, but there is still room for improvement.

REVIEW QUESTIONS

1. Why it is important for community health workers to be aware of the significant health problems of the various age groups in the United States?

2. What ages are included in the following two age groups: adolescents and young adults, and adults? What are the ages of the two subgroups of adults?

3. Why are the number of adolescents and young adults, living arrangements, and employment status such key demographic characteristics of young people in regard to community health? Briefly summarize the data available on these characteristics.

4. What are the leading causes of death for adolescents and young adults, and for adults?

5. What are the Youth Risk Behavior Surveillance System (YRBSS) and the Behavioral Risk Factor Surveillance System (BRFSS), and what type of data do they generate?

6. What are the behaviors that put each of these cohorts—adolescents, college students, and adults—at greatest risk?

7. How would you summarize the health profile of the two cohorts (adolescents and young adults, and adults) presented in this chapter?

ACTIVITIES

1. Obtain a copy of the most recent results of the Youth Risk Behavior Surveillance System (YRBSS) and the Behavioral Risk Factor Surveillance System (BRFSS) for your state. Review the data presented, and then prepare a two-page summary on the "Health Behavior Profile of the Adolescents and Young Adults and Adults" of your state.

2. Obtain data presenting the 10 leading causes of death according to age and race for the age groups presented in this chapter. Review the data, and prepare a summary paper discussing conclusions that can be drawn about race, the leading causes of death, and age.

3. Interview a small group (about 10) of adults (aged 45 to 64) about their present health status. Ask them questions about their health behavior and health problems. Then, summarize the data you collect in writing and compare it to the information in this chapter on this age group. How are the data similar? How do they differ?

4. Pick either adolescents and young adults or adults, and write a two-page paper that presents ideas on how the health profile of that age group can be improved in your state.

COMMUNITY HEALTH ON THE WEB

The Internet contains a wealth of information about community and public health. Increase your knowledge of some of the topics presented in this chapter by accessing the Jones & Bartlett Learning Web site at **http://health .jbpub.com/book/communityhealth/7e** and follow the links to complete the following Web activities.

- Youth Risk Behavior Surveillance System
- Vital Statistics
- Behavorial Risk Factor Surveillance System

REFERENCES

1. Snyder, T., and L. Shafer (1996). *Youth Indicators, 1996* (NCES 96-027). Washington, DC: U.S. Department of Education, National Center for Education Statistics.

2. MacKay, A. P., L. A. Fingerhut, and C. R. Duran (2000). *Health, United States, 2000 with Adolescent Health Chartbook*. Hyattsville, MD: National Center for Health Statistics.

3. American Medical Association (2000). *Talking to Your Teenagers 11-14: Discussion Guide*. Chicago: Author.

4. Seffrin, J. R. (1990). "The Comprehensive School Health Curriculum: Closing the Gap between State-of-the-Art and State-of-the-Practice." *Journal of School Health*, 60(4): 151-156.

5. Valois, R. F., W. G. Thatcher, J. W. Drane, and B. M. Reininger (1997). "Comparison of Selected Health Risk Behaviors between Adolescents in Public and Private High Schools in South Carolina." *Journal of School Health*, 67(10): 434-440.

6. Hobbs, F., and N. Stoops (2002). *Demographic Trends in the 20th Century* (Census 2000 Special Reports, Series CENSR-4). Washington, DC: U.S. Government Printing Office.

7. U.S. Bureau of the Census (1999). *Statistical Abstract of the United States, 1999*, 119th ed. Washington, DC: Author.

8. U.S. Census Bureau (2010). *The 2010 Statistical Abstract*. Available at http://www.census.gov/compendia/statab/2010edition.html.

9. MacKay, A., and C. Duran (2008). *Adolescent Health in the United States, 2007*. Hyatsville, MD: National Center for Health Statistics.

10. National Kids Count Program (2009). "Children in Single Parent Households. Annie E. Casey Foundation." Available at http://datacenter.kidscount.org.

11. Toossi, M. (2006). "A New Look at Long-Term Labor Force Projections to 2050." *Monthly Labor Review Online*, 129(11).

12. Toosi, M. (2009). "Labor Force Projections to 2018: Older Workers Staying More Active." *Monthly Labor Review Online*, 132(11).

13. Bureau of Labor Statistics (2010). "Labor Force Statistics from the Current Population Survey. United States Department of Labor." Available at http://data.bls.gov/cgi-bin/surveymost?ln.

14. National Center for Health Statistics (2010). *Health, United States, 2009 with Special Feature on Medical Technology*. Hyattsville, MD: Author.

15. National Center for Health Statistics (2009). *Health, United States, 2008 with Special Features on the Health of Young Adults*. Hyattsville, MD: Author.

16. National Center for Health Statistics (2009). "Deaths, Percent of Total Deaths, and Death Rates for the 15 Leading Causes of Death in 10-Year Age Groups." LCWK5, National Vital Statistics System. Available at http://www.cdc.gov/nchs/data/dvs/LCWK5_2006.pdf.

17. U.S. Department of Health and Human Services (2000). *Healthy People 2010: Leading Health Indicators*. Washington, DC: Author. Available at http://www.healthypeople.gov/Document/tableofcontents.htm#volume1.

18. Centers for Disease Control and Prevention (2010). "Youth Risk Behavior Surveillance—United States, 2009." *MMWR Surveillance Summaries*, 59(SS-5).

19. Centers for Disease Control and Prevention (2009). *Sexually Transmitted Disease Surveillance, 2008*. Atlanta, GA: U.S. Department of Health and Human Services.

20. Centers for Disease Control and Prevention (2010). *Sexually Transmitted Diseases Fact Sheets*. Available at http://www.cdc.gov/std/healthcomm/fact_sheets.htm.

21. Centers for Disease Control and Prevention (2008). "Subpopulation Estimates from the HIV Incidence Surveillance System—United States, 2006." *Morbidity and Mortality Weekly Report*, 57(36): 985-989.

22. Centers for Disease Control and Prevention (1996). "Tobacco Use and Usual Source of Cigarettes among High School Students—United States,1995." *Morbidity and Mortality Weekly Report*, 45(20): 413-418.

23. American Heart Association, American Cancer Society, Campaign for Tobacco-Free Kids, and American Lung Association (2006). *A Broken Promise to Our Children: The 1998 State Tobacco Settlement Eight Years Later*. Available at http://www.tobaccofreekids.org/reports/settlements/2007/fullreport.pdf.

24. Campaign for Tobacco-Free Kids (2009). "Congress, President Deliver Historic Victory for Children's Health by Increasing Tobacco Taxes to Fund SCHIP Program." February 4, 2009. Available at http://www.tobaccofreekids.org.

25. Centers for Disease Control and Prevention (1996). "Trends in Sexual Risk Behavior among High School Students—United States—1990, 1991, and 1993." *Morbidity and Mortality Weekly Report*, 44(7): 124-125, 131-132.

26. Centers for Disease Control and Prevention (2010). "Sexual Risk Behaviors." Available at http://www.cdc.gov/HealthyYouth/sexualbehaviors/index.htm.

27. Kost K., S. Henshaw, and L. Carlin (2010). *U.S. Teenage Pregnancies, Births and Abortions: National and State Trends and Trends by Race and Ethnicity*. Available at http://www.guttmacher.org/pubs/USTPtrends.pdf.

28. The National Campaign to Prevent Teen and Unplanned Pregnancy (2008). *Briefly . . . Unplanned Pregnancy in the United States*. Available at http://www.thenationalcampaign.org/nationa-data/unplanned-pregnancy-birth-rates.aspx.

29. Darroch, J. E., S. Singh, J. J. Frost, and the Study Team (2001). "Differences in Teenage Pregnancy Rates among Five Developed Countries: The Role of Sexual Activity and Contraceptive Use." *Family Planning Perspectives*, 33(6): 244-250, 281.

30. U.S. Department of Health and Human Services (2000). *Healthy People 2010: Understanding and Improving Health*. Washington, DC: U.S. Government Printing Office.

31. American College Health Association (2009). "National College Health Assessment Reference Group Executive Summary." Available at http://www.achancha.org/reports_ACHA-NCHAII.html.

32. Johnston, L. D., P. M. O'Malley, and J. G. Bachman (2010). *Monitoring the Future National Survey Results on Drug Use, 1975-2009. Vol. II: College Students and Adults Ages 19-50*. Bethesda, MD: National Institute on Drug Abuse.

33. U.S. Department of Education Statistics (2006). *Digest of Education Statistics: 2005*. Available at http://nces.ed.gov/programs/digest/.

34. Goldman, M. S., G. M. Boyd, and V. Faden, eds. (March 2002). "College Drinking, What It Is, and What to Do About It: A Review of the State of the Science" [Special issue]. *Journal of Studies on Alcohol* (Suppl. 14).

35. Centers for Disease Control and Prevention (2009). *Sexually Transmitted Disease Surveillance, 2008*. Atlanta, GA: Author.

36. Substance Abuse and Mental Health Services Administration (2010). SAMHSA National Registry of Evidence-Based Programs and Practices. Available at http://www.nrepp.samhsa.gov/.

37. Dusenbury, L., and M. Falco (1995). "Eleven Components of Effective Drug Abuse Prevention Curricula." *Journal of School Health*, 65: 420-425.

38. Joint Committee on National Health Education Standards (2007). *National Health Education Standards*, 2nd ed. Atlanta, GA: ACS.

39. Centers for Disease Control and Prevention (2008). *Health Education Curriculum Analysis Tool (HECAT)*. Atlanta, GA: Author. Available at http://www.cdc.gov/healthyyouth/HECAT/index.htm.

40. National Institute on Alcohol Abuse and Alcoholism (2007). *A Call to Action: Changing the Culture of Drinking at U.S. Colleges*. Washington, DC: Author.

41. Xu, J. Q., K. D. Kochanek, S. L. Murphy, and B. Tejada-Vera (2010). "Deaths: Final Data for 2007." *National Vital Statistics Reports*, 58(19). Hyattsville, MD: National Center for Health Statistics.

42. Heron M. (2010). "Deaths: Leading Causes for 2006." *National Vital Statistics Reports*, 58(14). Hyattsville, MD: National Center for Health Statistics.

43. American Cancer Society (2010). *Cancer Facts and Figures 2010*. Atlanta, GA: Author.

44. Mokdad, A. H., J. S. Marks, D. F. Stroup, and J. L. Gerberding (2004). "Actual Causes of Death in the United States, 2000." *Journal of the American Medical Association*, 291(10): 1238–1245.

45. American Heart Association (2010). "Obesity, Nutrition, and Physical Activity." Available at http://www.heart.org/obesitypolicy.

46. Odgen, C., and M. Carroll (2010). "Prevalence of Overweight, Obesity, and Extreme Obesity Among Adults: United States, Trends 1976–1980 Through 2007–2008." Available at http://www.cdc.gov/nchs/data/hestat/obesity_adult_07_08/obesity_adult_07_08.htm.

47. Centers for Disease Control and Prevention (2006). "Behavioral Risk Factor Surveillance System." Available at http://www.cdc.gov/brfss/index.htm.

48. Flegal, K., M. Carroll, C. Ogden, and L. Curtin (2010). "Prevalence and Trends in Obesity among US Adults, 1999–2008." *Journal of the American Medical Association*, 303(3): 235–241.

49. Centers for Disease Control and Prevention (2006). "Overweight and Obesity: Causes and Consequences." Available at http://www.cdc.gov/nccdphp/dnpa/obesity/contributing_factors.htm.

50. Pleis, J. R., J. W. Lucas, and B. W. Ward (2009). "Summary Health Statistics for U.S. Adults: National Health Interview Survey, 2008." National Center for Health Statistics. *Vital and Health Statistics*, 10(242). Available at http://www.cdc.gov/nchs/data/series/sr_10/sr10_242.pdf.

51. Manning, W. G., L. Blumberg, and L. H. Moulton (1995). "The Demand for Alcohol: The Differential Response to Price." *Journal of Health Economics*, 14(2): 123–145.

52. March of Dimes (2010). Drinking Alcohol During Pregnancy. Available at http://www.marchofdimes.com/professionals/14332_1170.asp.

53. Chen, Y. and T. Jianqiang (2010). *Seat Belt Use in 2009—Use Rates in the States and Territories*. Washington, DC: NHTSA National Center for Statistics and Analysis. Available at http://www.nhtsa.gov/Data/State+Data+Program+&+CODES.

54. Substance Abuse and Mental Health Services Administration (2006). *The NSDUH Report: Driving Under the Influence among Adult Drivers*. Available at http://www.oas.samhsa.gov/2K5/DUI/DUI.cfm.

55. American Heart Association (2010). "High Blood Pressure: The Silent Killer." Available at http://www.heart.org/HEARTORG/Conditions/HighBloodPressure/AboutHighBloodPressure/About-High-Blood-Pressure_UCM_002050_Article.jsp.

56. American Diabetes Association (2010). "All About Diabetes." Available at http://www.diabetes.org/diabetes-basics.

57. American Heart Association (2010). "About Cholesterol." Available at http://www.heart.org/HEARTORG/Conditions/Cholesterol/AboutCholesterol/AboutCholesterol_UCM_001220_Article.jsp.

58. U.S. Department of Health and Human Services (2008). *Dietary Guidelines for Americans, 2005*. Washington, DC: Author.

59. American Heart Association (2007). *Am I at Risk?* Dallas, TX: Author.

Chapter 9

Elders

Chapter Objectives

After studying this chapter, you will be able to:

1 Identify the characteristics of an aging population.

2 Define the following groups—*old, young old, middle old,* and *old old.*

3 Define the terms *aged, aging, elders, gerontology,* and *geriatrics.*

4 Refute several commonly held myths about the elder population.

5 Explain the meaning of an age pyramid.

6 List the factors that affect the size and age of a population.

7 Define fertility and mortality rates and explain how they affect life expectancy.

8 Explain the difference between support and labor-force ratios.

9 Describe older adults with regard to marital status, living arrangements, racial and ethnic background, economic status, and geographic location.

10 Explain how four health behaviors can improve the quality of later life.

11 Briefly outline elder abuse and neglect in the United States.

12 Identify the six instrumental needs of older adults.

13 Briefly summarize the Older Americans Act of 1965.

14 List the services provided for older adults in most communities.

15 Explain the difference between respite care and adult day care.

16 Identify the four different levels of tasks with which elderly persons need assistance.

SCENARIO

Carl and Sarah have been retired for about 5 years. Carl retired in good health after 35 years as an insurance agent, and Sarah stopped working outside the home after their children were grown and had families of their own. Upon retirement, they sold their home and paid cash for a condominium that had about half the square footage of their home. This relocation forced them to pare down their belongings to fit into their new and smaller surroundings. As a consequence, though, they felt less tied down to possessions and felt more freedom to do the traveling they had anticipated for several years. Although they now live on a fixed income, the profit from their home has allowed them to live out the retirement they had dreamed about, that is, having the financial resources to sign up for Exploritas (formerly called Elderhostel) programs in other cities and to visit or host their children and grandchildren over the holidays.

All is not completely rosy for Carl and Sarah, however. Though they enjoy their lives very much, they are faced with an increasing number of health problems. They have accepted this challenge and have begun to do brisk walking on a near daily basis. Also, Sarah has signed up for a yoga program. Carl joined a Tai Chi program at the senior center. They have also suffered the loss of good friends, several of whom have died, and their best friends and neighbors recently moved to be closer to their kids. Carl and Sarah are going to attend an orientation session at the local elementary school to help students read, in hopes of adding more meaning and purpose to their lives and to dwell less on their losses.

They look to the future with a mix of optimism and anxiety. The optimism is based on their consistent ability to meet the challenges of aging, even those losses that are very discouraging in the beginning. The anxiety is based on the unknown: What if their property taxes increase beyond what they can afford? What if their Medicare Part D provider continues to raise premiums, deductibles, and copayments? Many questions arise, with no definite answers. But Carl and Sarah feel up to the challenge and adventure of aging into the future and take satisfaction in looking back at lives well lived.

INTRODUCTION

The American population is growing older. The number of elders in America and their proportion of the total population increased dramatically during the twentieth century. In 1950, there were 12 million people (8% of the population) aged 65 years, and by 2008, that number had increased to 38.9 million. "They represented 12.8% of the U.S. population, over one in every eight Americans."[1] For the first time in U.S. history, a significant number of Americans will achieve elder status and, in doing so, live long enough to assume some responsibilities for the care of their aging parents. We need only to look around us to see the change that is taking place (see Figure 9.1). The number of gray heads in restaurants, malls, and movie theaters is increasing. Senior centers, retirement villages, and assisted living facilities are being built in record numbers. And today, more than ever before, many people belong to multigenerational families, where there are opportunities

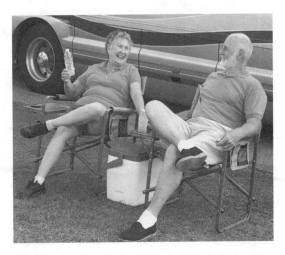

FIGURE 9.1

The number of elders in the United States is on the rise, and they are more energetic than previous cohorts.

to develop long-lasting relationships with parents, grandparents, and even great-grandparents. There are now families in which members of three successive generations receive monthly Social Security checks. In the twenty-first century, the economic, social, and health issues associated with the growing proportion of people older than age 65 in the United States have become major political concerns. In this chapter, we will define terminology, describe the demographics, and discuss the special needs of and community service for the aging.

Definitions

How old is old? The ageless baseball pitcher Satchel Paige once said, "How old would you be if you didn't know how old you was [sic]?" Although his English might be found wanting, Paige's point is important (see Figure 9.2). A person's age might depend on who measures it and how they define it. For example, whereas demographers might define old according to chronological years, clinicians might define it by stages of physiological development, and psychologists by developmental stages. Children might see their 35-year-old teacher as old, whereas the 35-year-old teacher might regard her 61-year-old principal as old. Age is and always will be a relative concept.

In the United States and other developed countries, people are considered *old* once they reach the age of 65. But because there are a number of people who are very active and healthy at age 65 and will live a number of productive years after 65, researchers have subdivided old into the *young old* (65–74), the *middle old* (75–84), and the *old old* (85 and over). Interestingly enough, it is this latter group, the old old, that makes up the fastest-growing segment of the elder population.

Also for the purposes of our discussion in this chapter, we use terms that are associated with aging. They include the following:

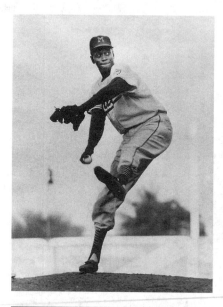

FIGURE 9.2

Some would say you are only as old as you think you are. (Satchel Paige remained active in professional baseball long after reaching the age at which others retired.)

aged   The state of being old. A person may be defined as aged on the basis of having reached a specific age; for example, 65 is often used for social or legislative policies, while 75 is used for physiological evaluations by geriatricians.[2]

aging   The changes that occur normally in plants and animals as they grow older. Some age changes begin at birth and continue until death; other changes begin at maturity and end at death.[2]

gerontology   The multidisciplinary study of the biological, psychological, and social processes of aging and the elderly.[3] Elie Metchnikoff, of the Pasteur Institute in Paris, first used the term in 1903 to describe the biological study of senescence (aging).[2]

geriatrics   The branch of medicine concerned with medical problems and care of the elderly.[3]

geriatrician   A physician specializing in the care of patients with multiple chronic diseases who may not be able to be cured but whose care can be managed.[3]

Many terms have been used to describe individuals who are 65 years of age and older, including seniors, "senior citizens, golden agers, retired persons, mature adults, elderly, aged, and old people. There is no clear preference among older people for any of these terms."[4] As Ferrini and Ferrini have stated, "Many gerontologists have chosen to adopt the term 'elder' to describe those 65 and older. This term is an attempt to redefine aging in a more positive way that connotes wisdom, respect, leadership, and accumulated knowledge."[4] We agree with Ferrini and Ferrini and the other gerontologists and will frequently use the term **elders** to designate those who have reached their 65th birthday.

elders
those 65 years of age
and older

MYTHS SURROUNDING AGING

Like other forms of prejudice and discrimination, **ageism** is the result of ignorance, misconceptions, and half-truths about aging and the elderly. Because most people do not interact with older people on a daily basis, it is easy to create a stereotypical image of elders based on the atypical actions of a few or negative images in the media.

ageism
prejudice and
discrimination against
the aged

When you think of older people, who comes to mind? Do you immediately think of a lonely man with a disheveled appearance sitting on a park bench or an older person lying in bed in a nursing home making incomprehensible noises? Or, do you think of Clint Eastwood and Sean Connery (each turned 80 years old in 2010) in an action-packed, high-suspense thriller?

Ferrini and Ferrini and Dychtwald and Flower have identified a number of commonly held myths about elders.[4,5] They are presented here to remind all that elders are not run-down, worn-out members of our society but are for the most part independent, capable, and valuable resources for our communities. Do not forget that several U.S. presidents have been eligible for Social Security and Medicare while in office. In 2010, the average age of a United States senator was 63 years, the oldest it has ever been.

Here are the myths and the reasons why they are only myths:

1. Myth: "After age 65 life goes steadily downhill."
   Truth: Any chronological age that defines old age is arbitrary. Nonetheless, many gerontologists are substituting age 85 for age 65 as the new chronological definition of old age.
2. Myth: "Old people are all alike."
   Truth: There are more differences among elders than any other segment of the U.S. population.
3. Myth: "Old people are lonely and ignored by their families."
   Truth: Elders are the least likely to be lonely of any age group; and those who live alone are likely to be in close contact, either in person, by e-mail, or by telephone, with close friends and/or their family.
4. Myth: "Old age used to be better."
   Truth: It is only in the last half of the twentieth century that a large portion of the U.S. population lived to be 65 years old. If people did live to be old, they were not treated any better than they are today.
5. Myth: "Old people are senile."
   Truth: Senility is the result of disease and only affects about 5% of elders living in noninstitutional settings.
6. Myth: "Old people have the good life."
   Truth: Though elders do gain certain advantages when they retire and when their children leave home, they still face a number of concerns, such as loss of loved ones, loss of health, and loss of value in society.
7. Myth: "Most old people are sickly."
   Truth: Most older people do have at least one chronic health problem, but the majority of elders live active lifestyles.
8. Myth: "Old people no longer have any sexual interest or ability."
   Truth: Sexual interest may or may not diminish with age, but there is an alteration in sexual response. Nonetheless, many elders in reasonably good health have active and satisfying sex lives.

9. Myth: "Most old people end up in nursing homes."
   Truth: Only approximately 4% of those above the age of 65 live in nursing homes, homes for the aged, or other group quarters. Only 1% of those aged 65 to 74 reside in such a place, though the percentage jumps to 19% for the oldest old (those 85 and older). However, this number is still well below half.
10. Myth: "Older people are unproductive."
    Truth: Older adults are more likely to be retired, but they are very likely to be productively engaged at home and in the community.

exploritas
education programs specifically for elders, held on college campuses or at a variety of sites around the world

Though a number of issues and concerns facing elders are presented later in this chapter, the majority of elders in the United States today are active and well (see Figure 9.3). In all parts of the country, many elders are still working. Many of the retired elders are (1) attending **Exploritas** (formerly called Elderhostel) programs, (2) remaining politically active (AARP, formerly called the American Association of Retired Persons, is one of the most active lobbying groups in the United States), and (3) volunteering countless hours as tutors at schools, workers for hospices and hospitals, advocates and companions for the mentally and physically ill, intake personnel at crisis centers, and members of community agency boards and churches, to name a few roles. Elders are an important part of society and play active roles in making communities work.

demography
the study of a population and those variables bringing about change in that population

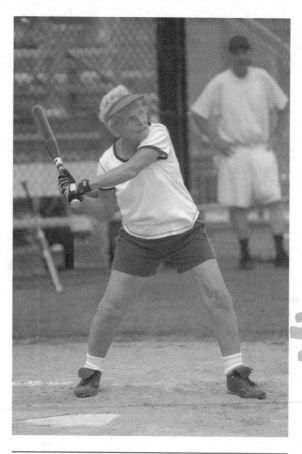

FIGURE 9.3
Many seniors are remaining active well after retirement age.

DEMOGRAPHY OF AGING

Demography is "the study of a population (an aggregate of individuals) and those variables bringing about change in that population."[2] The demography of aging is typically defined as a study of those who are 65 years and older and of the variables that bring about change in their lives. In the following paragraphs, we review some of the demographic features of the elder population, including size, growth rate, and the factors that contribute to this growth. We also discuss other demographic characteristics of this population, such as living arrangements, racial and ethnic composition, geographic distribution, economic status, and housing.

Size and Growth of the Elder Population

The aging of any population can be graphically illustrated with a symbolic age pyramid[6] (see Figure 9.4). The base of this pyramid represents the youngest and largest segment of the population. The sloping sides indicate higher mortality rates and limited life expectancy. Until the mid-1950s, the population pyramid for the United States was not so very different from the traditional age pyramid.

Since the mid-1950s, however, the shape of America's population pyramid has changed. As noted earlier in the chapter, both the number of elders and the proportion of the total population made up of elders grew significantly during the twentieth century. At the beginning of the twentieth century, only 1 in 25 Americans was over the age of 65 years. In 2008, that number had increased to 1 in

8.[1] Demographers' projections suggest that populations will continue to age, not only in this country, but in most other countries as well. In 2011, the *baby boom* generation began to turn 65, and by 2030, it is projected that 71.5 million people (1 in 5) will be age 65 or older.[1] The population aged 85 and older is currently the fastest-growing segment of the older population. It will double in size by 2030.[7] During this same time, it is expected that the percentage of people aged 18 and younger will decrease slightly to around 24%. These changes will alter the shape of the population pyramid and make it more like the shape of a population rectangle. Figure 9.5 shows the difference in the population pyramid of 2000 and the projections for 2030.

As one might guess, the projected growth of the elder population is expected to raise the **median age** of the U.S. population. In 2000, the median age was 35.3 years.[8] Projections put the median age at 36.9 years in 2010, and then continue up to 39 years by 2035 and stay right around that number until 2050.[8]

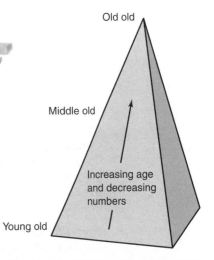

FIGURE 9.4
Symbolic age pyramid.

Factors That Affect Population Size and Age

Three factors affect the size and age of a population: its fertility rates, its mortality rates, and its gain or loss from migration of individuals into or out of that population.[2] Though one might assume that all populations will age with time, that is not necessarily true. In fact, a population could get younger with time.[2] If fertility rates and mortality rates are both high, life expectancy would be low, and the age of a population could grow younger. However, this has not been the case in the United States.

> **median age**
> the age at which half of the population is older and half is younger

Fertility Rates

The *fertility rate* is an expression of the number of births per 1,000 women of childbearing age (15–44) in the population during a specific time period. Fertility rates in the United States were at their highest at the beginning of the twentieth century. Those rates dipped during

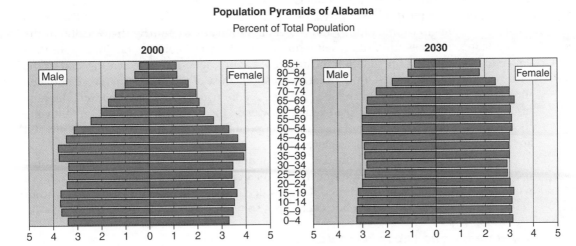

FIGURE 9.5
Population Pyramid for 2000 and the Projected Pyramid for 2030: Percent of Total Population.
Source: U.S. Census Bureau, Population Division, Interim State Population Projections, 2005.

the Depression years but rebounded after World War II. The period of consistently high fertility rates immediately following World War II has become known as the "baby boom years," hence the name *baby boomers* for those born between 1946 and 1964. During those years, 76 million babies were born. As the baby boomers continue to age, a "human tidal wave" (bulge) will continue to move up the U.S. age pyramid. In Figure 9.5, the baby boomers were included in the 36- to 54-year-olds in 2000 and in 2030 they will be ages 66 to 84 years old. American society has tried to adjust to the size and needs of the baby boom generation throughout the stages of the life cycle. Just as this generation had a dramatic impact on expanding obstetrics and pediatrics, creating split shifts for students in public schools, and disrupting government policy toward the Vietnam War, the baby boom cohorts will also place tremendous strain on programs and services (e.g., Social Security and Medicare) required by an elderly population. A window of opportunity now exists for planners and policymakers to prepare for the aging of the baby boom generation.[9]

Mortality Rates

The *mortality or death rate* (usually expressed in deaths per 100,000 population) also has an impact on the aging population. The annual crude mortality rate in the United States in 1900 was 1,720 per 100,000. Recent data show that that figure has dropped by half to 810.[10] The decrease in the annual mortality rate achieved over the twentieth century was the result of triumphs in medical science and public health practice.

Another demographic variable that interacts with the mortality rate is life expectancy. Although the mortality rate in the United States has been fairly constant for 20+ years, life expectancy has continued to increase. During the twentieth century, there was an overall jump in life expectancy at birth from 47.3 years in 1900 to 77.9 years in 2007.[10] The life expectancy of men and black Americans has always trailed those of women and white Americans, respectively. Whereas the increase in life expectancy in the first half of the twentieth century could be attributed to the decrease in infant and early childhood deaths, the increase in life expectancy since 1970 can be traced to the postponement of death among the middle-aged and elder population.

Migration

The movement of people from one country to another, *migration,* has also contributed to the aging of the population. **Net migration** is the population gain or loss from the movement of migrants in (immigration) and out (emigration) of a country. Historically, in the United States, net migration has resulted in population gain; more people immigrate than emigrate. The greatest immigration in the United States occurred between the end of the Civil War and the beginning of the Great Depression. Most of the immigrants were between the ages of 18 and 35 years—of childbearing age. As these immigrants had children, the population of the United States remained young. However, the decline in immigration following the Depression led to the aging of the American populace as the early immigrants grew old and were not replaced by younger immigrants.

net migration
the population gain or loss resulting from migration

Fortunately, however, the United States continued to absorb young immigrants during the closing decades of the twentieth century. As a consequence, the dependency ratio of workers to older adults in the United States is declining more slowly than in many other developed countries. The future, however, is not so bright. We turn to this topic next.

Dependency and Labor-Force Ratios

Other demographic signs of an aging population are changes in dependency and labor-force ratios. The **dependency ratio** is a comparison between those individuals whom society considers economically unproductive (the nonworking or dependent population) and those it considers economically productive (the working population). Traditionally, the productive and nonproductive populations have been defined by age; the productive population includes

dependency ratio
a ratio that compares the number of individuals whom society considers economically unproductive to the number it considers economically productive

those who are 19 to 64. The unproductive population includes both youth (0–19 years old) and the old (65+ years). When the dependency ratio includes both youth and old, it is referred to as a **total dependency ratio**. When only the youth are compared to the productive group, the term used is **youth dependency ratio**; when only the old are compared, it is called **old-age dependency ratio**.

Changes in dependency ratios "provide an indirect broad indication of periods when we can expect the particular age distribution of the country to affect the need for distinct types of social services, housing, and consumer products."[12] Thus, communities can refer to dependency ratio data as a guide for making the best social policy decisions and as a way to allocate resources. For example, leaders in a community with a relatively high youth dependency ratio compared to the old-age dependency ratio may want to concentrate community resources on programs such as education for the young, health promotion programs for children, special programs for working parents, and other youth-associated concerns. Communities with high old-age dependency ratios might increase programs for elders including programs to reengage retirees into **encore careers**.

The total dependency ratio (DR) is calculated by adding the number of youth and old, divided by the number of persons 20 to 64 years, times 100. In the twentieth century, the lowest DR (70.5) was recorded in 1900. The DR in 2010 was 67, but projections have it climbing to a peak of 85 in 2040 and staying steady through 2050[13] (see Figure 9.6). This increase over the next 30 to 40 years will be driven by the old-age dependency ratio and thus will guide future social policy.

Such an increase in the old-age dependency ratio provides an interesting political scenario because the costs to support youth and the old are not the same. Parents pay directly

total dependency ratio
the dependency ratio that includes both youth and old

youth dependency ratio
the dependency ratio that includes only youth

old-age dependency ratio
the dependency ratio that includes only the old

encore careers
when individuals transition out of their work careers and into jobs and volunteer opportunities in nonprofit and public sectors. Encore careers have a positive impact on society's greatest problems.[11]

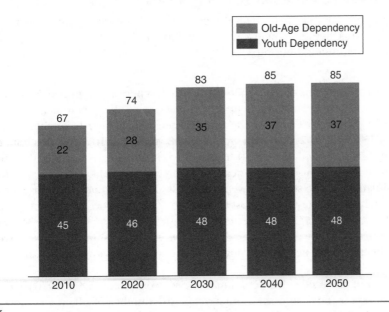

FIGURE 9.6

Dependency ratios for the United States: 2010 to 2050.

Note: Total dependency = ((Population under age 20 + Population aged 65 years and over) / (Population aged 20 to 64 years)) * 100.

Old-age dependency = (Population aged 65 years and over / Population aged 20 to 64 years) * 100.

Youth dependency = (Population under age 20 / Population aged 20 to 64 years) * 100.

Source: U.S. Census Bureau. (2010). "The Next Four Decades, The Older Population in the United States: 2010 to 2050, Current Population Reports" *Current Population Reports* (#P25-1138). Available at http://www.census.gov/newsroom/releases/archives/aging_population/cb10-72.html. Accessed November 30, 2010.

for most of the expenditures to support their children, with the primary exception being public education, which is paid for by taxes. In contrast, much of the support for elders comes from tax-supported programs such as Social Security, Medicare, and Medicaid. To meet the impending burden of the elderly, taxes will most certainly need to be raised or benefits reduced. Therefore, the two questions for the future are: Will the productive population be willing to pay increased taxes to support elders? Will services to the elderly be drastically reduced?

Although dependency ratio data clearly show one trend, they are merely an estimate and should not be the only accepted estimate. Actually, the dependency ratios presented in Figure 9.6 are based on the assumption that everyone of productive age supports all members of the nonproductive age group. Obviously, this is not the case. Many of those in the productive age group (for instance, homemakers, those who are unemployed, and those who are disabled) do not participate in the paid labor force. Conversely, many teenagers and elders do. Thus, dependency ratios, in some situations, could provide misleading figures for decision makers.

labor-force ratio
a ratio of the total number of those individuals who are not working to the number of those who are

Other experts believe that labor-force ratios also need to be considered. **Labor-force ratios** differ from dependency ratios in that they are based on the number of people who are actually working and those who are not, independent of their ages. When labor-force participation rates are used to calculate the labor-force ratios, it is projected that the burden of support for the labor force in the future will be somewhat lighter than that projected through dependency ratios. This is because of the fact that baby boomers plan to work longer than did members of the previous generations.[14] Nonetheless, under either method of calculation, the ratio of workers to dependants will be lower in the future than it is today.

Other Demographic Variables Affecting Elders

Other demographic variables that affect the community health programs of older Americans include marital status, living arrangements, racial and ethnic composition, geographic distribution, economic status, and housing.

Marital Status

Approximately three-fourths of elder men are married, whereas just over half of elder women are married. In addition, elder women are three times more likely than men to be widowed.[9] There are three primary reasons for these differences. First, men have shorter average life expectancies (75.7 years in 2010)[8] than women (80.8 years in 2010)[8] and thus tend to precede their wives in death. Second, men tend to marry women who are younger than themselves. Finally, men who lose a spouse through death or divorce are more likely to remarry than women in the same situation. These statistics reveal that most elderly men have a spouse for assistance, especially when health fails, whereas most women do not. However, "in many ways, the current generation of elderly women are pacesetters as they defy stereotypes of aging. Many have dealt with the shortage of men by developing new interests and friendships. For elderly women (and men) with protective social networks, living alone does not necessarily mean being lonely"[12] (see Figure 9.7).

The number of divorced elderly continues to rise, from almost 5% in 1970 to 9% in 2007.[15] As the baby boomers move into their older years, the number of divorced elders will grow two- to threefold. These divorced elders represent a new type of need group—those who lack the retirement benefits, insurance, and net worth assets associated with being married.

Living Arrangements

"Like marital status, the living arrangements of America's older population are important because they are closely linked to income, health status, and the availability of caregivers. Older persons who live alone are more likely to be in poverty than older persons who live with their spouses."[9] Two-thirds of noninstitutionalized elders live with someone else (spouse, relative, or other non-relatives), while the remainder live alone.[9] Of those living alone, women are much more likely (almost 2 to 1) to be living alone. The proportion of those living alone is projected to remain about the same, but the numbers are expected to increase dramatically over the next 20 years.[7] Reasons for these increased numbers revolve around the aging of the baby boomers and the improved economic status of the elderly, coupled with their strong desire to live as independently as possible.

Only a small percentage of the elderly population in the United States resides in nursing homes. About 1.8 million of those aged 65 years and older are in nursing homes, representing 5% of the elder population.[8] This percentage is down from previous years in part as a result of the increase in **assisted-living facilities**, which provide an alternative to long-term care in a nursing home. Of those who do live in nursing homes, older women at all ages have higher usage rates than men do. Approximately three-fourths of nursing home residents are women, and more than half of all nursing home residents are older than 85 years. As one might expect, the proportion of elders living in a nursing home increases with age.[9]

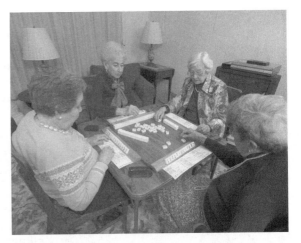

FIGURE 9.7

Elder women are three times more likely to be widowed than elder men are.

Racial and Ethnic Composition

As the elder population grows larger, it will also grow more diverse, reflecting the demographic changes in the U.S. population as a whole. In 2010, the elder population was predominately white. Of the total elder population in 2010, it was estimated that about 80% were white, 9% were black, 7% were of Hispanic origin, 3% were Asian, and Pacific Islanders, American Indians, and Alaska Natives were less than 1%.[1] By 2050, the white population is expected to decline to 58%, while Americans of Hispanic origin will increase to 15%, black Americans will increase to 11%, Asian Americans will increase to 8%, and Pacific Islanders, American Indians, and Alaska Natives will stay at less than 1% but still continue to grow in numbers.[1]

As the older population becomes more ethnically diverse, health professionals will need to become more knowledgeable about the cultural backgrounds of their elder clients. Additional knowledge and improved communication skills can lead to better adherence to health recommendations and to enhanced health outcomes.[16]

Geographic Distribution

In 2008, it was estimated that about two-fifths of America's elders lived in southern states (see Figure 9.8), and just more than half lived in the following 10 states: California, Florida, Illinois, Michigan, New Jersey, New York, North Carolina, Ohio, Pennsylvania, and Texas. Each of these states, as well as nine other states, had more than 1 million elders. California had the greatest number, while Florida had the greatest proportion.[1] Some states, including many in the Midwest, have a small total number of elders, but the elders make up a large percentage of their total population.

The populations of some states (such as Florida) "age" because of the inward migration of elders; others (such as the Farm Belt states) "age" because their young people leave. Still other states "age" because of low fertility or some combination of factors.[12]

From an ethnic and racial standpoint, the regional concentrations of the elderly are similar to the concentrations of the total population of each group.[12]

assisted-living facility a special combination of housing, personalized supportive services, and health care designed to meet the needs—both scheduled and unscheduled—of those who need help with activities of daily living

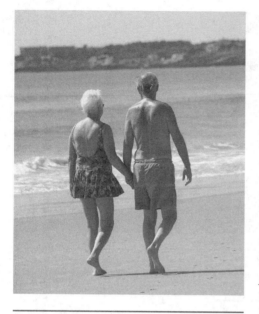

FIGURE 9.8

Many elders choose to spend their retirement years in states with warm weather.

Economic Status

The overall economic position of elders has improved significantly since the 1970s.[17] In 1970, about 25% of the elderly lived in poverty, whereas in 2006 the figure had dropped to just less than 9%.[9] Today, in fact, a smaller percentage of the elderly are impoverished than among those under age 18.[15]

When the sources of income of elders are examined, it is found that 37% of elder income comes from Social Security; almost equal percentages come from asset income (15%), pensions (18%), and earnings (28%); and a small percentage (2%) comes from other miscellaneous sources.[9] Because just more than one-fourth of elder income comes from work earnings, they are economically more vulnerable to circumstances beyond their control, such as the loss of a spouse; deteriorating health and self-sufficiency; changes in Social Security, Medicare, and Medicaid legislation; and inflation.

Housing

In general, most older Americans live in adequate, affordable housing.[9] Of the almost 3 million households headed by older Americans in 2007, 80% were owners and 20% were renters.[18] However, millions of elderly continue to live in housing that costs too much, is in substandard condition, or fails to accommodate their physical capabilities or assistance needs.[19] Characteristics of the homes of elders versus those of younger people are that elders have (1) older homes, (2) homes of lower value, (3) homes in greater need of repair, and (4) homes less likely to have central heating and air conditioning.[18]

For most elders, housing represents an asset because they have no mortgage or rental payments, or they can sell their home for a profit. But for others with low incomes, housing becomes a heavy burden. Approximately 30% of all elderly households pay more for housing than they can afford.[19] The cost of utilities, real estate taxes, insurance, repair, and maintenance have forced many to sell their property or live in a less-desirable residence.

A HEALTH PROFILE OF ELDERS

The health status of elders has improved over the years, both in terms of living longer and remaining functional. The percentage of chronically disabled older persons—those with impairments for 3 months or longer that impede daily activities—has been slowly falling. However, we do know that the most consistent risk factor of illness and death across the total population is age, and that in general, the health status of elders is not as good as their younger counterparts. In this section of the chapter, we examine some of the health concerns of aging, including mortality, morbidity, and health behaviors and lifestyle choices.

Mortality

In 2007, the top five causes of death for elders, in order of number of deaths, were heart disease, cancer, stroke, chronic lower respiratory disease (CLRD), and Alzheimer's disease.[20] These five causes of death were responsible for two-thirds of the deaths.[20] Over the past 50 years, the overall age-adjusted mortality rate for elders has continued to fall. The primary reason for this has been the declining death rates for heart disease and stroke. Despite such drops, heart disease remains the leading cause of death in this age group, and it is responsible

BOX
9.1

HEALTHY PEOPLE 2020: OBJECTIVES

Diabetes

Goal: Reduce the disease and economic burden of diabetes mellitus (DM) and improve the quality of life for all persons who have, or are at risk for, DM.

Objective: D 3 Reduce the diabetes death rate.

Target: 65.8 deaths per 100,000 population.

Baseline: 73.1 deaths per 100,000 population were related to diabetes in 2007 (age adjusted to the year 2000 standard population).

Target setting method: 10 percent improvement.

Data source: National Vital Statistics System (NVSS), CDC, NCHS.

Objective: D 11 Increase the proportion of adults with diabetes who have a glycosylated hemoglobin (HbA1c) measurement at least twice a year.

Target: 71.1 percent.

Baseline: 64.6 percent of adults aged 18 years and older with diagnosed diabetes had a glycosylated hemoglobin measurement at least twice in the past 12 months, as reported in 2008 (age adjusted to the year 2000 standard population).

Target setting method: 10 percent improvement.

Data source: Behavioral Risk Factor Surveillance System, CDC, NCCDPHP.

For Further Thought

If you were given the responsibility of getting people with diabetes to get regular HbA1c measurements, what community health activities would you use?

Source: U.S. Department of Health and Human Services, Office of Disease Prevention and Health Promotion (2010). *Healthy People 2020.* Available at http://www.healthypeople.gov/2020/default.aspx. Accessed December 2, 2010.

for almost one-third of the deaths.[20] Unlike the death rates for heart disease and stroke, the cancer death rate has stayed about the same in recent years. The biggest jump in death rates for elders has occurred with diabetes and CLRD (see Box 9.1).

Morbidity

"The quality of life in later years may be diminished if illness, chronic conditions, or injuries limit the ability of one to care for oneself without assistance. Older persons maintain their independence and eliminate costly caregiving services by, among other things, shopping on their own, cooking their meals, bathing and dressing themselves, and walking and climbing stairs without assistance."[17] Among Medicare enrollees aged 65 and older, about one in five men and one in three women are unable to perform at least one of five physical activities (walking two to three blocks; writing; stooping or kneeling; reaching up overhead; lifting something as heavy as 10 pounds).[9] Activity limitations increase with age, and women are more likely than men to have physical limitations.[9] The causes of this reduced activity can be classified into two types—chronic conditions and impairments.

Chronic Conditions

Chronic conditions are systemic health problems that persist longer than 3 months, such as hypertension, arthritis, heart disease, diabetes, and emphysema. "While not all chronic conditions are life threatening, they are a substantial burden on the health and economic status of individuals, their families, and the nation as a whole."[17] The actual number of chronic conditions increases with age; therefore, limitations from activities become increasingly prevalent with age. About one-third of elders reported a limitation of activity as a result of chronic conditions.[1] Furthermore, many chronic conditions can result in impairments, such as the loss of sight from diabetes. Chronic conditions of elders vary by gender and race. More men experience life-threatening acute illnesses (e.g., heart disease and hypertension-induced stroke), while more women experience physically limiting chronic illness (e.g., osteoporosis and arthritis).[9]

Impairments

Impairments are deficits in the functioning of one's sense organs or limitations in one's mobility or range of motion. Like chronic conditions, impairments are far more prevalent in older adults. The primary impairments that affect elders are sensory impairments (i.e., vision, hearing, postural balance, or loss of feeling in the feet), physical limitations, and memory impairments[21] (see Box 9.2). "Memory skills are important to general cognitive functioning, and declining scores on tests of memory are indicators of general cognitive loss for older adults. Low cognitive functioning (i.e., memory impairment) is a major risk factor for entering a nursing home."[22]

Sensory impairments increase with age and the prevalence of them will increase as life expectancy increases. Currently, one in six elders has impaired vision, one in four has loss of feeling in the feet, one in four has impaired hearing, and three in four have balance impairment.[22] The balance impairment may be in part why so many elders have physical limitations. *Physical limitations* refers to elders having difficulty performing any of these eight physical activities: (1) walking a quarter of a mile—about 3 city blocks; (2) walking up 10 steps without resting; (3) standing or being on their feet for about 2 hours; (4) sitting for about 2 hours; (5) stooping, bending, or kneeling; (6) reaching over their head; (7) using their fingers to grasp or handle small objects; or (8) lifting or carrying something as heavy as 10 pounds, such as a full bag of groceries.[23] Like sensory impairments, physical limitations increase with age. One in four elders aged 60–69 years has at least one physical limitation, while two in five of those 80 years of age and older have at least one.[23]

BOX 9.2 **HEALTHY PEOPLE 2020: OBJECTIVES**

Arthritis, Osteoporosis, and Chronic Back Conditions

Goal: Prevent illness and disability related to arthritis and other rheumatic conditions, osteoporosis, and chronic back conditions.

Objective: AOCBC 10 Reduce the proportion of adults with osteoporosis.

Target: 5.3 percent.

Baseline: 5.9 percent of adults aged 50 years and older had osteoporosis in 2005–08 (age adjusted to the year 2000 standard population).

Target setting method: 10 percent improvement.

Data source: National Health and Nutrition Examination Survey, CDC, NCHS.

For Further Thought

Have you seen any health care facilities in your community that have been advertising that they perform bone density testing? How is bone density measured? What are some community health activities that could be carried out in a community to reduce the proportion of adults with osteoporosis?

Source: U.S. Department of Health and Human Services, Office of Disease Prevention and Health Promotion (2010). *Healthy People 2020*. Available at http://www.healthypeople.gov/2020/default.aspx. Accessed December 2, 2010.

Like rates for chronic conditions, rates for impairments differ by gender and race. But unlike chronic conditions, impairments are affected by two other variables—previous income level and previous occupational exposure. The smaller the income and the more occupational exposure to health hazards, the greater the number of impairments.

Health Behaviors and Lifestyle Choices

There is no question that health behavior and social factors play significant roles in helping elders maintain health in later life. Some elders believe that they are too old to gain any benefit from changing their health behaviors. This, of course, is not true; it is never too late to make a change for the better.

In interviews, elders generally report more favorable health behaviors than their younger counterparts. They are less likely to (1) consume large amounts of alcohol, (2) smoke cigarettes, and (3) be overweight or obese. However, it should be noted that many of those who abused alcoholic beverages, smoked cigarettes, and were overweight or obese died before age 65 and thus were unavailable for interview.

Even though in general elders report better health behaviors than their younger counterparts, there is still room for improvement. The health behaviors that can most affect the health of elders are healthy eating, exercise, and immunizations. Healthy eating plays a major role in preventing or delaying the onset of chronic diseases. The dietary quality habits of elders are better than their younger counterparts, but they still leave room for improvement.[23]

The 1996 Surgeon General's Report on Physical Activity and Health—still the most definitive assessment of activity and age in the United States—reported that inactivity increased with age. Whereas a substantial majority of adults at all age levels did not achieve the recommended level of physical activity, the number of sedentary persons—those who engage in *no* discretionary physical activity at all—increased with age. Only 22% of those aged 65 and older report engaging in regular leisure-time physical activity, and that percentage drops to 10% for those aged 85 and older.[9]

The good news is that walking briskly (about twice as fast as a normal pace) for at least 30 minutes a day most days of the week is almost as beneficial for reducing the death rate as jogging up to 40 miles a week.[24] One study reported that walking 4 hours per week decreased the risk of future hospitalization for cardiovascular disease.[25] Another study reported that brisk walking 3 hours a week reduced the incidence of coronary events between 30% and 40%.[26]

Though aerobic conditioning has been considered the exercise of choice for improved cardiorespiratory function, other forms of exercise have proved beneficial as well. Tai chi[27] and resistance exercise,[28,29] for example, provide cardiorespiratory benefits. Resistance exercise, in fact, appears to reduce blood pressure level[30] and cholesterol level,[31,32] outcomes previously obtained primarily through aerobic exercise interventions.

Most people do not think of elders when they hear the word *immunizations.* "But for adults, especially those age 65 and older, getting immunized against certain diseases is important and can prevent thousands of deaths each year."[33] Influenza and pneumonia are the fifth leading cause of death in elders. Vaccinations against these diseases are recommended for elders, especially those who are at increased risk for complications from influenza and pneumonia. Influenza vaccinations are given annually, whereas pneumococcal vaccinations are usually given once in a lifetime, with possible revaccination with severe comorbidity after 5 years.

In large measure because of the onset of Medicare reimbursement, the pneumococcal vaccination rate increased dramatically, from 10% in 1989 to 57% in 2006.[9] Nonetheless, many elders remained unvaccinated, and there was considerable racial disparity. In 2006, 62% of whites received pneumonia vaccination, compared with 36% of blacks and 33% of Hispanics.[9]

Thanks once again to Medicare reimbursement, the influenza vaccination rate also increased dramatically, from 20% in 1989 to 64% in 2006.[9] Although this improvement is dramatic and gratifying to public health officials, almost a third of elders are still not getting an annual flu shot. And among older blacks, the influenza vaccination rate was about 20% lower than among older whites.[9]

Elder Abuse and Neglect

Reports of elder abuse and neglect have increased greatly in recent years. Perhaps a substantial part of the increase in these numbers was the result of all 50 states having passed some form of elder abuse prevention laws. Though the laws and definitions of terms vary from state to state, all states have set up reporting systems. Prior to the reporting systems, many incidences of abuse were never recorded. "Generally, adult protective service (APS) agencies receive and investigate reports of suspected elder abuse."[34] According to the first-ever National Elder Abuse Incidence Study, released in 1998, an estimated total of 551,000 elderly persons older than age 60 had experienced abuse (physical, emotional/psychological), neglect, or self-neglect in a domestic setting during the year of the study.[35] This study also revealed the following:

- Female elders are abused at a higher rate than are men.
- Elders 80 years and older are abused or neglected at two to three times the rate of their proportion of the elderly population.
- In almost 90% of all elder abuse and neglect incidents where a perpetrator is identified, the perpetrator is a family member, and two-thirds of the perpetrators are adult children or spouses.
- Victims of self-neglect are usually depressed, confused, or extremely frail.

Elder abuse and neglect are special problems for elders because they are (1) frail, (2) unable to defend themselves, (3) vulnerable to telemarketing scams and mail-order swindles, and (4) the most common victims of theft of their benefit checks. On a positive note, elder abuse is a problem that has responded well to community monitoring. However, there is still much need for improvement because one in four vulnerable elders is at risk of abuse and only a small portion of these incidents is detected and reported.[36]

INSTRUMENTAL NEEDS OF ELDERS

Atchley lists six instrumental needs that determine lifestyles for people of all ages.[37] These are income, housing, personal care, health care, transportation, and community facilities and services. However, the aging process can alter these needs in unpredictable ways. Whereas those elders in the young old group (65–74) usually do not experience appreciable changes in their lifestyles relative to these six needs, elders in the middle old group (75–84) and the old old group (85 and older) eventually do. The rest of this chapter explores these six needs, discusses their implications for elders, and describes community services for elders.

Income

Though the need for income continues throughout one's life, achieving elder status often reduces the income needs. Perhaps the major reduction occurs with one's retirement. Retirees do not need to purchase job-related items such as special clothing or tools, pay union dues, or join professional associations. Expenses are further reduced because retirees no longer commute every day, buy as many meals away from home, or spend money on business travel. Reaching elder status also usually means that children are grown and no longer dependent, and, as noted earlier, the home mortgage has often been retired. Taxes are usually lower because income is lower. In addition, many community services are offered at reduced prices for elders.

However, aging usually means increased expenses for health care and for home maintenance and repairs that aging homeowners can no longer do themselves. Despite these increased costs, the overall need for income seems to decrease slightly for people after retirement.

As noted earlier in this chapter, there are five sources of income for elders: Social Security, pensions (e.g., government employee pensions, private pensions, or annuities), earnings from jobs, income from assets (e.g., savings accounts, stocks, bonds, real estate), and other miscellaneous sources (e.g., public assistance for poor elders). Social Security benefits account for about two-fifths of income for elders; and asset income, pensions, and personal earnings each provide about one-fifth of total income. The average monthly Social Security benefit for a retired individual was about $1,170 at the beginning of 2010.[38] This amounts to an average of $14,040 per year. About 87% of all people older than age 65 years receive Social Security benefits.[39] Further, Social Security was the major source of income (providing at least 50% of total income) for about two-thirds of the recipients and it was 90% or more of the income for about one-third of the recipients.[39]

In recent years, the income of elders has improved significantly. When income and other assets of elders are combined, the economic status of elders and those younger than 65 is not that far apart. However, the fact remains that 9% of the elder population lives in poverty. Certain subgroups of elders have higher rates. Nonmarried women and minorities have the highest poverty rates, ranging from 12% to 23%. Married persons have the lowest poverty rates.[9]

Housing

Housing, a basic necessity for all, is a central concern for elders in terms of needs and costs. It is an important source of continuity for elders. A home is more than just a place to live. It is a symbol of independence; a place for family gatherings; a source of pleasant memories; and a link to friends, the neighborhood, and the community.[37]

When housing for the elderly is examined, four major needs are discussed. They include appropriateness, accessibility, adequacy, and affordability.[9] These needs are not independent of each other; in fact, they are closely intertwined. Elders may live in affordable housing, but the housing may not be appropriate for their special needs. Or, certain housing may be accessible to the elderly, but it may not be affordable, or there may not be an adequate number available to meet demand.

Housing requirements may change more rapidly than housing consumption during the course of retirement years as a result of changes in household composition, decreasing mobility, and/or increasing morbidity. Thus, the single biggest change in the housing needs of elders is the need for special modifications because of physical disabilities. Such modifications can be very simple—such as handrails for support in bathrooms—or more complex—such as chair lifts for stairs. Sometimes there is need for live-in help, while at other times disabilities may force seniors to leave their homes and seek specialized housing.

The decision to remove elders from their long-term residences is not easily made. Because of the psychological and social value of the home, changing an elder's place of residence has negative effects for both the elder and the family members who help make the arrangements for the move. Recognizing the importance of a home and independence, families often feel tremendous conflict and guilt in deciding to move an elder relative. If the elder does not adjust to the new situation, the guilt continues. Sometimes family members continue to question their decision even after the elder dies. Though moving an elder is very difficult, it is often best for all involved. For example, moving a frail person from a two-story to a one-story home makes good sense, and moving an elder from a very large home to a smaller home or an apartment is logical.

One of the biggest fears associated with relocating an elder is the move to group housing, especially a nursing home. The stereotype that many people have about group housing is not very positive, and most know it can be very expensive: approximately $74,000-plus per year in 2009 for a total care nursing home. However, just like any other consumer product, good group homes are available. There is some evidence that not-for-profit homes—which constitute about one-third of the nation's 17,000 nursing homes—may be more concerned about quality of care and less concerned about keeping costs down and profits up.[40]

Perhaps the ideal model for large-scale long-term care facilities, however, is the Eden Alternative, founded by William Thomas, M.D., in 1991. The basic premise of the Eden Alternative is that nursing homes should treat residents as people who need attentive care in a homelike setting. To accomplish this goal, nursing homes need to contain pets, plants, children, and other amenities that make life worth living.[41] Three hundred nursing homes around the country have incorporated the Eden Alternative into their facilities.

William Thomas, went one step further than the Eden Alternative; he created the Green House. These houses avoid the institutionalization of larger nursing homes—including those based on the Eden Alternative—by limiting residents in number to about 10 and creating a large home for them rather than a facility. The first Green House, about 6,400 square feet, was constructed in Tupelo, Mississippi, in 2003. Each resident had a private room and bath, and access to a central hearth where cooking and socializing was done. There was a surrounding garden for contemplative walks and for growing vegetables and flowers.

Green Houses promote autonomy. Residents get up, eat, and go to bed when they want. They decide on which foods to eat. Medications are locked in individual rooms, rather than distributed by a cart that is wheeled from room to room. There are few features that are different from the typical home. Green House workers are paid more and are better trained, but the extra costs are offset by employee empowerment that reduces staff turnover and additional training expenses.

People in the first 10 Green Houses were selected from nursing homes and represented a typical nursing home population. Of the first 40 residents selected, 12 had advanced dementia, and all Green House residents had the typical array of physical and cognitive limitations associated with the average nursing home resident.[16] One 2-year longitudinal study compared Green House residents to residents of traditional nursing home with the same owner. The Green House residents reported a higher quality of life, better emotional well-being, and a lower incidence of decline in late-loss activities of daily living (ADLs) functioning.[42]

In 2006, the Robert Wood Johnson Foundation provided a $10 million, 5-year grant to establish Green Houses around the United States and to allow other long-term care owners and administrators to replicate them through training support and up to $125,000 in predevelopment loans.

Over the next decade, most elders will not be fortunate enough to have a Green House available to them. To ease the stress and anxiety associated with the relocation of elders, the following are recommended:[43]

1. Inform the elder (and family members) that relocation stress is usually temporary.
2. Encourage the elder to endorse the move because those unwilling to move are most likely to experience stress.
3. Make a new environment predictable to the elder because it can help to reduce stress.
4. Keep those being moved and their families informed so that stress can be reduced.

retirement communities residential communities that have been specifically developed for those in their retirement years

The relocation of elders is not always traumatic or done against their will. Many elders are finding housing in communities that have been planned as **retirement communities**. Though these communities are available in all areas of the country, they are most popular in areas with temperate climates (see Figure 9.9). Some of the communities are built as private associations, while others are developed as special areas within larger, already established communities. Legally, the private associations are able to adopt by-laws that put restrictions on the residents, such as a minimum age to move into the area, no children under a certain age living in the residence, and no pets. Retirement communities usually offer a variety of housing alternatives ranging from home or condominium ownership to apartment living. Because these communities are developed to meet the needs of elders, special accommodations are usually made for socializing, recreation, shopping, transportation, and selected educational programs.

Two other housing options for elders are **continuing-care retirement communities (CCRCs)** and assisted-living residences. CCRCs guarantee the residents a lifelong residence and health care. They work in the following way: The retirees either purchase or term lease (sometimes lifelong) a living unit on a campus-like setting. The living unit could be a single-family dwelling, an apartment, or a room, as in a nursing home. In addition to the living units, the campus usually includes a health clinic and often has either a nursing home or health care center. These other facilities are available to the residents for an additional fee. Residents of the CCRCs can live as independently as they wish but have available to them a variety of services, including housekeeping, meals, transportation, organized recreational and social activities, health care, and security. Many living units are equipped with emergency call buttons.

CCRCs are a housing alternative for well-to-do seniors. Unfortunately, CCRCs are beyond the reach of many elders; the purchase or lifelong lease is more than $100,000, and the fee for many of the services is extra. Obviously, seniors who enter into contractual agreements for CCRCs should read their contracts carefully before signing them.

An assisted-living residence is a more recent housing option than CCRCs, but it includes many of the same concepts. It is a model of residential care that blends many of the characteristics of the nursing home and community-based long-term care. The Assisted Living Federation of America (ALFA) has defined assisted living "as a long-term care option that combines housing, support services and health care, as needed. Assisted living is designed for individuals who require assistance with everyday activities such as meals, medication management or assistance, bathing, dressing and transportation."[44] Such facilities may range from high-rise buildings to one-story Victorian mansions to large multi-acre campuses.[44] They are regulated in all 50 states and may be operated by nonprofit or for-profit companies. Most of these facilities offer a variety of amenities and personal care services, including the following:[44]

- Three meals a day served in a common dining area
- Housekeeping services
- Transportation
- 24-hour security
- Exercise and wellness programs
- Personal laundry services
- Social and recreational activities
- Staff available to respond to both scheduled and unscheduled needs

FIGURE 9.9
The number of planned retirement communities in the United States continues to increase.

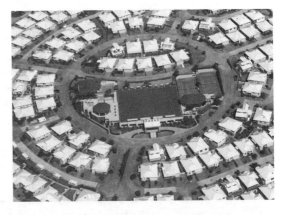

continuing-care retirement communities (CCRCs) planned communities for seniors that guarantee a lifelong residence and health care

- Assistance with eating, bathing, dressing, toileting, and walking
- Access to health and medical services, such as physical therapy and hospice
- Emergency call systems for each resident's apartment
- Medication management
- Care for residents with cognitive impairments

Costs for assisted living vary according to facility and parts of the county. "They offer a less-expensive, residential approach to delivering many of the same services available in skilled nursing, either by employing personal care staff or contracting with home health agencies and other outside professionals."[44] According to data collected by several different nonprofit senior living organizations, including ALFA, "the median rate for a private one-bedroom apartment in an assisted living residence is $2,575 per month."[44]

It has been estimated that there are about 36,000+ assisted-living facilities nationwide.[44] In a national study, about a fourth of the residents of these facilities received assistance with three or more activities of daily living, such as bathing, dressing, and mobility, and about one-third had moderate to severe cognitive impairment.[45]

Of all the housing problems that confront seniors, the availability of affordable housing is the biggest. Unfortunately, those seniors who are most in need of such housing are often frail and disabled, have low incomes, and live in rural areas. Until recently, many of the needs of this group of elders went unmet. However, during the Clinton presidency, funding was provided for the *Housing Security Plan for Older Americans* administered in the Office of Housing and Urban Development (HUD).[19] This plan embodied three overarching goals:

- "Help seniors remain in their homes and connected to their families and communities.
- Expand affordable housing opportunities for lower income seniors.
- Improve the range and coordination of affordable housing and supportive service combinations available to seniors."[19]

To reach these goals, HUD was working with older homeowners to help them convert the equity in their homes into funds for needed health and safety home improvements, including home rehabilitation loans through HUD's reverse mortgage program. HUD was also providing more money to help build more affordable rental housing for low-income elderly, in addition to helping finance the conversion of some existing housing units to assisted living residencies.[19] With each subsequent administration, however, presidential politics may (and usually does) change funding levels for programs such as this.

Personal Care

Although most elders are able to care for themselves, there is a significant minority of elders who require personal assistance for an optimal or even adequate existence. The size of this minority increases as the elders attain middle old (75–84) and old old (85+) status.

Four different levels of tasks have been identified with which seniors may need assistance:

1. Instrumental tasks—such as housekeeping, transportation, maintenance on the automobile or yard, and assistance with business affairs
2. Expressive tasks—including emotional support, socializing and inclusion in social gatherings, and trying to prevent feelings of loneliness and isolation
3. Cognitive tasks—assistance that involves scheduling appointments, monitoring health conditions, reminding elders of the need to take medications, and in general acting as a backup memory

4. Tasks of daily living—such as eating, bathing, dressing, toileting, walking, getting in and out of bed or a chair, and getting outside

Note that this last group of tasks, in addition to being a part of this listing, has special significance. These items have been used to develop a scale, called **activities of daily living (ADLs)**, to measure **functional limitations**. *Functional limitation* refers to the difficulty in performing personal care and home management tasks. However, ADLs do not cover all aspects of disability and are not sufficient by themselves to estimate the need for long-term care. As previously noted, some elders have cognitive impairments that are not measured by ADLs. An additional, commonly used measure called **instrumental activities of daily living (IADLs)** measures more complex tasks such as handling personal finances, preparing meals, shopping, doing housework, traveling, using the telephone, and taking medications.[17]

When elders begin to need help with one or more of these tasks, it is usually a spouse, adult children, or other family members who first provide the help, thus assuming the role of informal caregivers. An **informal caregiver** has been defined as one who provides unpaid care or assistance to one who has some physical, mental, emotional, or financial need that limits his or her independence. "There is wide latitude in the estimates of the number of informal caregivers in the U.S., depending on the definitions and criteria used."[46] Estimates range from about 6 to 52 million. An informal caregiver can be either a care provider or care manager. The **care provider** helps identify the needs of the individual and personally performs the caregiving service. Obviously, this can only be done if the person in need and the caregiver live in close proximity to each other. The **care manager** also helps to identify needs, but as a result of living some distance away or for other reasons, does not provide the service. The care manager makes arrangements for someone else (volunteer or paid) to provide the services.

With the aging of the population, it is now highly probable that many, if not most, adults can expect to have some responsibility as caregivers for their parents (see Figure 9.10). Their role may be as care provider, care manager, or in making the decision to relocate their parents by bringing them into their home, moving them to a smaller home or apartment, or moving them into a group home. This is a relatively new task because many of the elders of today did not have to care for their parents. Life expectancy was much shorter, and most did not live long enough to be cared for by their adult children.

Caregivers for elders face a number of problems, including decreased personal freedom, lack of privacy, constant demands on their time and energy, resentment that siblings do not share in the caregiving, and an increased financial burden. Many experience feelings of guilt for asking a spouse to help with the care of an in-law or in knowing that the end of caregiving responsibilities usually means either the elder person's death or placement in a group home. Caregivers often experience a change in lifestyle, especially associated with time for leisure and recreation. Caregiving can also lead to a negative impact on health.[15]

And yet even this onerous task of caregiving has its intimate qualities. One study of older caregivers reported that more than 70% of caregivers had positive feelings toward at least one aspect of caregiving for an older adult.[47] Some of the positive aspects included companionship, fulfillment, enjoyment, and the satisfaction of meeting an obligation. In addition, caregivers are typically not isolated in their role. One study reported that 88% of caregivers had social support from others who helped them with their caregiving responsibilities.[48]

The need for personal care for elders is projected to increase in the coming years. The primary responsibility for providing and financing this care will fall on the family. Because of the financial burden, more families will begin purchasing long-term health care insurance policies. These policies are very expensive if purchased after age 75 but do provide elders with sufficient income protection against the depletion of assets. However, the high premium

activities of daily living (ADLs) eating, toileting, dressing, bathing, walking, getting in and out of a bed or chair, and getting outside

functional limitations difficulty in performing personal care and home management tasks

instrumental activities of daily living (IADLs) more complex tasks such as handling personal finances, preparing meals, shopping, doing housework, traveling, using the telephone, and taking medications

informal caregiver one who provides unpaid assistance to one who has some physical, mental, emotional, or financial need limiting his or her independence

care provider one who helps identify the health care needs of an individual and also personally performs the caregiving service

care manager one who helps identify the health care needs of an individual but does not actually provide the health care services

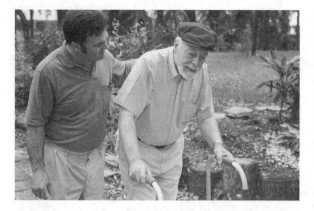

FIGURE 9.10

Adult children are gaining greater responsibility as caregivers.

and copayment costs of long-term care insurance policies mean that most Americans cannot afford them unless they are willing to purchase them when they are younger and the costs are considerably more modest. In actuality, though, most policies are bought by people later on in life, when the risk of needing long-term care is great. Not surprisingly, therefore, it is estimated that 50% of long-term care insurance policies lapse as a result of high premiums.[49] (See the discussion of long-term care insurance in Chapter 13.)

To assist caregivers, federal legislation was passed called the Older Americans Act Amendments of 2000 (Public Law 106-501). This law established the National Family Caregiver Support Program (NFCSP), which has been administered by the Administration on Aging (AoA) of the U.S. Department of Health and Human Services. It was modeled in large part after successful state long-term care programs in California, New Jersey, Wisconsin, Pennsylvania, and others and after listening to the needs expressed by hundreds of family caregivers in discussions held across the country. The program calls for all states, working in partnership with area agencies on aging and local community-service providers, to have the following five basic services for family caregivers:

- Information to caregivers about available services
- Assistance to caregivers in gaining access to services
- Individual counseling, organization of support groups, and caregiver training to assist them in making decisions and solving problems relating to their caregiving roles
- Respite care to enable caregivers to be temporarily relieved from their caregiving responsibilities
- Supplemental services, on a limited basis, to complement the care provided by caregivers

Further assistance for long-term care became available in January 2011. A part of the Patient Protection and Affordable Care Act (P.L. 111-148) signed into law by President Obama on March 23, 2010, was the community living assistance services and supports (CLASS) program. It is a voluntary program that employers can choose to offer employees. If offered, it will be a premium-funded (through payroll deductions) government insurance program in which all adult-age employees with functional limitations will become eligible for a cash benefit of not less than an average of $50 per day (to purchase nonmedical services and supports necessary to maintain community residence) after paying into the program for 5 years. Also, if offered by the employer, employees are automatically enrolled in the program, unless they choose to opt out.[50,51] The CLASS program was one of the last legislative efforts of the late Senator Edward Kennedy (D-MA) when he had it added to the health bill in the summer prior to his death.[50]

Health Care

Health care is a major issue for all segments of our society, particularly for elders. Although significant progress has been made in extending life expectancy, a longer life does not necessarily mean a healthier life. Health problems naturally increase with age. With these problems comes a need for increased health care services.

Elders are the heaviest users of health care services. Approximately 20% of elders have 10 or more visits a year to a physician, compared with 13% for all people in the United States.[8] They are also hospitalized more often and for longer stays. Although persons 65 years of age and older only represented approximately 13% of the total population in 2007, they accounted for almost 37% of the roughly 35 million patient discharges from nonfederal short-stay hospitals,[8] and they spend over twice as much per person on prescription drugs as those younger than 65 years of age. In addition, elders have higher usage rates for professional dental care, vision aids, and medical equipment and supplies than people younger than age 65. Usage of health care services increases with age, and much of the money spent on health care is spent in the last year of life.

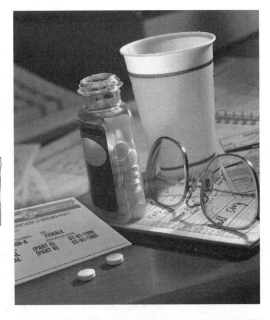

FIGURE 9.11

Medicare provides almost universal health insurance for elders.

Whereas private sources, such as employer-paid insurance, are the major sources of health care payment for people younger than age 65, public funds are used to pay for the majority of the health care expenses for elders. Medicare, which was enacted in 1965 and became effective July 1, 1966, provides almost universal health insurance coverage for elders. Medicare coverage, however, is biased toward hospital care, while chronic care health needs such as eyeglasses (see Figure 9.11), hearing aids, and most long-term services are not covered. In 2008, the Medicare program had 45.3 million enrollees and expenditures of just over $468 billion.[10] With the increasing cost of health care and the aging population, these numbers will only grow. Of those elders covered in 2008, less than 10% were covered by Medicare only, while the others were covered by both Medicare and a private insurance to supplement their Medicare coverage.[10] This private insurance is referred to as *Medigap* because it helps to fill the gaps in health care cost that Medicare leaves. In addition, Medicaid, a federal-state program that was also approved in 1965, helps to cover the health care costs of poor elders, primarily for nursing home care (continuing care), home health care, and prescription drugs. In 2006, almost 8 million elders were covered by Medicaid.[10] (See Chapter 13 for a complete discussion of Medicare, Medicaid, and Medigap.)

Over the years, a number of changes have been made in the Medicare program. One of the more significant changes took effect in January 2006. That is when Medicare Part D, a medication reimbursement program, was launched. This component of Medicare permitted Medicare enrollees to purchase prescription drug coverage. In 2008, 32.1 million elders were enrolled in this portion of Medicare (see Chapter 13 for more information on Medicare Part D).

All indications are that the health care costs for elders will continue to escalate because of the aging population and rising health care costs. In an effort to try to help offset the increasing costs of Medicare, a change was made to the premium structure for Medicare Part B (see Chapter 13 for a discussion of Part B). Beginning in 2007, about 4% of the enrollees— those with higher incomes (in 2010 >$85,000)—were charged higher premiums for Part B. The Patient Protection and Affordable Care Act (P.L. 111-148) signed into law in 2010 also has a number of changes for the Medicare program. Some that are associated with Medicare Part D took place almost immediately in 2010, whereas others were not due to be implemented fully until 2020. There were also a number of changes that are to take place in the 10 years in between (see Chapter 13 for the details). Even with all of these changes, more will have to come because of the 76 million people in the baby boom generation. The first of the baby boomers (those born in 1946) turned 65 years old, and thus became eligible for

Medicare in 2011. Therefore, future legislators will be forced to choose from among the following alternatives: (1) raising taxes to pay for the care, (2) reallocating tax dollars from other programs to pay for care, (3) cutting back on coverage presently offered, (4) offering care to only those who truly cannot afford it otherwise (also known as *means testing*), or (5) completely revamping the present system under which the care is funded.

In the meantime, the importance of instilling in Americans the value of preventing the onset of chronic diseases through healthy living cannot be overstated. Although it is not possible to prevent all chronic health problems, encouraging healthy behaviors is a step in the right direction.

Transportation

The National Institute on Aging estimates that 600,000 people aged 70 and older give up their driving each year. On average, elders live about 10 years after they stop driving.[52] There is little guidance, however, not only on when to stop driving, but also on how to compensate for no longer having personal control over one's transportation.

Transportation is of prime importance to elders because it enables them to remain independent. "Housing, medical, financial and social services are useful only to the extent that transportation can make them accessible to those in need."[53] The two factors that have the greatest effect on the transportation needs of elders are income and health status. Some elders who have always driven their own automobiles eventually find that they are no longer able to do so. The ever-increasing costs of purchasing and maintaining an automobile sometimes become prohibitive on a fixed income. Also, with age comes physical problems that restrict one's ability to operate an automobile safely. In addition, those with extreme disabilities may find that they will need a modified automobile (to accommodate their disability) or specialized transportation (e.g., a vehicle that can accommodate a wheelchair) to be transported.

With regard to transportation needs, elders can be categorized into three different groups: (1) those who can use the present forms of transportation, whether it be their own vehicle or public transportation, (2) those who could use public transportation if the barriers of cost and access (no service available) were removed, and (3) those who need special services beyond what is available through public transportation.[37]

The unavailability of transportation services has stimulated a number of private and public organizations that serve elders (e.g., churches, community services, and local area agencies on aging) to provide these services. Some communities even subsidize the cost of public transportation by offering reduced rates for elders. Although these services have been helpful to elders, mobility is still more difficult for elders than for other adults. Try to imagine what it would be like if you had to depend constantly on someone else for all your transportation needs.

To prepare professionals, family members, and concerned community members to have effective conversations about driver safety and community transportation issues with older adults, including alternatives to driving, there is a publication titled *Driving Transitions Education: Tools, Scripts, and Practice Exercises*. It was developed by the American Society on Aging and the National Highway Traffic Safety Administration and can be obtained free at www.nhtsa.dot.gov or by calling toll free 888-327-4236. For more information, visit www.asaging.org/drivewell.

The ideal solution to the transportation needs of elders, according to Atchley, would include four components: (1) fare reductions or discounts for all public transportation, including that for interstate travel, (2) subsidies to ensure adequate scheduling and routing of present public transportation, (3) subsidized taxi fares for the disabled and infirm, and

(4) funds for senior centers to purchase and equip vehicles to transport seniors properly, especially in rural areas.[37]

An innovative response to the challenge for older adults who give up driving is the Independent Transportation Network. Older adults who agree to stop driving trade in their cars, and the value is booked into an account from which they can draw to receive rides. About $8 is deducted for each car ride given by a paid driver, less when scheduling rides in advance or for sharing a ride.

The Independent Transportation Network program was started by Katherine Freund, whose son was hit by an elderly driver in Portland, Maine. Pilot programs are being started in several cities. For more information, contact www.itnportland.org.

Community Facilities and Services

As has been mentioned previously, one of the most common occurrences of the aging process is loss of independence. Even some of the most basic activities of adults become major tasks for elders because of low income, ill health, and lack of transportation. Because of the limitations of elders and the barriers they must face, they have special needs in regard to community facilities and services. If these needs are met, the lifestyles of elders are greatly enhanced. If not, they are confronted with anything from a slight inconvenience to a very poor quality of life.

With a view toward improving the lives of elders, Congress enacted the **Older Americans Act of 1965 (OAA)** and has amended it several times. Among the programs created by key amendments are the national nutrition program for elders, the State and Area Agencies on Aging, and other programs (e.g., the caregiver program discussed earlier) to increase the services and protect the rights of elders.

Though the initial act was important, the services and facilities available to elders were greatly improved after the passage of the 1973 amendments, which established the State Departments on Aging and Area Agencies on Aging. These systems inform, guide, and link older persons to available, appropriate, and acceptable services to meet their needs. The amendments were written to provide the state and area agencies with the flexibility to develop plans that allow for local variations. In 2010, there were 56 State Units on Aging (covering all 50 states and 6 territories). "Most states are divided into planning and service areas (PSAs), so that programs can be tailored to meet the specific needs of older persons residing in those areas. Area Agencies on Aging are the agencies designated by the state to be the focal point for OAA programs within a PSA."[53]

With each part of the country—and for that matter each community—having its own peculiarities, the services available to elders can vary greatly from one community to another. Even the names of the local agencies (few of which are called Area Agency on Aging) can vary a great deal, and it may require a phone call to the National Association of Area Agencies on Aging (202-872-0888) to locate your local Area Agency on Aging.

It is important to keep in mind, however, that the growth in our nation's elder population, combined with this population's financial ability to pay for service, has created an entrepreneurial atmosphere surrounding adult care services. In some larger communities, or in those communities with a large number of elder residents, the range of services can be astonishing. In the following text, we provide brief descriptions of facilities and services available in many communities.

Meal Service

The 1972 amendments to the Older Americans Act outlined a national nutrition program for elders and provided funds for communities to establish meal services. Today's meal services are

Older Americans Act of 1965 (OAA) federal legislation to improve the lives of elders

Meals on Wheels a community-supported nutrition program in which prepared meals are delivered to elders in their homes, usually by volunteers

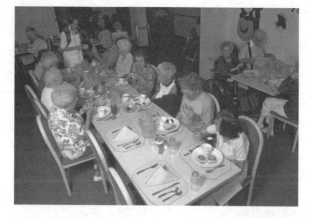

FIGURE 9.12
Congregate meal programs are not only valuable because of the enhanced nutrition but also because of the social interaction.

provided through home-delivered meal and congregate meal programs. The concept of the home-delivered meal programs (often known as **Meals on Wheels**) is the regular delivery of meals—usually once a day, five days per week—to elders in their homes. These meals are prepared in a central location, sometimes in a hospital, school, or senior center, and are delivered by community volunteers.

Congregate meal programs are provided for individuals who can travel to a central site, often within senior centers or publicly funded housing units. Usually, it is the noon meal that is provided. Generally, these meals are funded by federal and state monies and make use of commodity food services. In recent years, congregate meal programs seem to be gaining favor over home-delivered meal programs because they also provide social interaction (see Figure 9.12) and the opportunity to tie in with other social services.[37] However, there will always be a segment of the population requiring home-delivered meals because of their homebound status.

Both types of meal programs are strictly regulated by federal and state guidelines to ensure that the meals meet standard nutritional requirements. The cost of the meals varies by site and client income level. Elders may pay full price, pay a portion of the cost, or just make a voluntary contribution.

congregate meal programs
community-sponsored nutrition programs that provide meals at a central site, such as a senior center

Homemaker Service

For a number of elders, periodic homemaker services can be the critical factor enabling them to remain in their own homes. For these elders, physical impairment restricts their ability to carry out normal housekeeping activities such as house cleaning, laundry, and meal preparation. The availability of these services allows many elders to live semi-independently and delays their moving in with relatives or into group housing.

Chore and Home Maintenance Service

visitor services
one individual taking time to visit with another who is unable to leave his or her residence

Chore and home maintenance service includes such services as yard work, cleaning gutters and windows, installing screens and storm windows, making minor plumbing and electrical repairs, maintaining furnaces and air conditioners, and helping to adapt a home to any impairments seniors might have. This adaptation may include provisions for wheelchairs and installing ramps or special railings to assist elders to move from one area to another.

Visitor Service

homebound
a person unable to leave home for normal activities

Social interaction and social contacts are an important need for every human being, regardless of age. **Visitor services** amount to one individual taking time to visit with another person who is **homebound**, or unable to leave his or her residence. This service is usually done on a voluntary basis, many times with elders doing the visiting, and serves both the homebound and those who are institutionalized. It is not uncommon for church or social organizations to conduct a visitor program for homebound members.

adult day care programs
daytime care provided to elders who are unable to be left alone

Adult Day Care

Adult day care programs provide care during the daytime hours for elders who are unable to be left alone. These services are modeled after child day care. Most programs offer meals, snacks, and social activities for the clients. Some either provide or make arrangements for the clients to receive therapy, counseling, health education, or other health services. Other day care programs are designed for elders with special needs, such as Alzheimer clients, those who are blind, or veterans. Adult day care programs allow families to continue with daytime activities while still providing the primary care for a family member.

Respite Care

Respite care is planned, short-term care. Such care allows families who provide primary care for an elder family member to leave their elder in a supervised care setting for anywhere from a day to a few weeks. Respite services provide full care, including sleeping quarters, meals, bathing facilities, social activities, and the monitoring of medications.[2] This is the service most frequently requested by informal caregivers. (See the section on personal care earlier in chapter.) Such a program allows primary caregivers to take a vacation, visit other relatives, or be otherwise relieved from their constant caregiving responsibilities.

respite care
planned short-term care, usually for the purpose of relieving a full-time informal caregiver

Home Health Care

Home health care "is an important alternative to traditional institutional care. Services such as medical treatment, physical therapy, and homemaker services often allow patients to be cared for at lower cost than a nursing home or hospital and in familiar surroundings of their home."[17] These programs, run by official health agencies like the local health department, hospitals, or private companies, provide a full range of services, including preventive, primary, rehabilitative, and therapeutic services, in the client's home. The care is often provided by nurses, home health aides, and personal care workers (licensed health care workers). A decreasing percentage of home health care expenditures have been paid for by Medicare over the past decade, and a significant portion is being paid for by families out of pocket. However, starting in January 2011, working adults could participate in the community living assistance services and supports (CLASS) program (see discussion earlier in the chapter) if their employer offers the program. After paying the premiums for 5 years, the working adult would become eligible for a cash benefit to purchase nonmedical services and supports necessary to maintain a community residence. Other means of paying for this care could include long-term care insurance policies, Medicaid, or reimbursement by Medigap.

home health care services
health care services provided in the patient's place of residence

Senior Centers

The enactment of the Older Americans Act of 1965 provided funds to develop multipurpose senior centers, facilities where elders can congregate for fellowship, meals, education, and recreation. More recently, a number of communities have built additional senior centers with local tax dollars. There are about 13,000 senior centers in the United States and they are the most common community facility aimed at serving seniors.[34] However, they are found much less commonly in rural areas.

In addition to the traditional services (meals, fellowship, and recreation) offered at senior centers, some communities use the centers to serve as a central location for offering a variety of other senior services, including legal assistance, income counseling, income tax return assistance, program referrals, employment services, and other appropriate services and information.

Other Services

There are many other services available to seniors in some communities. Usually, larger communities and those with more seniors provide a greater variety of services. The types of services provided in any one community are limited only by the creativity of those providing the service. In some communities, "service packages" are being offered. Such packages allow seniors to pick several services they need and to pay for them as if they were a single service.

CHAPTER SUMMARY

- The median age of the U.S. population is at an all-time high and will continue to increase through the first third of this century.

- There are many myths about the elderly population.

- The increasing median age is affected by decreasing fertility rates, declining mortality rates, and the decline in immigration.

- We are now at a point in history when a significant portion of Americans will assume some responsibility for the care of their aging parents.

- One of the most common occurrences of the aging process is the reduction in independence.

- An aging population presents the community with several concerns, which means legislators and taxpayers will be faced with decisions about how best to afford the costs (Social Security, government employee pensions, Medicare, etc.) of an ever-increasing old-age dependency ratio.

- Communities will also need to deal with the special needs of income, housing, personal care, health care, transportation, and community facilities and services for elders.

- All projections indicate that the incomes of seniors will remain lower than those of the general population, that the need for affordable and accessible housing will increase, that there will be increased needs for personal services and care, that health care needs and costs will increase, and that the demand for barrier-free transportation will increase for elders.

- The growth in our nation's elder population, combined with this population's financial ability to pay for service, has created an entrepreneurial atmosphere surrounding adult care services.

REVIEW QUESTIONS

1. What are some signs, visible to the average person, that the U.S. population is aging?

2. What years of life are defined by each of the following groups—old, young old, middle old, and old old?

3. What is meant by the terms *aged, aging, elder, gerontology, geriatrician,* and *geriatrics*?

4. Why is there a myth that old people are sickly?

5. What are demographers? What do they do?

6. Why did a pyramid represent the age characteristics of the U.S. population of the 1950s, but in 2030 it will be a rectangle?

7. What are the three factors that affect the size and age of a population?

8. How have life expectancy figures changed over the years in the United States? What were the major reasons for the change in the first half of the twentieth century? The second half?

9. Why are dependency and labor-force ratios so important?

10. How are dependency and labor-force ratios calculated?

11. Are all elders the same with regard to demographic variables?

12. How do the income needs of people change in retirement?

13. Why do adults feel guilty when they have to relocate their aged parents?

14. What is the difference between a care provider and a care manager?

15. What are some of the major problems caregivers face?

16. Why are continuing-care retirement communities attractive to elders?

17. What is an assisted-living residence?

SCENARIO: ANALYSIS AND RESPONSE

1. Based on what you read in this chapter, how would you predict that Carl and Sarah's lives might progress over the next 20 years? Consider the six instrumental needs presented in the chapter.

2. What could Carl and Sarah have done when they were working to better plan for their retirement?

3. If you had to give Carl and Sarah two pieces of health care advice, what would they be?

18. What is the difference between activities of daily living and instrumental activities of daily living?

19. What are the most frequently occurring health problems of elders?

20. From what financial sources do elders normally pay for health care?

21. What is the community living assistance services and supports (CLASS) program? How does it work, and what will it provide?

22. What does the term *Medigap* mean?

23. How do income and health status affect the transportation needs of elders?

24. What is the ideal solution for the transportation needs of elders?

25. What are State Departments on Aging and Area Agencies on Aging?

26. Why is a visitor service so important for homebound and institutionalized persons?

27. What is the difference between adult day care and respite care?

ACTIVITIES

1. Make arrangements with a local long-term care facility to visit one of their residents. Make at least three 1-hour visits to a resident over a 6-week period of time. Upon completion of the visits, write a paper that answers the following questions:

   What were your feelings when you first walked into the facility?

   What were your feelings when you first met the resident?

   What did you learn about the elderly that you did not know before?

   What did you learn about yourself because of this experience?

   Did your feeling about the resident change during the course of your visits? If so, how?

   If you had to live in a long-term care facility, would you be able to adjust to it? What would be most difficult for you in your adjustment? What character traits do you have that would help you adjust?

2. Interview a retired person over the age of 65. In your interview, include the following questions. Write a two-page paper about this interview.

   What are your greatest needs as an elder?

   What are your greatest fears connected with aging?

   What are your greatest joys at this stage in your life?

   If you could have done anything differently when you were younger to affect your life now, what would it have been?

Have you had any problems getting health care with Medicare? If so, what were they?

Do you have a Medigap policy? If so, has your Medigap policy been worth the cost?

In what ways are you able to contribute to your community in retirement?

Are there any barriers to seeking volunteer opportunities in your community? What do you think about paid part-time work in retirement?

3. Spend a half-day at a local senior center. Then, write a paper that (a) summarizes your experience, (b) identifies your reaction (personal feelings) to the experience, and (c) shares what you have learned from the experience.

4. Review a newspaper obituary column for 7 consecutive days. Using the information provided in the obituaries: (a) demographically describe those who died, (b) keep track of what community services are noted, and (c) consider what generalizations can be made from the group as a whole.

COMMUNITY HEALTH ON THE WEB

The Internet contains a wealth of information about community and public health. Increase your knowledge of some of the topics presented in this chapter by accessing the Jones & Bartlett Learning Web site at **http://health.jbpub.com/book/communityhealth/7e** and follow the links to complete the following Web activities.

- AARP
- Administration on Aging
- National Institute on Aging

REFERENCES

1. Administration on Aging (2010). *A Profile of Older Americans: 2009*. Available at http://www.aoa.gov/AoAroot/Aging_Statistics/Profile/index.aspx.

2. U.S. Department of Health and Human Services (1986). *Age Words: A Glossary on Health and Aging* (NIH pub. no. 86-1849). Washington, DC: U.S. Government Printing Office.

3. Slee, D. A., V. N. Slee, and H. J. Schmidt (2008). *Slee's Health Care Terms*, 5th ed. Sudbury, MA: Jones & Bartlett.

4. Ferrini, A. F., and R. L. Ferrini (2000). *Health in the Later Years*, 3rd ed. Boston: McGraw-Hill Higher Education.

5. Dychtwald, K., and J. Flower (1989). *Age Wave: The Challenges and Opportunities of an Aging America*. Los Angeles: Jeremy P. Tarcher.

6. Thomlinson, R. (1976). *Population Dynamics: Causes and Consequences of World Demographic Change*. New York, NY: Random House.

7. U.S. Census Bureau (2010). *U.S. Population Projections*. Available at http://www.census.gov/population/www/projections/index.html.

8. U.S. Census Bureau (2010). *The 2010 Statistical Abstract: The National Data Book—Population*. Available at http://www.census.gov/compendia/statab/.

9. Federal Interagency Forum on Aging Related Statistics (2008). *Older Americans 2008: Key Indicators of Well-Being*. Available at http://www.agingstats.gov/main_site/default.aspx.

10. National Center for Health Statistics (2010). *Health, United States, 2009: With Special Feature on Medical Technology*. Hyattsville, MD: Author.

11. Freeman, M. (2007). *Encore: Finding Work That Matters in the Second Half of Life*. New York, NY: Public Affairs.

12. U.S. Bureau of the Census (1996). *65 in the United States* (Current Population Reports P23-190). Washington, DC: U.S. Government Printing Office.

13. Vincent, G. K., and V. A. Velkoff (2010). *The Next Four Decades—The Older Population in the United States: 2010 to 2050* (Current Population Reports P25-1138). Washington, DC: U.S. Census Bureau.

14. Mermin, G., et al. (2007). "Why Do Boomers Plan to Work Longer?" *Journal of Gerontology: Social Sciences*, 62B: S286–S294.

15. Hooyman, N., and H. Kiyak (2008). *Social Gerontology: A Multidisciplinary Perspective*, 8th ed. Boston: Allyn and Bacon.

16. Haber, D. (2005). "Cultural Diversity among Older Adults: Addressing Health Education." *Educational Gerontology*, 31: 683–697.

17. Kramarow, E. H., H. Lentzner, R. Rooks, J. Weeks, and S. Saydah (1999). *Health and Aging Chartbook: Health United States, 1999* (HHS pub. no. PHS-99-123-1). Hyattsville, MD: National Center for Health Statistics.

18. U.S. Census Bureau (2008). *American Housing Survey for the United States: 2007* (Current Housing Reports, Series H150/07). Washington, DC: U.S. Government Printing Office.

19. U.S. Department of Housing and Urban Development, Office of Policy Development and Research (1999). *Housing Our Elders*. Washington, DC: Author.

20. Xu, J. Q., K. D. Kochanek, S. L. Murphy, and B. Tejada-Vera (2010). "Deaths: Final data for 2007." *National Vital Statistics Reports*, 58(19). Hyattsville, MD: National Center for Health Statistics.

21. Dillon, C. F., et al. (2010). *Vision, Hearing, Balance, and Sensory Impairment in Americans Aged 70 and Over: United States 1999–2006* (NCHS Data Brief, no. 31). Hyattsville, MD: National Center for Health Statistics.

22. Federal Interagency Forum on Aging-Related Statistics (2001). *Older Americans 2000: Key Indicators of Well-Being*. Available at http://www.agingstats.gov/Agingstatsdotnet/Main_Site/Data/Data2000.aspx.

23. Haber, D. (2010). *Health Promotion and Aging: Practical Applications for Health Professionals*, 5th ed. New York, NY: Springer Publishing.

24. Blair, S., et al. (2001). "Physical Fitness and All-Cause Mortality: A Prospective Study of Healthy Men and Women." *Journal of the American Medical Association*, 262: 2395–2401.

25. LaCroix, A., et al. (1996). "Does Walking Decrease the Risk of Cardiovascular Disease Hospitalization and Death in Older Adults?" *Journal of the American Geriatrics Society*, 44: 113–120.

26. Manson, J., et al. (1999). "A Prospective Study of Walking as Compared with Vigorous Exercise in the Prevention of Coronary Heart Disease in Women." *New England Journal of Medicine*, 341: 650–658.

27. Lan, C., et al. (1999). "The Effect of Tai Chi on Cardiorespiratory Function in Patients with Coronary Artery Bypass Surgery." *Medical Science Sports Exercise*, 31: 634–638.

28. Tanassescu, M., et al. (2002). "Exercise Type and Intensity in Relation to Coronary Heart Disease in Men." *Journal of the American Medical Association*, 288: 1994–2000.

29. Vincent, K., et al. (2002). "Resistance Exercise and Physical Performance in Adults Aged 60 to 83." *Journal of the American Geriatrics Society*, 50: 1100–1107.

30. Kelley, G., and K. Kelley (2000). "Progressive Resistance Exercise and Resting Blood Pressure: A Meta-analysis of Randomized Controlled Trials." *Hypertension*, 35: 838–843.

31. Kraus, W., et al. (2002). "Effects of the Amount and Intensity of Exercise on Plasma Lipoproteins." *New England Journal of Medicine*, 347: 1483–1492.

32. Prabhakaran, B., et al. (1999). "Effect of 14 Weeks of Resistance Training on Lipid Profile and Body Fat Percentage in Premenopausal Women." *British Journal of Sports Medicine*, 33: 190–195.

33. Brooks, J. (May 2000). "Immunizations: Not Just for the Young." *Closing the Gap*, 10–12.

34. Administration on Aging (2006). "Elder Abuse Prevention." Available at http://www.aoa.gov/press/fact/alpha/fact_elder_abuse_pf.asp.

35. National Center on Elder Abuse, Administration on Aging (2005). *Fact Sheet: Elder Abuse Prevalence and Incidence*. Washington, DC: Author. Available at http://ncea.aoa.gov/AoARoot/AoA_Programs/Elder_Rights/Elder_Abuse/Index.aspx.

36. Cooper, C., et al. (2008). "The Prevalence of Elder Abuse and Neglect: A Systematic Review." *Age and Ageing*, 37(2): 151–160.

37. Atchley, R. C. (1994). *Social Forces and Aging: An Introduction to Social Gerontology*, 7th ed. Belmont, CA: Wadsworth.

38. Social Security Administration (2010). *Social Security Online: Questions?* Available at http://www.socialsecurity.gov/includes/topiclist.htm.

39. Social Security Administration (2010). *Fast Facts and Figures About Social Security, 2009*. Available at http://www.socialsecurity.gov/policy/docs/chartbooks/fast_facts/.

40. Harrington, C., et al. (2001). "Does Investor Ownership of Nursing Homes Compromise the Quality of Care?" *American Journal of Public Health*, 91: 1452–1455.

41. Thomas, W. (1995). *The Eden Alternative*. Acton, MA: VanderWyk & Burnham.

42. Kane, R., et al. (2007). "Resident Outcomes in Small-house Nursing Homes: A Longitudinal Evaluation of the Initial Green House Program." *Journal of the American Geriatrics Society*, 55: 832–839.

43. Borup, J. H. (1981). "Relocation: Attitudes, Information Network and Problems Encountered." *The Gerontologist*, 21: 501–511.

44. Assisted Living Federation of America (2010). "What Is Assisted Living?" Available at http://www.alfa.org/alfa/Assisted_Living_Information.asp?SnID=1383416766.

45. Hawes, C., M. Rose, and O. S. Phillips (1999). *A National Study of Assisted Living for the Frail Elderly. Executive Summary: Results of a National Survey of Facilities*. Available at http://aspe.os.dhhs.gov/daltcp/reports/facreses.htm.

46. Family Caregiver Alliance (2010). *Selective Caregiver Statistics*. Available at http://www.caregiver.org/caregiver/jsp/content_node.jsp?nodeid=439.

47. Cohen, C., et al. (2002). "Positive Aspects of Caregiving: Rounding Out the Caregiver Support System." *The Gerontologist*, 35: 489–497.

48. Penrod, et al. (1995). "Who Cares? The Size, Scope, and Composition of the Care Giver Support System." *The Gerontologist*, 35: 489–497.

49. Weiner, J., and L. Illston (1996). "Financing and Organization of Health Care." In R. Binstock and L. George, eds., *Handbook of Aging and the Social Sciences*, 4th ed. San Diego: Academic Press.

50. National Public Radio (2010). "Long-Term Care Program Debuts in New Health Law." Available at http://www.npr.org/templates/story/story.php?storyId=125461417.

51. Henry J. Kaiser Family Foundation (2010). *Focus on Health Reform: Summary of New Health Reform Law*. Available at: http://www.kff.org/healthreform/8061.cfm.

52. Foley, D., et al. (2002). "Driving Life Expectancy of Persons Aged 70 Years and Older in the United States." *American Journal of Public Health*, 92: 1284–1289.

53. Administration on Aging. (2007). "How to Find Help." Available at http://www.aoa.gov/eldfam/How_To_Find/Agencies/Agencies.asp.

Chapter 10

Community Health and Minorities

Chapter Objectives

After studying this chapter, you should be able to:

1 Explain the concept of diversity as it describes the American people.

2 Explain the impact of a more diverse population in the United States as it relates to community health efforts.

3 Explain the importance of the 1985 landmark report *The Secretary's Task Force Report on Black and Minority Health.*

4 List the racial and ethnic categories currently used by the U.S. government in statistical activities and program administration reporting.

5 List some limitations related to collecting racial and ethnic health data.

6 Identify some of the sociodemographic and socio-economic characteristics of minority groups in the United States.

7 List some of the beliefs and values of minority groups in the United States.

8 List and describe the six priority areas of the *Race and Health Initiative.*

9 Explain the role socioeconomic status plays in health disparities among racial and ethnic minority groups.

10 Define *cultural sensitivity* and *cultural and linguistic competence* and the importance of each related to minority community health.

11 Identify the three kinds of power associated with empowerment and explain the importance of each related to minority community health.

SCENARIO

Tom just returned from a cross-country business trip that took him from New York City to Miami, to San Antonio, to Los Angeles, and back to his Midwest hometown, Middletown, U.S.A. When his curious teenage children asked him to tell them about the people who live in the "big cities," he began by saying, "There seem to be more minorities and foreigners in the cities than before. I heard at least five or six different languages spoken. Signs in the hotels and in the storefronts are written in at least two, and sometimes three or four languages.

"Another thing that always amazes me is the number of ethnic restaurants. Here, we have just one Mexican, one Italian, and one Chinese restaurant, but in New York City and other big cities there are hundreds of restaurants serving foods from other cultures. I get the feeling that the United States is more culturally diverse than at anytime in its past, even when it was considered the 'melting pot' for the world's populations."

INTRODUCTION

majority
those with characteristics that are found in more than 50% of a population

minority groups
subgroups of the population that consist of fewer than 50% of the population

The strength and greatness of America lie in the diversity of its people. Over the centuries, wave after wave of immigrants has come to America to start new lives. They have brought with them many of their traditions and cultures. However, it is recognized that even as America rapidly becomes the world's first truly multiracial democracy, race relations remains an issue that too often divides the nation and keeps the American dream from becoming a reality for all Americans. In 1997, former President Bill Clinton announced "One America in the 21st Century: The President's Initiative on Race."[1] This initiative was a critical element in an effort to prepare the country to live as one America in the twenty-first century and was based on opportunity for all, responsibility for all, and one community for all Americans. The goal of Clinton's Initiative on Race was to strengthen our shared foundation as Americans so we can all live in an atmosphere of trust and understanding. Every American must invest in creating One America so that as a nation, people can effectively act together to fulfill the promise of the American dream in the twenty-first century. As we progress through the twenty-first century, we must continue to recognize that the strength and greatness of America lie in the diversity or differences of its people (see Figure 10.1). The failure to understand and appreciate these differences can have serious implications not only with race relations, but also when it comes to improving the health of diverse communities.

Today in the United States, the **majority** of Americans (66%) are referred to as "white, non-Hispanic." The remaining 34% of the U.S. population are members of what is traditionally viewed as racial or ethnic **minorities** (see Figure 10.2). Accordingly, **minority health** refers to the morbidity and mortality of American Indians/Alaska Natives, Asian Americans and Pacific Islanders, black Americans, and Hispanics in the United States. Current projections suggest that the U.S. population will become increasingly diverse. By 2050, nearly one-half of the U.S. population will be composed of racial minorities (see Figure 10.3).[2] The impact of a more diverse population in the United States in relation to community health efforts connected with minorities will be important based on what we learned about our past. "The

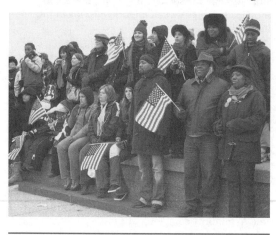

FIGURE 10.1

The strength and greatness of America lie in the diversity of its people.

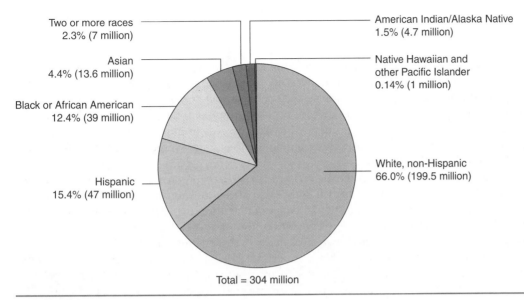

FIGURE 10.2

Percent distribution of U.S. population by race/ethnicity, 2008.

Note: Percentages do not add up to 100% due to rounding and because Hispanics may be any race and are therefore counted under more than one category.

Source: U.S. Census Bureau, National Population Estimates.

minority health
refers to the morbidity and mortality of American Indians/Alaska Natives, Americans of Hispanic origin, Asians and Pacific Islanders, and black Americans in the United States

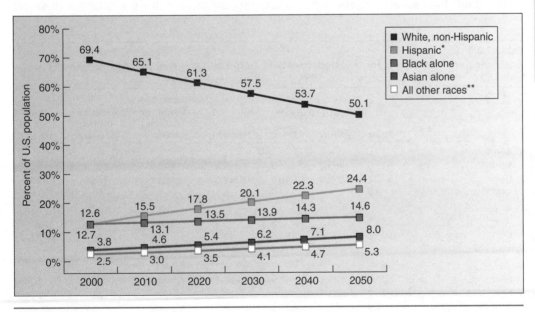

FIGURE 10.3

Projected U.S. population by race and Hispanic origin, selected years.

Note: Percentages for 2000 are actual.

*Hispanics can be of any race. Totals do not equal 100% for this reason.

**"All other races" includes American Indian and Alaska Native alone, Native Hawaiian and Other Pacific Islander alone, and two or more races.

Source: U.S. Census Bureau, Population Division (2004). *U.S. Interim Projections by Age, Sex, Race, and Hispanic Origin.* Available at http://www.census.gov/ipc/www/usinterimproj/. Accessed November 30, 2010.

health status of the nation as a whole has improved significantly during the twentieth century. Advances in medical technology, lifestyle improvements, and environmental protections have all led to health gains. Yet these changes have not produced equal benefit in some racial and ethnic populations. This is the continuing challenge to public health professionals and the standard we must keep in mind when measuring our progress: what is the health status of the least empowered among us?"[3] As the racial and ethnic minority groups currently experiencing poorer health status grow in proportion to the total U.S. population, the future health of all Americans will be influenced by the success in improving the health of these groups. The nature of health disparities among the least empowered (primarily minorities) is the main focus of this chapter.

A landmark 1985 report, *The Secretary's Task Force Report on Black and Minority Health,* first documented the health status disparities of minority groups in the United States.[4] This report provided substantial data documenting that minority populations, compared to the nation as a whole, experience higher rates of morbidity and mortality. Specifically, the report identified six causes of death that accounted for more than 80% of the excess mortality observed among black Americans, Hispanics, Asian Americans and Pacific Islanders, and Native Americans. These six causes were infant mortality, cancer, cardiovascular disease and stroke, diabetes, homicide and accidents, and chemical dependency. *The Secretary's Task Force Report on Black and Minority Health* contributed significantly to the development of a number of *Healthy People 2000* objectives.[5] Work toward these objectives via the community health initiatives concentrated on minority populations produced some measurable decreases in age-adjusted death rates for seven specific causes of death (see Table 10.1). In an attempt to further document racial and ethnic changes over time in important Health Status Indicators (HSI), the index of disparity is provided in Table 10.2 for 1990 and

Table 10.1
Age-Adjusted Death Rates for Selected Causes of Death by Race and Hispanic Origin, 1990 and 1998, and Percent Change from 1990 to 1998: United States

		Non-Hispanic			American Indian or Alaska Native	Asian or Pacific Islander	Ratio Highest/ Lowest[a]
	Total	White	Black	Hispanic			
Total deaths							
1990[b]	518.0	483.7	785.2	395.2	441.7	295.5	2.7
1998	471.7	452.7	710.7	342.8	458.1	264.6	2.7
Percent change, 1990–98	−8.9	−6.4	−9.5	−13.3	3.7	−10.5	
Heart disease							
1990[b]	151.3	145.3	211.8	101.5	106.0	78.0	2.7
1998	126.6	123.6	188.0	84.2	97.1	67.4	2.8
Percent change, 1990–98	−16.3	−14.9	−11.2	−17.0	−8.4	−13.6	
Stroke							
1990[b]	27.5	25.1	47.8	20.7	19.1	24.7	2.5
1998	25.1	23.3	42.5	19.0	19.6	22.7	2.2
Percent change, 1990–98	−9.0	−7.2	−11.1	−8.2	2.6	−8.1	
Lung cancer							
1990[b]	39.8	39.8	50.9	15.7	19.6	17.6	3.2
1998	37.0	38.3	46.0	13.6	25.1	17.2	3.4
Percent change, 1990–98	−7.0	−3.8	−9.6	−13.4	28.1	−2.3	
Female breast cancer							
1990[b]	23.0	23.0	27.3	14.0	9.9	9.9	2.8
1998	18.8	18.7	26.1	12.1	10.3	9.8	2.7
Percent change, 1990–98	−18.3	−18.7	−4.4	−13.6	4.0	−1.0	

Table 10.1   *(continued)*

	Total	Non-Hispanic White	Non-Hispanic Black	Hispanic	American Indian or Alaska Native	Asian or Pacific Islander	Ratio Highest/ Lowest[a]
Motor vehicle crash							
1990[b]	18.4	18.1	18.3	19.2	33.0	12.5	2.6
1998	15.6	15.7	17.2	14.9	31.8	8.6	3.7
Percent change, 1990–98	−15.2	−13.3	−6.0	−22.4	−3.6	−31.2	
Suicide							
1990[b]	11.5	12.5	7.0	7.2	12.4	6.0	2.1
1998	10.4	11.8	6.1	6.0	13.4	5.9	2.3
Percent change, 1990–98	−9.6	−5.6	−12.9	−16.7	8.1	−1.7	
Homicide							
1990[b]	10.2	4.1	39.6	17.5	11.1	5.2	9.7
1998	7.3	3.2	26.1	9.9	9.9	3.7	8.2
Percent change, 1990–98	−28.4	−22.0	−34.1	−43.4	−10.8	−28.8	

[a]Ratio of the highest race/ethnic-specific rate to the lowest race/ethnic-specific rate for each year.
[b]Age-adjusted death rates for 1990 were calculated based on population estimates for July 1, 1990. Rates published elsewhere for 1990 are based on the enumerated population on April 1, 1990, for the year in which the decennial census was taken. Rates for noncensus years are based on July 1 (midyear) populations. To measure changes over time, rates based on the July 1 populations are used.

Source: Keppel, K. G., J. N. Pearcy, and D. K. Wagener (January 2002). *Trends in Racial and Ethnic-Specific Rates for the Health Status Indicators: United States 1990–1998* (Healthy People Statistical Notes no. 23). Hyattsville, MD: National Center for Health Statistics.

Table 10.2
Index of Disparity among Five Racial/Ethnic Groups for the Health Status Indicators: United States, 1990, 1998, and Percent Change

	Index of Disparity 1990	Index of Disparity 1998	Percent Change 1990–98 Decrease	Percent Change 1990–98 Increase
Infant mortality rates	38.9	36.4	−6.4	
Low birth weight (percentage)	28.4	23.0	−19.0**	
No prenatal care in first trimester (percentage)	46.9	43.5	−7.2**	
Live birth rates for women aged 15–17 years	65.4	67.7		3.5**
Total death rates	27.9	25.8	−7.5**	
Heart disease death rates	31.1	30.9	−0.6**	
Stroke death rates	29.6	26.4	−10.8**	
Lung cancer death rates	39.0	35.4	−9.2**	
Female breast cancer death rates	34.3	33.6	−2.0	
Motor vehicle crash death rates	23.6	32.8		39.0**
Suicide death rates	28.2	33.8		19.9**
Homicide death rates	95.5	86.8	−9.1**	
Work-related injury death rates (1993–98)[a]	6.3	22.1		250.8[a]
Tuberculosis case rates	160.4	170.3		6.2[a]
Primary and secondary syphilis case rates	175.3	153.1	−12.7[a]	
Children under age 18 years in poverty (percentage)[b]	64.7	56.2	−13.1	
Percentage with poor air quality (1992–98)	31.1	29.5	−5.1[a]	

**The difference in the index of disparity is statistically significant at the 0.05 level.
[a]The statistical significance of the difference in the index of disparity was not tested. Methods for assessing the reliability of the underlying rates are not available.
[a]The index of disparity for work-related injury deaths is not strictly comparable with the index of disparity for the other indicators because the data are available for the following groups: white, black, Hispanic, American Indian, Aleut and Eskimo, and Asian or Pacific Islanders. Persons of Hispanic origin may be of any race.
[b]The index of disparity for the percentage of children in poverty is not strictly comparable with the index of disparity for the other indicators because the data are available for the following groups: white non-Hispanic, black, Hispanic, and Asian or Pacific Islander.

Source: Keppel, K. G., J. N. Pearcy, and D. K. Wagener (January 2002). *Trends in Racial and Ethnic-Specific Rates for the Health Status Indicators: United States 1990–1998* (Healthy People Statistical Notes no. 23). Hyattsville, MD: National Center for Health Statistics.

1998. The index of disparity summarizes differences among racial and ethnic minority groups' rates compared to the total group. "This statistic provides a basis for comparing the degree of difference in race and ethnic specific rates in 1990 with the disparity in race/ethnic rates in 1998."[6] As shown in Table 10.2, there was a decline in 12 of the 17 HSIs. However, in some instances the disparities remained the same or in some cases widened, as evidenced by an increase in 5 of the 17 HSIs.

In 1998, then-President Clinton declared that the United States would continue to commit to a national goal of eliminating racial and ethnic health disparities by the year 2010.[7] Following this announcement, the *Initiative to Eliminate Racial and Ethnic Disparities in Health,* or the *Race and Health Initiative,* was launched. The purpose of this national effort was to enhance efforts in (1) preventing disease, (2) promoting health, and (3) delivering care to racial and ethnic minority communities. One of the primary aims of this initiative consists of consultation and collaboration among federal agencies; state, local, and tribal governments; and community professionals to research and address issues of education, income, environment, and other socioeconomic factors that affect health outcomes. Accordingly, the *Race and Health Initiative* is a paramount part of *Healthy People 2020*'s broad health goal to "achieve health equity, eliminate disparities, and improve the health of all groups."[8] This initiative will be addressed in more detail after a brief discussion on how racial and ethnic populations are classified.

RACIAL AND ETHNIC CLASSIFICATIONS

It is standard practice for the federal government to describe participants and populations in terms of "race" or "ethnicity." The racial and ethnic categories are used in statistical activities and program administration reporting, including the monitoring and enforcement of civil rights. In the 1980s, the regulations used for the statistical classification of racial and ethnic groups by federal agencies were based on the 1978 publication by the Office of Management and Budget (OMB) of Directive 15 titled "Race and Ethnic Standards for Federal Statistics and Administrative Reporting."[9] This directive presented brief rules for classifying persons into four racial categories (American Indian or Alaska Native, Asian or Pacific Islander, black, and white) and two ethnic categories (of Hispanic origin or not of Hispanic origin) (see Appendix 2). It required the categorization of blacks and whites into one of the two ethnic categories. Directive 15 was not intended to be scientific or anthropological in nature, but rather a way to **operationalize** race and ethnicity. The operational definitions detailed in Directive 15 provided the standards by which federal government agencies collected and classified racial and ethnic data in the 1980s and 1990s.

In the early 1990s, this classification system came under increasing criticism from those who asserted that the minimum categories set forth in Directive 15 did not reflect the increasing diversity of our nation's population. In response to those criticisms, OMB committed to a comprehensive review process in the mid-1990s in collaboration with the Interagency Committee for the Review of the Racial and Ethnic Standards that would enhance the accuracy of the demographic information collected by the federal government. In 1997, revised standards were issued.[10] These revised standards were used in the year 2000 decennial census. (See Appendix 3 for a listing of the operational definitions that were used by the Bureau of Census to collect the 2000 decennial census.) One of the first federal programs to support and adopt the revised standards was the Department of Health and Human Services (HHS). In October 1997, the Secretary of the HHS issued a policy supporting the inclusion of the new revised federal standards for racial and ethnic data for employment in the HHS data systems and consequently in developing and measuring *Healthy People 2010* objectives.

The 1997 classification standards expanded race from four to five categories by separating the "Asian or Pacific Islander" category into two categories—"Asian" and "Native

operationalize (operational definition) provide working definitions

Hawaiian or Other Pacific Islander." Additionally, the term "Hispanic" was changed to "Hispanic or Latino" and "Negro" can be used in addition to "Black or African American." Finally, the reporting of more than one race for multiracial persons was strongly encouraged, along with specifying that the Hispanic origin question should precede the race question. The Census 2000 was the first to employ these changes. The Census 2010 form continues to illustrate these changes (see Figure 10.4). There are 15 checkbox response categories and 3 write-in areas on the Census 2010 questionnaire for indicating race and ethnicity. The Hispanic origin question (Question 8) is asked before the race question (Question 9), and "Asian and Pacific Islander" has been divided into two categories—"Asian" and "Native Hawaiian and Other Pacific Islander." There are six designated Asian and three specified Pacific Islander categories, as well as "Other Asian" and "Other Pacific Islander." Finally, the category "some other race," which was intended to gain responses such as Mulatto, Creole, and Mestizo, has a write-in area.

It is important to consider a couple of aspects related to the collecting of data on race and ethnicity. First, the categories of race are more of a social category than a biological one.[11] Although race historically has been viewed as a biological construct, it is now known to be more accurately characterized as a social category that has changed over time and varies across societies and cultures.[11,12] As you will read later in this chapter, numerous studies have shown

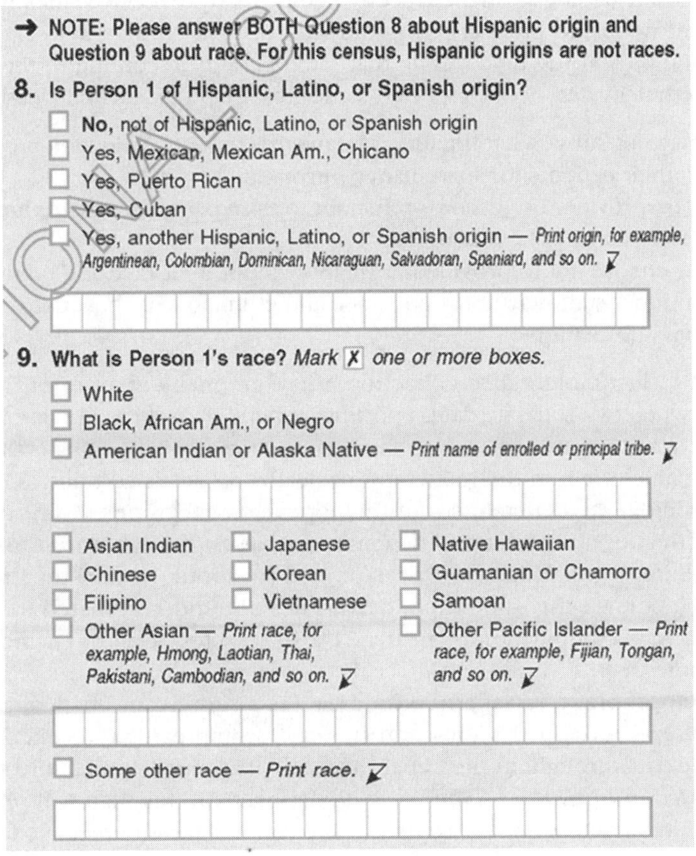
→ **NOTE: Please answer BOTH Question 8 about Hispanic origin and Question 9 about race. For this census, Hispanic origins are not races.**

8. Is Person 1 of Hispanic, Latino, or Spanish origin?

- ☐ **No,** not of Hispanic, Latino, or Spanish origin
- ☐ Yes, Mexican, Mexican Am., Chicano
- ☐ Yes, Puerto Rican
- ☐ Yes, Cuban
- ☐ Yes, another Hispanic, Latino, or Spanish origin — *Print origin, for example, Argentinean, Colombian, Dominican, Nicaraguan, Salvadoran, Spaniard, and so on.*

9. What is Person 1's race? *Mark ☒ one or more boxes.*

- ☐ White
- ☐ Black, African Am., or Negro
- ☐ American Indian or Alaska Native — *Print name of enrolled or principal tribe.*
- ☐ Asian Indian
- ☐ Chinese
- ☐ Filipino
- ☐ Other Asian — *Print race, for example, Hmong, Laotian, Thai, Pakistani, Cambodian, and so on.*
- ☐ Japanese
- ☐ Korean
- ☐ Vietnamese
- ☐ Native Hawaiian
- ☐ Guamanian or Chamorro
- ☐ Samoan
- ☐ Other Pacific Islander — *Print race, for example, Fijian, Tongan, and so on.*
- ☐ Some other race — *Print race.*

FIGURE 10.4
U.S. Census 2010 form questions for race and ethnicity.

Source: Courtesy of the U.S. Census Bureau.

that racial disparities in health generally do not mirror biologically determined differences in these groups.[13] Second, self-reported data regarding race and ethnicity may be unreliable because individuals of varied cultures and heritage and multiple races can have difficulty classifying their racial or ethnic identity on standardized forms. Third, many nonfederal health data systems do not collect self-reported race or ethnicity data, or in some cases, it may be uncertain who recorded the race and ethnicity data. For example, in a medical care setting the information may be entered by clerical staff or hospital personnel. This can make analyzing health information concerning the health status of minorities a challenging task.

HEALTH DATA SOURCES AND THEIR LIMITATIONS

The reporting of accurate and complete race and ethnicity data provides essential information to target and evaluate public health inventions aimed at minority populations.[14] However, because of the diversity in America's population, community health professionals and researchers have long recognized many crucial issues in the way that racial and ethnic variables are assessed in the collection, analysis, and dissemination of health information.[15] In the same manner, the HHS is aware of the serious gaps in its own information systems and databases regarding racial and ethnic data. For example, in a recent longitudinal study completed by the Centers for Disease Control and Prevention's National Electronic Telecommunications System for Surveillance, it was found that data regarding a patient's race and ethnicity were received in only one-half of the cases of selected notifiable diseases.[14] In comparison, data on age and sex were reported between 95% and 99% of the time during that same period. According to the authors of the study, race and ethnicity may not be reported by health care providers for at least four reasons:[14]

1. Providers may not know what the federal standards for data collection are about race and ethnicity on their patients for surveillance purposes.
2. If a health care provider forgets or is reluctant to ask a patient's racial/ethnic background, this information may not be recorded.
3. Patients may choose not to provide information about their race and ethnicity.
4. Clinical laboratory staff may not report race and ethnicity data because they do not have access to that information.

In addition to incomplete data collection, there are many cases of *bias analysis.* Bias analysis occurs when two separate data reporting systems are used to obtain rates by race and Hispanic origin. An illustration of analysis bias that is currently happening is the misreporting of race and Hispanic origin in the numerator of deaths on death certificates combined with the underreporting in the denominator of the population subgroups.[16] As a consequence of the combined effect of numerator and denominator biases, it has been estimated that death rates for the white population are overestimated by about 1% and by 5% for the black American population. At the same time, death rates are underestimated for the American Indian or Alaska Native population by nearly 21%, by 11% for Asian or Pacific Islanders, and by 2% for Hispanics.[16]

Collecting appropriate racial and ethnic data is a significant challenge facing public health. The HHS has developed a long-term strategy for improving the collection and use of racial and ethnic data throughout the department and its agencies and, more specifically, for the *Race and Health Initiative.*[17] The diversified aspects of this plan will require time and resources by the department and its agencies. One national health objective for 2020, which the HHS is overseeing, is the continued upgrading of data collection on race and ethnicity in public health surveys. In addition, the HHS continues to work with health data systems that do not collect self-reported race or ethnicity on individuals, to do so. Increasing both the reliability and amount of data will assist in monitoring and assessing the outcomes related to meeting the proposed goal of *Healthy People 2020* to "achieve health equity, eliminate disparities, and improve the health of all groups."[8] For example, the Office on Women's Health in the HHS publishes the *Health Disparities Profile*s online (www.healthstatus2010.com/owh/disparities/ChartBookData_search.asp) using standard data tables obtained from original data sources such as the CDC's National Vital Statistics System and the Behavioral Risk Factor Surveillance System. These tables display key health indicators at the state level for different racial and ethnic populations in each of the 50 states. Twenty-one health indicators are presented, which highlight some of the key areas related to health disparities among different populations. It can be used as a reference for policymakers and program managers to identify areas where major health disparities exist in each state.

Recognizing some of the limitations and gaps in collecting racial/ethnic data is important. Knowing that in some cases data are not available or the available data are not as precise as we would like, we present the best information about the community health issues faced by the primary minority groups. However, as you continue to read this chapter please be reminded of the limitations of the data on racial and ethnic minority groups. Finally, please note that throughout the remainder of the chapter we use the terms *Americans of Hispanic origin, Asian Americans, Pacific Islanders, black Americans, Native Americans,* and *white Americans,* unless there is a direct quotation or extrapolation from data or documents that use other terminology (e.g., *American Indians* in lieu of *Native Americans*).

Next, to gain a better understanding of minority groups in the United States, we briefly review several sociodemographic and socioeconomic characteristics along with broad general health beliefs for each group. These characteristics will eventually be used later in the chapter to discuss why health disparities exist in minority groups. Furthermore, all cultural and ethnic groups hold concepts related to health and illness and associated practices for maintaining well-being or providing treatment when it is indicated. However, caution is needed to avoid stereotyping. There is a considerable amount of heterogeneity within these groups, and therefore making summary statements of cultural beliefs is difficult and can be questionable. The world's 210 nations are well represented in the United States, and these diverse cultures are continually being integrated and intermixed. Additionally, members of a cultural or ethnic group who are younger or more **acculturated** into mainstream America society may not adhere to popular and folk health beliefs.

acculturated
cultural modification of an individual or group by adapting to or borrowing traits from another culture

AMERICANS OF HISPANIC ORIGIN

As we begin our discussion of Americans of Hispanic origin, readers are reminded that Hispanic origin is an ethnicity classification, not a race. The term *Hispanic* was introduced by the OMB in 1977, creating an ethnic category that included persons of Mexican, Puerto Rican, Cuban, Central America, South America, or some other Spanish origin.[9] In 1997, the term *Hispanic* was changed to "Hispanic or Latino."[10] For the purposes of data collection, the only ethnic distinction that the U.S. government makes is "Hispanic" or "non-Hispanic." Therefore, all Americans of Hispanic origin are also classified by a race. Nearly all Hispanics are classified as white Americans (96%) in the United States.

In 2008, Americans of Hispanic origin numbered approximately 47 million and constituted 15.4% of the total U.S. population, making them the largest minority group in the nation (see Figure 10.2). Since 1990, the Hispanic population has been the most rapidly growing ethnic group in the United States (see Figure 10.3). People of Mexican origin are the largest Hispanic group in the United States, representing nearly two-thirds of the country's Hispanic population.[2] Additionally, approximately 10% of Americans of Hispanic origin are of Puerto Rican background, with about 3% each of Cuban, Salvadoran, and Dominican origins. The remaining are of some other Central American, South American, or other Hispanic or Latino origins.

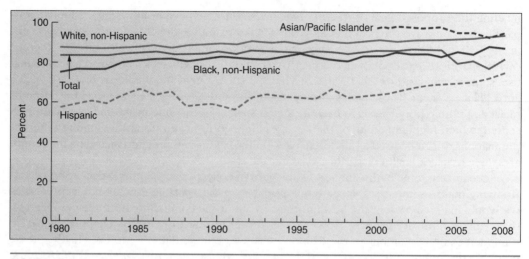

FIGURE 10.5

Percentage of adults ages 18 to 24 who have completed high school, by race and Hispanic origin, 1980 to 2008.

Note: Percentages are based only on those not currently enrolled in high school or below. Prior to 1992, this indicator was measured as completing 4 or more years of high school rather than the actual attainment of a high school diploma or equivalent.

Source: U.S. Census Bureau (2010). *Current Population Survey, School Enrollment Supplement.* Tabulated by the U.S. Department of Education, National Center for Education Statistics.

As mentioned earlier, disparities in health statistics among minorities can be traced to differences in education and income. A high school education is considered an essential basic training requirement to enter the labor force. The high school educational attainment level of Hispanic youth has been consistently lower when compared with other groups (see Figure 10.5).[18] However, the high school completion rate has increased over the last couple of decades, from 57% in 1980 to 75.5% in 2008. Linked with education is earning power. The median income of Hispanic families is significantly lower than that of Asian/Pacific Islanders and whites (see Figure 10.6).[19] Poverty rates for persons of Hispanic origin averaged 22%, nearly three times the rate for white Americans (see Figure 10.7).[20]

Traditional health beliefs of Mexican Americans and other Latin cultures include the "role of God."[21] Good health is seen as a matter of fortune or reward from God for good behavior. Maintaining harmony and balance with God is linked to the concept of good health, and warding off evil spirits is important to maintain this balance. *Curanderismo* is the most common form of Mexican American folk medicine.[21] A *curandera*'s, or healer's, ability includes a varied repertoire of religious belief systems (mainly Catholicism), herbal knowledge, witchcraft, and scientific medicine.

BLACK AMERICANS

Black Americans, or African Americans, are people having origins in any of the black racial groups from Africa. In 2008, black Americans numbered 39.7 million and constituted 12.4% of the population, making them the second largest minority group in the nation (see Figure 10.2). Even though black Americans live in all regions of the United States, more than one-half live in the southern regions of the United States. Black Americans have slightly lower high school graduation rates than white Americans (see Figure 10.5).[18] The median income for black Americans has consistently ranked below all racial and ethnic groups (see Figure 10.6),[19] and nearly one in four (24.7%) live in poverty,[20] more than three times the rates for whites (see Figure 10.7).

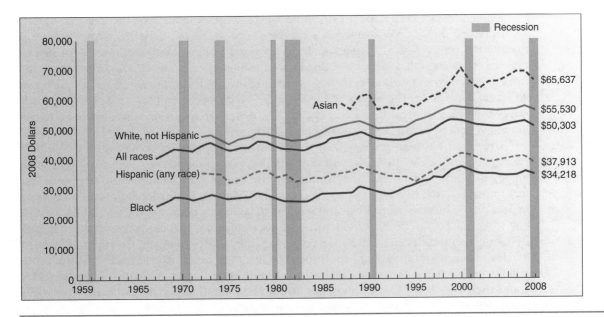

FIGURE 10.6

Real median income by race and Hispanic origin: 1967–2008. Note: Median household income data are not available prior to 1967. For information on recessions, see Appendix A.

Source: U.S. Census Bureau, *Current Population Survey, 1968 to 2009 Annual Social and Economic Supplements.* Washington, DC: U.S. Government Printing Office. Available at http://www.census.gov/prod/2009pubs/p60-236.pdf. Accessed November 30, 2010.

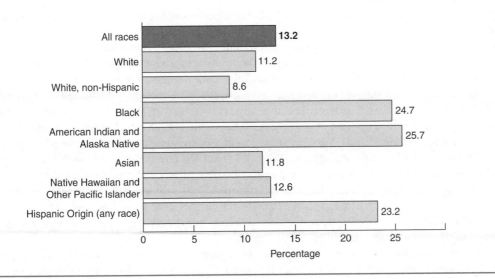

FIGURE 10.7

Poverty rates by race and Hispanic origin: 2008.

Note: Federal surveys now give respondents the option of reporting more than one race. Therefore, two basic ways of defining a race group are possible. A group such as Asian may be defined as those who reported Asian and no other race (the race-alone or single-race concept) or as those who reported Asian regardless of whether they also reported another race (the race-alone-or-in-combination concept). This figure shows data using the first approach (race alone).

Source: DeNavas-Walt, C., B. D. Proctor, J. C. Smith (2009). *U.S. Census Bureau, Current Population Reports, P60-236, Income, Poverty, and Health Insurance Coverage in the United States, 2008.* Washington, DC: U.S. Government Printing Office.

When discussing black American culture, it is important to mention the effect of slavery. Many cultural traits of black Americans can be traced to the period when slavery was practiced in the United States. Owners of slaves provided health care to their slaves for several reasons. "One was that slaves not be allowed to malinger; another concern was for the owner's property; a third concern was preventing disease from spreading; and a fourth was an actual concern for the health of the slaves."[22] These concerns plus the law that forbade slaves from providing health care to each other, under the threat of death, led to an underground system of health care by mostly untrained providers.

After the Civil War, poverty, discrimination, and poor living conditions led to a high prevalence of disease, disability, and death among black Americans.[23] Racial discrimination limited this group's access to adequate health care through the middle of the twentieth century, much as it did to education and voting rights. This discrimination continues to have an impact on the health status of black Americans today. Many black Americans still find it difficult to gain access to health care because of discrimination. Lacking access to more formalized American health care, first by slavery and then by segregation and discrimination, many black Americans implemented traditional health methods.[24] These traditional methods include curing illnesses with roots, herbs, barks, and teas by an individual knowledgeable about their use. Many black Americans continue to use traditional health methods today because they are acceptable, available, and affordable.

ASIAN AMERICANS AND PACIFIC ISLANDERS

As we begin our discussion of Asian Americans and Pacific Islanders, it is important to remind readers about the 1997 "Revisions to the Standards for the Classification of Federal Data on Race and Ethnicity." The most distinct change was separating Asian Americans and Pacific Islanders (see Figure 10.4 and Appendix 3).

In June 1999, former President Clinton signed Executive Order 13125 to improve the quality of life of Asian Americans and Pacific Islanders through increased participation in federal programs where they may be underserved (e.g., health, human services, education, housing, labor, transportation, and economic and community development).[25] One important goal of the order is collecting separate data on each group. Asian and Pacific Islanders are really two distinct groups, and combining the data tended to conceal substantial socioeconomic and health differences among these groups.[26] However, even by 2001, most federal agencies were still not collecting separate data on these two groups, citing methodological and funding constraints.[27] Accordingly, the following data on Asian Americans and Pacific Islanders are presented in aggregate, unless otherwise noted.

In 2008, Asians numbered approximately 13.6 million and constituted 4.4% of the population, and native Hawaiians and other Pacific Islanders numbered 1 million, or 0.14% of the population (see Figure 10.2). Asian American populations are generally concentrated in the western states, the Northeast, and parts of the South. Native Hawaiian and other Pacific Islanders (NHOPIs) live throughout the United States, but their populations are most concentrated in the western mainland states and Hawaii.[2]

When education and income are reported in aggregate for Asians and NHOPIs, they appear well off (see Figures 10.5 and 10.6). The high school completion rates of 18- through 24-year-olds and the median incomes were the highest compared with all other racial and ethnic groups. Unfortunately, these aggregated data mask the large variation within this population group.[28] According to Yoon and Chien, the education and income of Asians and NHOPIs form a *bipolar distribution* (skewed toward each extreme with few in the middle).[29] To better understand this concept, consider the following: Among people aged 25 years and older, Asians and NHOPIs are more likely than white Americans (42% vs. 28%) to have earned a college degree;

however, they are also more likely than white Americans (8% vs. 5%) to have less than a ninth-grade education.[30] Additionally, 33% of Asians and NHOPIs had incomes of $75,000 or more, compared with 29% of white families, while at the same time more Asians and NHOPIs had incomes under $25,000 than whites (21% vs. 19%). This deceptive view, formed by aggregate data only, has led to the myth that Asians and NHOPIs are a "model community" when in fact they suffer from as many disparities as other racial and ethnic minority groups.[29]

As mentioned previously, Asian Americans and Pacific Islanders are two discrete groups. Therefore, we now proceed with a brief overview of each. The term *Asian American* refers to people of Asian descent who are American citizens. Immigration is an integral part of Asian American community growth, as many are seeking better economic and employment opportunities and/or are reuniting with family members. They or their ancestors came from more than 20 different Asian countries, including Cambodia, China, India, Japan, Korea, Malaysia, Pakistan, the Philippine Islands, Thailand, and Vietnam.[30] Among these groups, the Chinese and Filipinos are the two largest subgroups. Even among those who have come from the same country, immigration to America may have occurred at different times, and thus there are generational differences. For example, some families may have immigrated well over a hundred years ago as laborers, while those coming today carry with them professional degrees.[31] These differences contribute to a substantial diversity in socioeconomic status among these groups, thus creating the myth discussed earlier that Asian Americans are a "model group."

Although variations among Asian Americans is the norm, many share similarities based on their religious background and the belief of equilibrium or balance.[32] The concept of balance is related to health, and imbalance is related to disease. This balance or imbalance is highly related to diet, which influences people's daily activities of living within their environment. Therefore, to achieve health and avoid illness, people must adjust to the environment in a holistic manner.

The term *Pacific Islander* (PI) includes peoples of Hawaii, Guam, Samoa, or other Pacific Islands and their descendants.[30] The Native Hawaiian population forms the majority of PIs. In contrast to Asian Americans, there is no large-scale immigration of PIs into the continental United States. Because Hawaii is the state in which the majority of PIs live, this will be our main focus. Similar to other minority groups, there are many health disparities among PIs.[33] Two key health issues for Native Hawaiians include health care allocation and the question of reimbursement for medical care.

Nearly 90% of Hawaii's land mass is federally designated as rural. Approximately 20% of Native Hawaiians live in rural Hawaii. However, the majority of the state's health care resources are fixed in the capital city of Honolulu. As a result of this imbalance of health care resource allocation, there is an inadequate number of health care professionals on the neighboring islands.[34] Additionally, transportation issues between the islands make it more difficult to access health care in Honolulu. Even public transportation on the separate islands is unreliable, so local access to medical care is challenging. The second medical care issue deals with the Native Hawaiian health belief, which suggests that the healer cannot be reimbursed directly for his or her therapeutic work. According to Blaisell,[35] such healer skill is not a question of learning but rather a question of righteousness. Therefore, it is not considered appropriate to be paid for doing what is right.

AMERICAN INDIANS AND ALASKA NATIVES

The American Indian and Alaska Native (AI/AN) population, the original inhabitants of America, numbered nearly 4.7 million in 2008, or 1.5% of the total population (see Figure 10.2). It has been estimated that prior to the arrival of European explorers, 12 million AI/ANs lived and flourished throughout what is now the United States. Exposure to diseases and ecological changes introduced by explorers and colonists decimated the AI/AN population.

Although many of the descendants were assimilated by intermarriages or successfully adapted to the new culture, as a group the AI/ANs became economically and socially disadvantaged, and this status is reflected in their relatively poor health status.[36,37] The 2008 average poverty rate for AI/ANs was 25.7%, which is the highest among all racial and ethnic groups (see Figure 10.7). Similarly, their median income and high school completion rates were among the lowest of any racial and ethnic group (see Figures 10.5 and 10.6).

Native Americans comprise many different American Indian tribal groups and Alaskan villages. Each of these tribes/villages has distinct customs, language, and beliefs. The majority, however, share the same cultural values that have been identified by Edwards and Egbert-Edwards:[38]

- Appreciation of individuality with emphasis upon an individual's right to freedom, autonomy, and respect.
- Group consensus in tribal/village decision making.
- Respect for all living things.
- Appreciation, respect, and reverence for the land.
- Feelings of hospitality toward friends, family, clanspeople, tribesmen, and respectful visitors.
- An expectation that tribal/village members will bring honor and respect to their families, clans, and tribes. Bringing shame or dishonor to self or tribe is negatively reinforced.
- A belief in a supreme being and life after death. Indian religion is the dominant influence for traditional Indian people.

Central to Native American culture is that the people "strive for a close integration within the family, clan and tribe and live in harmony with their environment. This occurs simultaneously on physical, mental, and spiritual levels; thus, individual wellness is considered as harmony and balance among mind, body, spirit and the environment."[38] This concept is not congruent with the medical model approach or public health approach that is generally accepted by the majority of Americans. As a result, in many Native American communities there is conflict between the medical/public health approach and the approaches used by Native American healers (see Table 10.3).[38] Providing appropriate health care for Native Americans usually involves resolving conflicts between the two approaches in such a way that they complement each other.

U.S. Government, Native Americans, and the Provision of Health Care

Though classified by definition and for statistical purposes as a minority group, Native Americans are unlike any other subgroup in the United States. Some (but not all) tribes are sovereign nations, based in part on their treaties with the U.S. government. Tribal sovereignty, which is

Table 10.3
A Comparison of Indian Medicine and Modern Medicine

Indian Medicine	Modern Medicine
Behavior-oriented	Complaint-oriented
Whole-specific	Organ-specific
Imbalance	Caused
Visionary diagnosis	Technical diagnosis
Wellness-oriented	Illness-oriented

Source: Garrett, J. T. (1990). "Indian Health: Values, Beliefs, and Practices." In M. S. Harper, ed., *Minority Aging: Essential Curricula Content for Selected Health and Allied Health Professionals* (HHS pub. no. HRS-P-DV90-4). Washington, DC: U.S. Government Printing Office.

perhaps the most important Native American issue, creates a distinct and special relationship between various tribes and the U.S. government. This sovereignty came about when the tribes transferred virtually all the land in the United States to the federal government in return for the provision of certain services. The U.S. government agreed to manage the land, water, agriculture, and mineral and timber resources, and to provide education and health services to tribe members. Each of these services is owed to them, and if they become indignant when people suggest they are getting them free, it is a rightful indignation.[39]

Provisions of education for Native Americans date back to the Civilization Act of 1819, while provisions for health services began in 1832.[36] The first medical efforts were carried out by Army physicians who vaccinated Native Americans against smallpox and applied sanitary procedures to curb other communicable diseases among tribes living in the vicinity of military posts. The health services provided for Native Americans after the signing of the early treaties were limited. It was common for the U.S. government, through the treaties, to impose time limits of 5 to 20 years on the provisions of health care.[40]

The original government agency overseeing the welfare of Native Americans was the Bureau of Indian Affairs (BIA). When this bureau was transferred from the War Department to the Department of the Interior in 1849, physician services were extended to Native Americans. Over the next 70+ years, health care services were continually improved, with the first Native American hospital built in 1882. However, comprehensive health services were still lacking. It was not until 1921, when the Snyder Act created the BIA Health Division, that more emphasis was given to providing health services to Native Americans. In 1954 with the passage of Public Law 83-568, known as the Transfer Act, the responsibility of health care for Native Americans was transferred from the Department of Interior's BIA to the Public Health Service (PHS). It was at this time that the Indian Health Service (IHS) was created. With this act, the health needs of Native Americans were finally met in a comprehensive way.

In keeping with the concept of tribal sovereignty, the Indian Self-Determination and Education Assistance Act (PL 93-63) of 1975 authorized the IHS to involve tribes in the administration and operation of all or certain programs under a special contract. It authorized the IHS to provide grants to tribes, on request, for planning, development, and operation of health programs.[36] Today, a number of programs are managed and operated under contract by individual tribes.[37]

Indian Health Service

The IHS, an agency within the HHS, is responsible for providing federal health services to Native Americans and Alaska Natives.[37] This agency is organized into 12 areas throughout the United States (see Figure 10.8) and operates hospitals, clinics and health stations, and a variety of other programs. The goal of the IHS is to raise the health status of American Indians and Alaska Natives to the highest possible level. To attain this goal, the IHS

1. Assists Indian tribes in developing their health programs through activities such as health management training, technical assistance, and human resource development
2. Facilitates and assists Indian tribes in coordinating health resources available through federal, state, and local programs, in operating comprehensive health care services and in health program evaluation
3. Provides comprehensive health care services, including hospital and ambulatory medical care, preventive and rehabilitative services, and development of community sanitation facilities
4. Serves as the principal federal advocate for Indians in the health field to ensure comprehensive health services for American Indian and Alaska Native people[37]

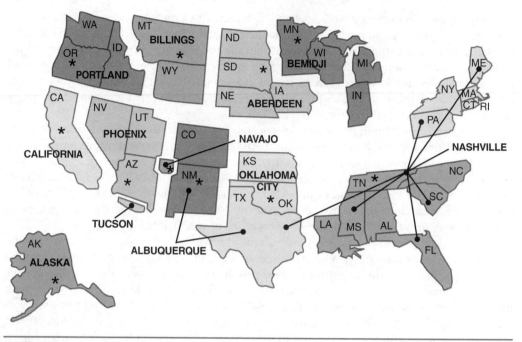

FIGURE 10.8

Indian Health Service (IHS) structure.

Note: Texas is administered by Nashville, Oklahoma City, and Albuquerque.

*Area office.

Source: U.S. Department of Health and Human Services (2000). "Regional Differences in Indian Health 1998–99." Indian Health Services, Program Statistics Team, 31. Available at http://www.ihs.gov/publicinfo/publications/trends98/region98.asp. Accessed December 17, 2010.

refugee
a person who flees one area or country to seek shelter or protection from danger in another

immigrant
individuals who migrate from one country to another for the purpose of seeking permanent residence

alien
a person born in and owing allegiance to a country other than the one in which he/she lives

illegal alien
an individual who entered this country without permission

REFUGEES: THE NEW IMMIGRANTS

In this section we introduce several new terms that describe people who have arrived in the United States relatively recently. Because of their status as new arrivals, these people sometimes share similar health problems. The first term, **refugees**, means people who flee one area, usually their home country, to seek shelter or protection from danger. Refugees arriving in the United States may be seeking political asylum, refuge from war, or escape from famine or other environmental disaster. The second term, **immigrants**, describes individuals who migrate here from another country for the purpose of seeking permanent residence and hopefully a better life. **Aliens** are people born in and owing allegiance to a country other than the one in which they live. Thus, aliens are not citizens and are only allowed to stay in a foreign country for a specified period of time defined by law or policy. Many aliens, including college students, although in the United States legally, are not permitted to work. Sometimes, however, they violate this provision and find employment illegally. Last, **illegal aliens** are those who enter this country without any permission whatsoever. Most of these illegal aliens have entered from Mexico simply by crossing the Rio Grande River at night.

Although all refugees who enter this country can be classified into one of the existing racial/ethnic categories used by our government, as a single group they present many special concerns not seen in minorities who are born and raised in the United States. Most of the refugees currently entering the United States arrive from *developing countries,* countries with meager economic resources. These refugees usually settle in urban areas, even though they may have a rural orientation. Many refugees are poor, have low levels of formal education, and have few marketable work skills. Many arrive with serious health problems, including undernourishment or starvation, physical and emotional injuries from hostile action or confinement in refugee camps, poor health care, and overcrowding.[41] A majority of the refugees are young, many of the women are of childbearing age, and most come from Latin American and Southeast Asian countries.

The arrival of such refugees places additional strains on both public and private health and social services. Some of the problems that have surfaced include the following:

- Lack of jobs to fit the skills of the refugees
- New competition for the lower socioeconomic groups in the United States for work and housing
- Strain on the budgets of the public education systems to meet the needs of the non-English-speaking refugee children
- Further burden on the human, health, and mental health services provided mostly by minority communities
- Cultural barriers to using the U.S. health care system, including lack of financial resources, cultural ignorance of health care providers, lack of bilingual health care workers, distrust and unfamiliarity with Western medicine, poor understanding of the etiology of certain diseases, difficulties of accessing services, and ignorance of available services

This immigration has resulted in growing backlash movements against refugees in some areas of the country. Examples include the "only English" movement and the Immigration Reform and Control Act of 1986 that requires employers to prove the identity and work authorization for every prospective employee—the logic of which is based on the perception of work as a privilege associated with citizenship and, by extension, with legal residence.[41]

The difficulties facing refugees in the United States, including finding employment and obtaining access to education and appropriate human, health, and mental health services, represent significant barriers to the social integration of refugees into American society. Like most of the other minority groups in the United States, refugees may become a part of those disadvantaged in this country. There is, however, one bright note to the increase of refugees in this country—the enrichment of the U.S. culture. Until 1970, the United States was primarily composed of only black and white Americans. In the last 40+ years, this country has been significantly enriched by the cultures of those coming from other countries, and, as noted earlier, the minority groups are the fastest-growing segments of the U.S. population.[42]

RACE AND HEALTH INITIATIVE

As mentioned previously, in 1998, former President Clinton committed the nation to an ambitious goal by the year 2010: Eliminate health disparities among racial and ethnic minority populations in six areas of health while maintaining the progress on overall health of the American people.[7] The *Race and Health Initiative*'s six priority areas are (1) infant mortality, (2) cancer screening and management, (3) cardiovascular disease, (4) diabetes, (5) HIV/AIDS, and (6) adult and child immunization.

The *Race and Health Initiative* reaffirms the government's extensive focus on minority health issues by emphasizing key areas that are representative of the larger minority health picture.[7] The six health issues account for a substantial burden of disease that is highly modifiable if appropriate interventions are applied. In addition, enough current data exist in each major area to be able to measure improvement and progress. Thus, the *Race and Health Initiative* is intertwined with *Healthy People 2020* and the goals of the nation for the next decade.[8]

It is important to note that *Healthy People 2020* will continue to pursue other areas of concern related to minority health that are not directly covered under these six major areas.

Similarly, we acknowledge that disparities exist in many other areas of minority health; however, this chapter presents data on the six health areas identified in the *Race and Health Initiative*. We begin by providing data documenting the disparities that exist in each of the categories, as well as data related to major risk factors that contribute to each of the conditions. As you continue to read, it is important not to stereotype any group, for it is known that each health concern cuts across all racial and ethnic groups.

Infant Mortality

As noted in Chapter 7, infant mortality is defined as the death of an infant before his or her first birthday. The infant mortality rate correlates highly to the general health and well-being of the nation. The United States made significant improvement in the twentieth century regarding infant health. However, whereas the vast majority of infants born in America today are healthy at birth, many are not. As a result, many industrialized nations report infant mortality rates that are better than those of the United States (see Figure 7.4). Additionally, infant mortality data within the United States are characterized by a long-standing and serious disparity among racial and ethnic minorities (see Figure 10.9). Infant death rates among black Americans, American Indians and Alaska Natives, and Americans of Hispanic origin have all been above the national average of approximately seven deaths per 1,000 live births. The greatest disparity exists for black Americans, whose infant death rate is more than two times that of white American infants.

There are many reasons associated with higher infant mortality rates among black Americans. Two of the more important explanations include lack of prenatal care and giving birth to low-birth-weight (LBW) babies. Prenatal care is crucial to maternal and infant health (see Chapter 7). Women who receive early and continuous prenatal health care have better pregnancy outcomes than women who do not. Black American, Native American, and Hispanic women are less likely to receive early and comprehensive prenatal care (see Figure 7.14).[43] In the same manner, black Americans and Native Americans are more likely to give birth to LBW babies (see Figure 10.10).

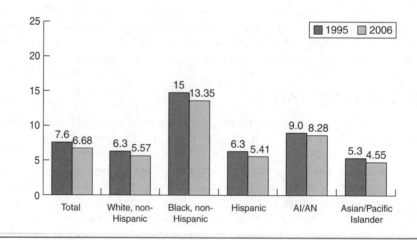

FIGURE 10.9

Infant mortality rates by race and Hispanic origin of mother: 1995 and 2006.

Source: Centers for Disease Control and Prevention, National Center for Health Statistics. *VitalStats*. Linked Birth and Infant Death Data. Available at http://www.cdc.gov/nchs/vitalstats.htm. Accessed December 14, 2010.

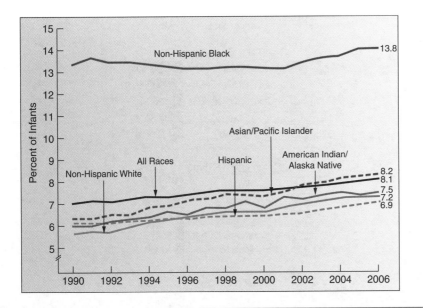

FIGURE 10.10

Percentage of infants born of low birth weight, by mother's race and Hispanic origin, 1990–2006.

Source: U.S. Department of Health and Human Services, Health Resources and Services Administration, Maternal and Child Health Bureau. *Child Health USA 2008-2009*. Rockville, Maryland: U.S. Department of Health and Human Services, 2009.

Cancer Screening and Management

Approximately 1.4 million new cases of invasive cancer are diagnosed in the United States annually.[44] Nearly one-third of those who develop cancer will die from it. Cancer is the second leading cause of death in the United States, accounting for more than 550,000 deaths annually (see Chapter 4 and Chapter 8). More than half of all new cancer cases annually are cancers of the lung, colon and rectum, breast, and prostate. From 2002 to 2006, cancer incidence rates per 100,000 population were highest among black Americans for lung, colon and rectum, and prostate cancers compared to white Americans, Asian/Pacific Islanders, American Indian/Alaska Natives, and Hispanics (see Figure 10.11). During the same period of time, cancer death rates per 100,000 population were highest among black Americans for lung, colon and rectum, and prostate cancers compared to white Americans, Asian/Pacific Islanders, American Indian/Alaska Natives, and Hispanics (see Figure 10.11). A number of these disparities in cancer incidence and death rates among minorities are attributed to lifestyle factors, late diagnosis, and access to health care.[45]

The good news is that cancer is preventable. *Primary cancer prevention* refers to preventing the occurrence of cancer. The American Cancer Society estimates that between 50% and 75% of cancer deaths in the United States are preventable through lifestyle behavior changes (i.e., avoiding smoking, avoiding excessive sun exposure, and eating nutritiously).[44] Smoking is the most preventable cause of lung cancer death in our society. The death rate for lung cancer is 20% higher in black Americans than in white Americans (see Figure 10.11). Paralleling this death rate is the fact that black Americans have a higher incidence of smoking than white Americans.

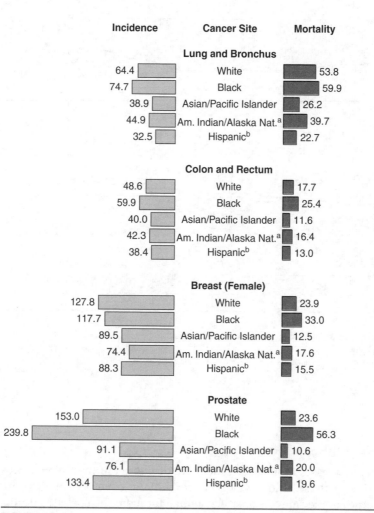

FIGURE 10.11

SEER cancer incidence and U.S. death rates, 2002-2006, by cancer site and race.

Source: Horner, M. J., L. A. G. Ries, M. Krapcho, et al. (eds). SEER Cancer Statistics Review, 1975-2006, based on November 2008 SEER data submission, posted to the SEER web site, 2009. Bethesda, MD: National Cancer Institute. Available at http://seer.cancer.gov/csr/1975_2006/. Accessed December 1, 2010.

Secondary cancer prevention refers to early detection of cancer through screening tests. The earlier a cancer is detected, the greater the chances the patient will survive. The racial/ethnic disparities in lower survival rates can partially be attributed to lower cancer screening rates among specific groups. Two cancers of significant interest are colorectal and breast. Colorectal cancer remains the second leading cause of cancer deaths in the United States and the leading cause of cancer deaths among nonsmokers. According to the CDC, 1,900 deaths could be prevented each year for every 10% increase in colonoscopy screening. Table 10.4 shows that underscreening persists for certain racial/ethnic groups when it comes to colorectal cancer screening.

Table 10.4
Percentage of Respondents Aged 50–75 Years Who Reported Receiving a Fecal Occult Blood Test (FOBT) within 1 Year, or a Lower Endoscopy* within 10 Years by Selected Characteristics

Characteristic	FOBT within 1 Yr		Lower Endoscopy within 10 Yrs		FOBT within 1 Yr or Lower Endoscopy within 10 Yrs	
	%	(95% CI§)	%	(95% CI)	%	(95% CI)
Overall	14.1	(13.8–14.4)	58.5	(58.1–59.0)	62.9	
(62.5–63.3)						
Race						
White	13.8	(13.5-14.1)	59.8	(59.4–60.2)	63.9	(63.5–64.4)
Black	17.2	(16.0–18.6)	56.6	(55.0–58.2)	62.0	(60.5–63.6)
Asian/Pacific Islander	13.5	(11.0–16.6)	51.1	(47.2–55.0)	55.5	(51.6–59.4)
American Indian/Alaska Native	15.1	(12.3–18.3)	50.7	(46.7–54.6)	54.4	(50.4–58.4)
Other	11.8	(9.7-14.1)	43.7	(40.6–46.9)	49.3	(46.1-52.6)
Ethnicity						
Hispanic	12.0	(10.5–13.7)	45.8	(43.6–48.0)	49.8	(47.6–52.0)
Non-Hispanic	14.3	(14.0–14.6)	59.8	(59.4–60.2)	64.2	(63.8–64.6)

*Sigmoidoscopy or colonoscopy.
†Percentages standardized to the age distribution in the 2008 BRFSS survey.
§Confidence interval.
¶General Educational Development certificate.

Source: Centers for Disease Control and Prevention (2010). "Vital Signs: Colorectal Cancer Screening Among Adults Aged 50-75 Years—United States, 2008." *Morbidity and Mortality Weekly Report*, 59: 1-9. Available at http://www.cdc.gov/mmwr/pdf/wk/mm59e0706.pdf. Accessed December 14, 2010.

Breast cancer is the second leading cause of cancer death among women. Most deaths from breast cancer can be reduced through early detection. Breast cancer survival rates are significantly increased if the cancer is detected early through monthly self-examination and/or periodic mammograms (breast X-rays). Despite the importance of mammography, it is underutilized as an early detection procedure by many minority women (see Box 10.1). The goal of *Healthy People 2020* is to have at least 81% of women from all racial or ethnic groups aged 50 and older receiving a mammogram within the preceding two years.[8]

Cardiovascular Diseases

Cardiovascular disease (CVD), primarily in the form of coronary heart disease and stroke, kills more Americans annually than any other disease. In fact, CVD claims more lives each year than the next five leading causes of death combined. Death rates from coronary heart disease and stroke vary widely among racial and ethnic groups (see Figures 10.12 and 10.13). Black Americans suffer disproportionately higher rates of death from coronary heart disease and stroke than do other racial and ethnic groups.

One of the major modifiable risk factors for coronary artery disease and stroke is hypertension. One in three adult Americans suffers from hypertension. The prevalence of hypertension varies noticeably according to race/ethnicity, with the highest prevalence among black Americans (see Figure 10.14).[46] In addition, black Americans tend to develop hypertension earlier in life than whites. The reasons for this are unknown. In fact, the cause of 90% to 95% of the cases of hypertension in all races and ethnic groups is unknown. Therefore, secondary prevention or screening for hypertension is essential. Hypertension is easily detected and normally controllable. However, because hypertension presents no symptoms, approximately one-third of people with high blood pressure do not know they have it.

BOX
10.1

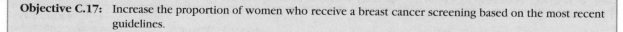

HEALTHY PEOPLE 2020: OBJECTIVE

Objective C.17: Increase the proportion of women who receive a breast cancer screening based on the most recent guidelines.

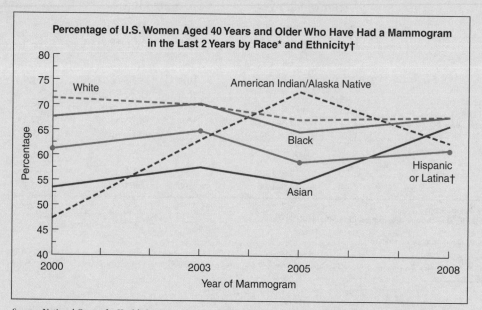

Percentage of U.S. Women Aged 40 Years and Older Who Have Had a Mammogram in the Last 2 Years by Race* and Ethnicity†

Source: National Center for Health Statistics (2010). *Health, United States, 2009 with Special Feature on Medical Technology.* (DHHS pub. No. 2010-1232). Hyattsville, MD. Available at http://www.cdc.gov/nchs/hus.htm. Accessed October 1, 2010.

For Further Thought

Research indicates that mortality resulting from breast cancer can be reduced through the use of mammography. Data for 2008 show that 68% of white and black women received mammograms, whereas American Indian/Alaska Native, Asian/Pacific Islander, and Hispanic women were less likely to have had a mammogram. What type of program could be implemented to further increase the percentage of these minority women who participate in mammograms?

Source: U.S. Department of Health and Human Services, Office of Disease Prevention and Health Promotion (2010). *Healthy People 2020.* Available at http://www.healthypeople.gov/2020/default.aspx. Accessed December 2, 2010.

Diabetes

Approximately 8.0% of children and adults (24 million people) in the United States have diabetes—a condition in which the body does not produce or properly use insulin.[47] The prevalence of diabetes has risen in recent years, and this trend is projected to continue. Furthermore, the prevalence of diabetes in people aged 20 years or older is varied in minority groups. Hispanics are 1.7 times more likely, black Americans 1.8 times more likely, and American Indians 2.2 times more likely to have diabetes than are whites of similar age (see Figures 10.15 and 10.16).

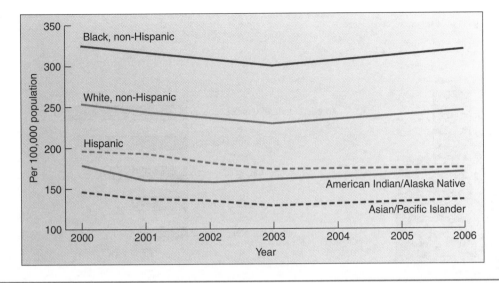

FIGURE 10.12

Heart disease deaths per 100,000 resident population (all ages), 2006.

Source: National Center for Health Statistics (2010). *Health, United States, 2009 with Special Feature on Medical Technology.* (DHHS pub. No. 2010-1232), Hyattsville, MD. Available at http://www.cdc.gov/nchs/hus.htm. Accessed October 1, 2010.

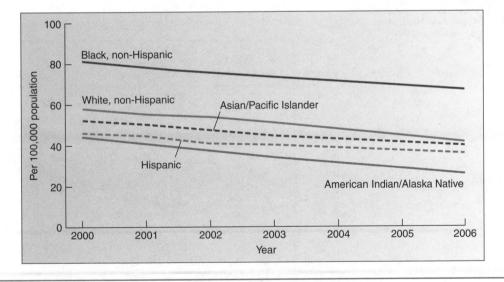

FIGURE 10.13

Cerebrovascular deaths per 100,000 resident population (all ages), 2006.

Source: National Center for Health Statistics (2010). *Health, United States, 2009 with Special Feature on Medical Technology.* (DHHS pub. No. 2010-1232), Hyattsville, MD. Available at http://www.cdc.gov/nchs/hus.htm. Accessed October 1, 2010.

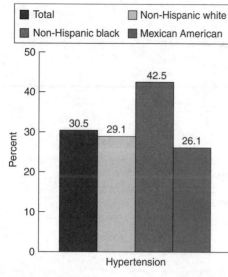

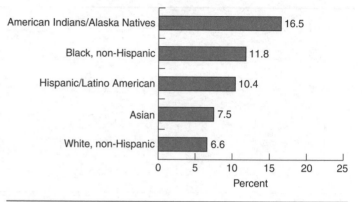

FIGURE 10.14

Age-adjusted prevalence of diagnosed or undiagnosed hypertension in adults, by race/ethnicity; United States, 1999–2006. 1 is the significant difference between non-Hispanic white and non-Hispanic black persons. 3 is the significant difference between non-Hispanic white and Mexican-American persons. Note: Persons of other race/ethnicity included in total.

Source: Centers for Disease Control and Prevention, National Center for Health Statistics. *National Health and Nutrition Examination Surveys, 1999–2006.* Available at http://www .cdc.gov/nchs/nhanes.htm. Accessed December 14, 2010.

FIGURE 10.15

Age-adjusted total prevalence of diabetes in people aged 20 years or older, by race/ethnicity: United States, 2007.

Source: National Institute of Diabetes and Digestive and Kidney Disease. National Diabetes Statistics, 2007 fact sheet. Bethesda, MD: U.S. Department of Health and Human Services, National Institutes of Health, 2008. Available at http://diabetes .niddk.nih.gov/dm/pubs/statistics/index.htm. Accessed November 30, 2010.

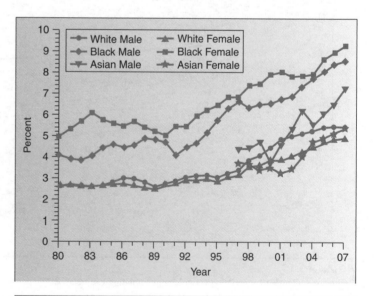

FIGURE 10.16

Age-adjusted percentage of civilian, noninstitionalized population with diagnosed diabetes, by race and sex, United States: 1980–2007.

Source: Centers for Disease Control and Prevention, National Diabetes Surveillance System, Available at http://www.cdc.gov/diabetes/statistics/prev/national/ figraceethsex.htm. Accessed November 30, 2010.

In 2007, diabetes contributed to nearly 3% of all deaths in the United States, making it the seventh leading cause of death in the United States.[48] Furthermore, the adjusted death rate for deaths related to diabetes has increased by approximately 40% in the last two decades. This increase in age-adjusted death rates occurred in all racial and ethnic groups. However, diabetes death rates do vary considerably among racial and ethnic groups. Compared to white non-Hispanics, diabetes death rates were nearly two and a half times higher among black Americans and American Indians, and nearly two times higher among Americans of Hispanic origin.[47]

In addition to causing death, other serious complications from diabetes include heart disease, stroke, blindness, and kidney disease. In fact, diabetes is the leading cause of new cases of blindness in people aged 20 to 74 and the leading cause of end-stage renal disease (ESRD), accounting for nearly half of all new cases. In 2006, more than 155,000 people with ESRD resulting from diabetes were living on chronic dialysis or with a kidney transplant.[47] Between 1980 and 2006, ESRD attributable to diabetes was greatest among black men and women and lowest among white women. Inpatient hospitalization care is one of the most expensive venues for diabetes care. Hospital admissions for long-term care of diabetes are highest among black Americans and Hispanics.

HIV Infection/AIDS

AIDS stands for *acquired immune deficiency syndrome*, a disorder first documented in the United States in 1981, through which the body's immune system is impaired to varying degrees. The cause of AIDS is a virus known as human immunodeficiency virus, or HIV. An HIV infection is a chronic condition that progressively damages the body's immune system, making an otherwise healthy person less able to resist a variety of infections and disorders. Currently, there is no known cure for HIV infection or AIDS and no vaccine to prevent it. Additionally, no major cure breakthroughs are expected for years to come.

At the end of 2006, an estimated 1.1 million persons in the United States were living with diagnosed or undiagnosed HIV.[48] At the end of 2007, the CDC estimates that 455,000 were living with AIDS in the United States. AIDS has had a disproportionate impact on racial and ethnic minority groups in the United States since the disease was first recognized in 1981. Through the end of 2007, well over half of all identified cases since 1981 were reported among racial and ethnic groups. In fact, the proportional distribution of AIDS cases among racial and ethnic groups has shifted since the beginning of the epidemic (see Figure 10.17). The proportion of cases has increased among black Americans and Hispanics and decreased among whites. In 2007, black Americans and Hispanics, who represented less than half of the population, accounted for more than one-half of the estimated number of HIV/AIDS cases diagnosed (see Figure 10.18). Consistent with the AIDS case rates are higher AIDS death rates for black Americans and Hispanics.[49]

Part of the reason for the disproportionate numbers of HIV and AIDS cases in black Americans and Americans of Hispanic origin has been attributed to a higher prevalence of unsafe or risky health behaviors (e.g., unprotected sexual intercourse and intravenous drug use), existing co-conditions (e.g., genital ulcer disease), and the lack of access to health care that would provide early diagnosis and treatment. A prevailing barrier to HIV/AIDS prevention may be that this condition is not being viewed as among the highest priorities in some minority communities when compared with other life survival problems.[50] With no cure for HIV/AIDS in sight, better health education to reduce and eliminate unsafe behaviors and increased access to medical resources for existing cases are essential to prevention.

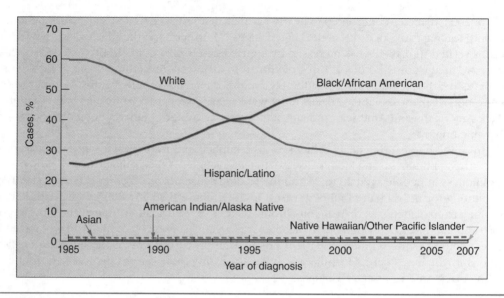

FIGURE 10.17

Percentages of AIDS cases among adults and adolescents, by race/ethnicity and year of diagnosis 1985–2007, United States and dependent areas.

Source: Centers for Disease Control and Prevention. "HIV/AIDS Surveillance in Adolescents and Young Adults through 2007."

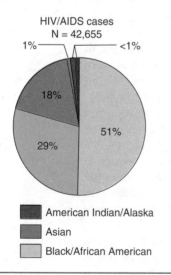

FIGURE 10.18

Percentage of HIV/AIDS cases and population by race/ethnicity, 2007, 34 states.

Note: Based on data from 35 areas with long-term, confidential, name-based HIV reporting.

Source: Centers for Disease Control and Prevention. "HIV/AIDS Surveillance in Adolescents and Young Adults through 2007."

Child and Adult Immunization Rates

As a result of widespread immunization practices, many infectious diseases that were once common have been significantly reduced. Childhood immunization rates provide one measure of the extent to which children are protected from dangerous vaccine-preventable illnesses. An important immunization rate for children aged 19 months to 35 months is the 4:3:1:3:3:1 vaccine series that includes DTP/DT/DTaP; poliovirus vaccine; measles, mumps, and rubella vaccine (MMR); *Haemophilus influenzae* type b vaccine; hepatitis B vaccine; and varicella vaccine. In 2008, coverage estimates for the 4:3:1:3:3:1 vaccine series did not vary significantly by race or ethnicity among children aged 19 months to 35 months, ranging from 76% for children of multiple races to 82% for Asians/Pacific Islanders, 78% for blacks, 76% for whites, and 78% for Hispanics.[51] The overall rise must continue to achieve the *Healthy People 2010* target of 90% coverage for all recommended childhood immunizations in all populations.[8]

Immunization does not end with childhood. It is important for adults, especially those 65 years and older, to become immunized against certain infectious diseases that can cause illness, disability, or death. Figure 10.19 shows the 2010 adult immunization schedule recommended by the CDC's National Immunization Program. Two important adult immunizations included on the schedule, as well as among the infectious disease objectives stated in *Healthy People 2020*, are immunizations for influenza and pneumoccocal diseases.[8] The goal is to

VACCINE ▼ / AGE GROUP ►	19–26 years	27–49 years	50–59 years	60–64 years	≥65 years
Tetanus, diphtheria, pertussis (Td/Tdap)*	Substitute one-time dose of Tdap for Td booster; then boost with Td every 10 years				Td booster every 10 years
Human papillomavirus*	3 doses (females)				
Varicella*	2 doses				
Zoster				1 dose	
Measles, mumps, rubella*	1 or 2 doses		1 dose		
Influenza*	1 dose annually				
Pneumococcal (polysaccharide)	1 or 2 doses			1 dose	
Hepatitis A*	2 doses				
Hepatitis B*	3 doses				
Meningococcal*	1 or more doses				

*Covered by the Vaccine Injury Compensation Program.

For all persons in this category who meet the age requirements and who lack evidence of immunity (e.g., lack documentation of vaccination or have no evidence of prior infection)

Recommended if some other risk factor is present (e.g., based on medical, occupational, lifestyle, or other indications)

No recommendation

VACCINE ▼ / INDICATION ►	Pregnancy	Immunocompromising conditions (excluding human immunodeficiency virus [HIV])	HIV infection CD4+ T lymphocyte count < 200 cells/µL	HIV infection CD4+ T lymphocyte count ≥ 200 cells/µL	Diabetes, heart disease, chronic lung disease, chronic alcoholism	Asplenia (including elective splenectomy and persistent complement component deficiencies)	Chronic liver disease	Kidney failure, end-stage renal disease, receipt of hemodialysis	Health-care personnel
Tetanus, diphtheria, pertussis (Td/Tdap)*	Td	Substitute one-time dose of Tdap for Td booster; then boost with Td every 10 years							
Human papillomavirus*		3 doses for females through age 26 years							
Varicella*	Contraindicated			2 doses					
Zoster	Contraindicated			1 dose					
Measles, mumps, rubella*	Contraindicated			1 or 2 doses					
Influenza*	1 dose TIV annually								1 dose TIV or LAIV annually
Pneumococcal (polysaccharide)	1 or 2 doses								
Hepatitis A*	2 doses								
Hepatitis B*	3 doses								
Meningococcal*	1 or more doses								

*Covered by the Vaccine Injury Compensation Program.

For all persons in this category who meet the age requirements and who lack evidence of immunity (e.g., lack documentation of vaccination or have no evidence of prior infection)

Recommended if some other risk factor is present (e.g., based on medical, occupational, lifestyle, or other indications)

No recommendation

FIGURE 10.19

Recommended adult immunization schedule, United States, 2010, by age group and medical condition.

Source: Centers for Disease Control and Prevention. Recommended adult immunication schedule—United States, 2010. *Morbidity and Mortality Weekly Report*, 58(1): 1–4.

increase the number of noninstitutionalized adults 65 and older who are immunized annually against influenza and who have ever received an immunization against pneumoccocal disease to 90%. Increased immunization rates of influenza and pneumoccocal diseases would significantly lower the number of infectious deaths caused in older adults. Annually, an estimated 50,000 adults older than 65 years die from influenza and pneumoccocal infections, making it the seventh leading cause of death among the elder population.[48] Immunization rates among nonminorities for influenza and pneumococcal infections are substantially lower than for white Americans (see Figures 10.20 and 10.21).[52] Therefore, even though these two immu-

---

FIGURE 10.20

Percentage of adults aged 65 and older who had received an influenza vaccination during the past 12 months, by race/ethnicity: United States, 2008.

Notes: Respondents were asked if they had received a flu vaccine sprayed in their nose (sometimes called by the brand name FluMist™) during the past 12 months, in addition to a question regarding receipt of a flu shot during the past 12 months. An error in calculating influenza vaccination rates occurred for the first quarter of 2005 to the first quarter of 2007. The effect of this error on estimates was small. Compared with the original estimates, corrected estimates are slightly higher, usually by no more than 0.3 percentage points. The error has been corrected for all estimates in this Early Release, and the correction of estimates had no perceptible impact on the graphs. Responses to these influenza vaccination questions cannot be used to determine when during the preceding 12 months the subject received the influenza vaccination. In addition, estimates are subject to recall error, which will vary depending on when the question is asked because the receipt of an influenza vaccination is seasonal. According to the recommendations of the Advisory Committee on Immunization Practices, all adults aged 50 years and over should receive an influenza vaccination (10). The analyses excluded 97 adults (2.1%) aged 65 years and over with unknown influenza vaccination status.

Data source: Based on data collected in the Sample Adult Core component of the 2008 National Health Interview Survey. Data are based on household interviews of a sample of the civilian noninstitutionalized population.

- For adults aged 65 years and over, the percentage of persons receiving an influenza vaccination during the past 12 months was 54.0% for Hispanic persons, 69.9% for non-Hispanic white persons, and 50.6% for non-Hispanic black persons.

- Hispanic persons and non-Hispanic black persons were less likely than non-Hispanic white persons to have received an influenza vaccination during the past 12 months.

Source: Centers for Disease Control and Prevention (2009). Summary Health Statistics for the U.S. Population: National Health Interview Survey, 2008.

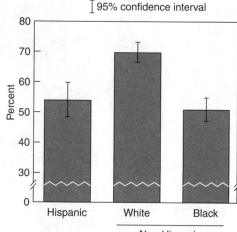

FIGURE 10.21

Percentage of adults aged 65 and older who had ever received a pneumococcal vaccination, by race/ethnicity: United States, 2008.

Note: The analyses excluded 181 adults (4.0%) aged 65 years and over with unknown pneumococcal vaccination status.

Source: Centers for Disease Control and Prevention (2009). Summary Health Statistics for the U.S. Population: National Health Interview Survey, 2008.

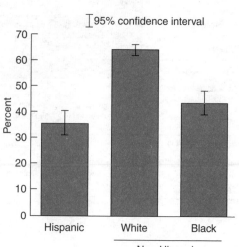

nization rates among all adults have shown a significant increase since 1990; to reach the goal of 90% by 2020, increased efforts must be focused on minority populations.[8]

SOCIOECONOMIC STATUS AND RACIAL AND ETHNIC DISPARITIES IN HEALTH

Preceding our discussion of the *Race and Health Initiative,* we acknowledged that disparities exist in many other areas of minority health. However, we limited our focus to the six health areas identified in the initiative. In like manner, there are many factors that contribute to these disparities. These include economics, education, and behavioral factors—such as lifestyle and health practices—as well as cultural, legal, and political factors (see Figure 10.22). We focus our discussion on **socioeconomic status** (SES), which has been considered the most influential single contributor to premature morbidity and mortality by many public health researchers.[13] However, it is important to emphasize that the association between SES and race

socioeconomic status relating to a combination of social and economic factors

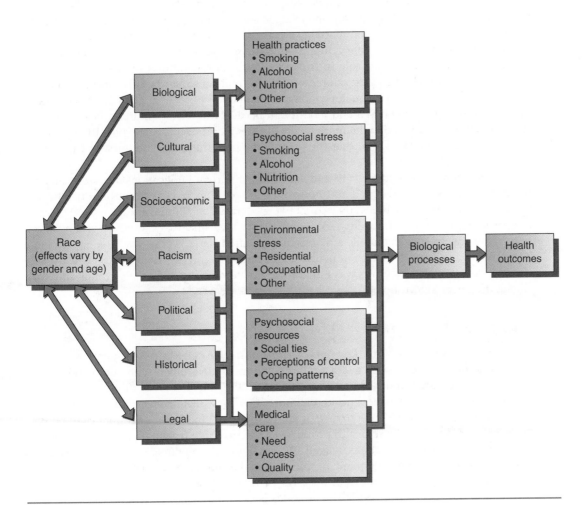

FIGURE 10.22

A framework for understanding the relationship between race and health.

Source: Centers for Disease Control and Prevention. Use of Race and Ethnicity in Public Health Surveillance. Summary of CDC/ASTDR Workshop. *Morbidity and Mortality Weekly Report*, 1993, 42(RR-10).

and ethnicity is complicated and cannot fully explain all disparities in health status. Furthermore, many of these factors are not always direct in nature—they are what are referred to as *indirect causal associations* or *intermediary factors*. For example, poverty by itself may not cause disease and death; however, by precluding adequate nutrition, preventive medical care, and housing, it leads to increased morbidity and premature mortality.

As we stated earlier, the categories of race are more of a social category than a biological one. Racial disparities in health generally do not reflect biologically determined differences.[13] In fact, biological differences between racial groups are small compared with biological differences within groups.[53] More than 90% of the differences in genetic makeup occur within racial and ethnic groups rather than between the groups. Such disparities in health status among minority groups are much better understood in terms of the groups' living circumstances.[54] A group's living circumstances may be referred to as its socioeconomic status (SES). Common SES factors studied include level of education, level of income, and poverty.

Public health research has long studied SES factors and their relationship to health. These studies have shown that better health is associated with more years of education and having more income, a more prestigious job, and living in superior neighborhoods. Similarly, elevated levels of morbidity, disability, and mortality are associated with less education, lower income, poverty, unemployment, and poor housing. An extensive amount of research documents that SES factors play a significant role in the association of race and ethnicity with health.[8] Furthermore, research in the last couple of decades indicates that the relationship between SES and health occurs at every socioeconomic level and for a broad range of SES indicators.[55] This relationship between SES and health can be described as a gradient. For example, research has documented that the more family income increases above the poverty threshold, the more health improves, and that the greater the gap in income, the greater the gap in health.

This gradient effect between SES and health has important implications that are related to the gap between the privileged and nonprivileged, or the "haves and have-nots." In the United States, many inequalities still exist between all racial and ethnic groups related to level of education, income, and poverty (see Figures 10.5, 10.6, and 10.7). Minority groups often occupy the lowest socioeconomic rankings in the United States. These low rankings become a significant community health concern when one recognizes that progress toward the *Healthy People 2010* objectives was found to be greatest among higher SES groups and least among the lower SES groups.[8]

EQUITY IN MINORITY HEALTH

One of the primary aims of the *Race and Health Initiative* consists of consultation and collaboration among federal agencies; state, local, and tribal governments; and community professionals to research and address issues of education, income, environment, and other socioeconomic factors that affect health outcomes. We know that many health problems faced by minorities are attributable not to race or ethnic origin but to social or economic conditions or disenfranchisement. These health problems are inseparable from a variety of other social problems, making simple solutions unlikely. We also know that multiple resources are required to resolve these social and economic problems, and that solutions to these problems for one group may not work for another. Americans of Hispanic origin, Asian Americans, Pacific Islanders, black Americans, and Native Americans each have unique cultural traditions that must be respected if the solutions are to be successful. In other words, we must operationally integrate an understanding of the culture of the target population; solutions must be *culturally sensitive*. In a more general sense, significant strides in the improvement of health in minority groups can be achieved if community health professionals become more culturally competent and are able to empower local communities.

Cultural Competence

In this chapter's introduction, we stated that the strength and greatness of America lies in the diversity of its people and their cultures. However, cultural differences can and do present major obstacles to implementing effective community health programs and services. The demographic shifts in minority populations and the resulting diversity in health providers treating more patients have increased interest among health professionals to increase culturally appropriate services that lead to improved outcomes, efficiency, and satisfaction for their clients.[56] This increased interest is not only being found among health care providers but also among patients, policymakers, educators, and accreditation and credentialing agencies. In March 2001, the HHS and the Office of Minority Health published standards for culturally and linguistically appropriate services (CLAS) in health care (see Box 10.2).[56] These criteria are the first comprehensive and nationally recognized standards of cultural and linguistic competence in health care service delivery that have been developed. In the past, national organizations and federal agencies independently developed their own standards and policies. The result was a wide spectrum of ideas about what constitutes culturally appropriate health services. The CLAS report went further and defined **cultural and linguistic competence** as

> **cultural and linguistic competence**
> a set of congruent behaviors, attitudes, and policies that come together in a system, agency, or among professionals, that enables effective work in cross-cultural situations

> A set of congruent behaviors, attitudes, and policies that come together in a system, agency, or among professionals that enables effective work in cross cultural situations. *Culture* refers to integrated patterns of human behavior that include language, thoughts, communications, actions, customs, beliefs, values, and institutions of racial, ethnic, religious or social groups. *Competence* implies having the capacity to function effectively as an individual and an organization within the context of the cultural beliefs, behaviors, and needs presented by consumers and their communities.[56]

Based on this definition, culture is a vital factor in both how community health professionals deliver services and how community members respond to community health programs and preventive interventions. In a society as culturally diverse as the United States, community health educators need to be able to communicate with different communities and understand how culture influences health behaviors.[57] It is important that community health promotion/disease prevention programs be understandable and acceptable within the cultural framework of the population to be reached. Lee has published the following list of 10 principles related to cultural competency that are considered important for community health practitioners to understand when planning and implementing health promotion/disease prevention programs:[58]

1. Having a self-understanding of race, ethnicity, and power
2. Understanding the historical factors that impact the health of minority populations, such as racism and immigration patterns
3. Understanding the particular psychosocial stressors relevant to minority participants (such as socioeconomic status and migration)
4. Understanding the cultural differences within minority groups
5. Understanding the minority client within a family life cycle and in an intergenerational conceptual framework
6. Understanding the differences between the "culturally acceptable" behaviors of psychopathological characteristics of different minority groups.

| BOX 10.2 | NATIONAL STANDARDS FOR CULTURALLY AND LINGUISTICALLY APPROPRIATE SERVICES IN HEALTH CARE |

1. Health care organizations should ensure that patients/consumers receive from all staff members effective, understandable, and respectful care that is provided in a manner compatible with their cultural health beliefs and practices and preferred language.
2. Health care organizations should implement strategies to recruit, retain, and promote at all levels of the organization a diverse staff and leadership that are representative of the demographic characteristics of the service area.
3. Health care organizations should ensure that staff at all levels and across all disciplines receive ongoing education and training in culturally and linguistically appropriate service delivery.
4. Health care organizations must offer and provide language assistance services, including bilingual staff and interpreter services, at no cost to each patient/consumer with limited English proficiency at all points of contact, in a timely manner during all hours of operation.
5. Health care organizations must provide to patients/consumers in their preferred language both verbal offers and written notices informing them of their right to receive language assistance services.
6. Health care organizations must assure the competence of language assistance provided to limited English proficient patients/consumers by interpreters and bilingual staff. Family and friends should not be used to provide interpretation services (except on request by the patient/consumer).
7. Health care organizations must make available easily understood patient-related materials and post signage in the languages of the commonly encountered groups and/or groups represented in the service area.
8. Health care organizations should develop, implement, and promote a written strategic plan that outlines clear goals, policies, operational plans, and management accountability/oversight mechanisms to provide culturally and linguistically appropriate services.
9. Health care organizations should conduct initial and ongoing organizational self-assessments of

CLAS-related activities and are encouraged to integrate cultural and linguistic competence-related measures into their internal audits, performance improvement programs, patient satisfaction assessments, and outcomes-based evaluations.
10. Health care organizations should ensure that data on the individual patient's/consumer's race, ethnicity, and spoken and written language are collected in health records, integrated into the organization's management information systems, and periodically updated.
11. Health care organizations should maintain a current demographic, cultural, and epidemiological profile of the community as well as a needs assessment to accurately plan for and implement services that respond to the cultural and linguistic characteristics of the service area.
12. Health care organizations should develop participatory, collaborative partnerships with communities and utilize a variety of formal and informal mechanisms to facilitate community and patient/consumer involvement in designing and implementing CLAS-related activities.
13. Health care organizations should ensure that conflict and grievance resolution processes are culturally and linguistically sensitive and capable of identifying, preventing, and resolving cross-cultural conflicts or complaints by patients/consumers.
14. Health care organizations are encouraged to regularly make available to the public information about their progress and successful innovations in implementing the CLAS standards and to provide public notice in their communities about the availability of this information.

Note: The standards are organized by three themes.
1. Culturally competent care (Standards 1–3)
2. Language access services (Standards 4–7)
3. Organizational supports for cultural competence (Standards 8–14)

Source: U.S. Department of Health and Human Services, Office of Minority Health (2001). *National Standards for Culturally and Linguistically Appropriate Services in Health Care: Final Report.* Washington, DC: Author.

7. Understanding the indigenous healing practices and the role of religion in the treatment of minority patients
8. Understanding the cultural beliefs of health and help-seeking patterns of minority individuals
9. Understanding the health service resources for minority patients
10. Understanding the public health policies and their impact on minorities and communities

For community health educators whose role is to educate groups and communities of diverse cultural backgrounds, cultural competence is critical (see Appendix 4). Additionally, successful community health intervention and educational activities should be firmly grounded in an understanding and appreciation of the cultural characteristics of the target group. *Healthy People 2020* is firmly devoted to the principle that "every person in every community across the Nation deserves equal access to comprehensive, culturally competent, community-based health care systems that are committed to serving the needs of the individual and promoting community health."[8]

Empowering the Self and the Community

Another principle deeply etched in *Healthy People 2020* with respect to achieving equity is the ideal that the "greatest opportunities for reducing health disparities are in *empowering* individuals to make informed health care decisions and in promoting community-wide safety, education, and access to health care."[8] One reason why minority groups lack the resources to eliminate community health problems is their lack of empowerment. To *empower* means to give power or authority; to enable or permit. With reference to our discussion, it means to enable people to work to solve their community health problems. Simply put, to acquire better health and health care services, a community must be empowered to do so.

Friedman identifies three kinds of power associated with empowerment—social, political, and psychological.[59] An increase in social power brings with it access to "bases" of production such as information, knowledge and skills, participation in social organizations, and financial resources. Increased productivity enables greater influence on markets, which in turn can influence change.

A social power-base is needed to gain political power. Political power is more than just being able to vote; it is also the power of voice and of collective action. In a democracy, seldom does a single voice effect change; it is the collective voice that can make things happen. The early labor movement in this country that led to the establishment of unions is a good example.

Psychological power is best described as an individual sense of potency demonstrated in self-confident behavior. It is often the result of successful action in the social and political domains. With the investiture of all three types of power, empowerment can take place. Empowerment replaces hopelessness with a sense of being in control and a sense that one can make a difference. Once people are empowered, the power then needs to be transferred to the communities. When communities are empowered, they can cause change and solve problems. See Chapter 5 for a discussion of community organization as a means of empowering a community.

The process of empowerment may seem abstract because of the theoretical concepts that are involved, but it is not. Follow the process in this example. A group of people, a community, lacks access to the appropriate health care. For this group to be empowered, they must build a foundation with social power. To do this, the group must gain access to the bases of production. They must acquire information about available health care programs and obtain the knowledge and skills to access care. Some in the group need to become members of social organizations that are concerned with health care (such as health departments or voluntary agencies), and the group has to obtain the necessary financial resources to enable them to be noticed in the marketplace as a consumer group. To gain such social power, it is imperative that the group be literate and have the appropriate education. Many groups never gain social power because they do not possess the education to access the bases of production.

When the group has attained social power, a subgroup is able to work toward political power. The subgroup can be heard in the marketplace with its vote and voice. Members of this subgroup can organize to present a united front for collective action. Minority groups have the potential to have a loud voice if united. Once united, they are in a position to influence decision makers at various governmental levels. In the specific case in which the goal is greater access to health care, this could mean getting the local health department to expand the types and numbers of available clinics.

Increased political power can lead to psychological power. Such power would give this particular group the confidence that the expansion of health department clinics is just the first of many achievements. Therefore, through this same process, other community improvements also can be made.

CHAPTER SUMMARY

- One of the great strengths of the United States has been, and remains, the diversity of its people.

- The federal government has recently categorized the U.S. population into five racial groups (American Indian or Alaska Native, Asian, black or African American, Native Hawaiian or Other Pacific Islander, and white) and two ethnic groups (Hispanic or Latino and non-Hispanic or non-Latino).

- The reporting of accurate and complete race and ethnicity data provides essential information to target and evaluate public health inventions aimed at minority populations.

- All cultural and ethnic groups hold concepts related to health and illness and associated practices for maintaining well-being or providing treatment when it is indicated.

- The *Race and Health Initiative* includes six priority areas: (1) infant mortality, (2) cancer screening and management, (3) cardiovascular disease, (4) diabetes, (5) HIV/AIDS, and (6) adult and child immunization. These key areas are representative of the larger minority health picture and account for a substantial burden of disease that is highly modifiable if the appropriate interventions are applied.

- Socioeconomic status (SES) has been considered the most influential single contributor to premature morbidity and mortality by many public health researchers. Research in the last couple of decades indicates that the relationship between SES and health occurs at every socioeconomic level and for a broad range of SES indicators. This relationship between SES and health can be described as a gradient.

- Significant strides in the improvement of health in minority groups can be achieved if community health professionals become more culturally sensitive and competent.

- Minority groups must be empowered to solve their own problems through the processes of social, political, and psychological empowerment.

REVIEW QUESTIONS

1. Why is it said that the United States was built on diversity?

2. What is the Office of Management and Budget's Directive 15?

3. Why is it important for community health workers to be aware of the significant health disparities among various minority groups in the United States?

SCENARIO: ANALYSIS AND RESPONSE

1. Do you agree with Tom when he says the United States is more culturally diverse than at any time in the past? Why or why not? Do you see this as a strength or weakness for the country?

2. What signs are there in your community that the United States is becoming more internationalized and that minority groups are growing?

3. What strengths do you see as a result of an increasingly diverse population in the United States? What weaknesses?

4. Do you agree with the major health priorities as outlined in the *Race and Health Initiative* regarding the community you live in? Why or why not?

4. What were the significant findings of the 1985 landmark report *The Secretary's Task Force Report on Black and Minority Health?*

5. List and explain the six priority areas in the *Race and Health Initiative.*

6. What role does socioeconomic status play in health disparities among racial and ethnic minority groups?

7. Why is it important for community health professionals and workers to be culturally sensitive and competent?

8. List each of the three kinds of power associated with empowerment. What is the importance of each in empowering individuals and communities?

ACTIVITIES

1. Using the most recent census report (available in your library or on the Web), create a demographic profile of the state and county in which you live. Locate the following information—population; racial/ethnic composition; percentage of people represented by the different age groups, gender breakdown, and marital status; and percentage of people living in poverty.

2. Make an appointment with an employee of the health department in your hometown. Find out the differences in health status between the racial/ethnic groups in the community among the race/ethnicity-specific morbidity and mortality data. Discuss these differences with the health department employee, and then summarize your findings in a one-page paper.

3. In a two- to three-page paper, present the proposal you would recommend to the President of the United States for closing the health status gap between the races and ethnic groups.

4. Identify a specific racial/ethnic minority group and select a health problem. Study the topic and present in a three-page paper the present status of the problem, the future outlook for the problem, and what could be done to reduce or eliminate the problem.

5. Write a two-page position paper on "Why racial/ethnic minority groups have a lower health status than the majority of white Americans."

COMMUNITY HEALTH ON THE WEB

The Internet contains a wealth of information about community and public health. Increase your knowledge of some of the topics presented in this chapter by accessing the Jones & Bartlett Learning Web site at **http://health.jbpub.com/book/communityhealth/7e** and follow the links to complete the following Web activities.

- Office of Minority Health
- Eliminating Racial and Ethnic Disparities in Health
- Indian Health Service

REFERENCES

1. The White House (1999). "One America in the 21st Century: The President's Initiative on Race." Available at http://www.ncjrs.gov/pdffiles/173431.pdf.

2. U.S. Census Bureau, Population Division (2004). "U.S. Interim Projections by Age, Sex, Race, and Hispanic Origin." Available at http://www.census.gov/ipc/www/usinterimproj/.

3. Centers for Disease Control and Prevention (1997). *Minority Health Is the Health of the Nation*. Washington, DC: U.S. Government Printing Office.

4. U.S. Department of Health and Human Services (1988). *Report of the Secretary's Task Force on Black and Minority Health*. Washington, DC: Author.

5. U.S. Department of Health and Human Services (1990). *Healthy People 2000: National Health Promotion Disease Prevention Objectives* (HHS pub. no. PHS 90-50212). Washington, DC: U.S. Government Printing Office.

6. Keppel, K. G., J. N. Pearcy, and D. K. Wagener (2002). *Trends in Racial and Ethnic-Specific Rates for the Health Status Indicators: United States 1990-1998* (Healthy People Statistical Notes no. 23). Hyattsville, MD: National Center for Health Statistics.

7. U.S. Department of Health and Human Services (2000). *Race and Health Initiative*. Available at http://raceandhealth.hhs.gov/.

8. U.S. Department of Health and Human Services, Office of Disease Prevention and Health Promotion (2010). *Healthy People 2020* Available at http://www.health.gov/2020/default.aspx.

9. Office of Management and Budget (1978). "Directive 15: Race and Ethnic Standards for Federal Statistics and Administrative Reporting." In *U.S. Department of Commerce, Office of Federal Statistical Policy and Standards, Statistical Policy Handbook*. Washington, DC: Author, 37-38.

10. Office of Management and Budget (1997). "Revisions to the Standards for the Classification of Federal Data on Race and Ethnicity." *Federal Register*.

11. Nelson, H., and R. Jurmain (1998). *Introduction to Physical Anthropology*, 4th ed. St. Paul, MN: West Publishing.

12. Williams, D. R., R. Lavizzo-Mourey, and R. C. Warren (1994). "The Concept of Race and Health Status in America." *Public Health Reports*, 109: 26-41.

13. Senior, P. A., and R. Bhopa (1994). "Ethnicity as a Variable in Epidemiological Research." *British Medical Journal*, 309: 327-330.

14. Centers for Disease Control and Prevention (1999). "Reporting Race and Ethnicity Data—National Electronic Telecommunications System for Surveillance, 1994-1997." *Morbidity and Mortality Weekly Report*, 48(15): 305-312.

15. Centers for Disease Control and Prevention (1993). "Use of Race and Ethnicity in Public Health Surveillance: Summary of the CDC/ATSDR Workshop." *Morbidity and Mortality Weekly Report*, 42(10): 1-17.

16. Rosenberg, H. M., J. D. Maurer, and P. D. Sorlie (1999). "Quality of Death Rates by Race and Hispanic Origin: A Summary of Current Research." *Vital Statistics Reports*, 2: 128.

17. U.S. Department of Health and Human Services (1999). "Improving the Collection and Use of Racial and Ethnic Data in HHS." Available at http://aspe.hhs.gov/datacncl/racerpt/index.htm.

18. U.S. Census Bureau (2010). *Current Population Survey, October Supplement*. Washington, DC: U.S. Department of Education, National Center for Education Statistics.

19. DeNavas-Walt, C., B. D. Proctor, and J. C. Smith (2009). *Income, Poverty, and Health Insurance Coverage in the United States: 2008*. Washington, DC: U.S. Government Printing Office.

20. U.S. Census Bureau (2009). *Current Population Survey, 2006-2008. Annual Social and Economic Supplements*. Washington, DC. U.S Government Printing Office.

21. Fishman, B., L. Bobo, K. Kosub, and R. Womeodu (1993). "Cultural Issues in Serving Minority Populations: Emphasis on Mexican Americans and African Americans." *American Journal of the Medical Sciences*, 306: 160-166.

22. U.S. Department of Health and Human Services (1993). "Advance Report of Final Mortality Statistics, 1990." *Monthly Vital Statistics Report*, 41(9): 42.

23. Satcher, D., and D. J. Thomas (1990). "Dimensions of Minority Aging: Implications for Curriculum Development for Selected Health Professions." In M. S. Harper, ed., *Minority Aging: Essential Curricula Content for Selected Health and Allied Health Professions* (HHS pub. no. HRS-P-DV 90-4). Washington, DC: U.S. Government Printing Office, 23-32.

24. Airhihenbuwa, C. O., and I. E. Harrison (1993). "Traditional Medicine in Africa: Past, Present and Future." In P. Conrad and E. Gallagher, eds., *Healing and Health Care in Developing Countries*. Philadelphia: Temple University Press.

25. President's Advisory Commission on Asian Americans and Pacific Islanders (2001). *A People Looking Forward: Action for Access and Partnerships in the 21st Century*. Interim Report to the President. Available at http://www.aapi/gov/intreport.htm.

26. President's Advisory Commission on Asian Americans and Pacific Islanders (2003). *Asian Americans and Pacific Islanders Addressing Health Disparities: Opportunities for Building a Healthier America*. Available at http://www.aapi.gov/Commission_Final_Health_Report.pdf.

27. Ghosh, C. (2003). "*Healthy People 2010* and Asian Americans/Pacific Islanders: Defining a Baseline of Information." *American Journal of Public Health*, 93: 2093-2098.

28. Mayeno, L., and S. M. Hirota (1994). "Access to Health Care." In N. W. S. Zane, D. T. Takeuchi, and K. N. J. Young, eds., *Confronting Critical Health Issues of Asian and Pacific Islander Americans*. Thousand Oaks, CA: Sage Publications.

29. Yoon, E., and E. Chien (1996). "Asian American and Pacific Islander Health: A Paradigm for Minority Health." *Journal of the American Medical Association*, 275: 736-737.

30. Humes, K., and J. McKinnon (2000). "The Asian and Pacific Islander Population in the United States." In U.S. Census Bureau, *Current Population Reports* (Series P20-529). Washington, DC: U.S. Government Printing Office.

31. Kitano, H. H. L. (1990). "Values, Beliefs, and Practices of Asian-American Elderly: Implications for Geriatric Education." In M. S. Harper, ed., *Minority Aging: Essential Curricula Content for Selected Health and Allied Health Professions* (HHS pub. no. HRS-P-DV 90-4). Washington, DC: U.S. Government Printing Office, 341-348.

32. Frye, B. A. (1995). "Use of Cultural Themes in Promoting Health among Southeast Asian Refugees." *American Journal of Health Promotion*, 9: 269-280.

33. Aiu, P. (June/July 2000). "Comparing Native Hawaiians' Health to the Nation." *Closing the Gap*, 8-9.

34. Jiang, S. (June/July 2000). "Correcting the Visions of Paradise." *Closing the Gap*, 4.

35. Blaisdell, R. K. (1989). "Historical and Cultural Aspects of Native Hawaiian Health." In E. Wegner, ed., *Social Process in Hawai'i*. Honolulu: University of Hawai'i Press, 32.

36. Garrett, J. T. (1990). "Indian Health: Values, Beliefs and Practices." In M. S. Harper, ed., *Minority Aging: Essential Curricula Content for Selected Health and Allied Health Professionals* (HHS pub. no. HRS-P-DV90-4). Washington, DC: U.S. Government Printing Office, 179-191.

37. U.S. Department of Health and Human Services, Indian Health Services, Program Statistics Team (2000). "Regional Differences in Indian Health 1998-99." Available at http://www.ihs.gov/publicinfo/publications/trends98/region98.asp.

38. Edwards, E. D., and M. Egbert-Edwards (1990). "Family Care and Native American Elderly." In M. S. Harper, ed., *Minority Aging: Essential Curricula Content for Selected Health and Allied Health Professions* (HHS pub. no. HRS-P-DV90-4). Washington, DC: U.S. Government Printing Office, 145-163.

39. Rhoades, E. R. (1990). "Profile of American Indians and Alaska Natives." In M. S. Harper, ed., *Minority Aging: Essential Curricula Content for Selected Health and Allied Health Professions* (HHS pub. no. HRS-P-DV90-4). Washington, DC: U.S. Government Printing Office, 45-62.

40. U.S. Department of Health and Human Services (1992). *Comprehensive Health Care Program for American Indians and Alaska Natives*. Washington, DC: U.S. Government Printing Office.

41. Uba, L. (1992). "Cultural Barriers to Health Care for Southeast Asian Refugees." *Public Health Reports*, 107(5): 544-548.

42. Sotomayor, M. (1990). "The New Immigrants: The Undocumented and Refugees." In M. S. Harper, ed., *Minority Aging: Essential Curricula Content for Selected Health and Allied Health Professions* (HHS pub. no. HRS-P-DV 90-4). Washington, DC: U.S. Government Printing Office, 627-637.

43. National Center for Health Statistics (2010). "Percentage of Mothers Receiving Late or No Prenatal Care by Race and Hispanic Origin, 2006." National Vital Statistics System. Available at http://www.cdc.gov/nchs/fastats/prenatal.htm.

44. National Cancer Institute (2010). *SEER Cancer Incidence and US Death Rates, 2002-2006 by Cancer Site and Race*. Available at http://seer.cancer.gov/csr/1975_2006/results_merged/topic_graph_rate_comparison.pdf.

45. Freeman, H. P. (2004). "Poverty, Culture, and Social Injustice: Determinants of Cancer Disparities." *CA: A Cancer Journal for Clinicians*, 54(2): 72-77.

46. Fryer, C. D., R. Hirsch, M. S. Eberhardt, S. S. Yoon, and J. D. Wright (2010). *Hypertension, High Serum Total Cholesterol, and Diabetes: Racial and Ethnic Prevalence Differences in U.S. Adults, 1999-2006* (NCHS Data Brief, no. 36). Hyattsville, MD: National Center for Health Statistics.

47. Centers for Disease Control and Prevention (2010). "National Diabetes Surveillance System." Available at http://www.cdc.gov/diabetes/statistics/index.htm.

48. Xu, J., K. Kochanek, S. Murphy, and B. Fejada-Vera (2010). "Deaths: Final Data for 2007." *National Vital Statistics Reports*, 58(19): 1-31.

49. Centers for Disease Control and Prevention (2009). HIV/AIDS Surveillance Report, 19: 1-37

50. Barrow, R. Y., L. M. Newman, and J. M. Douglas, Jr. (2008). "Taking Positive Steps to Address STD Disparities for African-American Communities." *Sexually Transmitted Diseases*, 35(12 Suppl) S1-S3.

51. Centers for Disease Control and Prevention (2010). "Vaccination Coverage among Children Aged 19 to 35 Months—United States, 1994-2008." National Immunization Program. NIS Data. Available at http://www.cdc.gov/vaccines/stats-surv/imz-coverage.htm.

52. Centers for Disease Control and Prevention (2010). "Influenza and Pneumococcal Vaccination Levels among Persons Aged 65 Years and Older, United States, 2005-2006." Available at http://www.cdc.gov/vaccines/stats-surv/imz-coverage.htm.

53. Shiver, M. D. (1997). "Ethnic Variation as a Key to the Biology of Human Disease." *Annals of Internal Medicine*, 127: 401-403.

54. Navarro, V. (1990). "Race or Class versus Race and Class: Mortality Differentials in the United States." *Lancet*, 336: 1238-1240.

55. Adler, N., and J. Ostrove (2000) "Socioeconomic Status and Health: What We Know and What We Don't." *Annals of the New York Academy of Sciences*, 896: 3-15.

56. Office of Minority Health (2001). "National Standards for Culturally and Linguistically Appropriate Services in Health Care—Final Report." Available at http://minorityhealth.hhs.gov/assets/pdf/checked/finalreport.pdf

57. Loustaunau, M. (2000). "Becoming Culturally Sensitive: Preparing for Service as a Health Educator in a Multicultural World." In S. Smith, ed., *Community Health Perspectives*. Madison, WI: Coursewise Publishing, 33-37.

58. Lee, E. (2000). *Working with Asian Americans*. New York: Guilford Press.

59. Friedmann, J. (1992). *Empowerment: The Politics of Alternative Development*. Cambridge, MA: Blackwell.

Community Mental Health

Chapter Objectives

After studying this chapter, you will be able to:

1 Define *mental health* and *mental disorders*.

2 Explain what is meant by the *DSM-IV-TR*.

3 Give an example of how cultural differences can
affect psychiatric diagnosis.

4 Identify the major causes of mental disorders.

5 Explain why mental health is one of the major community health problems in the United States.

6 Define *stress*, and explain its relationship to physical and mental health.

7 Briefly trace the history of mental health care in the
United States, highlighting the major changes both
before and after World War II.

8 Define the term *deinstitutionalization* and list and
discuss the propelling forces that brought it about.

9 Describe the movement toward community mental
health centers.

10 Identify the major mental and physical problems of
people who are homeless.

11 Describe mental health courts and the use of "legal
leverage" to compel treatment.

12 Define *primary*, *secondary*, and *tertiary prevention* as they relate to mental health care services
and give an example of each.

13 List and briefly describe the three basic approaches
to treatment for mental disorders.

14 Describe what "recovery" means for people with
mental illness in the United States, and for those in
less developed countries such as India or Tanzania.

15 Explain what is meant by psychiatric rehabilitation,
and list the kinds of services provided by effective
programs.

16 Define *self-help groups*, give examples, and explain how they are helpful to their members.

17 Identify key challenges presently faced by the mental health care system.

18 Explain the issues of managed care and parity in connection with health care services for people with mental illness.

SCENARIO

Maria Sanchez, her husband, and their three children had lived in their apartment building for about 2 years when they noticed a new person moving in on the floor below them. New families moved in from time to time, but this person didn't have a family and kept to herself. After asking around, Maria learned from a neighbor downstairs that the new person's name was Lynn and that she was not currently employed but hoped to find work soon, perhaps as a cashier or a custodian. Maria is annoyed that Lynn keeps her television on late into the night. She has been meaning to say something about it, but so far Lynn keeps to herself and Maria hasn't found her very friendly—Lynn tends to look away without saying anything when Maria passes her in the hallway. Maria also learned that Lynn was recovering from a recent bout of mental illness and that she was anxious about the demands of living independently once again.

Maria noticed that every few days a regular visitor arrived at the building in a van from the mental health center to spend an hour or so with Lynn in her apartment. Maria worries that people who see the mental health center van might think those in the van were visiting Maria's family. She knew that people with mental illness needed to live somewhere, but why did it have to be in her building? Would other recovering mental patients rent the next vacant apartment in her building? Would people begin loitering in front of the building or behaving strangely? Would Maria's children be safe? Would the reputation of their neighborhood begin to decline?

INTRODUCTION

Mental illness is one of the major health issues facing every community. It is the leading cause of disability in North America and Europe and costs the United States more than half a trillion dollars per year in treatment and other expenses (see Figure 11.1).[1] Approximately 26% of American adults (about 58 million people) have diagnosable mental or addictive disorders during a given year, and about 6% of adults in the United States have serious mental illness, that is, illness that interferes with some aspect of social functioning.[2] Only about one-third of those diagnosed with a mental disorder receive treatment.[3] Some of these people require only minimal counseling, followed by regular attendance of supportive self-help group meetings to remain in recovery, while others suffer repeated episodes of disabling mental illness. These individuals have conditions for which they require more frequent medical treatment and more significant community support. Finally, there are the most severely disturbed individuals, who require repeated hospitalization.

Tragic shootings at Virginia Tech and Northern Illinois Universities brought the issue of mental disorder in college students to national attention. Almost half of college students show a 12-month prevalence of some form of mental disorder (most often alcohol use disorder, at 20.37%), and less than 25% receive treatment (see Table 11.1).[4] A study of client problems seen by a university counseling center found that over a 13-year period, depression doubled and the number of suicidal students tripled.[5] Approximately 4 million children and adolescents suffer from a major mental illness that results in significant impairment at home, at school, and with peers.[6] While 1 in 10 youths has an impairing mental illness, only 1 in 5 receives mental health services in a given year.[7]

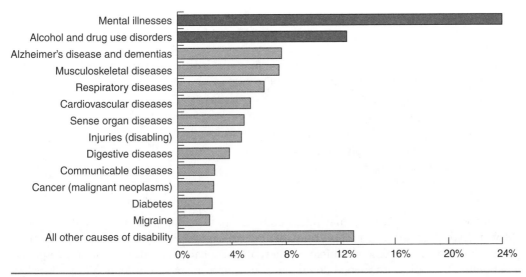

FIGURE 11.1

Causes of disability for all ages combined: United States, Canada, and western Europe, 2000.

Note: Measures of disability are based on the number of years of "healthy" life lost with less than full health (i.e., YLD: years lost due to disability) for each incidence of disease, illness, or condition.

Source: President's New Freedom Commission on Mental Health (2003). *Achieving the Promise: Transforming Mental Health Care in America.* Rockville, MD: Author, 20.

Because the needs of people with mental illness are many and diverse, the services required to meet these needs are likewise diverse and include not only therapeutic services but social services requiring significant community resources. As we explain, mental disorders and mental health care also occur in a diverse social, cultural, and economic context that has important ethical implications for diagnosis, treatment, and recovery.

mental health
emotional and social well-being, including one's psychological resources for dealing with day-to-day problems of life

Definitions

Mental health is the "state of successful performance of mental function, resulting in productive activities, fulfilling relationships with other people, and the ability to adapt to change and

Table 11.1
12-Month Prevalence of Mental Disorders in College Students and Non-College Attending Peers, in Percentage, Ages 18–25

Diagnostic Characteristic	In College	Not in College
Any psychiatric diagnosis	45.79	47.74
Any alcohol use disorder*	20.37	16.98
Any drug disorder*	5.08	6.85
Major depression	7.04	6.67
Bipolar disorder	3.24	4.62
Any anxiety disorder	11.94	12.66
Pathological gambling	0.35	0.23
Any personality disorder*	17.68	21.55

*Difference is statistically significant (p < .05).

Source: Adapted from Blanco, C., O. Mayumi, C. Wright, et al. (2008). "Mental Health of College Students and Their Non-College-Attending Peers." *Archives of General Psychiatry*, 65(12): 1429–1437.

to cope with adversity."[6] Characteristics of people with good mental health include possessing a good self-image, feeling right about other people, and being able to meet the demands of everyday life.

Good mental health can be expressed as emotional maturity. In this regard, adults who have good mental health are able to do the following:

1. Function under adversity
2. Change or adapt to changes around them
3. Maintain control over their tension and anxiety
4. Find more satisfaction in giving than receiving
5. Show consideration for others
6. Curb hate and guilt
7. Love others

mental illness
a collective term for all diagnosable mental disorders

"**Mental illness** is a term that refers collectively to all diagnosable mental disorders. **Mental disorders** are health conditions that are characterized by alterations in thinking, mood, or behavior (or some combination thereof) associated with distress and/or impaired functioning."[6] People with mental illness have organic or metabolic (biochemical) disorders that prevent them from functioning effectively and happily in society. Many people with mental illness can be treated successfully with medications and are thus able to live successfully in our communities.

mental disorders
health conditions characterized by alterations in thinking, mood, or behavior (or some combination thereof) associated with distress and/or impaired functioning

Classification of Mental Disorders

It is important to keep in mind that classification systems of human origin are imperfect attempts to arrange natural phenomena into carefully constructed, but sometimes arbitrary, categories. Such is the case with the classification of mental disorders, which are for the most part based on descriptions of behavioral signs and symptoms rather than definitive measurements involving the brain or another body system. The single most influential book in mental health is probably the *Diagnostic and Statistical Manual of Mental Disorders*, 4th edition, text revision (*DSM-IV-TR*; a new edition, *DSM-5*, is expected in 2013), published by the American Psychiatric Association.[8] It identifies the various mental disorders, provides descriptive information and diagnostic instructions for each, and has significant implications for who merits a diagnosis, whether a treatment should be reimbursed by insurance, the top priorities for mental health research, and what kinds of new therapeutic medications should be developed.

cultural competence
service provider's degree of compatibility with the specific culture of the population served, for example, proficiency in language(s) other than English, familiarity with cultural idioms of distress or body language, folk beliefs, and expectations regarding treatment procedures (such as medication or psychotherapy) and likely outcomes

Disorders classified in the *DSM-IV-TR* are listed in Table 11.2. One challenge in making these diagnoses is that nearly half of people with mental illness (46.4%) have more than one disorder,[2] a problem known as comorbidity. Depression and anxiety are separate categories in *DSM-IV*, for example, yet are found together in many individuals[9] and have similar genetic risk factors.[10] Language and cultural differences also complicate the application of *DSM* criteria. Given the same symptoms, for example, Latinos are more likely to be diagnosed with major depression than are whites or African Americans.[11] Lack of **cultural competence** (language proficiency, familiarity with cultural idioms of distress or body language) may lead a diagnostician to misinterpret as depression what is simply a Latino patient's subdued and discouraged demeanor and reluctance to disclose symptoms. The social context also affects diagnosis. Worldwide, for example, women are diagnosed with mood disorders more often than are men, but this difference is smaller in countries that have less traditional gender-role differences in employment opportunities, educational attainment, and control of fertility.[12] A final concern is that diagnosis with a mental disorder can stigmatize a person by imposing negative stereotypes, prejudice, and discrimination that the person often internalizes, reducing hope and self-esteem and hindering the person's efforts to recover.[13]

Table 11.2
Diagnostic Categories of Mental Disorders

Category	Example
Disorders usually first evident in infancy, childhood, or adolescence	Mental retardation; attention-deficit hyperactivity disorder
Organic mental disorders	Alzheimer's disease; dementia associated with alcoholism or chronic drug use
Psychoactive substance use disorders	Alcohol, nicotine, cocaine, or other drug dependence
Schizophrenia	Paranoid schizophrenia
Delusional (paranoid) disorder	Persecutory delusional (paranoid) disorder
Miscellaneous psychotic disorders	Brief reactive psychosis
Mood disorders	Major depression; bipolar disorder
Anxiety disorders	Panic disorder; obsessive compulsive disorder; post-traumatic stress disorder
Somatoform disorders	Conversion disorder; hypochondriasis
Dissociative disorders	Multiple personality disorder
Sexual disorders	Paraphilias (exhibitionism, fetishisms); sexual dysfunctions
Sleep disorders	Insomnia disorder; dream anxiety disorder
Impulse control disorders	Kleptomania; pathological gambling
Adjustment disorders	Anxious mood; withdrawal
Personality disorders	Avoidant; dependent; obsessive

Causes of Mental Disorders

Symptoms of mental illness can arise from many causes, and the comorbidity that exists among disorders suggests they are not discrete conditions, each with a specific cause. Instead, mental disorders can result from genetic influences on complex brain functions that control a person's thoughts and emotions,[14] physiologic disruptions in hormones such as testosterone and vasopressin,[15] intrauterine infections and malnutrition, maladaptive family functioning, and stress.

Two-thirds of mental retardation cases are traceable to environmental factors such as poor prenatal care, poor maternal nutrition, or maternal exposure to alcohol, tobacco, or other drugs; as such, they are preventable. For example, fetal alcohol spectrum disorder, a condition that includes mental deficiency, is the result of maternal (and fetal) exposure to excessive amounts of alcohol during gestation. One recent study revealed that an estimated 423,000 women used alcohol during their pregnancies, while 413,000 used cigarettes and 97,000 used at least one illicit drug.[16]

Mental disorders can also occur from postnatal exposure to physical, chemical, and biological agents, including secondhand cigarette smoke.[17] Brain function impairment can be caused by trauma, such as a car crash or bullet wound, or by disease, such as syphilis, cancer, or stroke. Mental impairment can also be caused by such environmental factors as chronic nutritional deficiency or by lead poisoning.

Psychological sources of mental disorders include maladaptive family functioning, which results from having a parent with mental illness, substance abuse, or criminality, and from experiencing violence, physical or sexual abuse, or neglect.[18] In addition, intimate partner violence against women is a common experience worldwide and a greater risk to women than is violence perpetrated by strangers.[19]

The prevalence of child abuse and neglect has reached epidemic proportions in the United States (see Figure 11.2). Each year there are more than 900,000 confirmed victims of maltreatment in the United States, according to the Children's Defense Fund.[20] It is estimated that 1 in 5 youths has some sort of diagnosable disorder. Furthermore, the prevalence of serious emotional disturbance in youth (9 to 17 years old) ranges from 5% to 13%. Thus, a

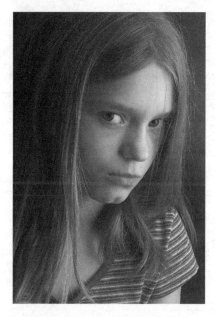

FIGURE 11.2

A dysfunctional family environment can increase one's risk for mental illness.

major depression
an affective disorder characterized by a dysphoric mood, usually depression, or loss of interest or pleasure in almost all usual activities or pastimes

minimum of 1 in 20 to a maximum 1 in 7.7 youths suffers from emotional disturbances that include functional impairment.[6,21] (See Figure 11.3.)

The negative influences of unhealthy neighborhoods, deviant peer groups (such as gangs), and challenging economic conditions or growing up in dysfunctional families may further increase the risk that these young people will develop mental disorders. Broken families add to the burden on our nation's mental health services, leading children's advocates to question the priorities of federal programs that provide more money to the states for foster care than for programs designed to strengthen families. The U.S. Department of Health and Human Services estimates that there were approximately 500,000 children in foster care in 2008.[20]

Two other populations at high risk for developing mental illness are citizens exposed to disasters and soldiers returning from combat zones. For example, 20% of Manhattan residents living near the World Trade Center at the time of the attacks of September 11, 2001, had symptoms consistent with post-traumatic stress disorder (PTSD) 5 to 8 weeks after the attack, and nearly 10% suffered from depression, which occurred most often in those who had suffered losses as a result of the attack.[22] The police officers and firefighters of New Orleans who responded following Hurricane Katrina were exposed to both physical injuries and illnesses and to psychological stressors. Approximately 19% of police officers and 22% of firefighters reported symptoms of PTSD, and 26% of police officers and 27% of firefighters reported symptoms of **major depression** (see Box 11.1).[23]

Military service in a combat zone increases one's risk of experiencing PTSD, major depression, or other mental health problems (see Figure 11.4). A 2006 study found a high rate of mental health services utilization among veterans of Operation Iraqi Freedom. The study noted that the prevalence rates of mental health problems were consistently higher

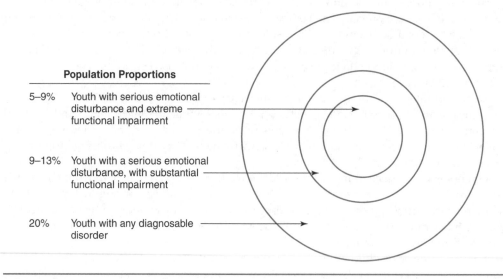

Population Proportions

5–9% Youth with serious emotional disturbance and extreme functional impairment

9–13% Youth with a serious emotional disturbance, with substantial functional impairment

20% Youth with any diagnosable disorder

FIGURE 11.3

Prevalence of serious emotional disturbance in 9- to 17-year-olds.

Source: Center for Mental Health Services (1996). *Mental Health, United States, 1996.* R. W. Mandersheid, and M. A. Sonnenschein, eds. (DHHS pub. no. SMA 96-3098). Washington, DC: U.S. Government Printing Office, 83.

BOX 11.1 — CRITERIA FOR MAJOR DEPRESSIVE EPISODE

A. Five (or more) of the following symptoms have been present during the same two-week period and represent a change from previous functioning. At least one of the symptoms is either (1) depressed mood or (2) loss of interest or pleasure.

Note: Do not include symptoms that are clearly due to a general medical condition, or mood-incongruent delusions or hallucinations.

(1) Depressed mood most of the day, nearly every day, as indicated by either subjective report (e.g., feels sad or empty) or observation made by others (e.g., appears tearful). Note: In children and adolescents, can be irritable mood

(2) Markedly diminished interest or pleasure in all, or almost all, activities most of the day, nearly every day (as indicated by either subjective account or observation made by others)

(3) Significant weight loss when not dieting or weight gain (e.g., a change of more than 5% of body weight in a month), or decrease or increase in appetite nearly every day. Note: In children, consider failure to make expected weight gains

(4) Insomnia or hypersomnia nearly every day

(5) Psychomotor agitation or retardation nearly every day (observable by others, not merely subjective feelings of restlessness or being slowed down)

(6) Fatigue or loss of energy nearly every day

(7) Feelings of worthlessness or excessive or inappropriate guilt (which may be delusional) nearly every day (not merely self-reproach or guilt about being sick)

(8) Diminished ability to think or concentrate, or indecisiveness, nearly every day (either by subjective account or as observed by others)

(9) Recurrent thoughts of death (not just fear of dying), recurrent suicidal ideation without a specific plan, or a suicide attempt or a specific plan for committing suicide

B. The symptoms do not meet criteria for a Mixed Episode.

C. The symptoms cause clinically significant distress or impairment in social, occupational, or other important areas of functioning.

D. The symptoms are not due to the direct physiological effects of a substance (e.g., a drug of abuse, a medication) or a general medical condition (e.g., hypothyroidism).

E. The symptoms are not better accounted for by bereavement, that is, after the loss of a loved one, the symptoms persist for longer than two months or are characterized by marked functional impairment, morbid preoccupation with worthlessness, suicidal ideation, psychotic symptoms, or psychomotor retardation.

Source: Adapted from American Psychiatric Association (2000). *Diagnostic and Statistical Manual of Mental Disorders*, 4th ed., text revision. Washington, DC: Author.

---

among those deployed to Iraq (19%) than those deployed to Afghanistan (11%). Thirty-five percent of veterans returning from Iraq accessed mental health services in the year after returning home.[24]

MENTAL ILLNESS IN AMERICA

Health and social statistics clearly indicate that mental illness constitutes one of our nation's most pervasive public health problems. In 2001, for example, the Number 2 and Number 3 leading causes of death in youth aged 15 to 24 were homicide (including legal intervention) and suicide, respectively (see Chapter 8).[25] Suicide in young people is associated with mood disorders[26] and PTSD.[27] One of the objectives of *Healthy People 2020* aimed at improving the mental health status of Americans is to reduce the suicide rate. From 2002 to 2006, little progress was made in reducing suicide

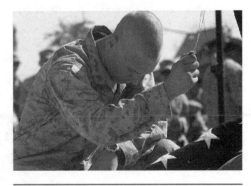

FIGURE 11.4

Military troops returning from duty in combat zones are heavy users of mental health services when these services are accessible.

rates in most population subgroups. Preventing suicide is difficult because the base rate of completed suicide is only 10.9 per 100,000 people.[28] Community-wide education campaigns can improve public knowledge and attitudes regarding suicide, but the durability of such changes is not known and educational efforts have shown no effects on help-seeking or suicidal behavior.[29]

The prevalence of alcohol, tobacco, and other drug abuse in this country is yet another social indicator of the mental illness problem. For example, in 2002 40% of the college-aged young adults and 28% of high school seniors interviewed had drunk at least five or more drinks in a row in the past 2 weeks, and the percentage of twelfth graders reporting the use of any illegal drug in the past 30 days increased to 25%.[30] These figures, which are discussed in more detail in Chapter 12, are further evidence that many of our youth lack the necessary psychological resources for coping with life's problems.

Stress: A Contemporary Mental Health Problem

Stress can be defined as one's psychologic and physiologic response to stressors—stimuli in the physical and social environment that produce feelings of tension and strain. Stress, as a contributor to mental health problems, is likely to remain important as life becomes increasingly complex. Even Americans who believe they have good mental health carry out their everyday activities under considerable stress. Stressors can be subtle—such as having to wait in line, getting stuck in traffic, or having to keep an appointment—or they can be major life events such as getting married or divorced or losing a loved one. Coping with a physical health problem such as hypertension, obesity, or other disease can increase stress and raise one's risk of developing a mental disorder. Whereas some exposure to stressors is good, perhaps even essential to a satisfying life, chronic exposure to stressors that exceed one's coping resources—biological, psychological, and social—can undermine one's health. Holmes and Rahe actually classified and ranked various stressors and found a relationship between these stressors and physical health.[31]

The process through which exposure to stressors results in health deficits has been described by Selye[32] and Sarafino.[33] According to Selye's model, which he called the **General Adaptation Syndrome (GAS)**, confrontation with a stressor results in a three-stage physiologic response: (1) an alarm reaction stage, (2) a stage of resistance, and finally (3) a stage of exhaustion (see Figure 11.5). In the alarm reaction stage, the body prepares to strongly resist the stressor. Various hormonal changes in the body increase the individual's heart rate, respiration, and blood pressure. This is the **fight or flight reaction**, a response that the body cannot maintain for very long. Continued presence of the stressor produces a stage of resistance. In this stage, the body tries to adapt to the stressor. The level of physiologic arousal declines

General Adaptation Syndrome (GAS) the complex physiological responses resulting from exposure to stressors

fight or flight reaction an alarm reaction that prepares one physiologically for sudden action

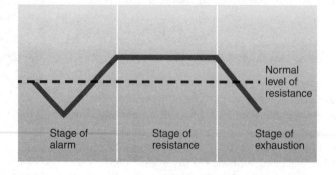

FIGURE 11.5
General Adaptation Syndrome.

somewhat but still remains above normal. During the stage of resistance, the body begins to replenish the hormones released in the alarm reaction stage, but the body's ability to resist new stressors is impaired. As a result, the person is increasingly vulnerable to certain health problems that are referred to as **diseases of adaptation**. Such diseases include ulcers, high blood pressure, coronary heart disease, asthma, and other diseases related to impaired immune function.[33] The third stage of Selye's GAS is the stage of exhaustion. Prolonged physiologic arousal produced by continual or repeated stress can deplete energy stores until one's physical ability to resist is very limited. During this stage, physiologic damage, physical diseases, mental health problems, and even death can occur.

Evidence suggests that stress can affect health either directly by way of physiologic changes in the body or indirectly through a change in a person's behavior. The clearest connection between stress and disease is demonstrated by the release of hormones by the endocrine system during the alarm reaction stage of the GAS. During this stage, both the cardiovascular and immune systems of the body are affected. Hormones produce fast or erratic beating of the heart, which can be fatal. The same hormones have been associated with increases in levels of blood lipids. High blood lipids cause a buildup of plaque on the blood vessel walls and greatly increase the likelihood of hypertension, stroke, and heart attack. The release of certain hormones also impairs the functioning of the immune system. These hormones reduce the activity of T cells and natural killer cells, making it more difficult for the immune system to fight cancer and other diseases.[34] Table 11.3 provides a list of psychophysiologic disorders that have been found to be associated with stress.

The indirect effects of stress on health occur when those who experience high levels of stress respond with unhealthy behaviors. For example, it has been shown that individuals under more stress drink more alcohol and smoke more cigarettes than those under less stress.[35,36] Use of these substances has been associated with higher risks for heart disease and cancer, as well as injury and death from unintentional injuries.

Relationships and other social resources can mediate the effects of stress. For example, people lacking support (in the form of marriage, church membership, social organization membership, and contacts with friends and relatives) face a greater risk than do others of experiencing mental illness, alcohol and drug abuse, suicide, illness, and mortality, independent of their overall health, socioeconomic status, smoking, drinking, obesity, and utilization of health care.[37]

Avoiding stressful situations is always preferable to managing stress. Effective time management, goal setting, and prioritizing tasks are ways individuals can reduce the stress that comes with approaching deadlines. Procrastination, on the other hand, can increase stress. Also, taking a realistic view of one's abilities and what one expects to accomplish is important. "Perfectionism leads to undue stress because perfection is an unattainable goal."[38]

Stress management is primarily a personal rather than a community health matter. Experts recommend a combination of physical, social, environmental, and psychological approaches to managing stress.[38] Physical approaches to stress reduction include good nutrition and

> **diseases of adaptation** diseases that result from chronic exposure to excess levels of stressors, which produce a General Adaptation Syndrome response

Table 11.3
Psychophysiological Disorders Associated with Stress

Allergies (asthma, tissue inflammation, rheumatoid arthritis)	Gastrointestinal problems (colitis, stomach ulcers)
Cancer	
Cardiovascular conditions	Headaches (muscle-contraction and migraine)
Coronary artery disease	Infectious diseases (colds and influenza)
Depression	Hypertension
Dysmenorrhea (painful menstruation)	Irritable bowel syndrome
Exhaustion	Skin disorders (eczema, hives, psoriasis)

adequate sleep and aerobic exercise. Healthy social interaction and optimizing environmental factors such as noise, lighting, and living space can also reduce one's stress. Finally, a variety of psychological techniques have proven effective in reducing stress for some people. These include guided imagery and visualization, biofeedback, progressive relaxation, and meditation and hypnosis.[38] Among the many resources available to help people deal with the stress in their lives is the American Institute of Stress Web site at www.stress.org.

Community support for those experiencing excessive stress in their lives can be found in local mental health associations, local offices of comprehensive mental health centers, and other more specialized agencies, such as A Better Way, for battered spouses and children. College and university counseling and psychological service centers provide help for students. Relief from stress for some might be as close as the nearest church, synagogue, or mosque. Religious leaders are often experienced in helping people suffering from stress; also, the social interactions available in these settings can be comforting. Finally, there are community service organizations such as Rotary, Kiwanis, Lions, and many others that provide opportunities for socialization. In a college or university setting, similar opportunities are available for joining in social or service clubs.

HISTORY OF MENTAL HEALTH CARE IN AMERICA

Before discussing our nation's current response to mental illness, we present a brief history of past efforts to confront this issue. The collective response to mental illness in America has been a cyclic phenomenon, marked by enthusiastic reform movements followed by periods of national ambivalence toward those suffering from mental disorders. The following reform movements we discuss began when an existing system for caring for those with mental illness became intolerable for society and ended when their economic burden became unbearable.

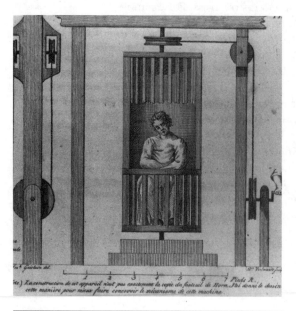

FIGURE 11.6

Treatment for mental illness in the eighteenth and nineteenth centuries was often inhumane and unsuccessful.

Mental Health Care before World War II

In Colonial America, when communities were sparsely populated, people experiencing mental illness were cared for by their families or private caretakers. Those "distracted" persons or "lunatics," as they were called, who were not cared for by their families usually became the responsibility of the local community. In the eighteenth century, as the size and complexity of communities grew, institutionalization of people with mental disorders first appeared. This often took place in undifferentiated poorhouses or almshouses where those who had mental retardation, those with physical disabilities, the homeless, and the otherwise deviant were also housed.[39]

As America's population grew in the late eighteenth and early nineteenth centuries, so did the number of people who were unable to live independently. Gradually, as the situation in the poorhouses and almshouses worsened, efforts were made to separate people by their type of disability. One of the first efforts was that of Dr. Thomas Bond, who in 1751 built Pennsylvania Hospital, the first institution in America specifically designed to care for those with mental illness.[40] Conditions in the hospital were harsh (see

Figure 11.6), and treatments, which consisted of "blood letting, blistering, emetics, and warm and cold baths," were unpleasant.[41]

The Moral Treatment Era

Philippe Pinel of France developed a more humane approach that he called *traitement moral*, or in English, **moral treatment**, based on the assumption that environmental changes could affect an individual's mind and thus alter behavior.[39] In America, William Tuke put moral treatment into practice beginning in 1792. This treatment was based on his belief that the causes of mental illnesses were moral deterioration, exemplified by "infidelity, overwork, envy, gluttony, drinking, sexual excesses, and the like."[41] In a peaceful rural setting, people with mental illness were removed from the everyday life stressors of their home environments and given "asylum" in a quiet country environment. They received a regimen of rest, light food, exercise, fresh air, and amusements. Although actual recovery rates are debatable, this approach, at the time, was deemed successful and became widely accepted as the ideal form of treatment for relatively well-to-do persons with mental illness in small, relatively homogeneous New England Protestant communities of that era.[42] The apparent successes of the moral treatment approach in the private sector led to attempts to adapt this model of mental health care to the public sector. However, by the 1840s, because of massive immigration and rapid urbanization, there was such a heterogeneous mass of people with

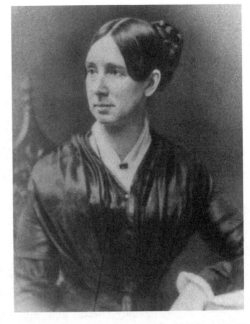

FIGURE 11.7
Dorothea Dix helped to establish public mental hospitals in many states.

mental illnesses that public asylums were soon overcrowded. The majority of those who were mentally and socially unfit again ended up in the urban almshouses, which were chronically underfunded and overpopulated. At this point, noted reformer Dorothea Lynde Dix (1802–1897) (see Figure 11.7) began a tireless campaign to establish public hospitals providing decent care to indigents with mental illness. When her lobbying for a federal law failed, Dix lobbied on a state-by-state basis. Her efforts were in most cases successful; all in all, Dix was personally involved in the founding of 32 public mental hospitals funded by individual states.[43]

moral treatment
treatment for mental illness based on belief that mental illness was caused by moral decay

The State Hospitals

The state mental hospitals were supposed to supply an environment in which medical care would be provided by professional staff, trained to work with each patient individually (see Figure 11.8). Initially, the upper limit of patients was set at 250 so that treatment could occur within the bonds of close personal relationships between caregiving staff members and patients, as prescribed in the methods of the moral treatment.

Unfortunately, even as new state hospitals continued to be built, the deterioration of those already in existence had begun. The chronic nature of mental illness was a large part of the problem. It became increasingly apparent that long-term or even lifetime stays were the norms for many patients.[43] "Maximum capacities" were quickly reached, exceeded, and repeatedly revised upward. The ability to provide personalized care was lost, as was the promise of significant medical treatment. Staff

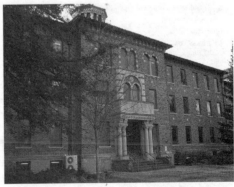

FIGURE 11.8
The state mental hospital was at one time viewed as the appropriate public response to the needs of those with mental illness.

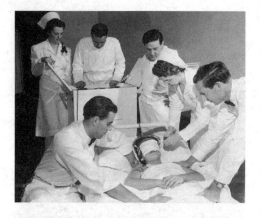

FIGURE 11.9
A team of doctors and nurses prepares to demonstrate the procedures involved in electroconvulsive therapy (shock treatment), 1942.

members were unable to reward patients for efforts at self-control, and physical restraints became more practical, especially in large wards.[40] As funding for these institutions became increasingly susceptible to state budget cuts, the level of care also diminished until all that remained was custodial care. The institutions at that point had become little more than places to "warehouse" people with mental illness. It became increasingly difficult to find dedicated staff to work at the unrewarding jobs in these institutions, and the turnover rate was high. Administration became more of a bureaucracy, and treatment and cure became almost nonexistent.

By 1940, the population in state mental institutions had grown to nearly one half million, many of whom were elderly and senile. Budget cuts continued, and caseloads per worker in the institutions became so large that only subsistence care was possible. In response to this situation, two new treatments began to gain prominence in psychiatric medicine—**electroconvulsive therapy (ECT)** and the lobotomy. In ECT, electric current is used to produce convulsions in the patient (Figure 11.9). The practice was introduced into the United States in 1939 and remains in use today because of its utility, cost-effectiveness, and short hospital stays.[44]

The **lobotomy**, where nerve fibers of the brain are severed by surgical incision, was first developed and used in dogs in Germany in 1890 and a couple of years later on patients with schizophrenia in Switzerland. Lobotomies were later popularized by a Portuguese neuropsychiatrist, Dr. Antônio Egas Moniz, and by American neurologist Walter Freeman. Freeman streamlined the procedure with his invention of the so-called ice-pick lobotomy, enabling him and other physicians to perform tens of thousands of lobotomies between 1939 and 1967.[45] The popularity of the lobotomy procedure grew after Moniz was awarded the Nobel Prize for Medicine and Physiology in 1949. However, later research found that following this irreversible operation only one-third of patients showed stable improvement, while another one-third became worse off. The appearance of new antipsychotic and antidepressive drugs in the 1950s made the widespread use of lobotomies unnecessary.[45]

Mental Health Care after World War II

In the postwar 1940s, a number of factors brought about greater federal involvement in mental health care. New feelings of optimism in the country, together with testimony before Congress by both military and civilian experts, soon resulted in the passage of the National Mental Health Act of 1946, which established the **National Institute of Mental Health (NIMH)**. Modeled after the National Cancer Institute, established in 1937, NIMH came under the umbrella of the National Institutes of Health. The purposes of the NIMH were (1) to foster and aid research related to the cause, diagnosis, and treatment of neuropsychiatric disorders; (2) to provide training and award fellowships and grants for work in mental health; and (3) to aid the states in the prevention, diagnosis, and treatment of neuropsychiatric disorders.[43] In 1950, a council of state governments suggested that more support was needed for research into the etiology of mental illness and treatment of those with mental illness so that these people could be discharged from mental institutions. During the early 1950s, public distress about the conditions in state mental hospitals continued to grow until the necessity of finding a new approach for caring for those with mental illness was clear and inescapable.[41]

electroconvulsive therapy (ECT) method of treatment for mental disorders involving the administration of electric current to induce a coma or convulsions

lobotomy surgical severance of nerve fibers of the brain by incision

National Institute of Mental Health (NIMH) the nation's leading mental health research agency, housed in the National Institutes of Health

Deinstitutionalization

The term **deinstitutionalization** has been used to describe the discharging of thousands of patients from state-owned mental hospitals and the resettling and maintaining of these discharged persons in less restrictive community settings. The magnitude of the process can be documented with the following statistics. In 1955, 322 state psychiatric hospitals served 558,922 resident patients.[46] By 1990, the number of patients had dropped to less than 120,000 (Figure 11.10), and by 2004 to less than 30,000.[46,47]

Deinstitutionalization, which began in the 1950s and continued through the 1980s, was not a preplanned policy. Rather, it was propelled by four forces that had been building up for more than half a century: (1) economics, (2) idealism, (3) legal considerations, and (4) the development and marketing of antipsychotic drugs.[41] Economically, there was not only a push, there was also a pull. The push was the states' need to reduce expenditures for mental hospitals so that more could be spent on the other three major state budgetary items—education, roads, and welfare. Meanwhile, a pulling economic force began to germinate with the prospect of profits from providing outpatient and inpatient services to those with mental illness. This prospect became brighter with changes in federal legislation (Medicare and Medicaid) enabling payment for these services with federal funds. (For more information about Medicare and Medicaid, see Chapter 13.)

In the early 1960s, questions began to be raised about the legality of keeping people locked up, especially if no real effort was being made to treat them. The American Bar Association published a study in 1961 of the laws relating to this issue. One of the points raised in its review was that people with mental disorders, even when institutionalized, had certain rights, including the right to treatment. The fundamental issue was "whether society, which is unable or unwilling to provide treatment, has the right to deprive a patient of his liberty on the sole grounds that he is in need of care."[46]

Over the ensuing decade, there was a subtle change in how the courts viewed civil commitment. There was more concern for the rights of individuals with mental illness—who

> **deinstitutionalization**
> the process of discharging, on a large scale, patients from state mental hospitals to less restrictive community settings

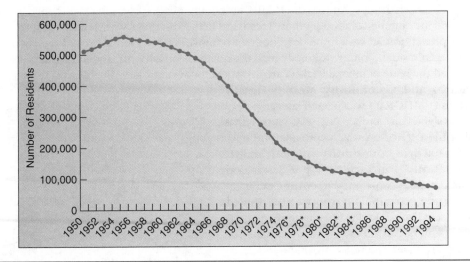

FIGURE 11.10

Number of resident patients in state and county mental hospitals at the end of the year, 1950–1994. Asterisk indicates linear interpolation.

Source: Frank, R. G., and S. A. Glied. Foreword by R. Carter. (2006). *Better but Not Well: Mental Health Policy in the United States Since 1950*, p. 55, figure 4.1 © 2006 The Johns Hopkins University Press, 55. Reprinted with permission of The Johns Hopkins University Press.

chlorpromazine (Thorazine)
the first and most famous antipsychotic drug, introduced in 1954 under the brand name Thorazine

Thorazine
(see *chlorpromazine*)

neuroleptic drugs
drugs that reduce nervous activity; another term for antipsychotic drugs

chemical straitjacket
a drug that subdues a mental patient's behavior

tardive dyskinesia
irreversible condition of involuntary and abnormal movements of the tongue, mouth, arms, and legs, which can result from long-term use of certain antipsychotic drugs (such as chlorpromazine)

Mental Retardation Facilities and Community Mental Health Centers (CMHC) Act
a law that made the federal government responsible for assisting in the funding of mental health facilities and services

were viewed as needing the courts' protection from inappropriate involuntary commitment—and less concern for society's right to be protected from these individuals.[41] Eventually, the test for involuntary civil commitment became one of whether these individuals could be considered dangerous to themselves or others.

Whereas economics, idealism, and legal considerations all helped to launch deinstitutionalization, another force expedited it—new antipsychotic drugs. The most widely used drug was **chlorpromazine**, introduced as **Thorazine** in 1954. Chlorpromazine was termed **neuroleptic** because it appeared to reduce nervous activity. When used in the institutional setting, the purpose of Thorazine and the other phenothiazines introduced later was to make patients more amenable to other forms of therapy. The drug did produce a remarkably calming effect in psychotic patients, and as a result, patients became more cooperative and hospital psychopathic wards became much quieter. So unusual were the effects of chlorpromazine that the drug in many cases became the only form of treatment provided. In these situations, a **chemical straitjacket** was said to have been substituted for a physical one.

In the haste to put this drug into use, some of its acute and chronic side effects were overlooked. Acute side effects (such as blurred vision, weight gain, and constipation) can cause compliance failures resulting in relapses or in attempts to self-medicate with other drugs, including drugs of abuse. Long-term use of chlorpromazine can result in deleterious consequences for the central nervous system. The most grave of these chronic side effects is **tardive dyskinesia**, the irreversible, involuntary, and abnormal movements of the tongue, mouth, arms, and legs.[40] Despite these deleterious effects, Thorazine and the other phenothiazines are still used extensively to treat psychotic patients.

Community Mental Health Centers

In 1961, the report of the Joint Commission on Mental Illness and Health (JCMIH) was released. The JCMIH, established in the 1950s, was made up of representatives of both the American Medical Association and the American Psychiatric Association along with members of several volunteer citizen groups. Among the JCMIH's recommendations was that acute mental illness be treated in community-based settings. Treatment in these settings was viewed as a form of secondary prevention, in which the development of more serious mental breakdowns would be prevented. President John F. Kennedy read the commission's report, and in February 1963, he addressed the issue of mental health care in a speech to Congress.[39] The **Mental Retardation Facilities and Community Mental Health Centers (CMHC)** Act was passed later that year and was signed on October 31, 1963. The original goal of the CMHC Act was to provide one fully staffed, full-time **community mental health center (CMHC)** in each of 1,499 designated catchment areas constituted to cover essentially 100% of the geographic territory in the United States (see Figure 11.11). Community mental health centers can meet the requirements for Medicare reimbursement by providing four core services: (1) outpatient services to older adults, children, and people with serious mental illness; (2) 24-hour-a-day emergency care; (3) day treatment or other partial hospitalization services; and (4) screenings to determine whether to admit patients to state mental facilities.[48] Although the CMHCs did provide mental health care

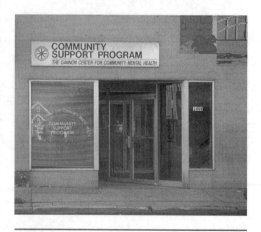

FIGURE 11.11
Between 1966 and 1989, 750 community mental health centers were established.

services to residents in the communities in which they were built, they did not live up to the expectation that they would also serve deinstitutionalized persons with chronic mental illness. The latter arrived in communities that in most cases could not provide the type of comprehensive social service network they needed. The necessary funding and services for this were simply not there.

Meanwhile, many older patients with chronic mental illness were never truly deinstitutionalized. Instead, they were **transinstitutionalized** to nursing homes, where the cost of their care was now paid for with federal, rather than state, funds and where the cost of the care turned out to be higher. In 1977, the NIMH responded to criticism that the CMHCs were not meeting the needs of deinstitutionalized people with chronic mental illness by creating the Community Support Program, which was the first recognition that the problems of people with chronic mental illness are—first and foremost—social welfare problems. This program offered grants to communities to develop needed social support systems to assist people with chronic mental illness with the resources necessary for successful independent living, namely, income, housing, food, medical care, transportation, vocational training, and opportunities for recreation.[49]

Despite all of the problems that have been attributed to deinstitutionalization, there have been some positive outcomes. One is that a majority of released mental patients surveyed have stated a preference for life in the community over life in an institution. Also, in some communities, halfway houses and support services were forthcoming once the need for these became clear. Finally, the quality of inpatient stays has improved and their duration has been shortened.

> **community mental health center (CMHC)** a fully staffed center originally funded by the federal government that provides comprehensive mental health services to local populations

> **transinstitutionalization** transferring patients from one type of public institution to another, usually as a result of policy change

MENTAL HEALTH CARE CONCERNS IN AMERICA TODAY

On balance, the experience of people with serious mental illness has improved in the 50 years since passage of the Community Mental Health Centers Act. Today nearly all of them live in the community, receive at least some treatment, have disability income, and enjoy civil liberties; some of them also lead productive lives.[47] However, specific challenges remain, including: (1) how to provide services to homeless people with serious mental illness and/or co-occurring substance use disorders, and (2) resolving the problem of the more than 1 million people with mental illness incarcerated in American jails and prisons.

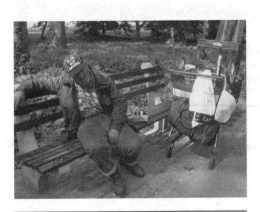

FIGURE 11.12

As many as two-thirds of all people with serious mental illness have experienced homelessness or been at risk for homelessness at some point in their lives.

Serious Mental Illness in People Who Are Homeless

More than 637,000 people are homeless during any given week in United States, and 2.1 million adults experience homelessness over the course of a year.[50] It is estimated that 80% of these homeless individuals are temporarily homeless, 10% are episodically homeless, and 10% are chronically homeless (see Figure 11.12).

Homeless people are more exposed to environmental factors such as extremes in temperature, moisture, burns, crowding, assaults, and motor vehicle-related injuries than are their domiciled counterparts. The effects of these environmental factors may be worsened by anxiety about where to find the next meal and safe shelter and, sometimes, by the effects of chronic alcohol or drug abuse.[51] About half of

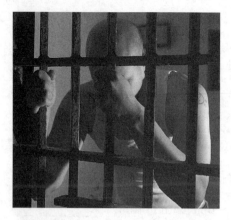

FIGURE 11.13

Many prison inmates with mental illness remain in prison years beyond their original sentence because they are unable to conform to good conduct requirements of the prison system.

all adults who are homeless have substance use disorders, and many have major depression and other co-occurring mental illness.[52]

Homeless people with mental illness generally have the same needs as other homeless people, and their most pressing need is safe, affordable housing. Successful interventions for homelessness require the provision of housing that these individuals choose and actually want to live in, and services they need.[53] If available at all, services to people who are homeless are often fragmented, although integration of medical, mental health, substance abuse, and housing services is possible.[54]

The New Asylums: Mental Health Care in Our Jails and Prisons

Given the cognitive and emotional deficits imposed by serious mental illness and the added risk of homelessness and other intense stressors, what relationship does serious mental illness have with other social problems, such as violent crime? On average, people with serious mental illness do perpetrate more violence than other people do, but a much bigger public health problem is that every year an estimated 35% of people with mental illness are victimized by violence.[55] Moreover, if people with mental illness are more likely to be violent, it isn't necessarily because of their mental illness because people with mental illness are also more likely to abuse substances and be poor, unemployed, uneducated, victimized, single or divorced, and have parents who themselves have arrest records. Controlling for these social context factors shows that having severe mental illness increases the risk of future violence only when accompanied by a history of past violence.[56]

That said, the criminal offender population does include many people who have serious mental illness. Some may originally have been arrested for relatively minor crimes, such as trespassing or stealing a bicycle, but remain in prison for years beyond their original sentence because they do not meet the good conduct guidelines required for release or parole (see Figure 11.13). Are local jails and state and federal prisons the most appropriate sites for housing and treating people with mental illness in this country? Although the answer is almost certainly no, data suggest that this is what occurs. According to a 2006 Department of Justice report, more than half of all prison and jail inmates have mental health problems.[57] This includes 705,600 inmates in state prisons, 70,200 in federal prisons, and 479,900 in local jails. These figures represent 56% of state prisoners, 45% of federal prisoners, and 64% of jail inmates (see Table 11.4). Furthermore, approximately 24% of jail inmates, 15% of state prisoners, and 10% of federal prisoners reported at least one symptom that meets the criteria for a psychotic disorder.[57]

Table 11.4
Prevalence of Mental Health Problems among Inmates in American Prisons and Jails, 2005

Mental Health Problem	State Prison Inmates		Federal Prison Inmates		Local Jail Inmates	
	Number	Percentage	Number	Percentage	Number	Percentage
Any mental health problem*	705,600	56.2	70,200	44.8	479,900	64.2
No mental health problem	549,000	43.8	86,500	55.2	267,600	35.8
Estimated number of inmates (June 30, 2005)	1,255,514	100.0	156,643	100.0	747,529	100.0

*Details do not add to totals because of rounding.

Source: James, D. J., and L. E. Glaze (2006). *Mental Health Problems of Prison and Jail Inmates.* Bureau of Justice Statistics Special Report (NCJ pub. no. 213600). Available at http://bjs.ojp.usdoj.gov/index.cfm?ty=pbdetail&iid=789. Accessed September 28, 2010.

A study published in 2004 revealed that rapid growth in the number of state prison facilities and the prison population has outstripped the slower growth of mental health services.[58] Thus, mental health services became less available to the prison population during that period, and even when services are available such care may amount to little more than medication without the supportive environment that is also needed to recover from mental illness. Incarceration can be countertherapeutic, particularly for minority women with schizophrenia or bipolar mood disorder, who face an elevated risk of sexual victimization in prison.[59] All of these problems come together in juvenile justice centers, where adolescents from diverse cultural backgrounds and with a variety of disorders, criminal convictions, and family problems receive little or no treatment, and sometimes only multiple forms of medication.[60]

In prison, severe mental illness (paranoid schizophrenia, **bipolar disorder**, or other serious mental disorder) may preclude inmates' compliance with their prescribed medication schedules. Without these medications, inmates with mental illness may be incapable of "good behavior," a prerequisite for parole or release. In fact, they may become candidates for placement in more isolated and restrictive prison units.[61]

For those whose mental illness is controlled with medication, and who remain on that medication, release is possible. Upon their release, these people are provided with enough medication for a short period (usually a 2-week supply). However, it can take up to 3 months to schedule an appointment with a physician to obtain a prescription for the needed medication. For this and other reasons, many of those released find it difficult to remain in compliance with their release documents. Whereas some, who are released directly to well-functioning community support programs or halfway houses, may experience extended periods of recovery, others find that it is all too easy to stop taking their medications. Their mental condition deteriorates, and their behavior becomes such that they end up back in prison.

For all these reasons, once released back into the community people with serious mental illness are more likely to commit another offense than are inmates without mental disorders, leading to recommendations that criminal justice practices with this population include "legal leverage" to compel treatment and special mental health courts.[62] Legal leverage applied to the patient to accept treatment may involve service providers taking control of the patient's disability income and/or suspending the patient's eligibility for subsidized housing.[63] Using such leverage is controversial, but with an increased risk of violence it represents an attempt to balance the values of civil rights and normalization with that of public safety. Mental health courts use judges who have special training and nonadversarial procedures that mandate treatment and rehabilitation of the individual rather than incarceration. Studies find increased amounts of treatment received by individuals diverted from criminal courts to mental health courts, improved functioning (e.g., less illicit drug use), less criminal recidivism even after court supervision ends,[64] and significant cost savings in comparison with criminal prosecution and incarceration.[65]

bipolar disorder
an affective disorder characterized by distinct periods of elevated mood alternating with periods of depression

Meeting the Needs of Those with Mental Illness: Prevention and Treatment

Meeting the needs of people with mental illness represents a significant challenge for many communities as they strive to provide effective and economical prevention and treatment services to this segment of the population.

Prevention

The basic concepts of prevention in community health are presented in Chapter 4. The concepts of primary, secondary, and tertiary prevention can be applied to community mental health. Application of prevention strategies is considered much more cost-effective than treatment.[66]

Primary prevention in community mental health has as its goal forestalling the onset of mental illness. Two examples are training in cognitive problem solving to prevent failure in school and social support groups for the newly widowed to prevent depression. Effective primary prevention reduces the incidence (rate of new cases) of mental illness in the community.

Secondary prevention, although not reducing the incidence of mental illness, can reduce its prevalence by shortening the duration of episodes, through case finding and prompt intervention. Employee assistance programs, juvenile delinquency diversion programs, and crisis intervention programs are all examples of secondary prevention of mental illness.

Tertiary prevention, treatment, and rehabilitation do not actually reduce the prevalence of mental illness in the community. Instead, they ameliorate the illness and prevent further problems for the individual and the community. Intensive community treatment programs, discussed later in connection with psychiatric rehabilitation, are examples of tertiary prevention.[66]

Preventive Services

Communities today are challenged with a difficult task in providing mental health care services for their members. These services need to be comprehensive, including primary, secondary, and tertiary prevention services.

psychotherapy
a treatment that involves verbal communication between the patient and a trained clinician

The task of providing primary prevention services falls mainly on the private voluntary agencies, such as the National Mental Health Association and its state and local affiliates. These agencies provide educational speakers, videos, books, and pamphlets about mental health, mental illness, and services. They also may offer workshops on stress management, self-esteem development, and coping-skills development. Some sponsor support groups for parents of children who are emotionally disabled or who suffer from some other behavioral disorder. These agencies also act as referral agencies for those in crisis.

The needs of those in the community who require mental health care (secondary prevention) are met by an assortment of providers, including treatment providers in private clinics, CMHCs, hospital emergency rooms, and social service providers in Social Security, welfare, veterans, and housing offices. For securing the necessary services, this hodgepodge of federal, state, and local offices and social programs is overwhelming even to someone in good mental health.

Although some would say that community mental health services are improving by and large, significant problems still remain. For example, a significant gap persists in the availability and quality of care for insured and uninsured patients. Continued federal and state budget constraints suggest that this gap will continue to widen.

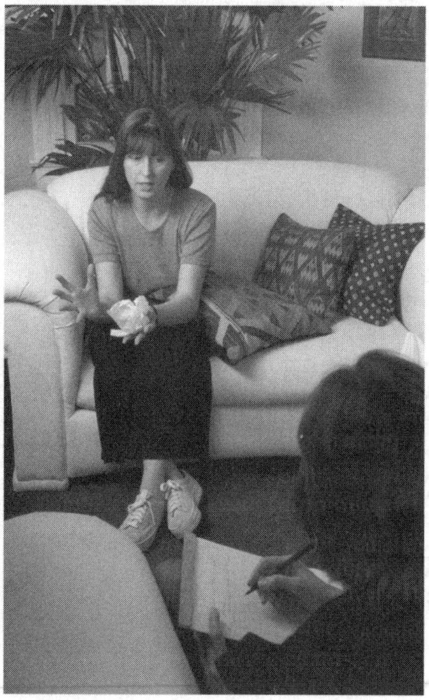

Treatment Approaches

Treatment goals for mental disorders are (1) to reduce symptoms, (2) to improve personal and social functioning, (3) to develop and strengthen coping skills, and (4) to promote behaviors that make a person's life better. The basic approaches to treating mental disorders include psychotherapy, psychopharmacology, and psychiatric rehabilitation.[6]

Psychotherapy

Psychotherapy, or psychosocial therapy, involves treatment through verbal communication (see Figure 11.14). There are numerous approaches to psychotherapy, including interpersonal, couple, group, and family formats. Psychodynamic psychotherapy examines current problems as they relate to earlier experiences, even from childhood, while cognitive psychotherapy focuses on current thinking patterns that are faulty or distorted. **Cognitive-behavioral therapy** focuses on how maladaptive feelings and behaviors are the result of distorted

FIGURE 11.14
Psychotherapy is usually only one of the services needed by persons who are suffering from mental illness.

thinking, and it uses structured procedures to promote new thought patterns and regular homework between sessions to practice more effective coping responses. Included in behavioral therapy are biofeedback, stress management, and relaxation training. In general, psychotherapy is most likely to be successful in less severe cases of emotional distress or when used in conjunction with other approaches (such as psychopharmacological therapy).

Psychopharmacology

Psychopharmacological therapy involves treatment with medications, a biological approach that is more "user friendly" than lobotomy or ECT. This treatment is based on the recognition that mental illnesses are medical illnesses just like hypothyroidism or diabetes and as such are treatable with drugs. Since the introduction of chlorpromazine in 1954, there has been a significant increase in the number and types of approved medications for the treatment of mental disorders. Conditions for which medications exist are schizophrenia, bipolar disorder, major depression, anxiety, panic disorder, and obsessive-compulsive disorder, although not everyone who has these disorders responds to medication.[67] Furthermore, because some of these drugs have serious side effects, and because of the nature of mental illness itself, almost half of patients may not cooperate fully in taking their medications.[68]

Another form of biomedical therapy is ECT, formerly known as shock therapy. In ECT, which was discussed earlier in this chapter, alternating electric current passes through the brain to produce unconsciousness and a convulsive seizure. This form of treatment is sometimes used for major depression, selected cases of schizophrenia, and overwhelming suicide ideation, especially when the need for treatment is seen as urgent. Contemporary ECT methods employ low doses of electric shock to the brain. General anesthetics are provided to reduce the unpleasant side effects.

Psychiatric Rehabilitation

One of the objectives of *Healthy People 2020* is to increase the proportion of adults with mental disorders who are receiving treatment (see Box 11.2). Unfortunately, the same force that

cognitive-behavioral therapy treatment based on learning new thought patterns and adaptive skills, with regular practice between therapy sessions.

psychopharmacological therapy treatment for mental illness that involves medications

---

BOX
11.2

HEALTHY PEOPLE 2020: OBJECTIVE

Mental Health and Mental Disorder Objectives

Objective MHMD-9: Increase the proportion of adults with mental disorders who receive treatment.

Targets and baselines:

Objective		2008 Baseline	2020 Target
MHMD-9.1	Adults aged 18 years and older with serious mental illness	58.7%	64.6%
MHMD-9.2	Adults aged 18 years and older with major depressive episode	68.3%	75.1%

Target setting method: 10% improvement.

Data source: National Survey on Drug Use and Health (NSDUH), SAMHSA.

For Further Thought

Just over half of adults with serious mental illness received treatment in 2008. What reasons do you think contribute to this statistic? Do you think the new Mental Health Parity and Addiction Act of 2008 (see page 330) will help to increase the proportion of those who receive treatment so that the *Healthy People 2020* target (10% increase) can be met? One third of adults with major depressive episodes do not receive treatment. How

would reaching the *Healthy People 2020* target (10% increase in the proportion of adults with major depression who receive treatment) affect the overall adult suicide rate?

Source: U.S. Department of Health and Human Services, Office of Disease Prevention and Health Promotion (2010). *Healthy People 2020.* Available at http://www.healthypeople.gov/2020/default.aspx. Accessed December 2, 2010.

recovery
outcome sought by most people with mental illness; includes increased independence, effective coping, supportive relationships, community participation, and sometimes gainful employment

psychiatric rehabilitation
intensive, individualized services encompassing treatment, rehabilitation, and support delivered by a team of providers over an indefinite period to individuals with severe mental disorders to help them maintain stable lives in the community

evidence-based practices
ways of delivering services to people using scientific evidence that shows that the services actually work

is driving most of the other types of health care decisions, namely, cost, also drives decisions about treatment for mental disorders. Thus, treatment goals are becoming more and more outcome based.

We have seen that mental disorders are widely prevalent and can begin in adolescence, or even earlier. They entail not only neurobiological lesions that produce distortions in thinking and feeling but also deficits in coping skills that damage relationships, and stigma that interferes with social acceptance. Mental disorders can last a lifetime, and most who have them simply live with their symptoms (e.g., people with schizophrenia learn to tolerate voices in their head) just as people with chronic arthritis or diabetes live with their disabilities. Thus, today the goal of treating mental disorders is most often one of "recovery" instead of cure. **Recovery** means progress toward financial and residential independence, coping effectively with symptoms, satisfaction with life, and basic "personhood"—that is, mental and physical well-being, supportive relationships, opportunities to spend time productively, and freedom to exercise the adult rights and privileges that come with community life.[69]

Recovery requires *change*, such as community participation in the form of work, volunteer activities, the forming of new relationships, and sometimes parenthood. Change is difficult and brings the risk of added stress, making daily pursuit of recovery a challenge to persons with mental illness and the providers who work with them. The current recovery-oriented services are collectively known as **psychiatric rehabilitation**.[70] Psychiatric rehabilitation arose in emulation of rehabilitation practices for people with physical and developmental disabilities (e.g., independent living, gainful employment) and its services often carry the modifier *support* (as in supported employment, supported housing, supported education) in keeping with patient self-determination. There is a strong emphasis on changing the environment through accommodations at work or school (e.g., extended time to complete tests and other assignments, use of aids such as tape recorders, and frequent breaks), and **evidence-based practices**, which are services supported by consistent evidence that they improve patient outcomes. In addition, staff represent diverse professional backgrounds (psychiatry, nursing, addictions, social work, and vocational services) and work collaboratively as an integrated team. Sometimes these team members are themselves recovering from mental illness, which brings a different perspective to the team's efforts.

One of the best-known and most successful models of psychiatric rehabilitation is the Madison (Wisconsin) Model, also called Assertive Community Treatment (ACT). ACT delivers intensive, individualized services encompassing treatment, rehabilitation, and support over an indefinite period. Active outreach is extended to individuals with severe mental disorders to help them maintain stable lives in the community (e.g., finding a place to live, learning self-care skills needed for independence, using public transportation).[49] Studies have shown that ACT reduces both hospital use and costs. As the Madison Model becomes disseminated into more communities and tested, the effectiveness of such structured, intensive services in promoting successful recovery will become clearer.[71]

Interestingly, recovery from disorders such as schizophrenia tends to be better (with longer remissions and fewer relapses) in the developing world, including Africa, India, and Indonesia, than in developed countries such as the United States, Canada, and Denmark.[72] Rather than being socially isolated, homeless, or in jail, for example, people in India who have schizophrenia are usually married and living with their families.[73] Non-Western cultures use less stigmatizing explanations for mental illness and prescribe a recovery process that includes collaborative roles for everyone—patient, family, and community. In Tanzania, for example, supernatural spirits are believed to cause mental illness, which is seen as a stern test by God that a faithful person should accept with patience and grace. A person with mental illness is not a source of embarrassment needing coercion but a family member or neighbor whose odd behavior is dealt with gently and, if possible, without confrontation.[74] The lesson in recovery provided by these "less developed" parts of the world is that mental disorders such as schizophrenia are not just "broken brains" but also culturally determined social and moral phenomena that involve all of us.

Self-Help Groups

Another approach or adjunct to successful treatment is **self-help groups**, comprising concerned members of the community who are united by a shared interest, concern, or deficit not shared by other members of the community. The shared characteristic is often stigmatizing or isolating and viewed as something not normal by the rest of the members of the community.[66] Self-help groups usually operate without professional leadership; instead, leadership responsibilities are often shared by members of the group. The roles of help-giver and help-receiver are entirely interchangeable. These groups serve to replace the community that was "lost" through stigmatization or isolation. Self-help groups supply feedback and guidance to their members based on the unique insights gained from their own recovery and provide their members with a philosophy and an outlook on their affliction.[66] Examples of self-help groups are the **National Alliance on Mental Illness (NAMI)**, Recovery, Inc., and Alcoholics Anonymous (AA). For more information on NAMI, see Box 11.3.

Mental health care in the United States faces a variety of challenges. Multiple services are needed by people with severe or comorbid disorders, and lack of some services (such as for addictions) limits the effectiveness of other services (e.g., ACT). Staff turnover is relatively high in behavioral health care,[75] and successful psychosocial rehabilitation requires sustained commitment by staff to the principles of evidence-based practice and patient recovery.[76] People with serious mental illness still face high rates of poverty, social disadvantage, and stigma, and substantial recovery (e.g., stable, gainful employment) is achieved by relatively few of them.[47] Related to all these problems are the immediate and longer-term needs of family members of people with mental illness for information, financial help, coping with stigma, and sometimes therapeutic support for themselves.[77]

The mental health care system is very decentralized and fragmented, with many different kinds of providers.[47] In 2006, there were about 350,000 licensed providers of mental health services (including psychiatrists, psychologists, social workers, psychiatric nurses, licensed

self-help groups groups of concerned members of the community who are united by a shared interest, concern, or deficit not shared by other members of the community (Alcoholics Anonymous, for example)

National Alliance on Mental Illness (NAMI) a national self-help group that supports the belief that major mental disorders are brain diseases that are of genetic origin and biological in nature and are diagnosable and treatable with medications

---

| BOX **11.3** | NATIONAL ALLIANCE ON MENTAL ILLNESS |

The National Alliance on Mental Illness (NAMI) "is the nation's largest grassroots mental health organization dedicated to improving the lives of persons living with serious mental illness and their families. Founded in 1979, NAMI has become the nation's voice on mental illness, a national organization including NAMI organizations in every state and in over 1,100 local communities across the country who join together to meet the NAMI mission through advocacy, research, support, and education."

According to its mission statement, "NAMI is dedicated to the eradication of mental illnesses and to the improvement of the quality of life of all whose lives are affected by these diseases." NAMI members, leaders, and friends share the agency's mission of "support, education, advocacy, and research for people living with

mental illness through various activities" that include maintaining a Web site and toll-free help line, sponsoring a Mental Illness Awareness Week, and maintaining a public education speakers bureau.

NAMI also provides a cadre of educational programs and a network of support groups. NAMI "advocates on the federal level to ensure nondiscriminatory and equitable federal and private-sector policies are in place as well as a commitment to research for the treatment and cures for mental illness." As with other voluntary health organizations, NAMI is involved in fund-raising, and does so with events such as NAMI Walks and an annual black-tie event, the Unmasking Mental Illness Science and Research Gala, held in Washington, DC.

More information about NAMI is available at their Web site: www.NAMI.org.

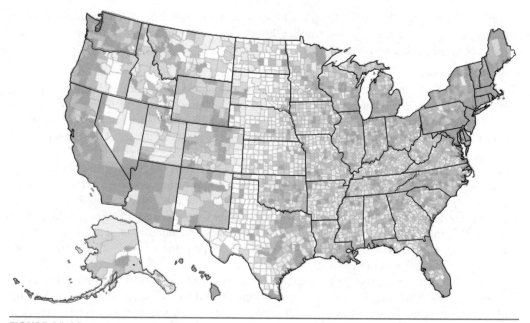

FIGURE 11.15

Number of mental health professionals, by county, among counties with mental health professionals. (The darker the shading, the higher the number of mental health professionals per 10,000 population.)

Source: Ellis, A., Konrad,T., Thomas, K., and Morrissey, J. (2009). "County-Level Estimates of Mental Health Professional Supply in the United States." *Psychiatric Services, 60:* 1315–1322. Reprinted with permission from Psychiatric Services (Copyright 2009). American Psychiatric Association.

counselors, and marital/family therapists) in the United States, but relatively few of them served rural and low-income counties (Figure 11.15).[78] Furthermore, about one-fifth of persons receiving treatment for mental disorders drop out prematurely, most after only one or two sessions. Those more likely to drop out have low incomes, lack of health insurance, and multiple (comorbid) disorders and are often ethnic minorities.[79]

General medical practitioners treat the largest number of people with mental disorders, with specialty mental health providers, human services, self-help groups, and various combinations serving the rest.[80] Patient sex, ethnicity, geography, immigration status, sexual orientation, and income are all related to the likelihood of receiving help from one kind of provider rather than another. Although the prevalence of depression is similar across different ethnic groups, for example, African Americans and Mexican Americans receive significantly less treatment for depression than do other groups.[81] The problem here may not be overt discrimination, but a lack of "cultural competence"[82] on the part of providers regarding their multicultural patients' attitudes toward medications and medication side effects (such as weight gain), and patients' misguided expectations of treatment in the context of particular religious, spiritual, or folk beliefs.

Finally, in addition to their often pronounced deficits in thinking and coping, people with serious mental disorders tend to be among the poorest members of society and typically live in neighborhoods where crime, illicit drugs, victimization, homelessness, unemployment, and social disorganization are rampant. It may be too much to expect that medications, psychotherapy, psychosocial rehabilitation, and other circumscribed supports and services are enough to overcome these systemic problems. From this vantage point, it is not the people with mental disorders who fail, but rather the communities and social systems they live in that have failed.

Federal Initiatives for Mental Health Care

Until recently, the federal government's leadership in community mental health has been spotty. Although federal funds have been made available for research, surveillance, and goal setting for mental health, there has been less support for prevention, early intervention, and treatment for those with mental illness. The "decade of the brain" culminated in 1999 when the U.S. Department of Health and Human Services issued *Mental Health: A Report of the Surgeon General*. This comprehensive report attempted to put mental health and mental illness "front and center" among America's public health problems. It was more than just a status report, although it provided many useful statistics. It was an excellent compilation of mental health care services, service needs, and barriers to receiving these services[2] In 2002, President George W. Bush created the New Freedom Commission on Mental Health. The commission's report, *Achieving the Promise: Transforming Mental Health Care in America*, is available at the commission's Web site, www.mentalhealthcommission.gov.[83] As its title indicates, the commission's report calls for a transformed mental health care system; it establishes six goals, with recommendations for achieving each goal. The commission envisions a mental health system in which (1) Americans understand that mental health is essential to overall health, (2) mental health care is consumer and family driven, (3) disparities in mental health services are eliminated, (4) early mental health screening, assessment, and referral to services are common practices, (5) excellent mental health care is delivered and research is accelerated, and (6) technology is used to access mental health care and information. The report does a good job of identifying the burden of mental illness and the challenges America faces in transforming the systems involved in intervention, prevention, and treatment of mental disorders. However, the report stops short of describing a road map or scheme for the transformation, and it certainly doesn't recommend the expenditure of any additional federal funds to achieve the stated goals.

Some of the existing federal resources devoted to mental health could be spent more effectively. The federal Medicaid program pays more than half of publicly funded mental health care, and its policies and regulations, which vary from state to state, affect what services are covered. Depending on individual state policies, Medicaid may pay for traditional services such as inpatient hospitalization but not newer approaches such as psychiatric rehabilitation. In addition, state policies may inadvertently punish people with mental illness who find jobs and reach a certain income level by revoking their eligibility for coverage under Medicaid, depriving them of financial help for expensive medications and other treatment services.[84]

COMMUNITY MENTAL HEALTH AND MANAGED CARE

Until deinstitutionalization began in the 1950s, the state hospital system served as the de facto social insurance program for mental illness in the United States.[47] With dramatic increases in all health care costs since then, managed care organizations (MCOs) have had a substantial impact on community mental health care. One effect has been to reduce the cost of mental health services.[2] This reduction is achieved by removing overutilization, such as unnecessary hospitalization. For MCOs, the cost of providing care is of prime importance, and in each case cost must be justified by an outcome that is effective. The risks of cost containment are that it will diminish either access to care or quality of care. In addition, CMHCs have undergone a wave of consolidations to achieve vast economies of scale in their overhead costs. Today these corporations are responsible for much larger populations and geographic expanses than was envisioned by the 1963 law's neighborhood-based definition of a community.

The term created by the managed care industry that applies to mental health and substance abuse care is **behavioral health care services**.[85] Under managed care programs,

behavioral health care services
the managed care term for mental health and substance abuse/dependence care services

medical services are provided only when a condition is serious enough that care is considered "medically necessary." Whether this requirement has been met may be difficult to determine in cases when a patient with mental illness presents with a "behavioral health" condition. Furthermore, in treating "behavioral health" problems, there is rarely a consensus among the stakeholders as to what constitutes a good outcome. We noted earlier the strong emphasis today on evidence-based practices, where only those interventions for which there is evidence of effectiveness are to be used.

parity
the concept of equality in health care coverage for people with mental illness and those with other medical illnesses or injuries

Another issue in mental health care coverage is parity. **Parity** refers to the effort to treat mental health care financing on the same basis as financing for general health care services. It took several decades of active lobbying to achieve parity in the coverage of mental illness and addictions. Some of the reason was a lack of clarity surrounding the diagnosis and treatment of mental disorders, some was the complexity and fragmentation of the mental health service system, but the delay also reflected the stigma attached to mental illness.[47] Managed care helped to make parity possible because a managed care system of financing controls provider services (and thus costs) rather than consumer demand. The Mental Health Parity and Addiction Act of 2008 mandates that any limits on the number of visits per year, annual or lifetime dollars spent, and any deductibles or copayments be the same for both mental and physical disorders. The act does not require health insurance plans to cover mental illnesses and addictions or, if they do, to cover every diagnosis in the *DSM-IV*. What it does require is that if there is coverage of mental health or substance abuse disorders, there must be parity with physical disorders in any limitations or restrictions in coverage.[86] Given the critical role played by intensive, team-delivered, and highly individualized services such as ACT and supported employment, the consequences of parity for recovery from serious mental illness through psychiatric rehabilitation remain to be seen.

It is difficult to determine how the nation, states, and local communities will respond to the needs of those with mental illness in the future. It will depend on economics, the degree to which taxpayers have been personally touched by mental illness, and the degree to which they are willing to tolerate the spectacle of homeless people with mental illness in their communities and in their jails and prisons. A key task facing communities is to find ways to unite formal services and informal supports to promote recovery by people who are coping with mental disorders.

CHAPTER SUMMARY

- Mental illness constitutes a major community health concern because of its prevalence and chronicity and because of the social, cultural, and economic attention and resources it demands from all of us.

- Americans are afflicted with a variety of mental disorders, caused by genetic factors, environmental factors, or a combination of both. These disorders, which can range from mild to severe, are often chronic and may limit the ability of some of those afflicted to live independently.

- Stress, resulting from social and environmental forces, can have a detrimental influence on both physical and mental health. Combat-zone military veterans and survivors of and responders to natural and humanmade disasters are at especially high risk for developing mental disorders.

- Over the years, society's response to the needs of those with mental illness has been characterized by long periods of apathy interrupted by enthusiastic movements for new and enlightened approaches to care.

- Deinstitutionalization, in which thousands of mental patients housed in state and county hospitals were discharged and returned to their communities, was the most prominent movement of the twentieth century. The origins of many of the current problems in community mental health care, such as a large number of homeless people and prison inmates with mental illness, can be traced to this movement.

- The basic concepts of prevention in community health (primary, secondary, and tertiary prevention) can be applied to the prevention and treatment of mental disorders.

- Among the most common treatment approaches are psychotherapy, including cognitive-behavioral therapy, and psychopharmacology, which is based on the use of medications. Self-help groups provide additional support to people at risk for relapse.

- People with severe mental illness generally pursue recovery rather than cure. Recovery entails adaptive change, including increased independence, effective coping, supportive relationships, community participation, and sometimes gainful employment.

- Psychiatric rehabilitation programs for those living in our communities with mental illness, such as the Madison Model, show promise that with community support, many individuals can achieve the level of recovery necessary for them to be integrated successfully into their communities.

- Important issues face those concerned with providing services for people with mental disorders. One is finding ways to provide a variety of easily accessible preventive, intervention, and treatment services to people from culturally diverse backgrounds, with multiple problems and few resources, in a climate of cost containment under managed care.

REVIEW QUESTIONS

1. What is meant by the term *mental health*?
2. What are the characteristics of a mentally healthy person?
3. What is a mental disorder?
4. What is the *Diagnostic and Statistical Manual of Mental Disorders*, 4th edition, text revision (*DSM-IV-TR*)? How do issues of comorbidity and cultural competence affect the use of *DSM-IV-TR*?
5. Name and give examples of the different causes of mental disorders.
6. What evidence is there that mental illness is one of our most pervasive public health problems in the United States?
7. What is stress? Give some examples of stressors.
8. How can stress cause physical illness?
9. What is the relationship between stress and mental health?
10. How were those with mental illness cared for in Colonial America?
11. What was included in Tuke's therapy known as "moral treatment"?
12. What role did Dorothea Dix play in the treatment of indigent people with mental illness?
13. How would you characterize the treatment of those with mental illness in state hospitals prior to World War II?
14. What piece of legislation resulted in the establishment of the National Institute of Mental Health, and what were the purposes of the institute?
15. Define the word *deinstitutionalization*. When did it start in the United States? What caused it?
16. What is a "chemical straitjacket"?
17. Why was there a movement toward community mental health centers in the early 1960s?
18. What services are provided by community mental health centers?

SCENARIO: ANALYSIS AND RESPONSE

1. Let's assume that Maria Sanchez is not alone in her concerns about Lynn, her new neighbor. Another neighbor, Paul, has called for a meeting of the residents to discuss this "new type" of resident. You are a resident too, and he is expecting you to attend. What is your response?
2. What worries might residents express regarding their new neighbor?
3. Would it make any difference to you whether Lynn found a job and was away at work during a good part of the day?
4. Do you suppose the landlord knew about Lynn's medical history when he or she rented the unit to her? Can landlords refuse to rent to someone like Lynn?
5. Are you aware of any federal laws, such as the Fair Housing Act or the Americans with Disabilities Act (ADA), that could bear on this matter?
6. If you were Maria, what would be your response? What would you do?

Source: Substance Abuse and Mental Health Services Administration Resource Center to Address Discrimination and Stigma. "Combating NIMBYism in Providing Housing to People Who Have Mental Illness." Available at http://www.stopstigma.samhsa.gov/archtel_pdfs/combatingNIMBY.pdf.

19. Why was the Community Support Program considered a novel approach?

20. Approximately what percentage of the homeless are living with mental illness? What percentage of state prison inmates have mental health problems?

21. How are legal leverage and mental health courts used to reduce the problem of people with mental illness ending up in jail or prison?

22. Describe primary, secondary, and tertiary prevention of mental illness and give an example of a service for each level of prevention.

23. What is involved in psychotherapy for mental illness? In cognitive-behavioral therapy? In psychopharmacological therapy?

24. What is meant by "recovery" from serious mental illness? How do psychiatric rehabilitation services such as Assertive Community Treatment promote recovery?

25. What are self-help groups? How do they increase treatment effectiveness?

26. What kinds of challenges do mental health care efforts face early in the twenty-first century?

27. What are some issues surrounding managed care for those with mental illness?

28. What does parity mean with regard to health care services for people with mental illness?

ACTIVITIES

1. Make a list of all the stressors you have experienced in the last 2 weeks. Select two of the items on the list and answer the following questions about them:

   Did you realize the stressor was a stressor when you first confronted it? Explain.

   What physiologic responses did you notice that you had when confronted with the stressor?

   Have you confronted the stressor before? Explain your answer.

   What stress mediators (coping responses) do you have to deal with each of the stressors?

   Do you feel you will someday fall victim to a disease of adaptation?

2. Using a local telephone book or one from your hometown, identify the organizations in the community that you believe would provide mental health services. Then, create a list of the agencies/organizations. Divide the list into three sections based on the type of service (primary, secondary, tertiary prevention) offered. If you are not sure what types of services are offered, call the agency/organization to find out. After you have com-

pleted your list, write a paragraph or two about what you feel to be the status of mental health care in your community.

3. Make an appointment with someone in the counseling and psychological service center on your campus for an orientation to the services offered by the center. Most mental health services range from stress management to test anxiety to individual counseling. Find out what your school has to offer and write a one-page summary of available services.

4. Call agencies or service groups in your community to find out what services are needed for people who are homeless. Also find out how serious the homeless situation is in the community and what plans there are to deal with the problem. Summarize your findings in a two-page paper. Agencies or services to call include the American Red Cross, the local police department, the Salvation Army, the local soup kitchen, a community mental health center, local hospitals, local homeless shelters, and other shelters.

5. Look through your local phone book or call the community information/crisis center to locate a mental health or substance abuse self-help group. Call the group's number and find out what kinds of open meetings or public education activities they have.

COMMUNITY HEALTH ON THE WEB

The Internet contains a wealth of information about community and public health. Increase your knowledge of some of the topics presented in this chapter by accessing the Jones & Bartlett Learning Web site at **http://health .jbpub.com/book/communityhealth/7e** and follow the links to complete the following Web activities.

- Center for Mental Health Services
- National Institute of Mental Health
- National Alliance on Mental Illness

REFERENCES

1. Eaton, W., S. Martins, G. Nestadt, O. Bienvenu, D. Clarke, and P. Alexandre (2008). "The Burden of Mental Disorders." *Epidemiologic Reviews*, 30: 1–14.

2. Kessler, R. C., W. T. Chiu, O. Demler, and E. E. Walters (2005). "Prevalence, Severity, and Comorbidity of Twelve-Month *DSM-IV* Disorders in the National Comorbidity Survey Replication (NCS-R)." *Archives of General Psychiatry*, 62(6): 617–627.

3. Kessler, R. C., O. Demler, R. G. Frank, M. Olfson, et al. (2005). "Prevalence and Treatment of Mental Disorders, 1990–2003." *New England Journal of Medicine*, 352: 2515–2523.

4. Blanco, C., O. Mayumi, C. Wright, et al. (2008). "Mental Health of College Students and Their Non-College-Attending Peers." *Archives of General Psychiatry*, 65(12): 1429–1437.

5. Benton, S. A., J. M. Robertson, W. C. Tseng, F. B. Newton, and S. L. Benton (2003). "Changes in Counseling Center Client Problems across 13 Years." *Professional Psychology: Research and Practice*, 34(1): 66-72.

6. U.S. Department of Health and Human Services (1999). *Mental Health: A Report of the Surgeon General*. Rockville, MD: Substance Abuse and Mental Health Services Administration.

7. Office of the Surgeon General, U.S. Department of Health and Human Services (3 January 2001). "Surgeon General Releases a National Action Agenda on Children's Mental Health." HHS News. Available at http://www.surgeongeneral.gov/news/pressreleases/pressrelease children.htm.

8. American Psychiatric Association (2000). *Diagnostic and Statistical Manual of Mental Disorders*, 4th ed., text revision. Washington, DC: Author.

9. Moffit, T., H. Harrington, A. Caspi, et al. (2007). "Depression and Generalized Anxiety Disorder." *Archives of General Psychiatry*, 64: 651-660.

10. Holden, C. (2010). "Experts Map the Terrain of Mood Disorders." *Science*, 327: 1068.

11. Minsky, S., W. Vega, T. Miskimen, et al. (2003). "Diagnostic Patterns in Latino, African American, and European American Psychiatric Patients." *Archives of General Psychiatry*, 60: 637-644.

12. Seedat, S., K. Scott, M., Angermeyer, M., et al. (2009). Cross-National Associations between Gender and Mental Disorders in the World Health Organization World Mental Health Surveys." *Archives of General Psychiatry*, 66(7): 785-795.

13. Yanos, P., D. Rowe, K. Markus, and P. Lysaker (2008). "Pathways between Internalized Stigma and Outcomes Related to Recovery in Schizophrenia Spectrum Disorders." *Psychiatric Services*, 59: 1437-1442.

14. Akil, H., S. Brenner, E. Kandel, et al. (2010). "The Future of Psychiatric Research: Genomes and Neural Circuits." *Science*, 327: 1580-1581.

15. Miller, G. (2010). "Beyond *DSM*: Seeking a Brain-Based Classification of Mental Illness." *Science*, 327: 1437.

16. Substance Abuse and Mental Health Services Administration (2006). *Results from the 2005 National Survey on Drug Use and Health: National Findings* (Office of Applied Studies, NSDUH Series H-30; DHHS pub. no. SMA 06-4194). Rockville, MD: Author. Available at http://www.oas.samhsa.gov/NSDUH/2k5NSDUH/2k5results.htm.

17. Hamer, M., E. Stamatakis, and G. Batty (2010). "Objectively Assessed Secondhand Smoke Exposure and Mental Health in Adults." *Archives of General Psychiatry*, 67(8): 850-855.

18. Green, J., K. McLaughlin, P. Berglund, et al. (2010). "Childhood Adversities and Adult Psychiatric Disorders in the National Comorbidity Survey Replication I." *Archives General Psychiatry*, 67: 113-123.

19. Garcia-Moreno, C., H. Jansen, M. Ellsberg, et al. (2006). "Prevalence of Intimate Partner Violence: Findings from the WHO Multi-Country Study on Women's Health and Domestic Violence." *Lancet*, 368: 1260-1269.

20. Children's Defense Fund (2005). *The State of Children in America's Union 2005*. Washington, DC: Author. Available at http://www .childrensdefense.org/child-research-data-publications/data/state-of-americas-children-2008-highlights.pdf.

21. Manderscheid, R. W., and M. A. Sonnenschein, eds. (1996). *Mental Health, United States, 1996* (DHHS pub. no. SMA 96-3098). Washington, DC: U.S. Government Printing Office.

22. Galea, S., J. Ahern, H. Resnick, D. Kilpatrick, M. Bucuvalas, J. Gold, and D. Vlahov (2002). "Psychological Sequelae of the September 11 Terrorist Attacks in New York City." *New England Journal of Medicine*, 346(13): 982-1087.

23. Centers for Disease Control and Prevention (2006). "Health Hazard Evaluation of Police Officers and Firefighters After Hurricane Katrina—New Orleans, Louisiana, October 17-28 and November 30-December 5, 2005." *Morbidity and Mortality Weekly Report*, 55(16): 456-458.

24. Hoge, C., J. Auchterlonie, and C. Milliken (2006). "Mental Health Problems, Use of Mental Health Services, and Attrition from Military Service After Returning from Deployment to Iraq and Afghanistan." *Journal of the American Medical Association*, 295(9): 1023-1032.

25. Miniño, A. M., M. Heron, and B. L. Smith (2006). "Deaths: Preliminary Data for 2004." *National Vital Statistics Report*, 54(19): 1-52.

26. Kessler, R., G. Borges, and E. Walters (1999). "Prevalence of and Risk Factors for Lifetime Suicide Attempts in the National Comorbidity Survey." *Archives of General Psychiatry*, 56(7): 617-626.

27. Wilcox, H., C. Storr, and N. Breslau (2009). "Posttraumatic Stress Disorder and Suicide Attempts in a Community Sample of Urban American Young Adults." *Archives of General Psychiatry*, 66(3): 305-311.

28. Centers for Disease Control and Prevention (2009). "National Suicide Statistics at a Glance." Available at http://www.cdc.gov/violenceprevention/suicide/statistics/trends01.html.

29. Dumesnil, H., and P. Verger (2009). "Public Awareness Campaigns about Depression and Suicide: A Review." *Psychiatric Servics*, 60(9): 1203-1213.

30. Johnston, L. D., P. M. O'Malley, J. G. Bachman, and J. E. Schulenbert (2006). *Monitoring the Future National Survey Results on Drug Use 1975-2005. Vol. I: Secondary School Students* (NIH pub. no. 06-5883). Rockville, MD: National Institute on Drug Abuse. Available at http://monitoringthefuture.org/pubs/monographs/vol1_2008.pdf.

31. Holmes, T. H., and R. H. Rahe (1967). "The Social Readjustment Rating Scale." *Journal of Psychosomatic Research*, 11: 213-218.

32. Selye, H. (1946). "The General Adaptation Syndrome and Disease of Adaptation." *Journal of Clinical Endocrinology and Metabolism*, 6: 117-130.

33. Sarafino, E. P. (1990). *Health Psychology: Biopsychological Interactions*. New York: John Wiley & Sons.

34. Schneiderman, N., G. Ironson, and S. D. Siegel (2005). "Stress and Health: Psychological, Behavioral, and Biological Determinants." *Annual Review of Clinical Psychology*, 1: 607-628.

35. Baer, P. E., L. B. Garmezy, R. J. McLaughlin, A. D. Pokorny, and M. J. Wernick (1987). "Stress, Coping, Family Conflict, and Adolescent Alcohol Use." *Journal of Behavioral Medicine*, 10: 449-466.

36. Conway, T. L., R. R. Vickers, H. W. Ward, and R. H. Rahe (1981). "Occupational Stress and Variation in Cigarette, Coffee, and Alcohol Consumption." *Journal of Health and Social Behavior*, 22: 155-165.

37. House, J. S., K. R. Landis, and D. Umberson (1988). "Social Relationships and Health." *Science*, 241: 540-545.

38. Payne, W. A., D. B. Hahn, and E. B. Lucas (2006). *Understanding Your Health*, 9th ed. New York: McGraw-Hill Higher Education.

39. Grob, G. N. (1994). *The Mad among Us: A History of the Care of America's Mentally Ill*. New York: The Free Press.

40. Johnson, A. B. (1990). *Out of Bedlam: The Truth about Deinstitutionalization*. New York: Basic Books, 306.

41. Gerhart, U. C. (1990). *Caring for the Chronic Mentally Ill*. Itasca, IL: F. E. Peacock, 5.

42. Mosher, L. R., and L. Burti (1989). *Community Mental Health*. New York: W. W. Norton.

43. Foley, H. A., and S. S. Sharfstein (1983). *Madness and Government*. Washington, DC: American Psychiatric Press.

44. Rosenbach, M., R. Hermann, and R. Dorwart (1997). "Use of Electroconvulsive Therapy in the Medicare Population between 1987 and 1992." *Psychiatric Services*, 48(12): 1537-1542.

45. El Hai, J. (2005). *The Lobotomist*. New York: John Wiley & Sons.

46. Grob, G. N. (1991). *From Asylum to Community*. Princeton, NJ: Princeton University Press.

47. Frank, R. G., and S. A. Glied (2006). *Better But Not Well*. Baltimore: Johns Hopkins University Press.

48. Centers for Medicare and Medicaid Services (2002). "Medicare Expands Crackdown on Waste, Fraud, and Abuse in Community Mental Health Centers [Press release]." Available at http://archive.hhs.gov/news/press/1998pres/980929.html.

49. Levine, M., P. A. Toro, and D. V. Perkins (1993). "Social and Community Interventions." *Annual Review of Psychology*, 44: 525–558.

50. U.S. Department of Health and Human Services, Substance Abuse and Mental Health Services Administration (2003). *Blueprint for Change: Ending Chronic Homelessness for Persons with Serious Mental Illnesses and/or Co-occurring Substance Use Disorders* (DHHS pub. no. SMA-04-3870). Rockville, MD: Author.

51. Fischer, P. J., R. E. Drake, and W. R. Breakey (1992). "Mental Health Problems among Homeless Persons: A Review of Epidemiological Research from 1980 to 1990." In R. H. Lamb, L. L. Bachrach, and F. I. Kass, eds., *Treating the Homeless Mentally Ill: A Report of the Task Force on the Homeless Mentally Ill*. Washington, DC: American Psychiatric Association, 75–93.

52. Schanzer, B., D. Boanerges, P. E. Shrout, and L. M. Caton (2007). "Homelessness, Health Status, and Health Care Use." *American Journal of Public Health*, 97(3): 464–469.

53. Gulcer, L., S. Tsemberis, A. Stefancic, and R. M. Greenwood (2007). "Community Integration of Adults with Psychiatric Disabilities and Histories of Homelessness." *Community Mental Health Journal*, 43(3): 211–228.

54. Gilmer, T., A. Stefancic, S. Ettner, W. Manning, and S. Tsemberis (2010). "Effect of Full-Service Partnerships on Homelessness, Use and Costs of Mental Health Services, and Quality of Life among Adults with Serious Mental Illness." *Archives of General Psychiatry*, 67(6): 645–652.

55. Choe, J., L. Teplin, and K. Abram (2008). "Perpetration of Violence, Violent Victimization, and Severe Mental Illness: Balancing Public Health Concerns." *Psychiatric Services*, 59: 153–164.

56. Elbogen, E. and S. Johnson (2009). "The Intricate Link between Violence and Mental Disorder." *Archives of General Psychiatry*, 66(2): 152–161.

57. James, D. J., and L. E. Glaze (2006). *Mental Health Problems of Prison and Jail Inmates* (NCJ pub. no. 213600). Available at http://bjs.ojp.usdoj.gov/content/pub/pdf/mhppji.pdf.

58. Mandersheid, R. W., A. Gravesande, and I. S. Goldstrom (2004). "Growth of Mental Health Services in State Adult Correctional Facilities, 1988 to 2000." *Psychiatric Services*, 55(8): 869–872.

59. Wolf, N., C. Blitz, and J. Shi (2007). "Rates of Sexual Victimization in Prison for Inmates with and without Mental Disorders." *Psychiatric Services*, 58: 1087–1094.

60. Moore, S. (10 August 2009). "Mentally Ill Offenders Strain Juvenile System." *New York Times*, A1.

61. Frontline (2005). *The New Asylums*, [PBS Video]. Boston: WGBH Educational Foundation. Available at http://www.pbs.org/wgbh/pages/frontline/shows/asylums.

62. Baillargeon, J., I. Binswanger, J. Penn, B. Williams, and O. Murray (2009). "Psychiatric Disorders and Repeat Incarcerations: The Revolving Prison Door." *American Journal of Psychiatry*, 166: 103–109.

63. Swanson, J., R. Van Dorn, J. Monahan, and R. Swartz (2006). "Violence and Leveraged Treatment for Persons with Mental Disorders." *American Journal of Psychiatry*, 163: 1404–1411.

64. McNiel, D. and R. Binder (2007). "Effectiveness of a Mental Health Court in Reducing Criminal Recidivism and Violence." *American Journal of Psychiatry*, 164: 1395–1403.

65. Kuehn, B. (2007). "Mental Health Courts Show Promise." *Journal of the American Medical Association*, 297(15): 1641–1643.

66. Levine, M., D. D. Perkins, and D. V. Perkins (2004). *Principles of Community Psychology: Perspectives and Applications*, 3rd ed. New York: Oxford University Press.

67. Gaynes, B., D. Warden, M. Trivedi, et al. (2009). "What did STAR*D Teach Us? Results from a Large-Scale, Practical, Clinical Trial for Patients with Depression." *Psychiatric Services*, 60: 1439–1445.

68. Sajatovic, M., M. Valenstein, F. Blow, D. Ganoczy, and R. Ignacio (2007). "Treatment Adherence with Lithium and Anticonvulsant Medications among Patients with Bipolar Disorder." *Psychiatric Services*, 58: 855–863.

69. Ware, N., K. Hopper, T. Tugenberg, et al. (2007). "Connectedness and Citizenship: Redefining Social Integration." *Psychiatric Services*, 58: 469–474.

70. Corrigan, P., K. Mueser, G. Bond, R. Drake, and P. Solomon (2008). *Principles and Practice of Psychiatric Rehabilitation: An Emprirical Approach*. New York: Guilford.

71. Salyers, M., and S. Tsemberis (2007). "ACT and Recovery: Integrating Evidence-Based Practice and Recovery Orientation on Assertive Community Treatment Teams." *Community Mental Health Journal*, 43: 619–641.

72. Hopper, K. (2004). "Interrogating the Meaning of "Culture" in the WHO International Studies of Schizophrenia." In J. Jenkins and R. Barrett, eds., *Schizophrenia, Culture, and Subjectivity: The Edge of Experience*. Cambridge, UK: Cambridge University Press, 62–86.

73. Miller, G. (2006). "A Spoonful of Medicine—and a Steady Diet of Normality." *Science*, 311: 464–465.

74. McGruder, J. (2004). "Madness in Zanzibar: An Exploration of Lived Experience." In J. Jenkins and R. Barrett, eds., *Schizophrenia, Culture, and Subjectivity: The Edge of Experience*. Cambridge, UK: Cambridge University Press, 255–281.

75. Woltmann, E. M., R. Whitley, G. J. McHugo, et al. (2008). "The Role of Staff Turnover in the Implementation of Evidence-Based Practices in Mental Health Care." *Psychiatric Services*, 59: 732–737.

76. Marshall, T., C. A. Rapp, D. R. Becker, and G. R. Bond (2008). "Key Factors for Implementing Supported Employment." *Psychiatric Services*, 59: 886–892.

77. Drapalski, A. L., T. Marshall, D. Seybolt, et al. (2008). "Unmet Needs of Families of Adults with Mental Illness and Preferences Regarding Family Services." *Psychiatric Services*, 59: 655–662.

78. Ellis, A., T. Konrad, K. Thomas, and J. Morrissey (2009). "County-Level Estimates of Mental Health Professional Supply in the United States." *Psychiatric Services*, 60: 1315–1322.

79. Olfson, M., R. Mojtabai, N. Sampson et al. (2009). "Dropout from Outpatient Mental Health Care in the United States." *Psychiatric Services*, 60: 898–907.

80. Wang, P., O. Demler, M. Olfson, et al. (2006). "Changing Profiles of Service Sectors Used for Mental Health Care in the United States." *American Journal of Psychiatry*, 163: 1187–1198.

81. Gonzalez, H., W. Vega, D. Williams, et al. (2010). "Depression Care in the United States." *Archives of General Psychiatry*, 67: 37–46.

82. Hernandez, N., T. Nesman, D. Mowery, et al. (2009). "Cultural Competence: A Literature Review and Conceptual Model for Mental Health Services." *Psychiatric Services*, 60: 1046–1050.

83. President's New Freedom Commission on Mental Health (2003). *Achieving the Promise: Transforming Mental Health Care in America*. Rockville, MD: Author.

84. Day, S. (2006). "Issues in Medicaid Policy and System Transformation: Recommendations from the President's Commission." *Psychiatric Services*, 57: 1713–1718.

85. Edmunds, M., R. Frank, M. Hogan, D. McCarty, R. Robinson-Beale, and C. Weisner, eds. (1997). *Managing Managed Care: Quality Improvement in Behavioral Health*. Washington, DC: National Academy Press.

86. Centers for Medicare and Medicaid Services (2010). "The Mental Health Parity and Addiction Equity Act." Available at https://www.cms.gov/HealthInsReformforConsume/04_TheMentalHealthParityAct.asp.

Chapter 12

Alcohol, Tobacco, and Other Drugs: A Community Concern

Chapter Outline

Chapter Objectives

After studying this chapter, you will be able to:

1 Identify personal and community consequences of alcohol and other drug abuse.

2 Describe the trends of alcohol and other drug use by high school students.

3 Define *drug use, misuse,* and *abuse.*

4 Define *drug dependence.*

5 List and discuss the risk factors for the abuse of alcohol and other drugs.

6 Explain why alcohol is considered the Number 1 drug abuse problem in America.

7 Describe the health risks of cigarette smoking.

8 Define the terms *over-the-counter* and *prescription drugs* and explain the purposes of these drugs and how they are regulated.

9 Define the terms *controlled substances* and *illicit (illegal) drugs* and provide examples.

10 Characterize recent trends in the prevalence of drug use among American high school seniors.

11 List and explain four elements of drug abuse prevention and control.

12 Give an example of primary, secondary, and tertiary prevention activities in drug abuse prevention and control programs.

13 Summarize the federal government's drug abuse control efforts.

14 List and describe an effective community and an effective school drug abuse prevention program.

15 List the five facets of a typical workplace substance abuse prevention program.

16 Name some voluntary health agencies and self-help support groups involved in the prevention, control, and treatment of alcohol, tobacco, and other drug abuse.

SCENARIO

Larissa started doing methamphetamine at 17. She had seen all of the TV ads about "your brain on drugs," but did not see herself in that role. She would sneak out to party with friends, at first on weekends, and then almost every night, and then every night. But that didn't make her an addict, she thought. She didn't sleep or eat much at home, but pretended to be asleep when her parents, who worked almost all of the time, were at home. If her parents left her food, she would put it in the garbage disposal so they would think she had eaten it. When they noticed her weight loss, she told them she had developed an eating disorder, but was correcting it.

Eventually meth became the most important thing in Larissa's life. She dropped out of school and moved in with her friend Dustin, who was cooking meth. The cooking made a mess and smelled, so she and Dustin kept moving to different motels. They even lived outside in the woods for a while. They had no money.

When Larissa became pregnant, she stopped using and moved back with her parents. Two months after her son Jarod was born, Larissa met Dustin and began using again. She left Jarod with her parents; she cared only about methamphetamine. She began injecting meth and developed abscesses on her arms. Dustin was gone a lot now, and she began to feel hopeless. She decided to end her life. One day, while Larissa was thinking about how to end her life, the police arrived and arrested her. She weighed 95 pounds and looked like a ghost. As she sat in jail, she realized that she was just the same as all of the other addicts she'd seen. She decided to enter a rehabilitation program.

INTRODUCTION

The use, misuse, and abuse of mind-altering substances undoubtedly predates our recorded history. It is perhaps part of human nature to wish to experience strange and unusual feelings or changes in mood and perceptions. Early civilizations may have used drugs as a vehicle to communicate with spirits. Even today, drugs are used for this purpose in some cultures.

For many Americans, drug-taking is experimental or social, a temporary departure from a natural, nondrugged physical and mental state. For many others, it is a misguided attempt to self-medicate or to cope with personal problems such as depression, loneliness, guilt, or low self-esteem. For a small but significant segment of the population, drug-taking ceases to be a matter of conscious choice; these people have become chronic drug abusers or drug dependent. In most cultures, chronic alcohol or other drug abuse or dependence is regarded as destructive behavior, both to oneself and to the surrounding community. Community members whose lives center around drug acquisition and use usually provide little benefit to their communities and often detract from their communities.

Scope of the Current Drug Problem in the United States

It is difficult to argue with those who state that the abuse of alcohol, tobacco, and other drugs is the nation's number 1 community health problem. More deaths, illnesses, and disabilities can be attributed to substance abuse than to any other preventable health condition.[1] One-fourth of the 2 million deaths each year are due to alcohol, tobacco, or illicit drug use (see Table 12.1). Estimates of the economic cost of substance abuse in the United States vary in range between $414 billion and $487 billion per year.[1,2] These estimates include direct costs (such as health care expenditures, premature death, and impaired productivity) and indirect costs, which include the costs of crime and law enforcement, courts, jails, and social work. Of the $487 billion annual drug bill, the cost of alcohol abuse and alcoholism is estimated at $220 billion, drug abuse at $110 billion, and smoking at $157 billion (see Table 12.1). Another study estimates that federal, state, and local governments spend $467.7 billion as a result of sub-

Table 12.1
The Annual Cost in Lives and Dollars Attributable to Alcohol, Tobacco, and Illicit Drug Abuse in the United States

Type of Drug	Estimated Number of Deaths Each Year	Economic Cost to Society (in Billions)
Alcohol	100,000	$220
Tobacco	430,000	$157
Illicit drugs	16,000	$110
TOTAL	546,000	$487

Sources: Horgan, C., K. C. Skwara, and G. Strickler (2001). *Substance Abuse: The Nation's Number One Health Problem.* Princeton, NJ: Robert Wood Johnson Foundation; and National Center on Addiction and Substance Abuse at Columbia University (2006). *The Commercial Value of Underage and Pathological Drinking to the Alcohol Industry: A CASA White Paper.* Available at http://www.casacolumbia.org/templates/Publications_Reports.aspx#r16. Accessed December 14, 2010.

stance abuse and addiction: $238.2 billion by federal, $135.8 by state, and $93.8 billion by local governments. This spending amounted to 10.7% of their entire $4.4 trillion budgets.[3] Clearly, the abuse of alcohol and other drugs is one of America's most expensive community health problems.

Those abusing alcohol and other drugs represent serious health threats to themselves, their families, and their communities. They are a threat to themselves and their families because they put themselves and their families at risk for physical, mental, and financial ruin. The habitual drug user may develop a psychological and/or **physical dependence** on the drug and thus experience great difficulty in discontinuing use, even in the face of deteriorating physical and mental health and erosion of financial resources. If the drug is an illegal one, its use constitutes criminal activity and may carry with it the added risks of arrest and incarceration.

Abusers of alcohol and other drugs represent a serious threat to the community because they have greater health care needs, suffer more injuries, and are less productive than those who do not. Community consequences range from loss of economic opportunity and productivity to social and economic destruction (see Table 12.2). Additionally, those who abuse drugs may perpetrate more violent acts that result in economic loss, injury, and death. The violence associated with the abuse of alcohol and other drugs is depicted in Figure 12.1.

physical dependence
a physiological state in which discontinued drug use results in clinical illness

Table 12.2
Personal and Community Consequences of Drug Abuse

Personal Consequences	Community Consequences
Absenteeism from school or work	Loss of productivity and revenue
Underachievement at school or work	Lower average SAT scores
Scholastic failure/interruption of education	Loss of economic opportunity
Loss of employment	Increase in public welfare load
Marital instability/family problems	Increase in number of broken homes
Risk of infectious diseases	Epidemics of sexually transmitted diseases
Risk of chronic or degenerative diseases	Unnecessary burden on health care system
Increased risk of accidents	Unnecessary deaths and economic losses
Financial problems	Defaults on mortgages, loans/bankruptcies
Criminal activity	Increased cost of insurance and security
Arrest and incarceration	Increased cost for police/courts/prisons
Risk of adulterated drugs	Increased burden on medical care system
Adverse drug reactions or "bad trips"	Greater need for emergency medical services
Drug-induced psychoses	Unnecessary drain on mental health services
Drug overdose	Unnecessary demand for medical services
Injury to fetus or newborn baby	Unnecessary use of expensive neonatal care
Loss of self-esteem	Increase in mental illness, underachievement
Suicide	Damaged and destroyed families
Death	

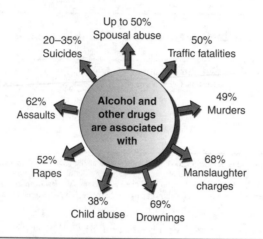

FIGURE 12.1

Violence associated with the use of alcohol and other drugs.

Source: National Clearinghouse for Alcohol and Drug Information (1995). *Making the Link* [Fact sheets]. Rockville, MD: Author.

According to the annual Monitoring the Future surveys on drug use among those in grades 8, 10, and 12, drug use declined steadily until 1992 and then rose again until 1996 or 1997, depending upon the grade. Overall illicit drug use began to decline gradually among eighth graders, while holding steady for older students, until 2002, when a general decline was noted.[4,5] The decline continued through 2008, but usage has still remained above the 1992 level (Table 12.3). For example, in 2008 the use of marijuana (in the past 30 days) was

Table 12.3
Percentage of High School Seniors Who Have Used Drugs

	Class of 1992			Class of 2008		
	Ever Used	**Past Month**	**Daily Use**	**Ever Used**	**Past Month**	**Daily Use**
Alcohol	87.5%	51.3%	3.4%	71.9%*	43.1%	2.8%
Cigarettes	61.8	27.8	17.2	44.7	20.3	11.4
Marijuana	32.6	11.9	1.9	42.6	19.4	5.4
Amphetamines	13.9	2.8	0.2	10.5	2.9	†
Methamphetamine	—	—	—	2.8	0.6	†
Inhalants	16.6	2.3	0.1	9.9	1.4	†
Cocaine	6.1	1.3	0.1	7.2	1.9	†
Tranquilizers	6.0	1.0	†	8.9	2.6	†
LSD	8.6	2.1	0.1	4.3	1.1	†
MDMA	—	—	—	6.2	1.8	†
Crack	2.6	0.6	0.1	2.1	0.8	†
PCP	2.4	0.6	0.1	1.8	0.6	†
Heroin	1.2	0.3	†	1.3	†	†

*More than just a few sips.
†Less than 0.05%.
— No data.

Sources: For 1992 data: Johnston, L. D., P. M. O'Malley, and J. G. Bachman (1993). National survey results from the Monitoring the Future study, 1975–1992. Volume I: Secondary School Students (NIH pub. no. 93-3597. Rockville, MD: National Institute on Drug Abuse.; and Johnston, L. D., P. M. O'Malley, J. G. Bachman, and J. E. Schulenbert (2009). Monitoring the Future National Survey Results on Drug Use 1975-2008, Volume I, Secondary School Students (NIH pub. no. 09-7402). Bethesda, MD: National Institute on Drug Abuse. Available at http://www.monitoringthefuture.org/pubs.html. Accessed December 15, 2010.

reported by 19.4% of high school seniors, compared with 22.4% in 2001, but only 11.9% in 1992. Use of any illicit drug other than marijuana (in the past 30 days) also showed a slight decline in recent years, from 11.0% in 2001 to 9.3% in 2008, but remained well above the 1992 figure of just 6.3%. Thirty-day use of one drug, MDMA (Ecstasy), declined significantly among high school seniors, however, from a high of 3.6% in 2000 to 1.8% in 2008.[5] It is interesting to note that college students report lower levels of usage of virtually all illicit drugs than high school seniors,[5] suggesting that drug-using high school seniors are less likely to attend college than their non-drug-using classmates.

When the words *drug abuse* are mentioned, most people think of illicit drugs, such as heroin, LSD, cocaine, and other illegal substances. Although the abuse of illicit drugs is certainly a major problem in America, abuse of alcohol and tobacco products are, perhaps, more serious challenges to America's health. Although the rate of cigarette smoking and alcohol consumption has declined among high school seniors since 1992, the rate of binge drinking (five or more drinks in a row) in the past 2 weeks (24.6%) remains high (see Figure 12.2).[5]

America has been trying to solve the problem of drug abuse for decades. Most adults who abuse drugs eventually "mature out" of the behavior, but there is a constant supply of potential drug users among America's children. This "generational forgetting" means that drug prevention education is never finished. Instead, drug prevention efforts must become a permanent part of our culture. That is, we must teach our children about the dangers of experimental drug use in the same way we teach them to look both ways before they cross the street.

Definitions

We begin a discussion of alcohol, tobacco, and other drugs as a community health problem by defining some terms. A **drug** is a substance, other than food or vitamins, that upon entering the body in small amounts alters one's physical, mental, or emotional state. **Psychoactive drugs** are drugs that alter sensory perceptions, mood, thought processes, or behavior.

In this chapter, the term **drug use** is a non-evaluative term referring to drug-taking behavior in general, regardless of whether the behavior is appropriate. **Drug misuse** refers primarily to the inappropriate use of legally purchased prescription or nonprescription drugs. For example, drug misuse occurs when one discontinues the use of a prescribed antibiotic before the entire prescribed dose is completed or when one takes four aspirin rather than two as specified on the label. **Drug abuse** can be defined in several ways depending upon the drug and the situation. Drug abuse occurs when one takes a prescription or nonprescription drug for a purpose other than that for which it is medically approved. For example, drug abuse occurs when one takes a prescription diet pill for its mood altering effects (stimulation). The abuse of legal drugs such as nicotine or alcohol is said to occur when one is aware that continued use is detrimental to one's health. Because illicit drugs have no approved medical uses, any illicit drug use is considered drug abuse. Likewise, the use of alcohol and nicotine by those under the legal age is considered drug abuse.

Drug (chemical) dependence occurs when a user feels that a particular drug is necessary for normal functioning. Dependence may be **psychological**, in which case the user experiences a strong emotional or psychological desire to continue use of the drug even though clinical signs of physical illness may not appear; or it can be physical, in which

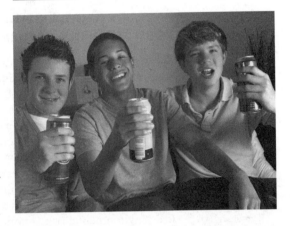

FIGURE 12.2
The prevalence of alcohol use among American high school seniors in the middle and late 1990s remained high, while cigarette smoking rose dramatically.

drug
a substance other than food that when taken in small quantities alters one's physical, mental, or emotional state

psychoactive drugs
drugs that alter sensory perceptions, mood, thought processes, or behavior

drug use
a non-evaluative term referring to drug-taking behavior in general; any drug-taking behavior

drug misuse
inappropriate use of prescription or nonprescription drugs

discontinuation of drug use results in clinical illness. Usually, both psychological and physical dependence are present at the same time, making the discontinuation of drug use very difficult. Such is frequently the case with cigarette smoking.

FACTORS THAT CONTRIBUTE TO ALCOHOL, TOBACCO, AND OTHER DRUG ABUSE

The factors that contribute to the abuse of alcohol, tobacco, and other drugs are many, and the decision to use drugs lies ultimately with the individual; it's a matter of choice. However, studies have determined that individuals are differentially at risk for engaging in drug-taking behavior.[6] Factors that increase the probability of drug use are called *risk factors;* those that lower the probability of drug use are called *protective factors.* People with a high number of risk factors are said to be vulnerable to drug abuse or dependence, while those who have few risk factors and more protective factors are said to be resistant to drug abuse.

Risk and protective factors can be either genetic (inherited) or environmental. Numerous studies have concluded that inherited traits can increase one's risk of developing dependence on alcohol, and it is logical to assume that susceptibility to other drugs might also be inherited. Environmental risk factors, such as one's home and family life, school and peer groups, and society and culture, have also been identified.

Inherited Risk Factors

The vast majority of the data supporting the notion that the risk of drug dependence can be inherited comes from studies on alcoholism. Evidence for the heritability of risk for alcoholism is provided by numerous studies,[7-9] which have been reviewed by Tabakoff and Hoffman[10] in the *Seventh Special Report to the U.S. Congress on Alcohol and Health,* from the Secretary of Health and Human Services.[11] Studies of alcoholics' families have found that there are at least two types of inherited alcoholism,[8] now referred to as Type I (or milieu-limited), and Type II (or male-limited) alcoholism.[11] These observational studies of alcoholics' families are supported by research using genetic and biological markers in animal models. Some of these markers predispose an individual biochemically to increased susceptibility to developing alcohol-related problems, while others may actually be protective in nature. For example, genes that code for enzymes that inhibit the normal metabolism of alcohol could cause one to respond positively to the effects of alcohol and thus to drink more, or respond negatively to alcohol and thus drink less or not at all.[10] A study has provided evidence in support of the idea that genes also influence cigarette smoking.[12] The heritability of susceptibility to other drugs is still under investigation.

Environmental Risk Factors

There are a great many environmental factors, both psychological and social, that influence the use and abuse of alcohol and other drugs. Included are personal factors such as the influences of home and family life, school and peer groups, and other components of the social and cultural environment.

Personal Factors

Personal factors include personality traits, such as impulsiveness, depressive mood, susceptibility to stress, or possibly personality disturbances. Some of these factors have been reviewed by Needle and colleagues.[13] Although models that involve personal factors provide frameworks for research and theorizing about the etiology of alcohol and drug abuse, they have their limitations. It is difficult to determine the degree to which these factors are inherited or are

---

drug abuse
use of a drug when it is detrimental to one's health or well-being

drug (chemical) dependence
a psychological and sometimes physical state characterized by a craving for a drug

psychological dependence
a psychological state characterized by an overwhelming desire to continue use of a drug

simply the product of the family environment. For example, one's choice to use alcohol or drugs in response to a stressful situation (and the outcome of that decision) could be the result of either inherited characteristics, learned behavior, or a combination of these factors.

Home and Family Life

The importance of home and family life on alcohol and drug abuse has been the subject of numerous studies, some of which have been reviewed by Meller[14] and by Needle and colleagues.[13] Research demonstrates that not all family-associated risk is genetic in origin. Family structure, family dynamics, quality of parenting, and family problems can all contribute to drug experimentation by children and adolescents (see Figure 12.3). Family turmoil (deaths and divorces) have been associated with the initiation of alcohol and other drug use.[13] In this sense, alcohol and drug use is a symptom of personal and/or family problems, not a cause.[15]

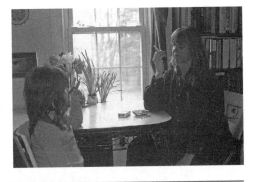

FIGURE 12.3
Influences of home and family life can affect one's decisions about alcohol, tobacco, and other drugs.

The development of interpersonal skills, such as communication skills, independent living skills, and learning to get along with others, is nurtured in the home. The failure of parents to provide an environment conducive to the development of these skills can result in the loss of self-esteem and increase in delinquency, nonconformity, and sociopathic behavior, all personal risk factors for alcohol and drug abuse.[11]

Finally, family attitudes toward alcohol and drug use influence adolescents' beliefs and expectations about the effects of drugs. These expectations have been shown to be important factors in adolescents' choices to initiate and continue alcohol use.[11] The age of first use of alcohol, tobacco, and illicit drugs is correlated to later development of alcohol and drug problems, especially if use begins before age 15.[16]

School and Peer Groups

Perceived and actual drug use by peers influences attitudes and choices by adolescents (see Figure 12.4). Some studies have shown that perceived support of drinking by peers is the single most important factor in an adolescent's choice to drink.[11] Peers can also influence expectations for a drug. Alcohol may be perceived as "a 'magic elixir' that can enhance social and physical pleasure, sexual performance and responsiveness, power and aggression and social competence."[11] It is interesting to note that these are precisely the mythical qualities about alcohol portrayed in advertisements for beer and other alcoholic beverages.

Sociocultural Environment

The notion of environmental risk includes the effects of sociocultural and physical settings on drug-taking behavior. The study of the effects of the physical and social environment upon the individual is termed *social ecology*.[17] Environmental risk for drug-taking can stem from one's immediate neighborhood or from society at large. For example, living in the inner city—with its sordidness, physical decay, and threats to personal safety—could set into motion a variety of changes in values and behaviors, including some related to alcohol or drug use.

Opportunities for community interventions exist, though. For example, federal, state, and local drug-prevention education programs, law enforcement successes, and treatment availability can

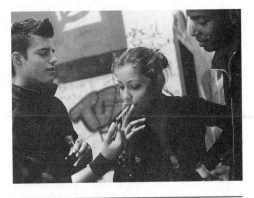

FIGURE 12.4
Peers can influence one's expectations of the effects of a drug.

improve the social environment and reduce the prevalence of drug abuse. Also, increasing taxes on tobacco products and alcoholic beverages and developing zoning ordinances that limit the number of bars and liquor stores in certain neighborhoods can be effective in reducing the alcohol, tobacco, and other drug problems in a community.

TYPES OF DRUGS ABUSED AND RESULTING PROBLEMS

Almost any psychoactive drug available is subject to abuse by at least some segment of the population. Classification systems of drugs of abuse are many, but none of them is perfect. Problems of classification arise because all drugs have multiple effects and because the legal status of a drug can depend upon its formulation and strength and, in some cases, upon the age of the user. In this chapter, our classification system includes legal drugs and illegal drugs. Legal (licit) drugs include alcohol, nicotine, and nonprescription and prescription drugs. Illegal (illicit) drugs can be classified further on the basis of physiological effects as stimulants, depressants, narcotics, hallucinogens, marijuana, and other drugs.

Legal Drugs

Legal drugs are drugs that can be legally bought and sold in the marketplace, including those that are closely regulated, like morphine; those that are lightly regulated, like alcohol and tobacco; and still others that are not regulated at all, like caffeine.

Alcohol

binge drinking
consuming five or more drinks in a row for males and four or more drinks in a row for females

Alcohol is the number 1 problem drug in America by almost any standard of measurement—the number of those who abuse it, the number of injuries and injury deaths it causes, the amount of money spent on it, and its social and economic costs to society through broken homes and lost wages. Alcohol is consumed in a variety of forms, including beer, wine, fortified wines and brandies, and distilled spirits. Although many people view distilled spirits as the most dangerous form of alcohol, it is now recognized that the form of alcohol involved in most heavy-episodic drinking is beer. Much of this beer is drunk by high school and college students, and much of this drinking is **binge drinking** (consuming five or more drinks on a single occasion for males and four or more drinks for females).

A major community health concern is underage drinking, that is, drinking by those younger than 21 years. An analysis has revealed that nearly 26% of underage drinkers meet clinical criteria for alcohol abuse or dependence, compared with 9.6% of adult drinkers.[2] Underage drinkers, many of them children and teenagers, can destroy their own lives and the lives of others through reckless driving, risky sexual behavior that can lead to disease transmission and unintentional pregnancies, and the commission of other violent and injurious acts. At issue is the fact that an estimated $22.5 billion, or 17% of all money spent on alcohol, can be accounted for by underage drinking.[2,18] The alcohol industry would take a huge hit if underage drinking were to stop. The industry relies on underage drinkers for two reasons: the amount of alcohol consumed by them and the fact that many pathological underage drinkers will become pathological adult drinkers, a group that accounts for $25.8 billion, or 20.1%, of the consumer expenditures for alcohol.[2,18]

Drinking by high school and college students continues to be very widespread despite the fact that it is illegal for virtually all high school students and for most college students to purchase these beverages. In 2008, 71.9% of high school seniors reported having drunk alcohol (more than a few sips) at least once in their lifetime, with 65.5% in the past year, and 43.1% in the past 30 days. More than one in four high school seniors reported having been drunk in the past 30 days.[5] Twenty-eight percent of high school seniors reported occasions of binge drinking at least once in the prior 2-week period. College students reported an even higher prevalence of binge drinking; 40% stated that they had consumed five or more drinks in a row in the past 2-week period. The rate of binge drinking among college students has not changed in the past 4 years.[5]

Most of those who experiment with alcohol begin their use in a social context and become light or moderate drinkers. Alcohol use is reinforcing in two ways: It lowers anxieties and produces a mild euphoria. For many people, alcohol use does not become a significant problem, but for about 10% of those who drink, it does. Some of these people become **problem drinkers**; that is, they begin to experience personal, interpersonal, legal, or financial problems because of their alcohol consumption. Still others lose control of their drinking and develop a dependence upon alcohol. Physical dependence on alcohol and the loss of control over one's drinking are two important characteristics of **alcoholism**. According to the *Journal of the American Medical Association:*

> *Alcoholism* is a primary, chronic disease with genetic, psychosocial, and environmental factors influencing its development and manifestations. The disease is often progressive and fatal. It is characterized by impaired control over drinking, preoccupation with the drug alcohol, use of alcohol despite adverse consequences, and distortions in thinking, most notably denial. Each of these symptoms may be continuous or periodic.[19]

The cost of alcohol abuse and alcoholism in the United States was estimated for 2005 to be $220 billion.[2] That is $740 for every man, woman, and child. To put it another way, it costs America $25 million every hour for alcohol-related problems. More than 60% of the cost is due to lost employment or reduced productivity, and 13% of the cost is due to medical and treatment costs. Health care costs for alcoholics are about twice those for nonalcoholics.[11]

Alcohol and other drugs are contributing factors to a variety of unintentional injuries and injury deaths. The risk of a motor vehicle crash increases progressively with alcohol consumption and **blood alcohol concentration (BAC)** (see Figure 12.5).

> Compared with drivers who have not consumed alcohol, the risk of a single-vehicle fatal crash for drivers with BAC's between 0.02 and 0.04 percent is estimated to be 1.4 times higher; for those with BAC's between 0.05 and 0.09 percent, 11.1 times higher; for drivers with BAC's between 0.10 and 0.14 percent, 48 times higher; and for those with BAC's at or above 0.15 percent, the risk is estimated to be 380 times higher.[20]

Young drivers are particularly at risk because they are inexperienced drivers and inexperienced drinkers. This combination can be deadly. One study found that 23% of drivers 16 to 20 years old who were involved in fatal motor vehicle crashes, and for whom any alcohol consumption is illegal, had alcohol in their blood.[20]

Despite these grim figures, significant progress has been made in reducing the overall rate of alcohol-related vehicle deaths. Between 1987 and 2007 this rate declined from 9.8 to 4.8 deaths per 100,000 people, meeting the *Healthy People 2010* objective. The *Healthy People 2020* objective, based on number of miles traveled, is to decrease the rate of alcohol-impaired driving (0.08 or greater blood-alcohol content) fatalities to 0.38 per 100 million miles traveled (see Box 12.1). Past success and the promise of future achievement of the target came through public policy changes—raising the minimum legal drinking age, strengthening and enforcing state license revocation laws, and lowering the BAC tolerance levels from 0.10% to 0.08% in some states—stricter law enforcement, and better education for those cited for driving while intoxicated.[21] In October 2000, President

problem drinker
one for whom alcohol consumption results in a medical, social, or other type of problem

alcoholism
a disease characterized by impaired control over drinking, preoccupation with drinking, and continued use of alcohol despite adverse consequences

blood alcohol concentration (BAC)
the percentage of concentration of alcohol in the blood

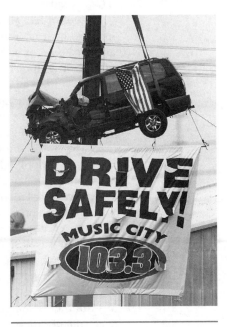

FIGURE 12.5
The risk of a motor vehicle crash increases progressively with alcohol consumption.

BOX 12.1	HEALTHY PEOPLE 2020: OBJECTIVES

Objective: SA-17 Decrease the rate of alcohol-impaired driving fatalities.

Target setting method: 5% improvement.

Data source: Analysis Reporting System (FARS), U.S. Department of Transportation.

Target and baseline:

Objective	2008 Baseline	2020 Target
	Per 100 million vehicle miles traveled	
SA-17 Decrease the rate of alcohol-impaired driving (0.08 or greater blood alcohol content) fatalities	0.40	0.38

For Further Thought

The reduction of alcohol-related vehicle deaths is one of the greatest success stories of public health during the twentieth century. What are some factors that have contributed to decreasing alcohol-related vehicle deaths? Similar success has not been achieved for substance abuse–related deaths or drug abuse–related emergency department visits overall. What explanation can you offer for this difference?

Source: U.S. Department of Health and Human Services, Office of Disease Prevention and Health Promotion (2010). *Healthy People 2020.* Available at http://www.healthypeople.gov/2020/default.aspx. Accessed December 2, 2010.

Clinton signed a bill that made 0.08% BAC the national standard. States that refused to impose the standard by 2004 would lose millions of dollars of federal highway construction money.[22] By the end of 2004, all 50 states, Puerto Rico, and the District of Columbia had adopted the 0.08% standard.[23]

Alcohol has also been found to increase one's risk for other types of unintentional injuries, such as drowning, falls, fires, and burns. Associations between unintentional injuries and the abuse of other drugs are less well documented, but given a knowledge of the effects of such drugs, one can assume that they increase neither the alertness nor the coordination of users.

Alcohol also contributes to intentional violence in the community. For example, 50% of spouse abuse, 49% of murders, 62% of assaults, 52% of rapes, 38% of child abuse cases, and 20% to 35% of suicides are traceable to alcohol consumption (see Figure 12.1).

"Alcohol is the number 1 rape drug," according to Henry Wechsler of the Harvard University School of Public Health.[24] The incidence of rape on college campuses is estimated at 35 per 1,000 female students, making rape the most common violent crime on American campuses. Yet, less than 5% of these rapes are reported to police. About half of the perpetrators and rape survivors on college campuses were drinking alcohol at the time of the assault. Ninety percent of college women who are raped know their assailants. A new law in Wisconsin was designed to protect women at risk of sexual assault by acquaintances at social gatherings where alcohol is served. A person convicted under the new law can be fined up to $100,000 and sentenced up to 25 years in prison. Wisconsin is the 50th state to enact such a law.[24]

Another community health problem resulting from pathological drinking is fetal alcohol spectrum disorder (FASD). FASD includes diagnoses such as fetal alcohol syndrome (FAS), fetal alcohol effects (FAE), alcohol-related birth defects (ARBD), and alcohol-related neurodevelopmental disorders (ARND). "Every year, about 40,000 babies are born with symptoms of prenatal alcohol exposure," according to a 2003 publication of the Substance Abuse and Mental Health Services Administration.[25] These babies cost society thousands of dollars over their lifetimes. Estimates vary greatly based upon estimated prevalence rates, from a low rate of 0.33 cases of FASD per 1,000 live births to 2.0 cases per 1,000. Costs can be attributable to medical treatment for pre- and postnatal growth defects requiring surgery; services for developmentally disabled children; home health care, special education, social services, training and supervision, and institutional care for affected individuals with mental retardation to age 65 years; and lost productivity. Estimates of the annual cost of FASD in the United States range from $0.5 million to $6 billion. Likewise, estimates for the lifetime costs for a specific individual with FASD range from $1 million to $5 million.[25] Clearly, this is a community health problem for which an ounce of prevention is worth a pound of cure. It is also clear that women of childbearing age who could become pregnant should exercise caution in their alcohol use.

Nicotine

Nicotine is the psychoactive and addictive drug present in tobacco products such as cigarettes, cigars, smokeless or "spit" tobacco (chewing tobacco and snuff), and pipe tobacco. For many years the enforcement of state laws prohibiting the sale of cigarettes and other tobacco products to minors was uneven. In other cases, cigarettes could easily be purchased by youth from vending machines. Thus, until recently many American youths have had ready access to tobacco products, and American tobacco companies made the most of this situation during the 1990s. With their seductive "Joe Camel" advertisements (now retired) and other similar youth-oriented marketing approaches, they made smoking highly attractive to today's youth. In a more recent effort to market cigarettes to children and adolescents, Reynolds Tobacco began selling candy-, fruit-, and liquor-flavored cigarettes. An agreement between Reynolds Tobacco and the attorneys general of 38 states to end the sale of these items was announced October 10, 2006.[26] The **Synar Amendment** is a federal law that requires all states to adopt legislation that prohibits the sale and distribution of tobacco products to people under age 18. States that do not comply with this regulation lose federal dollars for alcohol, tobacco, and other drug prevention and treatment programs.[27]

> **Synar Amendment** a federal law that requires states to set the minimum legal age for purchasing tobacco products at 18 years and requires states to enforce this law

On June 22, 2009, President Obama signed the Family Smoking Prevention and Tobacco Control Act into law, giving the Food and Drug Administration oversight over tobacco products. Beginning June 22, 2010, the tobacco industry must "halt the manufacture of its deceptively labeled 'light,' 'mild,' and 'low-tar' cigarettes."[28] It remains to be seen how effective this new law will be in lowering smoking rates among young Americans. Another proven way to reduce smoking rates is to increase taxes on cigarettes, thereby increasing the financial cost of smoking. The New York State legislature passed a bill on July 21, 2010, that will add another $1.60 in state taxes to every cigarette pack sold beginning July 1, raising the average price per pack in New York to $9.20. The price per pack in New York City will be about $11.00.[29] Perhaps, raising the cost of cigarettes in this manner will reduce smoking rates among young people.

The 30-day prevalence of cigarette smoking among high school seniors, which had declined to 27.8% in 1992 and then rebounded to 36.5% by 1997, reached a new low of 20.4% in 2008. The prevalence of daily smoking among high school seniors also declined in 2003, to 13.6%.[5] Although it is true that some of these students are light smokers (less than half a pack a day), studies show that many light smokers become heavy smokers (more than half a pack a day) as they become older. The prevalence of cigarette smoking in young adults (aged 19–28) seems to be related to college attendance. For college students, the 30-day prevalence of daily use of cigarettes was 9.2%; for young adults, it was 16.7%.[5]

BOX
12.2

TEN GREAT PUBLIC HEALTH ACHIEVEMENTS, 1900–1999:
RECOGNITION OF TOBACCO USE AS A HEALTH HAZARD

Less Smoke, More Prevention

During the twentieth century, smoking went from being an accepted norm to being recognized as the number 1 preventable cause of death and disability in the United States. Although substantial progress has been made and millions of lives have been saved, increased prevention efforts are needed to reduce the impact of tobacco use on public health.

> **SURGEON GENERAL'S WARNING: Smoking Causes Lung Cancer, Heart Disease, Emphysema, And May Complicate Pregnancy**

Each year, smoking kills more people than all of the following health hazards combined:

- AIDS
- Alcohol abuse
- Drug abuse
- Motor vehicle crash injuries
- Murders
- Suicides

Per capita consumption of cigarettes has decreased from a high of more than 4,000 cigarettes/year in the early 1960s to a low of 2,261/year in 1998, the lowest level seen since the early 1940s. Some of the changes appear to be associated with notable smoking and health events.

- 1964 Surgeon General's report
- Doubling of federal cigarette taxes
- Master Settlement Agreement
- Banning of tobacco advertising in many venues

During this century, smoking prevalence among adults aged 18 years decreased from approximately 40% in the mid-1960s to 25% in 1999, with the rate for men being approximately five percentage points higher than for women.

Source: Centers for Disease Control and Prevention (1999). Achievements in Public Health, 1990–1999: Tobacco Use—United States, 1900–1999. *Morbidity and Mortality Weekly Report*, 48(12): 241–242. Available at http://www.cdc.gov/mmwr/PDF/wk/mm4843.pdf. Accessed October 26, 2010.

The health consequences of tobacco use are familiar to all, even smokers (see Box 12.2). They include increased risks for heart disease, lung cancer, chronic obstructive lung disease, stroke, emphysema, and other conditions. Smoking accounted for an estimated 443,000 premature deaths per year in the United States and 5.4 million premature deaths per year worldwide.[30] By 2030, 8 million people are expected to die each year in the world and smoking could kill as many as 1 billion people during this century.[31] The economic costs of tobacco smoking in the United States are estimated at $193 billion, of which more than half is due to lost productivity; the remainder is attributable to medical costs.[30] A significant portion of the medical costs attributed to smoking (43%) are paid with government funds, including Medicaid and Medicare.[1] Inasmuch as tobacco use and nicotine addiction increase the cost of these programs, they clearly add to the economic burden on society.

environmental tobacco smoke (ETS) (secondhand smoke) tobacco smoke in the ambient air

Well-established research findings have demonstrated that one does not have to use tobacco products to be adversely affected. The 1986 Surgeon General's report on the effects of **environmental tobacco smoke (ETS) or secondhand smoke** indicated that adults and children who inhale the tobacco smoke of others (passive smoking) are also at increased risk for cardiac and respiratory illnesses.[32,33] These findings resulted in new smoking regulations in many indoor environments. Then, in December 1992, the Environmental Protection Agency (EPA) released the report *Respiratory Health Effects of Passive Smoking: Lung*

Cancer and Other Disorders.[34] This report stated that ETS is a human class A carcinogen (the same class that contains asbestos) and that it is responsible for 3,000 lung cancer deaths annually among nonsmoking Americans. Further, it stated that ETS exposure is causally associated with as many as 150,000 to 300,000 cases of lower respiratory infections (such as bronchitis and pneumonia) in infants and young children up to 18 months of age. The EPA study also found that ETS aggravates asthma in children and is a risk factor for new cases of childhood asthma.

The use of smokeless (spit) tobacco also carries with it serious health risks, including addiction, periodontal disease, and oral cancer. Approximately 3.9% of 12- to 17-year-old males and 10.3% of 18- to 25-year-old males reported using smokeless tobacco within the past 30 days in 2008.[35] This habit begins in high school, where in 2008, 5.5% of eighth-grade males, 8.2% of tenth-grade, males, and 11.8% of twelfth-grade males reported using smokeless tobacco in the past 30 days.[5]

Over-the-Counter Drugs

Over-the-counter (OTC) drugs are those legal drugs, with the exception of tobacco and alcohol, that can be purchased without a physician's prescription. Included in this category are internal analgesics such as aspirin, acetaminophen (Tylenol), and ibuprofen (Advil); cough and cold remedies (Robitussin, Contac); emetics; laxatives; mouthwashes; vitamins; and many others.[36] Thousands of different OTC products are sold by pharmacies, supermarkets, convenience stores, and in vending machines. These products are manufactured and sold to those who self-diagnose and self-medicate their own illnesses.

Over-the-counter drugs are carefully regulated by the **Food and Drug Administration (FDA)**, an agency of the Department of Health and Human Services. The FDA ensures the safety and effectiveness of these products when they are used according to their label directions. There is no person or agency that supervises the actual sale or use of these substances.

Naturally, some of these substances are misused and abused. Examples of misuse are not following the dosage directions or using the drugs after their expiration date. A specific example of OTC drug abuse is the taking of laxatives or emetics to lose weight or to avoid gaining weight. Other OTC drugs that are often abused are appetite suppressants (Dexatrim), stimulants (NōDōz), and nasal sprays (Neo-Synephrine). Recently, common cold OTC products that contain pseudoephedrine have been the target of thieves whose intent is to manufacture methamphetamine. This has led to tighter regulation that restricts the amounts that can be sold at one time.[37]

Most OTC drugs provide only symptomatic relief and do not provide a cure. For example, cough and cold remedies relieve the discomfort that accompanies a cold but do not in any way rid a person of the cold virus that is causing these symptoms. Therefore, a real danger of OTC drug misuse and abuse is that symptoms that should be brought to the attention of a physician remain unreported. Another danger is that those who abuse these drugs may become dependent, thus unable to live normally without them. Last, abuse of OTC drugs may establish a pattern of dependency that predisposes the abuser to developing dependent relationships with prescription drugs or illicit drugs.

Prescription Drugs

Because all prescription drugs have serious side effects for some people, they can be purchased only with a physician's (or dentist's) written instructions (prescription). Like OTC drugs, prescription drugs are carefully regulated by the FDA. More than 4,000 prescription drugs are listed in each annual edition of the *Physician's Desk Reference.*[38] The written prescription connotes that the prescribed drugs are being taken by the patient under the prescribing physician's supervision. Each prescription includes the patient's name, the amount to be dispensed, and the dosage.

over-the-counter (OTC) drugs (nonprescription drugs) drugs (except tobacco and alcohol) that can be legally purchased without a physician's prescription

Food and Drug Administration (FDA) a federal agency in the Department of Health and Human Services charged with ensuring the safety and efficacy of all prescription and nonprescription drugs

controlled substances
drugs regulated by the Comprehensive Drug Abuse Control Act of 1970, including all illegal drugs and prescription drugs that are subject to abuse and can produce dependence

Controlled Substances Act of 1970 (Comprehensive Drug Abuse Control Act of 1970)
the central piece of federal drug legislation that regulates illegal drugs and legal drugs that have a high potential for abuse

illicit (illegal) drugs
drugs that cannot be legally manufactured, distributed, or sold, and that usually lack recognized medicinal value. Drugs that have been placed under Schedule I of the Controlled Substances Act of 1970

Nonetheless, prescription drugs are also subject to misuse and abuse. Types of misuse include those previously cited for the OTC drugs and also the giving of one person's prescription drug to another. Furthermore, certain prescription drugs such as stimulants (amphetamines), depressants (Valium), and pain relievers such as narcotics (morphine, codeine) have a higher potential for abuse than others. Because prescription drugs are usually stronger or more concentrated than OTC drugs, there is a greater risk of developing dependence or taking an overdose from these drugs. Those who develop dependence may try to obtain duplicate prescriptions from other physicians or steal the drugs from hospital dispensaries or pharmacies.

One serious consequence of the misuse of prescription drugs, in addition to becoming dependent, is the development of drug-resistant strains of pathogens. When patients fail to complete the entire antibiotic treatment (i.e., 3 days of a 10-day prescription), some of the bacteria survive and multiply, reinfecting the body with drug-resistant organisms. Thus, succeeding treatments are less effective. When this strain of the disease is transmitted to another, the antibiotic treatment fails. New drugs are then needed to treat these patients. As drug misuse continues to occur, bacteria become resistant to multiple drugs. Multidrug-resistant tuberculosis (MDR-TB) is an example. Another example is the growing number of reports of community-associated methicillin-resistant *Staphylococcus aureus* (CA-MRSA) infections. These are bacterial infections of the skin or other organs that are resistant to some antibiotics.[39] The prevalence of MDR-TB and the increase in the incidence of CA-MRSA point both to the dangers of drug misuse and the need to continue to develop new antibiotics for the treatment of bacterial infections.

In recent years, the number of deaths from unintentional drug overdoses has risen to unprecedented levels. During 1999–2006, fatal poisonings involving opioid analgesics (painkillers) more than tripled in the United States and accounted for almost 40% of all poisoning deaths in 2006. Opioid analgesics include such drugs as oxycodone, hydrocodone, fentanyl, propoxyphene, as well as methadone. Although some of these deaths can be attributed to drugs prescribed for the decedent, at least some of these deaths occurred in people who obtained the opioid analgesics illegally.[40] With the 26,400 such deaths reported in 2006, drug overdoses ranked second only to motor vehicle crash deaths among leading causes of unintentional injury deaths in the United States.[41] Prescription drug abuse puts an additional strain on our already overburdened emergency departments (EDs). About half of the 2 million ED visits involving drugs in 2008 were for legal drugs used nonmedically and for illegal drugs.[41] The estimated number of ED visits involving the nonmedical use of opioid analgesics increased 104% between 2004 and 2008.[42]

Controlled Substances and Illicit (Illegal) Drugs

Controlled substances are those regulated by the **Controlled Substances Act of 1970** (CSA), officially called the **Comprehensive Drug Abuse Control Act of 1970**. Many of the drugs discussed next belong to Schedule I under this act because they have a high potential for abuse and have no accepted medical uses and, hence, no acceptable standards of safe use. These are considered **illicit (illegal) drugs**. They cannot be cultivated, manufactured, bought, sold, or used within the confines of the law. Well over 100 drugs are listed in this category, including heroin, methaqualone, marijuana (see Figure 12.6), LSD, psilocybin, mescaline, MDMA, and DMT.[43]

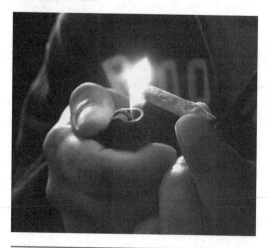

FIGURE 12.6
Marijuana is the nation's most popular illicit drug.

Other drugs, which do have medical uses, are placed in Schedules II to V of the act, depending upon their potential for abuse and risk of causing dependence. Included in Schedule II is a variety of very powerful compounds that have specific medical uses but have a high risk for potential abuse. Included in this category are many opium derivatives, such as morphine, fentanyl, and methadone. Also included in Schedule II are the stimulants amphetamine and methamphetamine, certain depressants such as amobarbital, pentobarbital, secobarbital, and phencyclidine, and several other drugs. Schedule III drugs have medical uses and exhibit a lower risk of potential abuse than Schedule II drugs. Included are less concentrated forms of certain Schedule II drugs and also many of the anabolic steroids. Schedule IV drugs exhibit even less potential for abuse than Schedule III drugs. Included are many milder stimulants and depressants. Schedule V drugs are primarily very dilute concentrations of opium or opiates used in such medicines as cough syrups.[43]

The **Drug Enforcement Administration (DEA)**, under the Department of Justice, has the primary responsibility of enforcing the provisions of the Controlled Substances Act. Once a drug is placed in Schedule I of the CSA, it becomes the primary responsibility of the DEA to interdict the trafficking (manufacturing, distribution, and sales) of the substance. The only sources of these drugs are illegal growers and manufacturers. Schedule II to V substances often reach the street illegally, either by illegal production (in clandestine labs) or by diversion of legally manufactured prescription drugs.

Drug Enforcement Administration (DEA) the federal government's lead agency with the primary responsibility for enforcing the nation's drug laws, including the Controlled Substances Act of 1970

Marijuana

Marijuana is the most abused illicit drug in the United States. "Pot" and the related products, hashish and hash oil, are derived from the hemp plant, *Cannabis sativa*. The products are most commonly used by smoking but can also be ingested. Although marijuana abuse has declined, it remains a concern for several reasons. First, it is illegal, and therefore brings the user into contact with those involved in illegal activities. Second, the act of smoking is detrimental to one's health. Third, marijuana smoking often occurs in conjunction with the drinking of alcohol or the use of other drugs. The effects of **polydrug use** (the use of more than one drug at a time) may be more serious than those of single-drug use. Last, as is true of all drugs, the adolescent who uses marijuana is delaying the accomplishment of developmental tasks such as attaining an adult self-identity, achieving independence, and developing the interpersonal skills necessary for successful independent living.

marijuana dried plant parts of the hemp plant, *Cannabis sativa*

polydrug use concurrent use of multiple drugs

In a 2008 survey, the percentage of high school seniors who reported having smoked marijuana at least once in their lives was 42.6%. Also, 19.4% reported having smoked marijuana in the past 30 days.[5] As with many of the other drugs, the prevalence of marijuana use has waxed and waned over the past 30 years. The perceived risk of use is one of the factors that seems to contribute to the level of use. In 1992, when 76.5% of high school seniors felt there was great risk associated with regular marijuana use, the 30-day use prevalence was 11.9%. In 2008, when 51.7% of seniors felt there was great risk associated with regular marijuana use, the 30-day use prevalence was 19.4%.[5] Another measurement of students' attitudes is disapproval rates. National anti-drug-use campaigns directed at youth, aimed at increasing disapproval rates, may be working. Although still lower than their highest levels in the early 1990s, disapproval rates for trying marijuana once or twice edged upward in eighth, tenth, and twelfth graders since their lowest levels in the mid-1990s.[5] One of the objectives of *Healthy People 2020* is to increase the proportion of adolescents (eighth, tenth, and twelfth graders) who disapprove of trying marijuana or hashish once or twice. The target is set at 10% improvement (see Box 12.3).

The acute health effects of marijuana use include reduced concentration, slowed reaction time, impaired short-term memory, and impaired judgment. Naturally, these effects can have serious consequences for someone operating a motor vehicle or other machinery or can

BOX
12.3

HEALTHY PEOPLE 2020: OBJECTIVES

Objectives SA-3.4, SA-3.5, and SA-3.6: Increase the proportion of adolescents who disapprove of trying marijuana or hashish once or twice—eighth graders, tenth graders, and twelfth graders.

Target setting method: 10% improvement.

Data source: Monitoring the Future Study, NIH, National Institute of Drug Abuse (NIDA).

Targets and baselines:

Objective	2009 Baseline	2020 Target
	Percentage	
SA-3.4 Eighth graders	75.3	82.8
SA-3.5 Tenth graders	60.1	66.1
SA-3.6 Twelfth graders	54.8	60.3

For Further Thought

Attitudes and beliefs are often key factors influencing drug-taking behavior among adolescents. Studies have shown that when there is a high level of disapproval of marijuana use by adolescents, the prevalence of marijuana use declines. Conversely, an increase in marijuana use occurs when there is an apparent decline in those expressing strong disapproval of use. How strong are prevailing feelings of disapproval of marijuana use in your community? Do adolescents in your community feel that it is "OK" to try marijuana once or twice?

Source: U.S. Department of Health and Human Services, Office of Disease Prevention and Health Promotion (2010). *Healthy People 2020.* Available at http://www.healthypeople.gov/2020/default.aspx. Accessed December 2, 2010.

even result in a medical emergency. Marijuana use in combination with other drugs can be especially dangerous because drugs in combination may affect the brain differently. In 2007, marijuana, used alone or with one or more other drugs, was involved in an estimated 308,547 emergency department visits.[44]

amotivational syndrome
a pattern of behavior characterized by apathy, loss of effectiveness, and a more passive, introverted personality

The chronic effects of smoking marijuana include damage to the respiratory system by the smoke itself and, for some, the development of a controverisal condition known as **amotivational syndrome**. Amotivational syndrome has been described as a chronic apathy toward maturation and the achievement of the developmental tasks listed previously (e.g., developing skills for independent living, setting and achieving goals, and developing an adult self-identity). There is also evidence now that long-term marijuana users experience physiological and psychological withdrawal symptoms. Although these "unpleasant behavioral symptoms are less obvious than those for heroin or alcohol, they are significant and do perhaps contribute to continued drug use."[45] Further evidence of the dependence-producing nature of marijuana is the number of persons seeking admission to treatment programs. Between 1994 and 2004, the proportion of admissions to treatment programs for marijuana abuse rose 9%. Nearly 16% of those entering drug abuse treatment programs are admitted for marijuana abuse; this was more than for any other single drug except alcohol.[46] Finally, one of the chief concerns with marijuana is that those who smoke marijuana are more likely to use other, more addictive drugs. For example, 89% of those who use cocaine first used cigarettes, alcohol, and marijuana.[47]

narcotics
drugs derived from or chemically related to opium that reduce pain and induce stupor, such as morphine

Narcotics: Opium, Morphine, Heroin, and Others

Opium and its derivatives, morphine and heroin, come from the oriental poppy plant, *Papaver somniferum.* These **narcotics** numb the senses and reduce pain. As such, they have a high potential for abuse. The narcotic that is most widely abused is heroin, a derivative of morphine. In 2008, about 3.8 million (1.5%) of the 250 million noninstitutionalized people older than the age of 12 reported the use of heroin in their lifetime, while 453,000 (0.2%) reported use in the past year.[35] This estimate is low because this survey undoubtedly missed a great many addicts who may be homeless and living in shelters. Use in the past year among high school seniors was 0.7% in 2008, only slightly higher than the 0.6% level in 1992.[5]

Opium poppies do not grow in the continental United States. Heroin arrives in the United States from four geographic areas: Southwest Asia, Southeast Asia, Mexico, and South America. Most of the heroin available in the United States now enters across our southwestern border. Although significant amounts of heroin reaching the United States originate in South America, the proportion of heroin seizures in which the heroin originated in Mexico has grown. Mexican heroin production has increased in recent years, and the influence of Mexican drug trafficking organizations is expanding.[48]

Heroin remains the number 1 illicit narcotic of abuse and the third leading cause of drug-related emergency department visits after cocaine and marijuana.[44] Historically, heroin has been the leading cause of unintentional narcotic-induced drug deaths. Now, however, heroin has been overtaken by other synthetic opioids, including methadone, as the leading cause of narcotic-induced overdose drug deaths. Together, these substances accounted for more than 15,000 poisoning deaths in the United States in 2006.[40]

Narcotics produce euphoria, analgesia, and drowsiness. They reduce anxiety and pain without affecting motor activity the way alcohol and barbiturates do. If use continues, the body makes physiological adjustments to the presence of the drug. This **tolerance** means that larger and larger doses are required to achieve the same euphoria and numbing as the initial dose. Whereas tolerance develops rapidly to the euphoric effects, the depressing effects on respiration may continue to increase with dose level, increasing the risk of a fatal overdose. As the cost of the drug habit becomes higher, the abuser usually attempts to quit. This results in withdrawal symptoms because the body has become physically dependent upon the drug. Heroin addicts have a difficult time changing their lifestyle for several reasons. First, there is the addiction itself, both physical and psychological. Often, there are underlying psychosocial problems as well, such as poor self-image, lack of job skills, and absence of supporting family and friends. Addicts usually mistrust official programs set up to help them. They are usually in poor health mentally and physically. Because the duration of action of heroin is only 4 to 5 hours, the addict is usually too concerned with finding the next dose or recovering from the previous one to be productive in the community.

The community is affected by more than just the loss of productivity. The addict must obtain money to purchase heroin, and the price of the habit can be very high—as much as $200 per day. The money is usually obtained illegally through burglaries, thefts, robberies, muggings, prostitution (male and female), and selling drugs. If a prostitute can make $50 dollars a trick, he or she needs to turn at least four tricks a day just to maintain the habit. The result is not only a deteriorating community but also epidemics of sexually transmitted diseases, such as gonorrhea, syphilis, chlamydia, herpes, and AIDS. Because most heroin addicts inject the drug, there are also epidemics of bloodborne diseases, such as those caused by HIV and hepatitis viruses. In this way, drug abuse increases the burden on community health resources. Addicts who turn to dealing drugs to support their habit do even more damage because they increase the availability of the drug and may introduce it to first-time users. There is an additional burden on the criminal justice system when these addicts are arrested, prosecuted, incarcerated, and rehabilitated.

Cocaine and Crack Cocaine

Cocaine is the psychoactive ingredient in the leaves of the coca plant, *Erythoxolyn coca*, which grows in the Andes Mountains of South America. Cocaine is a **stimulant**; that is, it increases the activity of the central nervous system. For centuries, natives of the Andes Moun-

tolerance
physiological and enzymatic adjustments that occur in response to the chronic presence of drugs, which are reflected in the need for ever-increasing doses

cocaine
the psychoactive ingredient in the leaves of the coca plant, *Erythoxolyn coca*, which, when refined, is a powerful stimulant/euphoriant

stimulant
a drug that increases the activity of the central nervous system

hallucinogens
drugs that produce profound distortions of the senses

synesthesia
impairment of mind characterized by a sensation that senses are mixed

amphetamines
a group of synthetic drugs that act as stimulants

methamphetamine
the amphetamine most widely abused

tains have chewed the leaves to improve stamina during work and long treks. In its more purified forms, as a salt (white powder) or dried paste (crack), cocaine is a powerful euphoriant/stimulant and very addictive.

Cocaine use among high school seniors peaked in 1985, when 6.7% reported use within the past 30 days. By 1992 this figure had dropped to only 1.3%, but by 1999 those reporting use in the past 30 days had doubled to 2.6%.[4,5] The 2008 30-day prevalence rate among high school seniors was 1.9%. Estimates for 2008 indicated that as many as 2.2 million Americans had used cocaine or crack in the past 30 days.[35] Therefore, cocaine remains a serious drug problem in the United States.

Hallucinogens

Hallucinogens are drugs that produce illusions, hallucinations, and other changes in one's perceptions of the environment. These effects are due to the phenomenon known as **synesthesia**, a mixing of the senses. Hallucinogens include both naturally derived drugs such as mescaline, from the peyote cactus, and psilocybin and psilocin, from the *Psilocybe* mushroom; and synthetic drugs, such as lysergic acid diethylamide (LSD). Although physical dependence has not been demonstrated with the hallucinogens, tolerance does occur. Though overdose deaths are rare, "bad trips" (unpleasant experiences) do occur, and a few people have experienced permanent visual disturbances. Because there are no legal sources for these drugs, users are always at risk for taking fake, impure, or adulterated drugs.

Stimulants

As previously mentioned, stimulants are drugs that increase the activity level of the central nervous system. Examples include the amphetamines, such as amphetamine itself (bennies), dextroamphetamine (dexies), methamphetamine (meth), and dextromethamphetamine (ice); methylphenidate (Ritalin); and methcathinone (cat). These drugs cause the release of high levels of the neurotransmitter dopamine, which stimulates brain cells. Tolerance builds quickly, so abusers must escalate their doses rapidly. Chronic abusers can develop tremors and confusion, aggressiveness, and paranoia. The long-term effects include permanent brain damage and Parkinson's disease–like symptoms.[49]

Amphetamines are Schedule II prescription drugs that have been widely abused for many years. Increased regulatory efforts in the 1970s probably contributed to the rise in the cocaine trade in the 1980s. When cocaine abuse declined in the late 1980s, there was a resurgence of amphetamine abuse, primarily **methamphetamine**, also known as "crystal," "crank," "speed," "go fast," or just "meth." At first, the clandestine labs that produced methamphetamine, and those abusing the substance, were concentrated primarily in the southwestern states. However, by 1995 production and abuse had spread to the Midwest, and by 1999 methamphetamine abuse had become the fastest growing drug threat in America. The popularity of amphetamines has declined since its peak in 2001. In 2008, 2.9% of high school seniors reported abusing amphetamines and 0.6% reported abusing methamphetamine in the past 30 days.[5] In 2008, the DEA seized 1,540 kilograms of methamphetamine and recorded 6,783 clandestine lab incidents, including labs, Dumpsters, chemcials and glassware, and equipment (see Figures 12.7 and 12.8).[50]

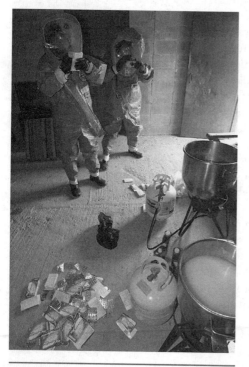

FIGURE 12.7
Dismantling a clandestine methamphetamine lab is hazardous work.

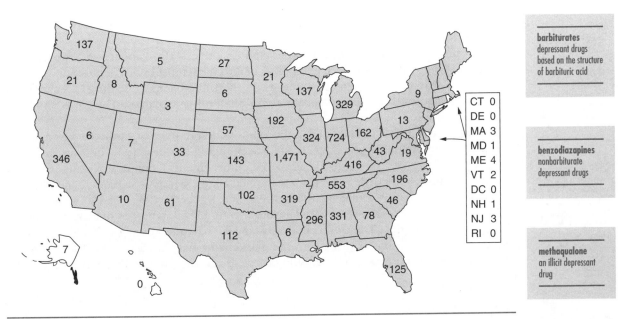

CT	0
DE	0
MA	3
MD	1
ME	4
VT	2
DC	0
NH	1
NJ	3
RI	0

FIGURE 12.8

Total of all clandestine laboratory incidents involving methamphetamine (including labs, dump sites, and chemicals, glassware, or equipment), calendar year 2008.

Source: Drug Enforcement Administration, Department of Justice (2010). "Maps of Methamphetamine Lab Incidents." Available at http://www.usdoj.gov/dea/concern/map_lab_seizures.html. Accessed December 14, 2010.

barbiturates
depressant drugs based on the structure of barbituric acid

benzodiazapines
nonbarbiturate depressant drugs

methaqualone
an illicit depressant drug

depressants
drugs that slow central nervous system activity, for example, alcohol, barbiturates, benzodiazepines

Methylphenidate (Ritalin) is a Schedule II drug used to treat attention-deficit hyperactivity disorder. Though not produced in clandestine labs, the drug is often diverted from its intended use and abused by those for whom it was not prescribed.

Depressants

Barbiturates, **benzodiazapines**, **methaqualone**, and other **depressants** slow down the central nervous system. They are attractive to some people because, like alcohol, among the first effects of taking these drugs are the lowering of anxiety and the loss of inhibitions. These effects produce the feeling of a "high," even though these drugs depress the central nervous system. As one continues to use these drugs, tolerance develops, and the user experiences the need for greater and greater doses to feel the same effects that the previous dose provided. Strong physical dependence develops so that abstinence results in severe clinical illness; thus, abusers of these substances must often rely on medical assistance during detoxification and recovery.

Club Drugs and Designer Drugs

Club drugs is a term for a number of illicit drugs, primarily synthetic, that are most commonly encountered at nightclubs and raves (all-night dance parties). These drugs include MDMA, ketamine, GHB, GBL, Rohypnol, LSD, PCP, methamphetamine, and others. Because these drugs are illegal, there is no guarantee of their safety or even their identity. Also, these drugs are often taken in combination with alcohol or other drugs. As a result, the number of emergency reports for many of these club drugs quadrupled between 1994 and 1998.[51] MDMA, also known as "Ecstasy," is the most popular of the club drugs. Use of MDMA rose sharply among eighth, tenth, and twelfth graders through 2001 and then declined sharply. Five percent of high school seniors surveyed in 2008 had taken MDMA at least once, 4.3% in the past year.[5]

club drugs
a general term for those illicit drugs, primarily synthetic, that are most commonly encountered at night clubs and "raves" (examples include MDMA, GHB, GBL, LSD, PCP, ketamine, Rohypnol, and methamphetamine)

Rohypnol (flunitrazepam)
a depressant in the benzodiazapine group that has achieved notoriety as a date-rape drug

designer drugs
drugs synthesized illegally that are similar to, but structurally different from, known controlled substances

Long-term effects of MDMA are still under evaluation, but there is evidence that the drug causes brain damage.[51]

Rohypnol (flunitrazepam) is another club drug that is also known as a "date-rape" or "predatory" drug. This drug, which exhibits all of the characteristics of a depressant, is a legal prescription drug in more than 50 countries. In the United States, the drug is regarded as more dangerous, and thus less medically useful than other sedatives. Thus, it is an illegal (Schedule I) drug.

Designer drugs is a term coined in the 1980s to describe drugs synthesized by amateur chemists in secret laboratories. By constantly changing the design of their drugs, these chemists hoped to stay one step ahead of law enforcement. Examples of designer drugs included MDMA (3,4-methylenedioxy-methamphetamine), synthetic narcotics, and dissociative anesthetics such as PCP (angel dust) and ketamine. Under the Controlled Substance Act of 1970, only those drugs that were listed as illegal were illegal, whereas similar, but slightly altered, drugs were not. The Controlled Substances Analogue Act of 1986 was enacted to reduce the flow of designer drugs into the market and make it easier to prosecute those involved in manufacturing and distributing these drugs. Designer and club drugs are still a problem.

anabolic drugs
compounds, structurally similar to the male hormone testosterone, that increase protein synthesis and thus muscle building

Anabolic Drugs

Anabolic drugs are protein-building drugs. Included are the anabolic/androgenic steroids (AS), testosterone, and human growth hormone (HGH). These drugs have legitimate medical uses, such as the rebuilding of muscles after starvation or disease and the treatment of dwarfism. But they are sometimes abused by athletes and body builders as a shortcut to increasing muscle mass,

inhalants
breathable substances that produce mind-altering effects

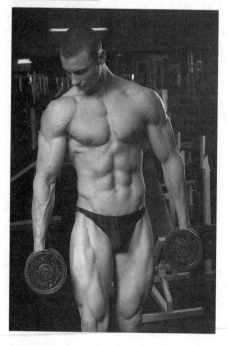

strength, and endurance. Abuse of steroids is accompanied by numerous acute and chronic side effects for men, including acne, gynecomastia (the development of breasts), baldness, reduced fertility, and reduction in testicular size. Side effects for women are masculinizing: development of a male physique, increased body hair, failure to ovulate (menstrual irregularities), and a deepening of the voice. Long-term abuse of anabolic steroids can result in psychological dependence, making the discontinuation of use very difficult.[52]

In the late 1980s, it became apparent that increasing numbers of boys and young men of high school and college age were taking anabolic steroids as a shortcut to muscle building or to maturity (see Figure 12.9). Because of these trends in the abuse of anabolic steroids, these drugs were placed in Schedule III of the Controlled Substance Act in 1990. Abuse of steroids increased during the 1990s but has leveled off recently. As with other drugs discussed earlier, "steroids" sold on the Internet may not be authentic. Purchasing such substances online is certainly an example of the phrase "Buyer, beware."

Inhalants

Inhalants are a collection of psychoactive, breathable chemicals. They include paint solvents, motor fuels, cleaners, glues, aerosol sprays, cosmetics, and other types of vapor. Because of their easy availability and low cost, they are often the drug of choice for the young. The primary effect of most of the inhalants is depression. As with alcohol, the user may at first experience a reduction of anxieties and inhibitions, making the user feel high. Continued use may result in hallucinations and loss

FIGURE 12.9
Abuse of anabolic drugs carries the risk of serious acute and chronic health problems.

of consciousness. Many of these chemicals are extremely toxic to the kidneys, liver, and nervous system. The use of inhalants by youth results from boredom and perhaps peer pressure and represents a maladaptation to these conditions.

PREVENTION AND CONTROL OF DRUG ABUSE

The prevention and control of alcohol and other drug abuse require a knowledge of the causes of drug-taking behavior, sources of illicit drugs, drug laws, and treatment programs. Also required are community organizing skills, persistence, and cooperation among a vast array of concerned individuals and official and unofficial agencies.

From a community health standpoint, drug abuse tends to be a chronic condition. Thus, the activities of drug abuse and prevention agencies and organizations can be viewed as chronic disease-prevention activities. This approach, involving three different levels of prevention, was first discussed in Chapter 4 and is discussed next in relation to drug abuse prevention and control.

Levels of Prevention

Drug abuse prevention activities can be viewed as primary, secondary, or tertiary depending upon the point of intervention. *Primary prevention* programs are aimed at those who have never used drugs, and their goal is to prevent or forestall the initiation of drug use. Drug education programs that stress primary prevention of drug and alcohol use are most appropriate and successful for children at the elementary school age. In a broader sense, almost any activity that would reduce the likelihood of primary drug use could be considered primary prevention. For example, raising the price of alcohol, increasing cigarette taxes, arresting a neighborhood drug pusher, or destroying a cocaine crop in Bolivia could be considered primary prevention if it forestalled primary drug use in at least some individuals.

Secondary prevention programs are aimed at those who have begun alcohol or other drug use but who have not become chronic abusers and have not suffered significant physical or mental impairment from their drug or alcohol abuse. Alcohol and other drug abuse education programs that stress secondary prevention are often appropriate for people of high school or college age. They can be presented in educational, workplace, or community settings.

Tertiary prevention programs are designed to provide drug abuse treatment and aftercare, including relapse prevention programs. As such, they are usually designed for adults. Tertiary programs for teenagers are far too uncommon. Tertiary prevention programs may receive clients who "turn themselves in" for treatment voluntarily, but more often than not their clients are referred by the courts.

Elements of Prevention

Four basic elements play a role in drug abuse prevention and control. These are (1) education, (2) treatment, (3) public policy, and (4) enforcement. The goals of education and treatment are the same: to reduce the demand for drugs. Likewise, setting effective public policy and law enforcement share the same goal: to reduce the supply and availability of drugs in the community.

Education

The purpose of **drug abuse education** is to limit the demand for drugs by providing information about drugs and the dangers of drug abuse, changing attitudes and beliefs about drugs, providing the skills necessary to abstain from drugs, and ultimately changing drug abuse behavior. Education, principally a primary prevention activity, can be school-based or

drug abuse education providing information about drugs and the dangers of drug abuse, changing attitudes and beliefs about drugs, providing the skills necessary to abstain from drugs, and ultimately changing drug abuse behavior

community-based. Examples of school-based drug abuse prevention programs are Here's Looking at You, 2000 and Project DARE (Drug Abuse Resistance Education). For these programs and other school-based programs to be successful, other community members such as parents, teachers, local business people, and others must visibly support the program. Examples of community-based programs are the American Cancer Society's Great American Smokeout; Race Against Drugs (RAD), a nationwide program that links drug abuse prevention with motor sports; and the Reality Check Campaign, a program to boost awareness of the harmful effects of marijuana smoking among youth.

Treatment

treatment
(for drug abuse and dependence) care that removes the physical, emotional, and environmental conditions that have contributed to drug abuse and/or dependence

The goal of **treatment** is to remove the physical, emotional, and environmental conditions that have contributed to drug dependency. Like education, treatment aims to reduce demand for drugs. It also aims to save money. Consider the money saved on law enforcement, medical costs, and lost productivity when treatment is successful. It is estimated that for every $1 spent on treatment, between $5 and $7 are saved.[53,54] Treatment for drug abuse occurs in a variety of settings and involves a variety of approaches. Treatment may be residential (inpatient) or nonresidential (outpatient). Under managed care, "behavioral health care" guidelines usually limit inpatient care to 28 days, after which the care may continue on an outpatient basis. In drug abuse treatment, what happens after the initial treatment phase is critical. **Aftercare**, the continuing care provided the recovering former drug abuser, often involves peer group or self-help support group meetings, such as those provided by Alcoholics Anonymous (AA) or Narcotics Anonymous (NA). Despite frequent relapses, treatment for drug dependence is viewed as an important component of a community's comprehensive drug abuse prevention and control strategy.

aftercare
the continuing care provided the recovering former drug abuser

Beginning January 1, 2010, The Mental Health Parity and Addiction Equity Act of 2008 (MHPAEA) took effect. This new law "requires group health plans and health insurance issuers to ensure that financial requirements (such as co-pays, deductibles) and treatment limitations (such as visit limits) applicable to mental health or substance use disorder are no more restrictive than the predominant requirements or limitations applied to substantially all medical/surgical benefits."[55] Implementation of the provisions of this law should improve substance abuse treatment options for many people.

Public Policy

public policy
the guiding principles and courses of action pursued by governments to solve practical problems affecting society

Public policy embodies the guiding principles and courses of action pursued by governments to solve practical problems affecting society. Examples include passing drunk-driving laws or zoning ordinances that limit the number of bars in a neighborhood and enacting ordinances that regulate the type and amount of advertising for such legal drugs as alcohol and tobacco. Public policy should guide the budget discussions that ultimately determine how much a community spends for education, treatment, and law enforcement. Further examples of public policy decisions are restrictions of smoking in public buildings, the setting of 0.08% blood alcohol concentration as the point at which driving becomes illegal, and zero tolerance laws for BACs for minors. Setting the level of state excise taxes on alcohol and tobacco is also a public policy decision.

Law Enforcement

law enforcement
the application of federal, state, and local laws to arrest, jail, bring to trial, and sentence those who break drug laws or break laws because of drug use

Law enforcement in drug abuse prevention and control is the application of federal, state, and local laws to arrest, jail, bring to trial, and sentence those who break drug laws or break laws because of drug use. The primary roles of law enforcement in a drug abuse prevention and control program are to (1) control drug use, (2) to control crime, especially crime related to drug use and drug trafficking—the buying, selling, manufacturing, or transporting of illegal drugs, (3) to prevent the establishment of crime organizations, and (4) to protect neighborhoods.[56] Law enforcement is concerned with limiting the supply of drugs in the community by interrupting the source, transit, and distribution of drugs. There are law enforcement agencies at all levels of government. The principal agencies are discussed next.

Governmental Drug Prevention and Control Agencies and Programs

Governmental agencies involved in drug abuse prevention, control, and treatment include a multitude of federal, state, and local agencies. At each of these levels of government, numerous offices and programs aim to reduce either the supply of or the demand for drugs.

Federal Agencies and Program

Our nation's anti-drug efforts are headed up by the White House **Office of National Drug Control Policy (ONDCP)**, which annually publishes a report detailing the nation's drug control strategy and budget. The 2010 National Drug Control Strategy will endeavor to accomplish the following:[57]

> **Office of National Drug Control Policy (ONDCP)** the headquarters of America's drug control effort, located in the executive branch of the U.S. government, headed by a director appointed by the president

- Strengthen efforts to prevent drug use in communities
- Seek early intervention opportunities in health care
- Integrate treatment for substance use disorders into health care, and expand support for recovery
- Break the cycle of drug use, crime, delinquency, and incarceration
- Disrupt domestic drug trafficking and production
- Strengthen international partnerships
- Improve information systems for analysis, assessment, and local management

The National Drug Control Strategy Goals to be attained by 2015 are the following:

Goal 1: Curtail illicit drug consumption in America

1a. Decrease the 30-day prevalence of drug use among 12- to 17-year-olds by 15%
1b. Decrease the lifetime prevalence of eighth graders who have used drugs, alcohol, or tobacco by 15%
1c. Decrease the 30-day prevalence of drug use among young adults aged 18–25 by 10%
1d. Reduce the number of chronic drug users by 15%

Goal 2: Improve the public health and public safety of the American people by reducing the consequences of drug abuse

2a. Reduce drug-induced deaths by 15%
2b. Reduce drug-related morbidity by 15%
2c. Reduce the prevalence of drugged driving by 10%

Sixty-four percent of the National Drug Control budget is aimed at reducing the supply of drugs; 36% is aimed at reducing the demand for drugs (see Figure 12.10). Domestic law enforcement and treatment will each receive about 25% of the budget; 24% will be spent on interdiction, 15% on international support, and 11% on prevention (Figure 12.11).

The National Drug Control Strategy budget request for the fiscal year (FY) 2011 is $15.55 billion.[57] The department scheduled to receive the largest portion of funds in FY 2011 is the Department of Health and Human Services (the National Institute on Drug Abuse and the Substance Abuse and Mental Health Services Administration). The Department of Homeland Security is slated for the second-largest portion, followed by the Department of Justice. The remainder of the funding is spread over the Departments of Defense, State, Education, Veterans Affairs, Treasury, Transportation, and the Office of National Drug Control Policy.

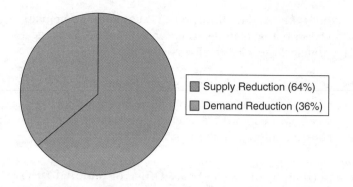

FIGURE 12.10

Federal drug control spending for fiscal years 2009–2011; supply reduction vs. demand reduction.

Source: Office of the National Drug Control Policy, The White House (2010). *National Drug Control Safety 2010.* Washington, DC: The White House. Available at http://www.whitehousedrugpolicy.gov/strategy. Accessed December 22, 2010.

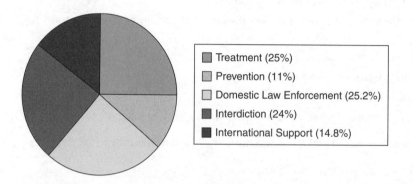

FIGURE 12.11

Federal drug control spending by function for fiscal years 2009–2011.

Source: Office of the National Drug Control Policy, The White House (2010). *National Drug Control Safety 2010.* Washington, DC: The White House. Available at http://www.whitehousedrugpolicy.gov/strategy. Accessed December 22, 2010.

Department of Health and Human Services

The Department of Health and Human Services (HHS) receives the largest portion of the federal drug budget, more than $4.28 billion in FY 2011.[57] This money is spent on drug prevention education, treatment programs, and research into the causes and physiology of drug abuse. The preponderance of these funds is spent to reduce the demand for drugs. The approach of HHS to the drug problem is broad and includes research, treatment, and educational activities.

The misuse and abuse of tobacco, alcohol, and other drugs are addressed primarily as lifestyle problems, that is, as health promotion issues—like physical fitness and nutrition. As such, HHS recognizes that the problems of drug misuse and abuse are complex—involving inherited, environmental, social, and economic causes. Therefore, the solutions are also viewed as being complex. The typical approach involves the application of the three levels of prevention—primary, secondary, and tertiary. It also recognizes the importance of incorporating the three primary prevention strategies of education, regulation, and automatic protection. These are discussed in greater detail in Chapter 15.

The HHS has published health status, risk reduction, and service and protection objectives on the use of tobacco, alcohol, and other drugs in *Healthy People 2020* (see Boxes 12.1

and 12.2). These objectives are but two examples of objectives that set the direction and standards for success of all our national drug control efforts.

The lead agency within HHS is the **Substance Abuse and Mental Health Services Administration (SAMHSA)**. Within SAMHSA, there are three centers: the Center for Substance Abuse Prevention (CSAP), the Center for Substance Abuse Treatment (CSAT), and the Center for Mental Health Services (CMHS). In addition to SAMHSA, there are two other important agencies that deal with the problems of alcohol and other drugs: the National Institute on Drug Abuse and the Food and Drug Administration (see Chapter 2 for more information on these agencies).

The **National Institute on Drug Abuse (NIDA)** is the largest institution in the world devoted to drug abuse research. At NIDA, research efforts are aimed at understanding the causes and consequences of drug abuse and at evaluating prevention and treatment programs. Within NIDA are several important divisions and centers, such as the Division of Clinical Research, the Division of Epidemiology and Prevention Research, the Division of Preclinical Research, the Division of Applied Research, the Medications Development Division, and the Addiction Research Center. These agencies conduct research and publish articles on the causes, prevention, and treatment of tobacco, alcohol, and other drug abuse.

Another important agency in HHS is the Food and Drug Administration (FDA). As stated earlier, the FDA is charged with ensuring the safety and efficacy of all prescription and non-prescription drugs. The FDA dictates which drugs reach the market and how they must be labeled, packaged, and sold. The FDA is more concerned with drug misuse than abuse.

Department of Homeland Security

Shortly following the terrorist attacks on the World Trade Center and the Pentagon on September 11, 2001, President George W. Bush authorized the establishment of the Department of Homeland Security (DHS). Subsequently, a number of federal agencies involved in drug control activities were transferred into this new department, which is scheduled to receive the second-largest portion of funding from the National Drug Control Budget ($3.8 billion).[57] Those agencies receiving funds are Immigration and Customs Enforcement, Customs and Border Protection, Counternarcotics Enforcement, and the United States Coast Guard. In the current environment, in which protection from terrorist acts is DHS's primary concern, the prevention and control of drug trafficking seem somewhat less urgent by comparison. Nonetheless, it is part of the mission of these agencies. For example, Immigration and Customs Enforcement works to prevent the immigration to this country of criminals, including those involved in drug trafficking. Customs and Border Protection works with the Immigration and Customs Enforcement to protect our borders from external threats, including illegal drugs (see Figure 12.12). The United States Coast Guard helps to interdict illegal drug trafficking in our coastal waters.

Department of Justice

The third-largest portion of federal spending for drug control, $3.45 billion in FY 2011, goes to the Department of Justice (DOJ).[57] The DOJ addresses the supply side of the drug trade most directly by identifying, arresting, and prosecuting those who break drug laws. It tries to protect the welfare of society by incarcerating the most serious offenders, deterring others from becoming involved in drug trade, and providing a clear picture to all of the cost of drug trade and abuse. Regarding the latter, the DOJ indirectly contributes to reducing the demand for drugs.

The DOJ's budget is large because, in addition to its enforcement responsibilities, the department maintains prisons and prisoners. The DOJ employs not only those who manage the penal system, but also many

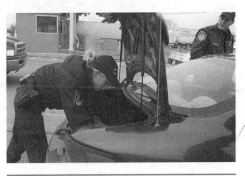

FIGURE 12.12

Customs agents assist in the arrest and prosecution of those involved in drug trafficking.

Substance Abuse and Mental Health Services Administration (SAMHSA) the agency within the Department of Health and Human Services that provides leadership in drug abuse prevention and treatment. It houses the Center for Substance Abuse Prevention and the Center for Substance Abuse Treatment

National Institute on Drug Abuse (NIDA) the federal government's lead agency for drug abuse research, one of the National Institutes of Health

marshals, attorneys, and judges. The single largest portion of the DOJ's budget goes to the Bureau of Prisons. The DOJ also operates treatment, education, and rehabilitation programs in these prisons.

Within the DOJ are several important drug-fighting agencies. The lead agency in this respect is the Drug Enforcement Agency (DEA), which investigates and assists in the prosecution of drug traffickers and their accomplices in the United States and abroad and seizes the drugs as well as the assets on which they depend. The DEA employs more than 7,000 special agents and support personnel.

Three other important agencies in the DOJ that are involved in the prevention and control of drug abuse are the Federal Bureau of Investigation (FBI), the Office of Justice Programs (OJP), and the **Bureau of Alcohol, Tobacco, Firearms, and Explosives (ATF)**. The FBI investigates multinational organized-crime networks that control the illegal drug market. The OJP provides leadership to federal, state, local, and tribal justice systems by disseminating knowledge and practices and providing grants for the implementation of these crime-fighting strategies. The OJP does not directly carry out law enforcement and justice activities, but it works with the justice community to identify crime-related challenges and to provide information, training, coordination, and innovative strategies and approaches for addressing these challenges.[58] The ATF has a wide range of responsibilities. One of its responsibilities is to protect our communities from the illegal diversion of alcohol and tobacco products. ATF partners with communities, industries, law enforcement, and public safety agencies to safeguard the public through information sharing, training, research, and use of technology.[59]

Bureau of Alcohol, Tobacco, Firearms, and Explosives (ATF) the federal agency in the Department of Justice that regulates alcohol and tobacco

Other Federal Agencies

Other federal agencies involved in drug abuse prevention and control are the Departments of State, Defense, Veterans Affairs, and Education. The State Department, through various diplomatic efforts, including "drug summits," attempts to achieve a reduction in the production and shipment of illicit drugs into this country. The Defense Department assists foreign allies to control the cultivation of illegal drug crops and the production of illegal drugs. Funding slated for the Department of Veteran Affairs is aimed primarily at the treatment of drug-related health problems of veterans.

The Department of Education (DE) launched a program to support drug-free schools and communities in the late 1980s. The effort was aimed at encouraging schools to adopt clear "no drug use" policies and to provide a message that both communities and schools do not condone or approve of alcohol or drug use by minors. A handbook titled *What Works: Schools Without Drugs* was prepared and distributed to schools and communities.[60] The Department of Education continues to participate in the federal drug prevention effort. The National Drug Control budget for the Department of Education for fiscal year 2011 is $283 million.[57]

State and Local Agencies and Programs

Whereas considerable economic resources can be brought to bear on the drug problem at the federal level, it is becoming increasingly clear that to achieve success, the drug war in America must be fought at the local level—in homes, neighborhoods, and schools. State support usually comes in the form of law enforcement expertise in education and mental health, the coordination of local and regional programs, and sometimes funding initiatives. It is usually up to local citizens to put these state initiatives into action or to begin initiatives of their own.

State Agencies

State agencies that address drug abuse prevention and control issues include the offices of the governor, as well as state departments of health, education, mental health, justice, and law enforcement. Sometimes there is an umbrella agency that coordinates the activities of these various offices and departments; other times there is not. To review agencies involved in the prevention and control of drug abuse and drug dependence problems in your state, visit your state government's homepage and search using the terms "drug abuse prevention agencies" or "drug abuse prevention programs." (You can usually find your state government's homepage by typing "www.nameofyourstate.gov," or "www.postalcodeforyourstate.gov." For example, www.texas.gov/ will take you to the Texas government's homepage; www.in.gov/ will take you to the homepage of the Indiana state government.) Searching these sites in this way will reveal the agencies involved in drug abuse prevention at the state level.

The role of these state-level agencies is evident from their titles. Some state agencies provide actual services; others provide statistics or other information. Still others provide expertise or serve as a conduit for federal funding aimed at local (city or county) governments.

The role of state government is to promote, protect, and maintain the health and welfare of its citizens. Thus, each state has its own laws regulating the sale of tobacco, alcohol, and prescription drugs. States issue licenses to doctors, dentists, pharmacists, liquor stores, and taverns. Each state also passes laws and sets the penalties for the manufacture, sale, and possession of illicit drugs such as marijuana. For example, in California, possession of 28.5 grams (1 ounce) of marijuana or less is a misdemeanor but not an arrestable offense; it carries a $100 fine. Possession of more than 28.5 grams is also a misdemeanor, punishable by 6 months in jail and a $500 fine. In Utah, however, possession of less than 1 ounce of marijuana is a misdemeanor punishable by 6 months in jail and a $1,000 fine. Possession of more than 1 pound is a felony punishable by 5 years in jail and a $5,000 fine.[61]

In some cases, states have passed laws that conflict with federal laws. For example, some states have decriminalized marijuana cultivation and possession for medical use. In Hawaii, patients with a signed statement from their physician affirming that they suffer from a certain medical condition are protected under law. These patients must be on a state-run registry that issues identification cards. They are then permitted to cultivate up to seven marijuana plants (only three mature plants) and to be in possession of no more than 1 ounce of usable marijuana. These people could still be arrested by the DEA and prosecuted under federal law.

Local Agencies

Agencies of local governments that are involved in drug abuse prevention and control include mayors' offices, police and sheriffs' departments, school corporations, health departments, family services offices, mental health services, prosecutors' offices, the juvenile justice system, judges and courts, drug task forces, and so on. In some communities, there is a community drug task force or coordinating council that includes both government officials and representatives of nongovernmental agencies. Such task forces or councils might include local religious leaders, representatives from local industry (both labor and management), health care providers, and members from local voluntary agencies. The task of these organizations is usually to prioritize problems faced by the community and decide on approaches to solving them. The goal is to develop a coordinated and effective effort to resolve the issue. Sometimes a solution might involve selecting an approach that has been used with success in another community or school system.

Nongovernmental Drug Prevention and Control Agencies and Programs

Many nongovernmental programs and agencies make valuable contributions to the prevention and control of drug abuse in America. Among these are community- and school-based programs, workplace programs, and voluntary agencies.

FIGURE 12.13

Use of appropriate language can be the difference between success and failture of a community drug prevention program.

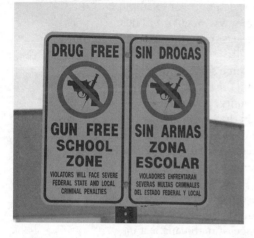

Community-Based Drug Education Programs

Community-based drug education can occur in a variety of settings, such as child care facilities, public housing, religious institutions, businesses, and health care facilities. Information about the abuse of alcohol, tobacco, and other drugs can be disseminated through television and radio programs, movies, newspapers, and magazines.

Community-based drug education programs are most likely to be successful when they include six key features:[62]

1. A comprehensive strategy
2. An indirect approach to drug abuse prevention
3. The goal of empowering youth
4. A participatory approach
5. A culturally sensitive orientation
6. Highly structured activities

Community-based drug education programs that address broader issues (e.g., coping and learning skills) are most effective, as are those embedded in other existing community activities (see Figure 12.13). Participation can be increased by planning drug education programs around sporting or cultural events. Culturally sensitive programs are crucial for reaching minorities in the community. Use of the appropriate language, reading level, and spokespersons can mean the difference between success or failure of a program.

In the past 30 years, a great many drug abuse prevention education programs have been conceived and tested. Some of these have been scientifically proven to be effective. The Substance Abuse and Mental Health Services Administration in the U.S. Department of Health and Human Services has a searchable database of successful programs linked to its Web site.[63]

An example of a community-based program with a record of success is *Across Ages.*

Across Ages is a school- and community-based drug prevention program for youth 9 to 13 years, that seeks to strengthen the bonds between adults and youth and provide opportunities for positive community involvement. The unique and highly effective feature of Across Ages is the pairing of older adult mentors (age 55 and above) with young adolescents, specifically youth making the transition to middle school. The program employs mentoring, community service, social competence training, and family activities to build youths' sense of personal responsibility for self and community.[64]

Across Ages has been able to demonstrate success in the following areas: decreased substance use, decrease in tobacco and alcohol use, increased problem-solving ability, increased school attendance, decreased suspensions from school, improved attitude toward adults, and improved attitude toward school and the future.[64]

School-Based Drug Education Programs

Most health educators believe that a strong, comprehensive school health education program (see Chapter 6)—one that occupies a permanent and prominent place in the school curriculum—is the best defense against all health problems, including drug abuse. However, many schools lack these strong programs and, in their absence, substitute drug education programs developed specifically for school use.

One such program is the Drug Abuse Resistance Education (DARE) program, which began in Los Angeles. In the DARE program, local police enter the classroom to teach grade-school children about drugs. While imparting some knowledge, the program's primary approach is to change attitudes and beliefs about drugs. It is also successful in improving children's images of the police themselves. Unfortunately, although very popular in many communities, DARE programs have been unable to demonstrate any real success in reducing actual drug use.[65]

An example of a program from the CSAP list that has been scientifically proven to be effective is Project ALERT. Project ALERT reduced students' initiation of marijuana use by 30%, decreased current marijuana use by 60%, reduced past-month cigarette use by 20% to 25%, decreased regular and heavy smoking by 33% to 55%, and substantially reduced students' pro-drug-use attitudes and beliefs.[64]

Student assistance programs (SAPs) are school-based programs modeled after employee assistance programs in the workplace. They are aimed at identifying and intervening in cases of drug problems. **Peer counseling programs** are also present in some schools. In these programs, students talk about mutual problems and receive support and perhaps learn coping skills from peers who have been trained in this intervention activity and do not use drugs.

Workplace-Based Drug Education Programs

In September 1986, concern about widespread drug use in the workplace led then President Ronald Reagan to sign Executive Order 12564, proclaiming a Drug Free Federal Workplace.[66] The rationale for the order signed in September 1986 was cited in the document itself: the desire and need for the well-being of employees, the loss of productivity caused by drug use, the illegal profits of organized crime, the illegality of the behavior itself, the undermining of public confidence, and the role of the federal government as the largest employer in the nation to set a standard for other employers to follow in these matters. It had also become apparent to all that drug abuse is not just a personal health problem and a law enforcement problem, but that it also is a behavior that affects the safety and productivity of others, especially at work. Studies have shown that substance abusers (1) are less productive, (2) miss more work days, (3) are more likely to injure themselves, and (4) file more workers' compensation claims than their non-substance-abusing counterparts.

The Drug Free Federal Workplace order required federal employees to refrain from using illegal drugs, and it required agency heads to develop plans for achieving drug-free workplaces for employees in their agencies. The order further required the setting up of drug testing programs and procedures and employee assistance programs that would include provisions for rehabilitation.[66] Similar workplace substance abuse programs, which include drug testing, soon spread to the private sector so that by the mid-1990s, such programs were in place in more than 80% of American companies.[67]

A typical workplace substance abuse prevention program has five facets.[68] The first is a formal written substance abuse policy that reflects the employer's commitment to a drug-free workplace. The second is an employee drug education and awareness program. Third is the supervisor training program. Fourth is the **employee assistance program (EAP)** to help those who need counseling and rehabilitation. The last component is a drug testing program. Large companies are more likely than small companies to have the major components of a drug-free workplace program.

Although a substantial part of the problem can be attributed to alcohol consumption, illicit drug use remains a problem in many workplaces. Though it is true that the prevalence of illegal drug abuse in the unemployed adult population is nearly twice that of the employed adult population, nearly 73% of all the illegal users are employed.[35] Fortunately, the prevalence of workplace drug use has declined significantly, in part because of the proliferation of workplace drug abuse and prevention programs that include drug testing. In 1987, the first year of workplace drug testing, 18.1% of all tests were positive;[69] by 1998, this figure had

student assistance programs (SAPs) school-based drug education programs to assist students who have alcohol or other drug problems

peer counseling programs school-based programs in which students discuss alcohol and other drug-related problems with peers

employee assistance program (EAP) a workplace drug program designed to assist employees whose work performance is suffering because of a personal problem such as alcohol or other drug problems

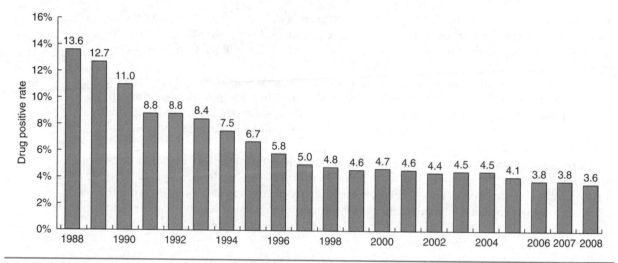

FIGURE 12.14

Drug positivity rates for combined U.S. workforce, 1988 through 2008.

Source: The Quest Diagnostics Drug Testing Index® (2010), from Quest Diagnostics Incorporated. Available at http://www.questdiagnostics.com. Accessed December 22, 2010. Reprinted with permission.

dropped below 5%, where it has remained. In 2008, only 3.6% of all workplace drug tests were positive (see Figure 12.14).[70]

Voluntary Health Agencies

Drug prevention and control programs are carried out at the local level with the cooperation and effort of many community members. Some of these programs are of local origin, whereas others have received national recognition and even endorsement. The people who actually deliver drug abuse prevention programs include teachers, community health educators, social workers, law enforcement officers, and volunteers.

The programs presented vary greatly in their message and approach. Some programs seek to educate or provide knowledge, others seek to change beliefs or attitudes about alcohol or other drug use, while still others seek to alter behavior by providing new behavior skills. Studies have shown that programs incorporating all these approaches are most successful.

A large number of voluntary health agencies have been founded to prevent or control the social and personal consequences of alcohol, tobacco, and other drug abuse. Among these are such agencies as Mothers Against Drunk Driving (MADD), Students Against Destructive Decisions (SADD), Alcoholics Anonymous (AA), Narcotics Anonymous (NA), the American Cancer Society (ACS), and many others. Each of these organizations is active locally, statewide, and nationally.

An important function of community leaders is to encourage parents, school officials, members of law enforcement, businesses, social groups, community health workers, and the media to work together in an effort to reduce the abuse of alcohol, tobacco, and other drugs. Every approach should be used, including seeking favorable legislation and judicial appointments, fairness in advertising, school and community education and treatment, and law enforcement. Only through citizen support and vigilance can there be a reduction in the threat that alcohol and other drugs pose to our community.

CHAPTER SUMMARY

- The abuse of alcohol, tobacco, and other drugs is a major community health problem in the United States.

- Alcohol, tobacco, and other drug abuse affects not only individuals but also communities, where it results in a substantial drain both socially and economically.

- Investigations into the causes of drug experimentation, drug abuse, and drug dependence indicate that both inherited and environmental factors contribute to the problem.

- Rates of tobacco, alcohol, and other drug use rose during the 1990s. After peaking in 1998, use of these drugs began to level off and decline.

- Chronic alcohol and tobacco use results in the loss of billions of dollars and thousands of lives in America each year.

- The misuse and abuse of prescription and nonprescription drugs remain a problem of concern.

- There are four principal elements of drug abuse prevention and control—education, treatment, public policy, and law enforcement.

- Prevention activities can be categorized as primary, secondary, and tertiary prevention.

- There are substantial federal, state, and local efforts to reduce the use, misuse, and abuse of drugs in the United States.

- Federal agencies involved include the Departments of Health and Human Services, Homeland Security, Justice, and many others.

- Efforts at the state level vary from state to state but usually include attempts to coordinate federal and local efforts.

- Drug testing in the workplace reveals a decline in illicit drug use in the workplace since testing began in 1987.

- Alcohol, tobacco, and other drug abuse continues to cause injuries and lost productivity in the American workplace.

- A typical workplace substance abuse prevention program has five components: A written policy, a drug education program, a supervisor training program, an employee assistance program, and a drug testing program.

- A large number of voluntary health agencies are involved in drug abuse prevention and control activities.

REVIEW QUESTIONS

1. What are some personal consequences resulting from the abuse of alcohol and other drugs?

2. What are some community consequences resulting from the abuse of alcohol and other drugs?

3. What are the recent trends in drug use by high school seniors?

SCENARIO: ANALYSIS AND RESPONSE

Please reread the scenario at the beginning of this chapter. How would you respond to the following questions?

1. Re-examine Table 12.2. Which of the personal consequences of drug use were evident in Larissa's story?

2. Re-examine Figure 12.1. Which of the violent acts was mentioned or inferred in the scenario?

3. Which of the factors discussed in this chapter that contribute to drug abuse could have contributed to Larissa's drug dependence?

4. Methamphetamine has become a nationwide problem. Figure 12.8 is a map showing the number of incidents involving methamphetamine clandestine laboratories in each state. Which states appear to have the most serious methamphetamine problem? Is methamphetamine a widespread problem in your state? Have you heard about any meth lab busts in your community?

5. Child maltreatment, a serious problem in the United States, is discussed in Chapter 15. Larissa left her baby with her parents. How many grandparents in the United States are forced into raising their children's children? If Larissa had had no parents, what do you think would have happened to her baby?

6. What state or local agencies are available to help Larissa get into and stay in recovery?

4. What do you feel is our most serious drug problem? Why?

5. Explain the differences among drug use, misuse, and abuse.

6. How are physical and psychological dependence different?

7. What are the two sources of risk factors that contribute to substance abuse?

8. Name the four categories of environmental risk factors that contribute to substance abuse and give an example of each.

9. What are the two major types of abused drugs? Give examples of each.

10. Why is alcohol considered the number 1 problem drug in America?

11. In what forms do Americans consume nicotine, and in what groups of people do we see the heaviest users?

12. What agency regulates over-the-counter and prescription drugs? What two characteristics must a drug have to be approved for sale?

13. How can misuse of prescription drugs become a risk to your health?

14. What is the most commonly abused illicit drug? Why is this drug a concern?

15. What are controlled substances? Give some examples.

16. What are the side effects for both men and women that result from the use of anabolic drugs?

17. What are the four elements of drug prevention and control?

18. What are primary, secondary, and tertiary prevention strategies for the drug problem?

19. Describe the roles of each of the following federal departments in controlling drug abuse: Health and Human Services, Homeland Security, and Justice.

20. What role do state governments play in preventing and controlling drug abuse? Local governments?

21. What is Across Ages? What does it do? What is Project ALERT? What does it do?

22. How would you respond to the statement "Most drug abusers are unemployed"?

23. What are the names of four voluntary agencies and self-help groups involved in the prevention, control, and treatment of alcohol, tobacco, and other drug abuse?

Activities

1. Schedule an appointment with the vice president of Student Affairs, the Dean of Students, or the alcohol and drug abuse prevention educator on your campus to find out more about drug (including alcohol) problems. Find

out what the greatest concerns are and how the administration is trying to deal with the issues.

2. Make an appointment with the health educator or another employee in your local health department to find out more about the existing alcohol, tobacco, and other drug problems in the community. Collect the same information as noted in the first activity, except find information for the community, not the campus.

3. Find six articles that appeared in your local paper during the past 2 weeks that deal with drugs. Find two that related to problems at the national or international level, two at the state level, and two at the local level. Summarize each and present your reaction to these articles in a written paper.

4. Conduct a survey of at least 100 students on your campus. Try to get a random sample of people. Interview these people and find out what they think are the major drug problems on your campus and how they might be solved. Feel free to include other questions on your survey. Summarize the results in a two-page paper.

5. Attend a meeting of a community group that is involved in the prevention and control of drug abuse (e.g., local drug task force, AA, a smoking cessation group, MADD, or SADD). In a two-page paper, summarize the meeting and share your reaction to it.

Community Health on the Web

The Internet contains a wealth of information about community and public health. Increase your knowledge of some of the topics presented in this chapter by accessing the Jones & Bartlett Learning Web site at **http://health.jbpub.com/book/communityhealth/7e** and follow the links to complete the following Web activities.

• National Clearinghouse for Alcohol and Drug Information
• MADD
• Office on Smoking and Health

References

1. Horgan, C., K. C. Skwara, and G. Strickler (2001). *Substance Abuse: The Nation's Number One Health Problem*. Princeton, NJ: Robert Wood Johnson Foundation.

2. National Center on Addiction and Substance Abuse at Columbia University (2006). *The Commercial Value of Underage and Pathological Drinking to the Alcohol Industry: A CASA White Paper*. Available at http://www.casacolumbia.org/templates/Publications_Reports.aspx#rib.

3. National Center on Addiction and Substance Abuse at Columbia University. (2009). *Shoveling Up II: The Impact of Substance Abuse on Federal, State and Local Budgets*. Available at http://www.casacolumbia.org/articlefiles/380=ShovelingUpII.pdf.

4. Johnston, L. D., P. M. O'Malley, and J. G. Bachman (1993). *Monitoring the Future National Survey Results on Drug Use, 1975–1992*.

Volume I: Secondary School Students (NIH pub no. 93-3597). Bethesda, MD: National Institute on Drug Abuse.

5. Johnston, L. D., P. M. O'Malley, J. G. Bachman, and J. E. Schulenbert (2009). *Monitoring the Future National Survey Results on Drug Use 1975-2008, Volume I, Secondary School Students* (NIH pub. no. 09-7402). Bethesda, MD: National Institute on Drug Abuse. Available at http://www.monitoringthefuture.org/pubs/monographs/vol1_2008.pdf.

6. Glantz, M., and R. Pickens (1992). "Vulnerability to Drug Abuse: Introduction and Overview." In M. Glantz and R. Pickens, eds., *Vulnerability to Drug Abuse*. Washington, DC: American Psychological Association.

7. Cotton, N. S. (1979). "The Familial Incidence of Alcoholism: A Review." *Journal of Studies on Alcohol*, 40: 89-116.

8. Cloninger, C. R., M. Bohman, and S. Sigvardsson (1981). "Inheritance of Alcohol Abuse." *Archives of General Psychiatry*, 38: 861-868.

9. Schuckit, M. A., S. C. Risch, and E. O. Gold (1988). "Alcohol Consumption, ACTH Level, and Family History of Alcoholism." *American Journal of Psychiatry*, 145(11): 1391-1395.

10. Tabakoff, B., and P. L. Hoffman (1988). "Genetics and Biological Markers of Risk for Alcoholism." *Public Health Report*, 103(6): 690-698.

11. U.S. Department of Health and Human Services (1990). *Seventh Special Report to the U.S. Congress* (DHHS pub. no. ADM-90-1656). Washington, DC: U.S. Government Printing Office.

12. Zickler, P. (2000). "Evidence Builds That Genes Influence Cigarette Smoking." *NIDA Notes*, 15(2): 1-2.

13. Needle, R., Y. Lavee, S. Su, et al. (1988). "Familial, Interpersonal, and Intrapersonal Correlates of Drug Use: A Longitudinal Comparison of Adolescents in Treatment, Drug-Using Adolescents Not in Treatment, and Non-Drug-Using Adolescents." *International Journal of Addictions*, 239(12): 1211-1240.

14. Meller, W. H., R. Rinehart, R. J. Cadoret, and E. Troughton (1988). "Specific Familial Transmission in Substance Abuse." *International Journal of Addictions*, 23(10): 1029-1039.

15. Shedler, J., and J. Block (1990). "Adolescent Drug Use and Psychological Health: A Longitudinal Inquiry." *American Psychologist*, 45(5): 612-630.

16. Horgan, C., K. C. Skwara, and G. Strickler 2001. *Substance Abuse: The Nation's Number One Health Problem*. Princeton, NJ: Robert Wood Johnson Foundation, 30.

17. Dembo, R., W. R. Blount, J. Schmeidler, and W. Burgos (1986). "Perceived Environmental Drug Use Risk and the Correlates of Early Drug Use or Nonuse among Inner-City Youths: The Motivated Actor." *International Journal of Addictions*, 21(9-10): 977-1000.

18. Foster, S. E., R. D. Vaughan, W. H., Foster, J. A. and Califano, Jr. (2006). "Estimate of the Commercial Value of Underage Drinking and Adult Abusive and Dependent Drinking to the Alcohol Industry." *Archives of Pediatrics and Adolescent Medicine*, 160(5): 473-478.

19. Morse, R. M., and D. K. Flavin (1992). "The Definition of Alcoholism." *JAMA*, 268(8): 1012-1014.

20. National Institute on Alcohol Abuse and Alcoholism (January 1996). "Drinking and Driving." *Alcohol Alert*, 31(362): 1-4.

21. U.S. Department of Health and Human Services, Public Health Service (2000). *Healthy People 2010: Understanding and Improving Health*. Washington, DC: U.S. Government Printing Office.

22. Hunt, T. (4 October 2000). "Tough Standard Set for Drunken Driving." *USA Today*, 4A.

23. Insurance Institute for Highway Safety, Highway Loss Data Institute (2007). "DUI/DWI Laws as of March 2007." Available at http://www.iihs.org/laws/state_laws/dui.htm.

24. Cole, T. B. (2006). "Rape at U.S. Colleges Often Fueled by Alcohol." *JAMA*, 296(5): 504-505.

25. Lupton, C. (2003). "The Financial Impact of Fetal Alcohol Syndrome." Substance Abuse and Mental Health Services Administration, FASD Center for Excellence. Available at http://fasdcenter.samhsa.gov/publications/cost.cfm?&print=y.

26. Office of New York Attorney General Eliot Spitzer (11 October 2006). "Attorneys General and R. J. Reynolds Reach Historic Settlement

to End the Sale of Flavored Cigarettes [Press release]." Available at http://www.oag.ny.gov/media_center/2006/oct/oct11a_06.html.

27. Department of Health and Human Services (August 1993). "Substance Abuse Prevention and Treatment Block Grants: Sale or Distribution of Tobacco Products to Individuals Under 18 Years of Age: Proposed Rule." *Federal Register Part II*, 45: 96.

28. American Lung Association, (2009). "President Obama Signs Bill Granting the U.S. FDA Regulatory Control over Tobacco Products." Available at http://www.lungusa.org/press-room/press-releases/pres-obama-signs-bill-for-fda-tobacco-control.html.

29. Confessore, N. (21 June 2010). "Cigarette Tax Increased to Keep State Running." *New York Times*. Available at http://www.nytimes.com/2010/06/22/nyregion/22budget.html.

30. American Cancer Society. (2010). *Cancer Facts and Figure—2010*. Atlanta, GA: Author.

31. World Health Organization. (2008). *WHO Report on the Global Tobacco Epidemic, 2008: The MPOWER Package*. Geneva: Author.

32. U.S. Department of Health and Human Services, Public Health Service, Centers for Disease Control (1986). *The Health Consequence of Involuntary Smoking. A Report of the Surgeon General* (DHHS pub. no. CDC-87-8398). Washington, DC: U.S. Government Printing Office.

33. Byrd, J. C., R. S. Shapiro, and D. L. Schiedermayer (1989). "Passive Smoking: A Review of Medical and Legal Issues." *American Journal of Public Health*, 79(2): 209-215.

34. Environmental Protection Agency (1991). *Respiratory Health Effects of Passive Smoking: Lung Cancer and Other Disorders* (EPA/600/6-90/006F). Washington, DC: Indoor Air Quality Clearinghouse.

35. Department of Health and Human Services, Substance Abuse and Mental Health Services Administration (2009). *Results from the 2008 National Survey on Drug Use and Health: National Findings*. Available at http://www.oas.samhsa.gov/nsduh/2k8nsduh/2k8Results.pdf.

36. Physicians' Desk Reference. (2009). *2010 PDR for Nonprescription Drugs, Dietary Supplements, and Herbs*. Montvale, NJ: PDR Network. Available at http://www.pdr.net.

37. U.S. Department of Justice, Drug Enforcement Administration (2006). *Pseudoephedrine Notice*. Office of Diversion Control. Available at http://www.azpharmacy.gov/pdfs/pseud.Notice.pdf.

38. Physicians' Desk Reference. (2009). *2010 Physicians' Desk Reference, 64th ed*. Montvale, NJ: PDR Network. Available at http://www.pdr.net.

39. Centers for Disease Control and Prevention (2006). "MRSA (Methicillin-Resistant *Staphylococcus aureus*)." Available at http://www.cdc.gov/ncidod/diseases/submenus/sub_mrsa.htm.

40. Warner, M., L. J. Chen, and D. M. Makuc (2009). *Increase in Fatal Poisonings Involving Opioid Analgesics in the United States, 1999-2006* (NCHS data brief, no. 22). Hyattsville, MD: National Center for Health Statistics.

41. Centers for Disease Control and Prevention (2010). "CDC's Issue Brief: Unintentional Drug Poisoning in the United States." Available at http://www.cdc.gov/HomeandRecreationalSafety/Poisoning/brief.htm.

42. Centers for Disease Control and Prevention (2010). "Emergency Department Visits Involving Nonmedical Use of Selected Prescription Drugs—United States, 2004-2008. *Morbidity and Mortality Weekly Report*, 59(23): 705-709.

43. Federal Register, Code of Federal Regulations, Food and Drugs, Part 1308. *Schedules of Controlled Substances*, Rev. April 1, 1998. Washington, DC: Author.

44. Substance Abuse and Mental Health Services Administration, Office of Applied Studies (2010). *Drug Abuse Warning Network, 2007: National Estimates of Drug-Related Emergency Department Visits* (DAWN Series D-28, DHHS Pub. no. (SMA) 06-4143). Rockville, MD: Author. Available at https://dawninfo.samhsa.gov/pubs/edpubs/default.asp.

45. Zickler, P. (2000). "Evidence Accumulates That Long-Term Marijuana Users Experience Withdrawal." *NIDA Notes*, 15(1).

46. Substance Abuse and Mental Health Services Administration, Office of Applied Studies (2008). *Treatment Episode Data Set (TEDS). Highlights—2006. National Admissions to Substance Abuse Treatment Services* (DASIS Series: S-40, DHHS pub no. (SMA) 08-4313). Rockville, MD: Author. Available at http://www.oas.samhsa.gov/teds2k6highlights/teds2k6highWeb.pdf.

47. Center for Addiction and Substance Abuse at Columbia University (1994). *Cigarettes, Alcohol, Marijuana: Gateways to Illicit Drug Use.* New York: Author.

48. Department of Justice, National Drug Intelligence Center (2010). *National Drug Threat Assessment 2010* (Product no. 2006-Q0317-003, October 2006). Johnstown, PA: Author. Available at http://www.usdoj.gov/ndic/topics/ndtas.htm.

49. Volkow, N. D. (2005). "Message from the Director: Communities across the country are trying to respond to increased abuse of methamphetamine, a powerfully addictive stimulant." National Institute of Drug Abuse. Available at http://www.drugabuse.gov/about/welcome/messagemeth405.html.

50. Drug Enforcement Administration, Department of Justice, (2010). "Stats & Facts. National Statistics." Available at http://www.justice.gov/dea/statistics.html.

51. National Institute on Drug Abuse, National Institutes of Health (2010). "MDMA (Ecstasy)." *NIDA Infofacts.* Available at http://www.drugabuse.gov/infofacts/ecstasy.html.

52. National Institute on Drug Abuse, National Institutes of Health (2009). "Steroids (Anabolic and Androgenic)." *NIDA InfoFacts.* Available at http://www.drugabuse.gov/PDF/Infofacts/Steroids09.pdf.

53. Center for Substance Abuse Prevention, Substance Abuse and Mental Health Services Administration (1997). *A Look at Successful and Cost-Effective State Treatment Programs: Treatment Works Fact Sheet.* Rockville, MD: Author.

54. Yates, B. T. (1999). Measuring and Improving Cost, Cost-Effectiveness, and Cost-Benefit for Substance Abuse Treatment Programs (NIH pub. no. 99-4518). Bethesda, MD: National Institutes of Health.

55. Centers for Medicare and Medicaid Services (2010). "The Mental Health Parity and Addiction Equity Act." Available at https://www.cms.gov/HealthInsReformforConsume/04_TheMentalHealthParityAct.asp.

56. Bureau of Justice Statistics (1992). *Drugs, Crime and the Justice System 1992.* Washington, DC: U.S. Government Printing Office.

57. Office of National Drug Control Policy, The White House (2010). *National Drug Control Strategy 2010.* Washington, DC: The White House. Available at http://www.whitehousedrugpolicy.gov/strategy.

58. U.S. Department of Justice, Office of Justice Programs (n.d.). "About OJP." Available at http://www.ojp.usdoj.gov/about/about.htm.

59. U.S Department of Justice, Bureau of Alcohol, Tobacco, Firearms, and Explosives (n.d.). "ATF's Mission." Available at http://www.atf.gov/about/mission/.

60. U.S. Department of Education (1987). *What Works: Schools without Drugs.* Washington, DC: U.S. Government Printing Office.

61. NORML (National Organization for the Reform of Marijuana Laws) (n.d.). Home page. Available at http://www.norml.org.

62. Brown, M. E. (1993). "Successful Components of Community and School Prevention Programs." *National Prevention Evaluation Report: Research Collection,* 1(1): 4–5.

63. Substance Abuse and Mental Health Services Administration (2010). "National Registry of Evidence-Based Programs and Practices." Available at http://nrepp.samhsa.gov/.

64. Across Ages: An Intergenerational Mentoring Approach to Prevention (n.d.). "Goals and Objectives." Available at http://www.acrossages.org/.

65. Lynam, D. R., R. Milich, R. Zimmerman, S. P. Novak, T. K. Logan, C. Martin, C. Leukefeld, and R. Clayton (1999). "Project DARE: No Effects at 10-Year Follow-up." *Journal of Consulting and Clinical Psychology,* 67(4): 590–593.

66. Drug-Free Federal Workplace (Executive Order 12564) (17 September 1986). *Federal Register,* 51(180).

67. American Management Associates (1996). *AMA Survey: Workplace Drug Testing and Drug Abuse Policy.* New York: Author.

68. U.S. Department of Labor (1991). *What Works: Workplaces without Alcohol or Other Drugs* (pub. no. 282-148/54629). Washington, DC: U.S. Government Printing Office.

69. SmithKline Beecham Clinical Laboratories (29 February 1996). "Drug Detection in the Workplace in 1995 Declines for the Eighth Straight Year [Press release]." Collegeville, PA: Author.

70. Quest Diagnostics (2009). *Drug Testing Index: New Hair Data Validate Sharp Downward Trend in Cocaine and Methamphetamine Positivity in General U.S. Workforce, According to Quest Diagnostics Drug Testing Index.* Available at http://www.questdiagnostics.com/employer solutions/dti/2009_11/dti_index.html.

Chapter 13

Health Care Delivery in the United States

Chapter Objectives

After studying this chapter, you will be able to:

1 Define the term *health care system*.

2 Trace the history of health care delivery in the United States from colonial times to the present.

3 Discuss and explain the concept of the spectrum of health care delivery.

4 Distinguish between the different kinds of health care, including population-based public health practice, medical practice, long-term practice, and end-of-life practice.

5 List and describe the different levels of medical practice.

6 List and characterize the various groups of health care providers.

7 Explain the differences among allopathic, osteopathic, and nonallopathic providers.

8 Define *complementary* and *alternative medicine*.

9 Explain why there is a need for health care providers.

10 Prepare a list of the different types of facilities in which health care is delivered.

11 Explain the differences among private, public, and voluntary hospitals.

12 Explain the difference between inpatient and outpatient care facilities.

13 Briefly discuss the options for long-term care.

14 Explain what the Joint Commission does.

15 Identify the major concerns with the health care system in the United States.

16 Explain the various means of reimbursing health care providers.

Chapter Objectives (*cont.*)

17 Briefly describe the purpose and concept of insurance.

18 Define the term *insurance policy*.

19 Explain the insurance policy terms *deductible*, *co-insurance*, *copayment*, *fixed indemnity*, *exclusion*, and *pre-existing condition*.

20 Explain what is meant when a company or business is said to be self-insured.

21 List the different types of medical care usually covered in a health insurance policy.

22 Briefly describe Medicare, Medicaid, and Medigap insurance.

23 Briefly describe the Children's Health Insurance Program (CHIP).

24 Briefly explain long-term care health insurance.

25 Define *managed care*.

26 Define the terms *health maintenance organization (HMO)*, *preferred provider organization (PPO)*, and *exclusive provider organization (EPO)* and *point-of-service option*.

27 Identify the advantages and disadvantages of managed care.

28 Define consumer-directed health plans and give several examples.

29 Provide a brief overview of the Affordable Care Act passed in 2010.

SCENARIO

Chad had adapted well and was enjoying his first year in college. He liked his classes and professors, had made friends quickly, and enjoyed the freedom that came with living in a resident hall on a college campus. What he missed was being a part of a formal athletic team because while in high school he was a three-sport letterman. However, he was enjoying participation in the campus intramural program and found the competition to be reasonably good. He played on a flag football team in the fall and was now member of a pretty good basketball team.

Chad was an aggressive player and didn't mind trying to drive to the basket when the odds were against him or scrambling for a loose ball on the floor. It was during the seventh game of the year, when his team was playing the other undefeated team in the league, that his aggressive play got the best of him. He was under the basket going after a rebound against a much taller player. He got the ball, but when he came down his foot landed on top of his opponent's and he "rolled" his ankle. He also heard a strange sound when it happened—like something popped in his ankle. The intramural staff responded quickly with some first aid and information on the Recreational Sports Department's protocol for injuries. The intramural supervisor told Chad that the campus health center was closed but that he would be happy to call 911 for him. Chad wasn't sure if he wanted 911. He thought that he would just go home, "ice it down," take some aspirin, and see how things were in the morning. He could then decide whether he would go to the campus health center, the hospital emergency room, the local orthopedic walk-in clinic, the "doc-in-the-box" emergi-center, or just make an appointment with his own family doctor back home.

INTRODUCTION

The process by which health care is delivered in the United States is unlike the processes used in other countries of the world. Other developed countries have national health insurance run or organized by the government and paid for, in large part, by general taxes. Also, in these countries almost all citizens are entitled to receive health care services, including routine and basic health care.[1] Health care in the United States is delivered by an array of **providers**, in a variety of settings, under the watchful eye of regulators, and paid for in a variety of ways. Because of this process, many question the notion that the United States has a health care delivery system (see Figure 13.1). That is, "[a]lthough these various individuals and organizations are generally referred to collectively as 'the health care delivery system,' the phrase suggests order, integration, and accountability that do not exist. Communication, collaboration, or systems planning among these various entities is limited and is almost incidental to their operations."[2] Whether or not health care delivery in the United States should be called a "system," there is a process in place in which health care professionals, located in a variety of facilities, provide services to deal with disease and injury for the purpose of promoting, maintaining, and restoring health to the citizens. In this chapter, we outline the history of health care delivery in the United States, examine the structure of health care, and describe how our unique system functions. And finally, we discuss health care reform in the United States.

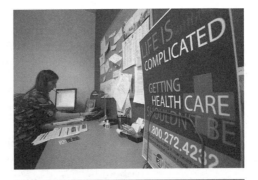

FIGURE 13.1
Do we really have a health care system?

providers
health care facilities or health professionals that provide health care services

A BRIEF HISTORY OF HEALTH CARE DELIVERY IN THE UNITED STATES

For as long as humankind has been concerned with disease, injury, and health, there has always been a category of health care in which people have tried to help or treat themselves. This category of care is referred to as *self-care* or *self-treatment*. For example, in most American homes, there are usually provisions to deal with minor emergencies, nursing care, and the relief of minor pains or ailments. This type of care continues today. The following discussion of the history of health care in the United States does not include self-care because it is assumed that most people would engage in some type of self-care prior to seeking professional help. Instead, we review the development of professional care provided by those trained to do so.

As might be assumed with the birth of a new country, from colonial times through the latter portion of the nineteenth century, health care and medical education in the United States lagged far behind their counterparts in Great Britain and Europe. During this period of time anyone, trained or untrained, could practice medicine. Much of the early health care was provided by family members and neighbors and consisted of home and folk remedies that had been handed down from one generation to another. When a person did receive training as a physician, it was nothing like the rigorous training that a physician goes through today. The early medical education in the colonies was not grounded in science, but rather was experience based.[1] Prior to 1870, medical education was provided primarily through an apprenticeship with a practicing physician who may have been trained in the same way.[3] Consequently, medical care was primitive and considered to be more a trade than a profession.[1] In addition, most of the health care was provided in the patient's home and not in an office or clinic.

There were some hospitals during these early years, but they were located primarily in large cities and seaports such as New York, Philadelphia, and New Orleans. However, the hospitals were much different from the hospitals of today and served more in a social welfare function than as places to receive health care. They were not very clean, and unhygienic practices prevailed. The forerunner of today's hospital and nursing home was the *almshouse* (also called a *poorhouse*).[1] Almshouses were run by the local government primarily to provide food, shelter, and basic nursing care for indigent people (i.e., the elderly, homeless, orphans, the ill, and the disabled) who could not be cared for by their own families.[1] In addition to almshouses, local government also operated *pesthouses*, which served as a place to isolate people who had contracted an infectious disease such as cholera, smallpox, or typhoid.[1]

In the late nineteenth century, formal health care gradually moved from the patient's home to the physician's office and into the hospital. The primary reason for this change was the building and staffing of many new hospitals. It was felt that patients could receive better care in a setting designed for patient care, staffed with trained people, and equipped with the latest medical supplies and instruments. In addition, physicians could treat more patients in a central location because of the reduced travel time.

It was also during the latter portion of the nineteenth century that the scientific method began to play a more important role in medical education and health care. Medical procedures backed by scientific findings began to replace "rational hunches," "good ideas," and "home remedies" as the standards for medical care. With the acceptance of the germ theory of disease and the identification of infectious disease agents, there was real hope for the control of communicable diseases, which were the leading health problems of that period.

At the beginning of the twentieth century, although communicable diseases were still the leading causes of death, mortality rates were beginning to decline. Most of the decline can be attributed to improved public health measures. Yet, at the end of World War I, mortality rates spiked not only in the United States but also worldwide because of the 1918–1919 influenza pandemic. This deadliest pandemic in history killed as many as 100 million people. Shortly after the pandemic in the early 1920s, a major shift took place in the United States as chronic diseases moved past communicable diseases as the leading causes of death.

At the same time that chronic diseases were pushing to the top of the list of causes of death, much change was taking place in health care. New medical procedures such as X-ray therapy, specialized surgical procedures, and chemotherapy were developed, group medical practices were started, and new medical equipment and instruments (such as the electrocardiograph to measure heart function) were invented. The training of doctors and nurses also improved and became more specialized. By 1929, the United States was spending about 3.9% of its gross domestic product (GDP) on health care, which means that 3.9% of all goods and services produced by the nation that year were associated with health care.

Even with some of these "new" advances in the practice of medicine, U.S. medicine was still limited pretty much to two parties—patients and physicians. "Diagnosis, treatment, and fees for services were considered confidential between patients and physicians. Medical practice was relatively simple and usually involved long-standing relationships with patients and, often, several generations of families. Physicians collected their own bills, set, and usually adjusted their charges to their estimates of patients' ability to pay. This was the intimate physician-patient relationship the professional held sacred."[4]

By the early 1940s, the United States was again at war. World War II affected health care in the United States in a variety of ways. One consequence of the war that would have a lasting impact on health care was employers' use of health insurance to lure workers to their companies. Because of the large number of men and women in the armed services, there was a shortage of workers to fill the jobs back home. Also, because of the need for resources for the war effort, the U.S. government put restrictions on the wages that companies could pay their employees. However, there were no restrictions on the health care insurance that employers could provide for their employees. Thus, companies began using health insurance to recruit and retain workers, and as a result employer-provided health insurance took a foothold at this time.

Also as a result of World War II, huge technical strides were made in the late 1940s and 1950s as medical procedures and processes developed during the war found applications in civilian medicine. However, adequate health facilities to treat long-term diseases were lacking in many areas of the country. The **Hospital Survey and Construction Act of 1946**, better known as the **Hill-Burton Act** (after the authors of the legislation), provided substantial funds for hospital construction. The infusion of federal funds helped to remedy the serious hospital shortage caused by the lack of construction during the Depression and World War II. The Hill-Burton Act was primarily a federal-state partnership. State agencies were given grants to determine the need for hospitals and then were provided with seed money to begin construction of the facilities.[5] However, the major portion of construction dollars came from state and local sources.[6] Through the years, the Hill-Burton Act has been amended several times to help meet health care needs in the United States. Funds have been made available for additional construction, modernization, and replacement of other health care facilities and for comprehensive health planning.

With improved procedures, equipment, and facilities and the increase in noncommunicable diseases, the cost of health care began to rise. As the cost of health care rose, it became too expensive for some people. Concerns were expressed about who should receive health care and who should pay for it. The debate over whether health care is a basic right or a privilege in America began in earnest. By the end of the 1950s, there remained an overall shortage of quality health care in America. There was also a maldistribution of health care services—metropolitan areas were being better served than the less-developed rural areas.

In the 1960s, there was an increased interest in health insurance, and it became common practice for workers and their bargaining agents to negotiate for better health benefits (see Figure 13.2). Undoubtedly, some employers preferred to increase benefits rather than to raise wages. Few then could foresee the escalation in health care costs for Americans. Thus, the **third-party payment system** for health care became solidified as the standard method of payment for health care costs in the United States. The third-party payment system gets its name from the fact that the insurer—either government or a private insurance company (third party)—reimburses (pays the bills) to the provider (second party) for the health care given to the patient (first party).[7] (A detailed explanation of the third-party payment system is presented later in this chapter.) More recently, when some speak of the third-party payment system, they add a fourth party—the purchaser of the insurance, usually an employer. It should be noted that the government and private insurers pay the medical bills with tax dollars and collected premiums, respectively—not with their own funds.

With the growth of the third-party system of paying for health care, the cost of health care rose even more rapidly than before because patients enjoyed increased access to care without or little out-of-pocket expenses. However, those without insurance found it

Hospital Survey and Construction Act of 1946 (Hill-Burton Act) federal legislation that provided substantial funds for hospital construction

third-party payment system a health insurance term indicating that bills will be paid by the insurer and not the patient or the health care provider

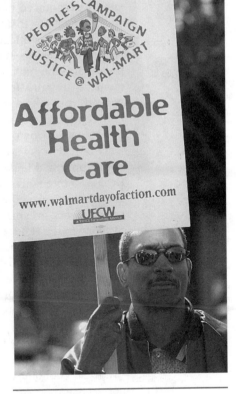

FIGURE 13.2
Health benefits have become an important part of the total compensation package for workers.

increasingly difficult to afford care. When the Democrats regained the White House in the 1960s, they led a federal policy change to increase citizen access to health care, which culminated in 1965 with the authorization of Medicare and Medicaid by Titles XVIII and XIX, respectively, of the Social Security Act. (These programs, which were enacted to help provide care for the elderly, the disabled, and the poor, are also discussed later in this chapter.) Also in the 1960s, the federal government increased funding for medical research and technology to support transplants and life extension.

By the late 1960s and early 1970s, it had become apparent that the Hill-Burton Act had stimulated not only the growth of health care facilities, but also the demand for health care services. With this growth came a continuing rise in health care costs and a need for better planning in health care delivery.

Among the early attempts at planning were the 1964 amendments to the Hill-Burton Act. The amendments called for comprehensive planning on a regional level. Their purpose was to make more efficient use of federal funds by preventing the duplication of facilities. However, they depended on good faith efforts and could not be enforced. It soon became evident that more powerful legislation was needed to control costs and to coordinate and control rapid growth in health care facilities.

Another attempt was made to encourage better planning 2 years later. The Comprehensive Health Planning and Public Service Amendments of 1966 authorized funds for state- and area-wide Comprehensive Health Planning Agencies. These too failed because they had no teeth. Then, in 1974, Public Law 93-641 was passed. This law, known as the National Health Planning and Resources Development Act of 1974, combined several pieces of previous legislation to put teeth into comprehensive planning efforts. There were high hopes and expectations that these pieces of legislation would provide reason and order to the development and modification of health care services.[8] This legislation led to the formation of Health Systems Agencies throughout the entire country. Their purpose was to cut costs by preventing the building of "unnecessary" facilities or the purchase of unnecessary equipment. Although some money may have been saved, the Health Systems Agencies were viewed by some as yet another unnecessary government bureaucracy, and when the late President Reagan took office in 1980, he, along with Congress, eliminated this program.

Before leaving our health care discussion of the 1970s, it should be noted that another piece of legislation was passed that did not seem all that important at the time but that would have a profound impact on the way health care was delivered later. This legislation was the Health Maintenance Organization (HMO) Act of 1973. This act "provided both loans and grants for the planning, development, and implementation of combined insurance and health care delivery organizations and required that a minimum prescribed array of services be included in the HMO arrangement."[4]

The 1980s brought many changes to the health care industry, the most notable of which was probably the deregulation of health care delivery. In 1981, with Ronald Reagan in the White House, it was announced that the administration would let the competitive market, not governmental regulation, shape health care delivery.[9] Open competition is a philosophy of allowing consumers to regulate delivery by making choices about where and from whom they receive their care. In theory, those who provide good care will get more patients and in turn be able to offer the care at a lower price. In other words, the resulting competition would help squeeze out costly waste and ineffective care.[10]

Some economists, however, do not believe that the health care system behaves like a normal market. For example, it is not likely that an ill patient seeking medical care will shop for a less expensive physician. Physicians do not advertise the cost of their services. Also, it is the physician who tells the patient which hospital to go to and when to check in and out, due to the admitting privileges that physicians have. In addition, providers tend to offer more and more services to entice the market to "shop with us," which in effect drives up health care spending. For these reasons, the competitive market approach is of questionable value in lowering health care costs.

The 1980s also saw a proliferation of new medical technology (e.g., MRIs and ultrasound). Along with this new technology have come new health care issues such as medical ethics (e.g., prolonging life and ending life) and more elaborate health insurance programs (e.g., policies that cover specific diseases such as cancer and AIDS, home care, and rehabilitation).

Many of the concerns of the 1980s continued into the 1990s. The 1992 presidential campaign again brought attention to America's problems with health care delivery. Bill Clinton, then governor of Arkansas, based his election campaign strategy on being a new kind of Democrat—one who could take on the nation's domestic ills. He saw health care as one of those ills because the present system failed to cover all, and its spiraling costs threatened to bankrupt the government and cripple American industry.

Shortly after being elected president, Mr. Clinton appointed the first lady, Hillary Rodham Clinton, to head a committee to develop a plan to overcome the shortcomings of the health care system. By the fall of 1993, the committee had completed a plan that the president then presented to a joint session of Congress in front of a national television audience. This detailed plan, referred to informally as the president's Health Security Plan and formally as the **American Health Security Act of 1993**, was over 1,500 pages in length. The focal point of the plan was to provide universal coverage. President Clinton's health care plan was much discussed in Congress in 1994; however, opposition kept it from ever reaching the floor for a vote before Congress adjourned. This was the sixth time in U.S. history that the concept of universal coverage was defeated. Although the plan was never approved, the pressures generated by the plan transformed the private health care system in the United States.

In the mid- to late 1990s, rapid changes occurred in the organization and financing of health care. These changes can be summed up in two words—managed care. **Managed care** "is a system of health care delivery that (1) seeks to achieve efficiency by integrating the basic functions of health care delivery, (2) employs mechanisms to control (manage) utilization of medical services, and (3) determines the price at which the services are purchased, and consequently, how much the providers get paid."[1]

With the advent of managed care, the increase of health care costs slowed in the mid-1990s; in fact, the actual growth for several years was almost flat. Even so, both the percentage of the GDP and the dollars spent on health care continued to inch up. In 1996, for the first time in history, the total health care bill for the United States topped $1 trillion ($1,039 billion, 13.6% of the GDP).[11] In 2010, health care expenditures were projected at $2.6 trillion (17.3% of the GDP).[12] Put another way, approximately one-sixth of all the output of the United States in 2010 was spent on health care. Health care is the one segment of the U.S. economy that continues to grow consistently faster than the cost of inflation (see Table 13.1). Ever-newer technology, ever-increasing demands for the best care, growing medical liability, new diagnostic procedures, the lengthening of life spans, the development of new drugs (e.g., Viagra), and newly identified diseases put great demands on the system.

By the mid- to late 1990s, managed care had become the dominant form of health care financing and delivery, but it became apparent that support for it, with some exceptions, was not deep.[13] In addition, it was obvious that the slowdown in health care costs, which was attributed to managed care, would be just a one-time savings if other measures were not taken. President Clinton saw this as an opportunity to again seek health care reform.

This time then President Clinton treaded carefully, offering small but politically popular programs like health care coverage for uninsured children (see the discussion of CHIP later in this chapter) and a mandatory minimum hospital stay for childbirth to counter the so-called drive-by deliveries created by managed care.[14] So, in 1996, through an executive order and

American Health Security Act of 1993 the comprehensive health care reform introduced by then President Clinton, but never enacted

managed care "a system of health care delivery that (1) seeks to achieve efficiency by integrating the basic functions of health care delivery, (2) employs mechanisms to control utilization of medical services, and (3) determines the price at which the services are purchased and how much the providers get paid."

Table 13.1

Consumer Price Index and Average Annual Percentage of Change for All Items and Selected Items: United States, Selected Years 1960–2009

[Data are based on reporting by samples of providers and other retail outlets.]

Year	All Items	Medical Care	Food	Apparel	Housing	Energy
1960	29.6	22.3	30.0	45.7	—	22.4
1970	38.8	34.0	39.2	59.2	36.4	25.5
1980	82.4	74.9	86.8	90.0	81.1	86.0
1990	130.7	162.8	132.4	124.1	128.5	102.1
2000	172.2	260.8	167.8	129.6	169.6	124.6
2009	214.5	375.6	217.9	120.1	217.1	193.1

—, Data not available.

Note: 1982–1984 = 100.

Source: U.S. Department of Labor, Bureau of Labor Statistics (2010). Consumer Price Index. Available at http://www.bls.gov/cpi/tables.htm. Accessed December 15, 2010.

with an amendment by way of a second executive order in 1997, President Clinton created the Advisory Commission on Consumer Protection and Quality in the Health Care Industry.[15] Formally, "the Commission was charged to advise the President on changes occurring in the health care system and, where appropriate, to make recommendations on how best to promote and ensure consumer protection and health care quality."[15] Informally, this meant creating a "consumer bill of rights" and conducting a comprehensive review of the quality of health care in the nation. In 2002, both the House and the Senate passed differing versions of the Patient's Bill of Rights, but no compromise could be worked out. Ultimately, the states took the lead in patient rights area, with many passing their own version of a Patient's Bill of Rights.[4]

The most notable change to U.S. health care during the presidency of George W. Bush was the passage of the Medicare Prescription Drug, Improvement, and Modernization Act of 2003 (MMA). The most visible components of the MMA have been the voluntary outpatient prescription drug benefit for people on Medicare, know as Part D (see the discussion of Medicare Part D later in the chapter), and health savings accounts (HSAs). HSAs are tax-free savings accounts that can be used to pay for near-term medical expenses incurred by individuals, spouses, and dependants and to save for future longer-term costs.[16] (HSAs are also discussed in greater detail later in the chapter.)

Throughout the early part of the twenty-first century, both consumers and health care providers agreed that health care delivery in the United States needed to be changed. The Institute on Medicine (IOM) claimed that "health care today harms too frequently and routinely fails to deliver its potential benefits."[17] Further, the health care system suffered from lack of coordinated, comprehensive services, resulting in both the wasteful duplication of efforts and unaccountable gaps in care.[17] In its reports, the IOM outlined a number of recommendations for changing health care delivery in the United States. These recommendations, combined with the release of the World Health Organization's report *The World Health Report 2000—Health Systems: Improving Performance*, in which the U.S. health system was ranked thirty-seventh out of 191 countries,[18] provide some direction for changing the way health care was delivered.

Because of the great concern for health care reform, much attention was given to the topic during the presidential debates in 2008. In fact, all major candidates outlined plans for change if elected. As it is now known, when President Obama took office one of the top issues on his agenda for change was health care reform. However, one of the first pieces of legislation signed into law by President Obama was the Children's Health Insurance Program (CHIP) Reauthorization Act of 2009 (*Note:* CHIP was formerly known as the State Children's Health Insurance Program [SCHIP]). This law expanded CHIP to approximately 4.1 million uninsured children and was funded by a 62-cent increase in the federal tax on cigarettes.

It took another year before more comprehensive health care reform was passed. In March 2010, President Obama signed into law two bills—the Patient Protection and Affordable Health Care Act (PPACA) (Public Law 111-148) and the Health Care and Education Reconciliation Act of 2010 (HCERA) (Public Law 111-152). These two acts were consolidated with other approved legislation and are now referred to as the "Affordable Care Act." This act introduced many changes to health care delivery in the United States that will have great impact on health care delivery for years to come. Portions of this act went into effect in 2010 and the last portion will go into effect in 2020. A more complete presentation of the act comes in the last part of this chapter.

HEALTH CARE SYSTEM: STRUCTURE

The structure of the health care system of the United States is unique in the world. In the sections that follow, we examine the spectrum of health care delivery and describe the various types of health care providers and the facilities in which health care is delivered.

The Spectrum of Health Care Delivery

Because health care in the United States is delivered by an array of providers in a variety of settings, reference is sometimes made to the spectrum of health care delivery (see Table 13.2). The *spectrum of health care delivery* refers to the various types of care. Within this spectrum, four levels of practice have emerged: population-based public health practice, medical practice, long-term practice, and end-of-life practice.

Population-Based Public Health Practice

Population-based public health practice incorporates interventions aimed at disease prevention and health promotion, specific protection, and a good share of case findings.[19,20] A primary component of population-based public health practice is education. If people are going to behave in a way that will promote their health and the health of their community, they first must know how to do so. Health education not only provides such information but also attempts to empower and motivate people to put this information to use by discontinuing unhealthy behaviors and adopting healthy ones. Though much of public health practice takes place in governmental health agencies, it also takes place in a variety of other settings (such as voluntary health agencies, social service agencies, schools, businesses and industry, and even in some traditional medical care settings).[19]

> **population-based public health practice** incorporates interventions aimed at disease prevention and health promotion, specific protection, and a good share of case findings

Medical Practice

Medical practice means "those services usually provided by or under the supervision of a physician or other traditional health care provider."[19] Such services are offered at several different levels. You may remember that in Chapter 4 we used the terms *primary, secondary,* and *tertiary* as they related to levels of prevention. These terms have a similar meaning here, but they are now applied to health care delivery rather than prevention.

Primary Medical Care

Primary care is "front-line" or "first-contact" care. "The unique characteristic of primary care is the role it plays as a regular or usual source of care for patients and their families."[2] Formally, **primary care** has been defined as "clinical preventive services, first-contact treatment

> **primary care** "clinical preventive services, first-contact treatment services, and ongoing care for commonly encountered medical conditions"

Table 13.2
The Spectrum of Health Care Delivery

Level of Practice	Description	Examples of Delivery Settings
Population-based public health practice	Practice aimed at disease prevention and health promotion that shapes a community's overall health; emphasizes education and prevention	Public, community, and school health programs; public health clinics
Medical practice		
Primary care	Clinical preventive services, first-contact treatment services, and ongoing care for commonly encountered medical conditions; emphasizes prevention, early detection, and routine care	Primary care provider offices; public clinics; managed care organizations; community mental health centers
Secondary care	Specialized attention and ongoing management for common and less frequently encountered medical conditions, including support services for people with special challenges due to chronic or long-term conditions	
Acute care	Short-term, intense medical care that may require hospitalization	Emergency rooms; urgent/emergent care centers; outpatient/inpatient surgical centers; hospitals
Subacute care	After acute care, need for more nursing intervention	Special subacute units in hospitals (e.g., transitional care units); skilled nursing facilities; home health care
Tertiary care	Subspecialty referral care requiring highly specialized personnel and facilities	Specialty hospitals (e.g., psychiatric, chronic disease) and general hospitals with highly specialized facilities
Long-term practice		
Restorative care	Intermediate follow-up care such as surgical post-operative care	Home health; progressive and extended care facilities; rehabilitation facilities that specialize in therapeutic services; halfway houses
Long-term care	Care for chronic conditions; personal care	Nursing homes; facilities for the mentally retarded or emotionally disturbed; geriatric day care centers
End-of-life practice	Care provided to those who have less than six months to live	Hospice services provided in a variety of settings

Sources: Cambridge Research Institute (1976). *Trends Affecting the U.S. Health Care System.* Washington, DC: U.S. Government Printing Office; U.S. Public Health Service (1994). *For a Healthy Nation: Return on Investments in Public Health.* Washington, DC: Author; Turnock, B. J. (2009). *Public Health: What It Is and How It Works,* 4th ed. Sudbury, MA: Jones & Bartlett Learning; Shi, L., and D. A. Singh (2010). *Essentials of the U.S. Health Care System,* 2nd ed. Sudbury, MA: Jones & Bartlett Learning.

services, and ongoing care for commonly encountered medical conditions."[19] Eighty percent of medical care is primary care.[19] Primary care includes routine medical care to treat common illnesses or to detect health problems in their early stages, and thus includes such things as semiannual dental checkups; annual physical exams; health screenings for hypertension, high blood cholesterol, and breast or testicular cancer; and sore throat cultures. Primary care usually is provided in practitioners' offices, clinics, and other outpatient facilities by physicians, nurse practitioners, physician assistants, and an array of other individuals on the primary care team. Primary care is the most difficult for the poor and uninsured to obtain (see Box 13.1).

Secondary Medical Care

Secondary medical care is "specialized attention and ongoing management for common and less frequently encountered medical conditions, including support services for people with special challenges due to chronic or long-term conditions."[19] This type of care is usually provided by physicians, ideally upon referral from a primary care source.[19]

secondary medical care "specialized attention and ongoing management for common and less frequently encountered medical conditions, including support services for people with special challenges due to chronic or long-term conditions"

BOX 13.1

HEALTHY PEOPLE 2020: OBJECTIVES

Access to Health Services

Goal: Improve access to comprehensive, quality health care services.

Objective: AHS-3, Increase the proportion of persons with a usual primary care provider.

Target: 83.9 percent.

Baseline: 76.3 percent of persons had a usual primary care provider in 2007.

Target setting method: 10 percent improvement.

Data source: Medical Expenditure Panel Survey (MEPS), AHRQ.

Objective: AHS-5.1 (all ages), Increase the proportion of persons who have a specific source of ongoing care.

Target: 95.0 percent.

Baseline: 86.4 percent of persons of all ages had a specific source of ongoing care in 2008.

Target setting method: 10 percent improvement.

Data source: National Health Interview Survey (NHIS), CDC, NCHS.

Objective: AHS-5.3 (adults aged 18 to 64 years), Increase the proportion of persons who have a specific source of ongoing care.

Target: 89.4 percent.

Baseline: 81.3 percent of persons aged 18 to 64 years had a specific source of ongoing care in 2008.

Target setting method: 10 percent improvement.

Data source: National Health Interview Survey (NHIS), CDC, NCHS.

For Further Thought

Why is it so important for the United States to reach the three objectives stated above? What impact would reaching these objectives have on the cost of health care in the United States? Provide a rationale for your response.

Source: U.S. Department of Health and Human Services, Office of Disease Prevention and Health Promotion (2010). *Healthy People 2020.* Available at http://www.healthypeople.gov/2020/default.aspx. Accessed December 2, 2010.

Tertiary Medical Care

Tertiary medical care "is even more highly specialized and technologically sophisticated medical and surgical care than secondary medical care for those with unusual or complex conditions (generally no more than a few percent of the need in any service category)."[19] This care is not usually performed in smaller hospitals; however, it is provided in specialty hospitals, academic health centers, or on specialized floors of general hospitals. Such facilities are equipped and staffed to provide advanced care for people with illnesses such as cancer and heart disease, and procedures such as heart bypass surgery.

tertiary medical care specialized and technologically sophisticated medical and surgical care for those with unusual or complex conditions (generally no more than a few percent of the need in any service category)

Long-Term Practice

Long-term practice can be divided into two subcategories—restorative care and long-term care.

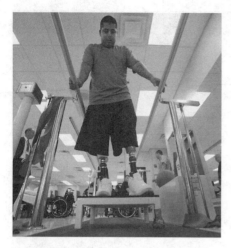

FIGURE 13.3
Restorative care can follow either secondary or tertiary care.

Restorative Care

Restorative care is the health care provided to patients after surgery or other successful treatment, during remission in cases of an oncogenic (cancerous) disease, or when the progression of an incurable disease has been arrested. This level of care includes follow-up to secondary and tertiary care, rehabilitative care, therapy, and home care (see Figure 13.3). Typical settings for this type of care include both inpatient and outpatient rehabilitation units, nursing homes, assisted-living facilities, halfway houses, and private homes.

Long-Term Care

Long-term care includes the different kinds of help that people with chronic illnesses, disabilities, or other conditions that limit them physically or mentally need. In some situations time-intensive skilled nursing care is needed, while some people just need help with basic daily tasks like bathing, dressing, and preparing meals. This type of care is provided in various settings such as nursing homes, facilities for the mentally and emotionally disturbed, assisted-living facilities, and adult and senior day care centers, but often long-term care is used to help people live at home rather than in institutions.

End-of-Life Practice

The final level of practice in the health care delivery is end-of-life practice. **End-of-life practice** is usually thought of as those health care services provided to individuals shortly before death. The primary form of end-of-life practice is hospice care. **Hospice care** "is a cluster of special services for the dying. It blends medical, spiritual, legal, financial, and family support services. The venue can vary from a specialized facility to a nursing home to the patient's own home."[21] The most common criterion for admission to hospice care is being terminally ill with a life expectancy of less than 6 months. The first hospice program in the United States was established in 1974.[22] In 2007, there were 3,255 Medicare-certified providers and suppliers of hospice services in the United States, compared with 164 in 1985.[23]

Types of Health Care Providers

To offer comprehensive health care that includes services at each of the levels just mentioned, a great number of health care workers are needed. In 2008, the number of civilians employed in the health service industry was 14.5 million. These 14.5 million represented approximately 1 of every 10 (10.4%) employed civilians in the United States.[23]

Despite the large number of health care workers, the demand for more is expected to continue to grow. "Employment growth is expected to be driven by technological advances in patient care, which permit a greater number of health problems to be treated, and by an increasing emphasis on preventive care. In addition, the number of older people, who are much more likely than younger people to need nursing care, is projected to grow rapidly."[24] Due to the continuing geographic maldistribution of health care workers, the need will be greater in some settings than in others. The settings of greatest need will continue to be the rural and inner-city areas (see Box 13.2).

In 2008, just more than two-fifths (41.3%) of all health care workers were employed in hospitals, more than one-fourth (25.6%) work in outpatient health care settings (i.e., offices and clinics of physicians, dentists, chiropractors, optometrists, and other health practitioners, and outpatient care centers), about one-sixth (16.3%) in nursing and residential care facilities, while the remaining one-sixth (16.7%) work in home health care or other settings.[23] As changes have come to the way health care is offered, the proportions of health care workers

restorative care care provided after successful treatment or when the progress of an incurable disease has been arrested

long-term care different kinds of help that people with chronic illnesses, disabilities, or other conditions that limit them physically or mentally need

end-of-life practice health care services provided to individuals shortly before death

hospice care a cluster of special services for the dying that blends medical, spiritual, legal, financial, and family support services

BOX 13.2	HEALTHY PEOPLE 2020: OBJECTIVES

Access to Health Services

Goal: Improve access to comprehensive, quality health care services.

Objective: AHS-4 (Developmental), Increase the number of practicing primary care providers.

Objective: AHS-4.1 (Developmental), Medical doctors

Target: TBD

Baseline: TBD

Target setting method: TBD

Potential data source: American Medical Association (AMA), Masterfile, AMA.

Objective: AHS-4.2 (Developmental), Doctors of osteopathy

Target: TBD

Baseline: TBD

Target setting method: TBD

Potential data source: American Osteopathic Association (AMA), Masterfile, AOA.

Objective: AHS-4.3 (Developmental), Physician assistants

Target: TBD

Baseline: TBD

Target setting method: TBD

Potential data source: American Academy of Physician Assistants (AAPA) Census, AAPA.

Objective: AHS-4.4 (Developmental), Nurse practitioners

Target: TBD

Baseline: TBD

Target setting method: TBD

Potential data source: National Provider Identifier (NPI) Registry, CMS.

TBD = To be determined

For Further Thought

What impact would reaching these objectives have on access to health care in the United States especially in the rural and inner-city areas? Provide a rationale for your response.

Source: U.S. Department of Health and Human Services, Office of Disease Prevention and Health Promotion (2010). *Healthy People 2020.* Available at http://www.healthypeople.gov/2020/default.aspx. Accessed December 2, 2010.

by setting have also changed, with fewer persons working in hospitals (in 1970, 63% worked in hospitals), and more employed in nursing homes and ambulatory care settings (such as surgical and emergency centers). This trend is expected to continue in the future, with special needs in the area of long-term care workers to meet the needs of the aging baby boom generation.

There are well over 200 different careers in the health care industry. To help simplify the discussion of the different types of health care workers, they have been categorized into six different groups—independent providers, limited care providers, nurses, nonphysician practitioners, allied health care professionals, and public health professionals.

Independent Providers

independent providers
health care professionals with the education and legal authority to treat any health problem

Independent providers are those health care workers who have the specialized education and legal authority to treat any health problem or disease that an individual has. This group of workers can be further divided into allopathic, osteopathic, and nonallopathic providers.

Allopathic and Osteopathic Providers

allopathic providers
independent providers whose remedies for illnesses produce effects different from those of the disease

Allopathic providers are those who use a system of medical practice in which specific remedies for illnesses, often in the form of drugs or medication, are used to produce effects different from those of diseases. The practitioners who fall into this category are those who are referred to as Doctors of Medicine (MDs). The usual method of practice for MDs includes the taking of a health history, a physical examination—perhaps with special attention to one area of the complaint—and the provision of specific treatment, such as antibiotics for a bacterial infection or a tetanus injection and sutures for a laceration.

osteopathic providers
independent health care providers whose remedies emphasize the interrelationships of the body's systems in prevention, diagnosis, and treatment

Another group of physicians that provides services similar to those of MDs are **osteopathic providers**—Doctors of Osteopathic Medicine (DOs). At one time, MDs and DOs would not have been grouped together because of differences in their formal education, methods, and philosophy of care. While the educational requirements and methods of treatment used by MDs have remained essentially consistent over the years, those of DOs have not. The practice of osteopathy was started in 1874 by Andrew Taylor Still, MD, DO, who was dissatisfied with the effectiveness of nineteenth-century medicine.[25] The distinctive feature of osteopathic medicine is the recognition of the reciprocal interrelationship between the structure and function of the body. The actual work of DOs and MDs is very similar today. Both types of physicians use all available scientific modalities, including drugs and surgery, in providing care to their patients. Both can also serve as primary care physicians (about one-third of MDs[1] and more than three-fifths of DOs are primary care physicians)[25] or as board-certified specialists. Their differences are most notably the DOs' greater tendency to use more manipulation in treating health problems and the DOs' perception of themselves as being more holistically oriented than MDs. Few if any patients today would be able to tell the difference between the care given by a DO and a MD.

intern
a first-year resident

The educational requirements for MD and DO degrees are very similar. Both educational programs generally accept students into their classes after they have completed a bachelor's degree. Medical education takes 4 years to complete. The first 2 years include course work in the sciences, while the final 2 years emphasize clinical experiences and rotations through the specialty areas of medicine. At the end of the second year of medical school and again at the end of the fourth year, medical students take the first two parts of their licensing examination. During the fourth year of medical school, the students apply for entrance into a medical residency program. It is during their residency program that the physicians receive the training to specialize in a particular field of medicine. The residency programs typically range in length from 3 (such as in family medicine) to 5 (such as in pathology) years. The first year of a residency is referred to as the *internship year,* and the physicians are referred to as **interns** or first-year **residents**. During this year, the interns can only practice medicine under the guidance of a licensed physician. Upon successful completion of the internship year, the interns are then eligible to sit for the third part of the licensing examination. If they pass the exam, they are then entitled to practice medicine without the supervision of another licensed physician. At this point, almost all interns will complete the remaining years of residency (and are referred to generically as residents) to be eligible to sit for the board specialty examinations. Passing this examination will make them "board certified" in their specialty. A list of such medical care specialties and subspecialties is presented in Box 13.3.

resident
a physician who is training in a specialty

BOX 13.3	LISTING OF MEDICAL SPECIALTIES AND SUBSPECIALTIES

Allergy and immunology (immune systems)
Anesthesiology (administer drugs for pain during surgery)
Cardiology (heart and circulatory system)
Colon and rectal surgery
Dermatology (skin)
Emergency medicine
Family medicine (general family health)
   Geriatric medicine (care of elderly)
   Sports medicine
Hospitalist (in-patient medicine)
Internal medicine
   Cardiovascular medicine
   Clinical cardiac electrophysiology
   Critical care medicine
   Diagnostic laboratory immunology
   Endocrinology (diabetes and metabolism)
   Gastroenterology (digestive organs)
   General practice (usually just for adults)
   Geriatric medicine (care of elderly)
   Hematology (blood, spleen, and lymph glands)
   Infectious disease
   Medical oncology (cancer)
   Nephrology (kidney)
   Neurology
   Pulmonary disease (lungs)
   Rheumatology (joints, muscle, bones, and tendons)
Nuclear medicine (use radioactive substances to diagnose, research, and treat disease)
Obstetrics and gynecology (female reproductive system, the fetus, and the newborn)
   Gynecologic oncology
   Maternal-fetal medicine
   Reproductive endocrinology
Ophthalmology (eye)
Otolaryngology (ear and throat)
Otorhinolaryngology (ear, nose, and throat)
Pathology
   Blood banking/transfusion medicine
   Cytopathology (tumors)
   Dermatopathology
   Forensic pathology (cause of death)

   Hematology
   Immunopathology
   Medical microbiology
   Neuropathology
   Pediatric pathology
Pediatrics (children)
   Adolescent medicine (adolescents and young adults)
   Diagnostic laboratory immunology
   Neonatal–prenatal medicine (problems of the fetus and newborns)
   Pediatric cardiology
   Pediatric critical care
   Pediatric emergency medicine
   Pediatric endocrinology
   Pediatric gastroenterology
   Pediatric hematology-oncology
   Pediatric infectious disease
   Pediatric nephrology
   Pediatric rheumatology
   Pediatric sports medicine
Physical medicine and rehabilitation
   Pain medicine
   Sports medicine
Plastic and reconstructive surgery
Preventive medicine
   Aerospace medicine
   Occupational medicine
   Public health and general preventive medicine
Psychiatry
Radiology (radiation to diagnose and treat disease)
   Diagnostic radiology
   Radiation oncology
Surgery
   Colon and rectum surgery
   General vascular surgery
   Hand surgery
   Orthopedic (bones and joints)
   Pediatric surgery
   Surgical critical care
   Thoracic surgery (chest area)
Urology (genitals and urinary tract)

With so many specialties and subspecialties, health care experts are worried that not enough primary care physicians (which includes general practice/family medicine, internal medicine, obstetrics/gynecology, and pediatrics) will be trained. There are some data to support this claim. In 1949, 59% of active doctors of medicine (MDs and DOs) practiced as primary care physicians. This percentage dropped to approximately 39% by 1990. However, the percentage has remained fairly stable since 1990. In 2007, the figure was 39.1%.[23] This stabilizing effect may in part be because of the managed care movement and its need for primary care practitioners and not specialists.

Nonallopathic Providers

Nonallopathic providers are identified by their nontraditional means of providing health care. Some have referred to much of the care provided by these providers as complementary/

nonallopathic providers independent providers who provide nontraditional forms of health care

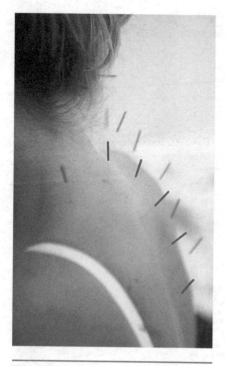

FIGURE 13.4

Many people seek out nontraditional means of health care, such as acupuncture.

chiropractor
a nonallopathic, independent health care provider who treats health problems by adjusting the spinal column

complementary/ alternative medicine (CAM)
a group of diverse medical and health care systems, practices, and products that are not presently considered to be a part of conventional medicine

alternative medicine (CAM) or complementary/integrative medicine. Included in this group of providers are chiropractors, acupuncturists (see Figure 13.4), naturopaths (those who use natural therapies), herbalists (those who use herbal brews for treating illness), and homeopaths (those who use small doses of herbs, minerals, and even poisons for therapy).

The best-known and most often used nonallopathic providers in the United States are **chiropractors**. The underlying premise of the care provided by chiropractors is that all health problems are caused by misalignments of the vertebrae in the spinal column. The chiropractic (done by hand) approach to the treatment is (1) the identification of the misalignment through X-rays, and (2) the realignment of the bones through a series of treatments called "adjustments."

Chiropractors are educated in 4-year chiropractic colleges. The Council on Chiropractic Education accredits colleges of chiropractic medicine in the United States. As with allopathic and osteopathic programs, students usually enter chiropractic programs after earning a bachelor's degree. Those who graduate from chiropractic colleges earn a Doctor of Chiropractic (DC) degree. Chiropractors are licensed in all 50 states and must pass either a state licensing examination or an examination given by the National Board of Chiropractic Examiners.

As noted earlier, much of the care provided by nonallopathic providers is often referred to as **complementary/alternative medicine (CAM)** or *complementary/integrative medicine*. CAM has been defined as "a group of diverse medical and health care systems, practices, and products that are not presently considered to be a part of conventional medicine."[4] When used together with conventional medicine, a therapy is identified as *complementary*. An example of a complementary medicine is "using accupuncture in addition to usual care to help lessen pain."[26] When a therapy is used in place of a conventional medicine, it is labeled as *alternative*. "An example of an alternative therapy is using a special diet to treat cancer instead of undergoing surgery, radiation, or chemotherapy that has been recommended by a conventional doctor."[26] When mainstream medical therapies are combined with CAM therapies for which there is some high-quality scientific evidence of safety and effectiveness, it is referred to as *integrative medicine*.[26] CAM is one of the fastest growing areas of health care today. Data indicate that approximately 38% (83 million) of adults and 11% (8.5 million) of children in the United States reported using CAM in the past year,[27] although the percentage changes depending on what is considered CAM. The percentage of use is highest when the definition of CAM includes prayer specifically for health reasons. Even with its popularity, Americans paid for most CAM out of pocket (approximately $34 billion in 2007[28]). Nearly two-thirds of the total out-of-pocket costs that adults spent on CAM were for self-care purchases of CAM products, classes, and materials, while the remaining portion was spent on practitioner visits. Despite this emphasis on self-care therapies, adults made more than 354 million visits to CAM practioners.[28] "Private health insurance plans may offer coverage of certain CAM therapies, such as chiropractic and massage. Overall, however, coverage of CAM therapies is relatively limited—compared with coverage of conventional therapies. One factor is a lack of scientific evidence regarding the cost-effectiveness of CAM therapies. As consumer interest in CAM grows, more insurance companies and managed care organizations may consider offering coverage of CAM therapies shown to be safe and effective."[26] (See Box 13.4.)

BOX 13.4	A NOTE ABOUT SAFETY AND EFFECTIVENESS OF CAM

Rigorous, well-designed clinical trials for many CAM therapies are often lacking; therefore, the safety and effectiveness of many CAM therapies are uncertain. The National Center for Complementary and Alternative Medicine (NCCAM) is sponsoring research designed to fill this knowledge gap by building a scientific evidence base about CAM therapies—whether they are safe, whether they work for the conditions for which people use them, and, if so, how they work.

As with any medical treatment, there can be risks with CAM therapies. These general precautions can help to minimize risks:

- Select CAM practitioners with care. Find out about the practitioner's training and experience.
- Be aware that some dietary supplements may interact with medications or other supplements, may have side effects of their own, or may contain potentially harmful ingredients not listed on the label. Also keep in mind that most supplements have not been tested in pregnant women, nursing mothers, or children.
- Tell all your health care providers about any complementary and alternative practices you use. Give them a full picture of what you do to manage your health. This helps ensure coordinated and safe care. For tips about talking with your health care providers about CAM, see NCCAM's Time to Talk campaign at nccam.nih.gov/timetotalk/.

Source: National Center for Complementary and Alternative Medicine, National Institutes of Health (2010). CAM Basics. Available at http://nccam.nih.gov/health/whatiscam/. Accessed September 29, 2010.

There are literally hundreds of systems, approaches, and techniques that fall within the CAM rubric. CAM practices are often grouped into broad categories, such as natural products (e.g., herbal medicines also known as botanicals), mind-body medicine (e.g., meditation, yoga, acupuncture, hypnotherapy, tai chi), manipulative and body-based practices (e.g., spinal manipulation and massage therapy), and other CAM practices (movement therapies [i.e., Pilates], traditional healers, manipulation of energy fields [i.e., magnet therapy], and whole medical systems [i.e., Ayurvedic medicine, homeopathy, naturopathy]).[29]

"Although alternative approaches use a wide range of techniques, most share a number of common features. These include:

1. A focus on disease prevention and health maintenance
2. A holistic approach in which the whole person—mind, emotions, and spirit—is considered
3. The use of natural processes and materials in healing
4. A focus on the cause of the disease rather than symptoms
5. A consideration of lifestyle and emotional issues
6. A belief that the body has an innate ability to heal itself when it is brought into balance and harmony"[27]

Limited (or Restricted) Care Providers

Much health care is provided by **limited (or restricted) care providers** who have advanced training, usually a doctoral degree, in a health care specialty. Their specialty enables them to provide care for a specific part of the body. This group of providers includes but is not limited to dentists (teeth and oral cavity), optometrists (eyes, specifically refractory errors), podiatrists (feet and ankles), audiologists (hearing), and psychologists (mind).

limited (restricted) care providers health care providers who provide care for a specific part of the body

Nurses

We have categorized nurses into a group of their own because of their unique degree programs, the long-standing tradition of nursing as a profession, and their overall importance in the health care industry. It has been estimated that there are a little over 4 million individuals who work in the nursing profession. These include registered nurses, licensed practical

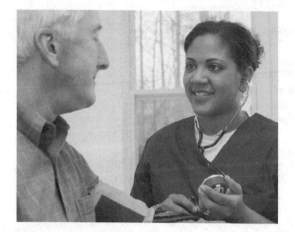

FIGURE 13.5
There is still a need for more nurses.

nurses, and ancillary nursing personnel such as nurse's aides.[23] Nurses outnumber physicians, dentists, and every other single group of health care workers in the United States.[23] Even with such numbers, the need for nurses will continue (see Figure 13.5). The nurse "shortage is driven by a broad set of factors related to recruitment and retention—among them, fewer workers, an aging workforce, and unsatisfying work environments—that have contributed to a different kind of shortage that is more complex, more serious, and expected to last longer than previous shortages."[30]

Training and Education of Nurses

Nurses can be divided into subcategories based on their level of education and type of preparation. The first are those who are prepared as licensed practical nurses. Once they complete their 1 to 2 years of education in a vocational, hospital, or associate degree program and pass a licensure examination, these nurses are referred to as **licensed practical nurses (LPNs)**, or *licensed vocational nurses* (LVNs) in some states,[31] and are able to work under the supervision of physicians or registered nurses. The duties of LPNs vary depending on their work setting. In a hospital, LPNs usually perform routine duties and provide nontechnical bedside nursing care. In a nursing home, they may handle a more broad range of duties, including routine and more complex nursing procedures such as treating bedsores, preparing and giving injections, and inserting catheters. In outpatient settings, LPNs may perform a variety of clinical and clerical duties depending on the size and nature of the practice, and in home health care their duties may range from education to routine nursing care to use of technical equipment.[31] Not too many years ago it was thought that LPNs would be phased out and replaced with more qualified nurses. In 2008, there were 753,600 LPNs or LVNs working in the United States, and that number was projected to grow by 21% to 909,200 by 2018.[32]

A second group of nurses is *registered nurses*. **Registered nurses (RNs)** are those who have successfully completed an accredited academic program and a state licensing (registration) examination. The three typical educational paths to registered nursing are a bachelor's degree (BSN), an associate degree (ADN), and a diploma from an approved nursing program.[33] ADN programs take about 2 to 3 years to complete and are typically offered by community or junior colleges. Diploma programs are offered by hospitals and last about 3 years. RNs holding BSN degrees are referred to as **professional nurses** and are considered to have been more thoroughly prepared for additional activities involving independent judgment. Of the employed registered nurses, 60% worked in hospitals, about 8% in offices of physicians, 5% in home health care services, 5% in nursing care facilities, and 3% in employment services. The remainder worked mostly in government agencies, social assistance agencies, and educational services.[33] In 2008, there were 2.6 million RNs working in the United States, and that number was projected to grow by 22% to 3.2 million in 2018.[33]

Advanced Practice Nurses

With advances in technology and the development of new areas of medical specialization, there is a growing need for specialty-prepared advanced practice nurses (APNs). Many professional nurses continue their education and earn master's and doctoral degrees in nursing. The master's degree programs are aimed primarily at specialties such as nurse practitioners (NPs) (e.g., pediatric nurse practitioners and school nurse practitioners), clinical

licensed practical nurse (LPN) those prepared in 1- to 2-year programs to provide nontechnical bedside nursing care under the supervision of physicians or registered nurses

registered nurse (RN) one who has successfully completed an accredited academic program and a state licensing examinationn

professional nurse a registered nurse holding a bachelor of science degree in nursing (BSN)

nurse specialists (CNSs), certified registered nurse anesthetists (CRNAs), and certified nurse midwives (CNMs). These APNs are qualified to conduct health assessments, diagnose and treat a range of common acute and chronic illnesses, and manage normal maternity care. Not only do they provide high-quality care in a cost-effective manner, but they are also considered primary care providers in chronically medically underserved inner-city and rural areas. Like other nurses, the demand for APNs is also expected to increase, especially as a greater portion of the population gains access to health care and more of the population becomes enrolled in managed care. In 2008, the number of RNs prepared to practice in at least one advanced practice role was estimated to be 250,527, or 8.2% of the total RN population.[34] The largest portion of these APNs were nurse practitioners (see Figure 13.6).

The relatively few nurses who hold doctorate degrees in nursing are highly sought after as university faculty. Nurses with doctorates teach, conduct research, and otherwise prepare other nurses or hold administrative (leadership) positions in health care institutions.

Nonphysician Practitioners

Nonphysician practitioners (NPPs) (also known as nonphysician clinicians [NPCs] or midlevel providers or physician extenders) constitute a relatively new classification of health care workers. This group is composed of those "clinical professionals who practice in many of the areas in which physicians practice, but do not have an MD or a DO degree."[1] NPPs are middle-level health workers with training and skills beyond those of RNs and less than those of physicians.[31] This group typically includes the just discussed nurse practitioners and certified midwives as well as physician assistants (PAs).[1] Because the former two were just presented as part of the section on advanced practice nurses, we discuss only PAs here.

Physician assistant programs began in response to the shortage of primary care physicians. PAs' academic programs usually last 2 years and are offered in a variety of formats, including diploma and certificate programs, or as associate, bachelor's, or master's degrees.

nonphysician practitioners (NPPs) clinical professionals who practice in many of the areas similar to those in which physicians practice, but do not have an MD or DO degree

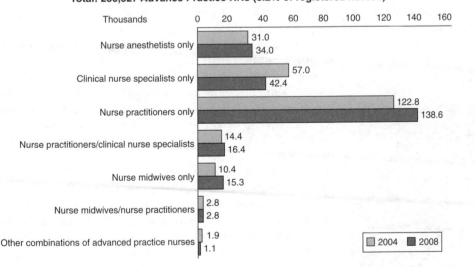

Total: 250,527 Advance Practice RNs (8.2% of registered nurses)

Thousands		2004	2008
Nurse anesthetists only		31.0	34.0
Clinical nurse specialists only		57.0	42.4
Nurse practitioners only		122.8	138.6
Nurse practitioners/clinical nurse specialists		14.4	16.4
Nurse midwives only		10.4	15.3
Nurse midwives/nurse practitioners		2.8	2.8
Other combinations of advanced practice nurses		1.9	1.1

FIGURE 13.6
Registered nurses prepared for advanced practice, 2004–2008.

Source: U.S. Department of Health and Human Services, Health Resources and Services Administration (2010). *The Registered Nurse Population: Findings from the 2008 National Sample Survey of Registered Nurses.* Available at http://bhpr.hrsa.gov/healthworkforce/rnsurvey. Accessed September 29, 2010.

After completion of the program or degree, PAs must pass a national certifying examination. PAs always work under the direct supervision of a licensed physician (thus the name *physician extenders*). They carry out many of the same duties that are thought of as the responsibilities of physicians, such as taking medical histories, examining patients, ordering and interpreting laboratory tests and X-rays, counseling patients, making preliminary diagnoses, treating minor injuries, and, in most states, prescribing medications.[31]

Allied Health Care Professionals

allied health care professionals health care workers who provide services that assist, facilitate, and complement the work of physicians and other health care specialists

Allied health describes a large group of health-related professions that fulfill necessary roles in the health care delivery system. These **allied health care professionals** assist, facilitate, and complement the work of physicians, dentists, and other health care specialists. These health care workers provide a variety of services that are essential to patient care. Often they are responsible for highly technical services and procedures. Allied health care professionals can be categorized into several groups.[4] They include (1) laboratory technologists and technicians (e.g., medical technologists, emergency medical technicians, nuclear medicine technicians, operating room technicians, dental technicians and hygienists, and radiographers [X-ray technicians]); (2) therapeutic science practitioners (e.g., occupational, physical, radiation, and respiratory therapists and speech pathologists); (3) behavioral scientists (e.g., health education specialists, social workers, and rehabilitation counselors); and (4) support services (e.g., medical record keepers and medical secretaries). The educational backgrounds of allied health workers range from vocational training to master's degrees. Many of these professionals also must pass a state or national licensing examination before they can practice.

The demand for allied health care workers in all of the areas previously noted is expected to continue well into the twenty-first century. The primary reasons for this are the growth of the entire health care industry and the impending arrival of the baby boomers as senior citizens.

Public Health Professionals

public health professional a health care worker who works in a public health organization

A discussion about health care providers would be incomplete without the mention of a group of health workers who provide unique health care services to the community—**public health professionals**. They support the delivery of health care by such hands-on providers as public health physicians, dentists, nurses, and dieticians who work in public health clinics sponsored by federal, state, local, and voluntary health agencies (see Figure 13.7). Examples of other public health professionals are environmental health workers, public health administrators, epidemiologists, health education specialists, public health nurses and physicians, biostatisticians, the Surgeon General, and the research scientists at the Centers for Disease Control and Prevention. Public health professionals often make possible the care that is practiced in immunization clinics, nutritional programs for women, infants, and children (WIC), dental health clinics, and sexually transmitted disease clinics. School nurses are also considered public health professionals. Public health services are usually financed by tax dollars and, although available to most taxpayers, serve primarily the economically disadvantaged.

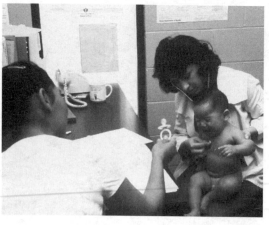

FIGURE 13.7
Public health professionals make up a key component of the health care system.

Health Care Facilities and Their Accreditation

Health care is provided in a variety of settings in the United States. The major settings and the accreditation of these facilities are discussed in the sections that follow.

Health Care Facilities

Health care facilities are the physical settings in which health care is actually provided. They include a wide variety of settings but can be divided into two large categories of inpatient and outpatient care facilities. *Inpatient care facilities* include any in which a patient stays overnight, such as a hospital. *Outpatient care facilities* refer to any facility in which the patient receives care and does not stay overnight.

Inpatient Care Facilities

The primary inpatient care facilities are hospitals, nursing homes, and assisted-living facilities. Because nursing home and assisted-living facilities were discussed in Chapter 9, we discuss only hospitals here. Hospitals vary in size, mission, and organizational structure. The major purpose of hospitals is to provide secondary and tertiary care.

Hospitals can be categorized in several different ways; one way is by hospital ownership (see Figure 13.8 and Table 13.3). A **private (proprietary or investor-owned) hospital** is one that is owned as a business for the purpose of making a profit. "Most for-profit hospitals belong to one of the large hospital management companies that dominate the for-profit hospital network."[4] Recently, a new type of for-profit hospital has been popping up in the United States: the **specialty hospital**. These are hospitals that provide mainly one type of medicine—usually surgery, either cardiac or orthopedic; most are owned, at least in part, by the physicians who practice in them.[4] A lot of controversy surrounds these hospitals. Larger general hospitals, which are losing patients and revenue to the specialty hospitals, say that these specialty hospitals are just a "grab for money" by the physicians who own them. Physicians say specialty hospitals allow them to practice medicine the way it should be practiced, without answering to a hospital administrator who is trying to cut corners to make a profit. Currently, specialty hospitals make up about 2% of all hospitals in the United States, with more being planned for construction in the near future.[35]

A second type is a **public hospital**. These hospitals are supported and managed by governmental jurisdictions and are usually found in larger cities. Public hospitals can be operated by agencies at all levels of government. Hospitals operated by the federal government include

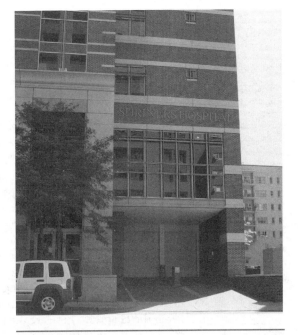

FIGURE 13.8
Hospitals are often categorized by ownership.

private (proprietary) or investor-owned hospitals for-profit hospitals

specialty hospital a hospital that provides mainly one type of medicine, is for-profit, and is owned at least in part by the physicians who practice in it

public hospitals hospitals that are supported and managed by governmental jurisdictions

Table 13.3
Hospitals According to Ownership: United States, 2008

Type	Number
All hospitals	5,815
Federal	213
Nonfederal community hospitals	5,010
Private or proprietary or investor-owned (for-profit)	982
Public (state or local)	1,105
Voluntary (not-for-profit)	2,923
Other (e.g., psychiatric, long-term care, prisons, college infirmaries)	592

Source: Adapted from American Hospital Association (2009). "Fast Facts on US Hospitals." Available at http://www.aha.org/aha/resource-center/Statistics-and-Studies/fast-facts.html. Accessed September 29, 2010.

voluntary hospitals
nonprofit hospitals administered by not-for-profit corporations or charitable community organizations

military hospitals (e.g., Walter Reed Army Hospital and the Bethesda Naval Hospital) and the many hospitals run by the Veterans Administration and Indian Health Service. There are also hospitals that are owned or partially financed by states and local governments. Examples include university hospitals, state mental hospitals, and local city and county hospitals.

Voluntary hospitals make up the third category of hospitals. These are nonprofit hospitals administered by not-for-profit corporations or religious, fraternal, and other charitable community organizations. These hospitals make up about one-half of all hospitals in the United States. Examples of this latter group are the Southern Baptist hospitals, the many Shriners' hospitals, and many community hospitals. In recent years, voluntary hospitals have been expanding their scope of services and many now include wellness centers, stress centers, chemical dependency programs, and a variety of satellite centers.

A second way of classifying hospitals is by dividing them into *teaching* and *nonteaching hospitals.* Teaching hospitals have, as a part of their mission, the responsibility to prepare new health care providers. These hospitals are typically aligned with medical schools, universities, and medical residency programs. However, a number of hospitals not affiliated with medical schools provide medical residency programs, clinical education for nurses, allied health personnel, and a wide variety of technical specialties.

full-service hospitals
hospitals that offer services in all or most of the levels of care defined by the spectrum of health care delivery

A third means of categorizing hospitals is by the services offered. **Full-service hospitals**, or general hospitals, are those that offer care at all or most of the levels of care discussed earlier in the chapter. These are the most expensive hospitals to run and are usually found in metropolitan areas. **Limited-service hospitals** offer the specific services needed by the population served, such as emergency, maternity, general surgery, and so on, but they lack much of the sophisticated technology available at full-service hospitals. This type of hospital is more common in rural areas. Many limited-service hospitals were once full-service hospitals but have become limited-service hospitals because of the low volume of patients, a shortage of health care personnel, and financial distress.

limited-service hospitals
hospitals that offer only the specific services needed by the population served

Clinics

When two or more physicians practice as a group, the facility in which they provide medical services is called a *clinic.* Some clinics are small, with just a few providers, while others are very large with many providers, such as the Mayo Clinic in Rochester, Minnesota, or the Cleveland Clinic in Cleveland, Ohio. Some clinics provide care only for individuals with special health needs such as treatment of cancer or diabetes or assistance in family planning; others accept patients with a wide range of problems. A misconception held by many is that clinics are not much different from hospitals. One big difference is that clinics do not have inpatient beds, and hospitals do. Some clinics do have an administrative relationship with inpatient facilities so that if a person needs to be admitted to a hospital, it is a relatively simple process; other clinics may be free-standing, or independent of all other facilities.

medically indigent
those lacking the financial ability to pay for their own medical care

Although many of the clinics are run as either for-profit or not-for-profit facilities, some are also funded by tax dollars. These clinics have been created primarily to meet the needs of the **medically indigent**—those lacking the financial ability to pay for their own medical care. Most of these clinics are located in large urban areas or rural areas that are underserved by the private sector. Two examples of this type of clinic are *public health clinics* and *community health centers.* The former are usually a part of a local health department (LHD). The scope of health care services offered by LHDs varies greatly. These services can range from prevention-oriented programs, such as immunizations and well-baby care, to complete personal health services such as those offered at private-sector clinics. Community health centers have been around since the late 1960s, known initially as *neighborhood health centers.* Today, the 1,100 community health centers operate under the auspices of the Bureau of Primary Health Care, which is part of the U.S. Department of Health and Human Services.[1] The importance of community health centers to the primary health care needs of the underserved populations in the United States is huge.[4] This fact was reinforced by the Obama administration in 2009 when $2 billion of the Recovery Act funds were earmarked for (1) major construction and renovation projects at 85 community health centers, (2) support for the adoption of electronic medical records and other health information technology systems in the centers, and (3) increased services.[36]

Outpatient Care Facilities

Often the terms *outpatient care facilities* and *ambulatory care facilities* have been used interchangeably. However, in the strict sense there is a difference. *Ambulatory care facilities* refer to those facilities into which a patient can physically walk, whereas *outpatient care facilities* are ones that do not include an overnight stay regardless of how the patient got into the facility. Thus, the term *outpatient care facilities* is a more inclusive term. Because of the variety of outpatient care services offered throughout the United States and the variety of arrangements for ownership of the services (i.e., hospitals, hospital systems, physician groups, and for-profit or not-for-profit chains) it is difficult to identify all possible outpatient care facilities. "For example, agencies providing home health services can be freestanding, hospital based, or nursing home based; physician practices, in many instances, are merging with hospitals, and hospitals and freestanding surgical centers often compete against each other for various types of surgical procedures."[1]

What is known is that today, care and procedures that once were performed only on an inpatient basis are increasingly being performed in a variety of outpatient settings.[22] In fact, today the majority of all surgical procedures are performed on an outpatient basis.[4] The growth and movement of services to outpatient care facilities have resulted from a combination of new medical and diagnostic procedures, technological advances, consumer demand for user-friendly environments, the reimbursement process, and financial mandates from insurance companies and government.[4] The types of outpatient care facilities found in communities are health care practitioners' offices, clinics, primary care centers, retail clinics, urgent/emergent care centers, ambulatory surgery centers, and freestanding service facilities (see Figure 13.9).

Probably the outpatient care facilities with which people have the most familiarity are health care practitioners' offices that house private practices. In 2007, there were more than 994,321,000 patient visits to physician offices in the United States.[23]

Because it is very expensive to set up a private practice, it is increasingly common to see more than one practitioner sharing both an office and staff. These practices are often referred to as *group practices* to distinguish them from *solo (single practitioner) practices.*

Primary care centers present another way to offer primary care in addition to the more traditional physician office mode. Though they may appear to be just another physician's office or group practice, many of these facilities are owned by hospitals and also include laboratory, radiology, and pharmacy services. "In hospital-operated facilities, staff physicians are commonly employees of the owner hospital, or, in the case of a teaching facility, physicians may be jointly compensated through a medical school–affiliated faculty practice group and the hospital."[4] In some parts of the country, depending on licensing procedures, it may be common to see nurse practitioners and physician assistants, under physician supervision, as the primary care practitioners in these facilities.[4]

Some of the most recent additions to outpatient care facilities are retail clinics found in pharmacies (CVS and

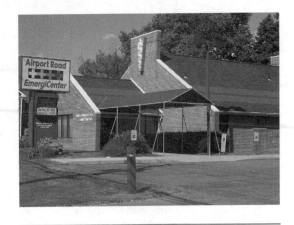

FIGURE 13.9

Many outpatient care facilities provide medical services safely and efficiently without the overhead of a hospital.

Walgreens), supermarkets, and retail stores (i.e., Walmart and Target). The services offered are limited, but they "represent an entrepreneurial response to consumer demand for fast, affordable treatment of easy-to-diagnose, acute conditions."[4] The facilities are often operated by an outside company, maybe even a hospital, and are generally staffed by nurses, nurse practitioners, and physician assistants. Initially, payment at these clinics was out of the pocket of the consumer, but the concept has caught the eye of insurers as a lower cost way of providing acute care, and thus many insurers now have contracts with the clinics.[4] Employers like the idea too and waive the copay when employees use them,[4] and some employers have even set up similar "Quick Clinics" within their own facility. Response to these clinics has been good from the insurers and consumers, but some in the medical community question the quality of care received.

Urgent/emergent care centers have been around in the United States since the early 1970s. They "fill gaps in the delivery system created by the rigidity of private physician appointment and unavailability during nonbusiness hours. The centers also can provide a much more convenient and user friendly alternative to a hospital emergency department during hours when private physicians are not available."[4] Urgent/emergent care centers often provide quicker service with less paperwork, particularly for those with cash or credit cards. These facilities (often not much larger than a fast-food restaurant) have sometimes been referred to as "Docs in a Box"! These facilities are not appropriate for all emergency cases. A majority of patients with life-threatening conditions are still taken to hospital emergency rooms, where top-of-the-line, advanced life support equipment and emergency physicians are on staff. Although emergency rooms are expensive for hospitals to maintain, they obviously perform a needed service.

Ambulatory surgery centers do not perform major surgery, such as heart transplants, but perform same-day surgeries where a hospital stay following the surgery is not needed. As noted earlier, today the majority of all surgical procedures are performed in these types of facilities.[4] The factors that have promoted the increase in ambulatory surgical procedures as alternatives to inpatient surgery include the development of new, safe, and faster-acting general anesthetics; advances in surgical equipment and materials; development of noninvasive or minimally invasive surgical and nonsurgical procedures; and reduced coverage by insurance companies for hospital stays.

One area of tremendous growth in outpatient care facilities in recent years has been in the development of freestanding, non-hospital-based, specialty facilities. Often, these facilities offer a single service, such as dialysis for individuals with kidney failure, or several similar services, such as those found in a diagnostic imaging center. In this latter example, the services often included are simple radiograph technology (X-rays) and computed tomography (CT) and magnetic resonance imaging (MRI), which are used for viewing the body's anatomical structures in several planes. These technologies are ideal for ambulatory facilities because of their noninvasive nature and profitability.

Even though convenience and cost are often the reasons for the development of new outpatient care facilities, the establishment of a new outpatient care facility in a community is not always received with enthusiasm. In previously underserved communities, fast-growing communities, or communities with many temporary residents such as resort communities, they have been well received. However, in stable or shrinking communities where there is an adequate number of health providers, the arrival of a new freestanding ambulatory care facility is sometimes viewed as unfriendly competition. In some of these cases the "unfriendly competition" has come from outside for-profit health care companies, but a more recent trend has been physicians breaking away from voluntary (independent or not-for-profit) hospitals where they once performed the procedures in the hospital's outpatient facility to create their own facilities in which to perform the procedures. The primary reasons for this trend are physicians wishing to have control over how the facility is run (i.e., the times and days procedures are scheduled, who is hired to work in the facilities) and to receive a greater share of the profits.

Rehabilitation Centers

Rehabilitation centers are health care facilities in which patients work with health care providers to restore functions lost because of injury, disease, or surgery. These centers are sometimes part of a clinic or hospital but may also be freestanding facilities. Rehabilitation centers may operate on both an outpatient and an inpatient basis. Those providers who commonly work in a rehabilitation center include physical, occupational, and respiratory therapists as well as exercise physiologists.

rehabilitation center a facility in which restorative care is provided following injury, disease, or surgery

Long-Term Care Options

Not too many years ago, when the topic of long-term care was mentioned, most people thought of nursing homes and state hospitals for the mentally ill and emotionally disabled. Today, however, the term *long-term care* includes not only the traditional institutional residential care, but also special units within these residential facilities (such as for Alzheimer patients), halfway houses, group homes, assisted-living facilities, transitional (step-down) care in a hospital, day care facilities for patients of all ages with health problems that require special care, and personal home health care. Many of these options were discussed in Chapter 9 because elders are the biggest users of long-term care, but other users include those with disabilities or chronic conditions, and those with acute and subacute conditions who are unable to care for themselves.

One area of long-term care that has received special attention in recent years is home health care. The demand for home health care has been driven by the restructuring of the health care delivery system, technological advances that enable people to be treated outside a hospital and to recover more quickly, and the cost containment pressures that have shortened hospital stays. Home health care should not be confused with home care. *Home care* is a more inclusive term and "denotes a range of services provided in the home, including skilled nursing and therapies, personal care, and even social services, such as meals, and home modifications"[37] (see Chapter 9 for a discussion of personal care). **Home health care** involves providing health care via health personnel and medical equipment to individuals and families in their places of residence, for the purpose of promoting, maintaining, or restoring health or to maximize the level of independence while minimizing the effects of disability and illness, including terminal disease. Home health care can be either long term, to help a chronically ill patient avoid institutionalization, or it can be short term to assist a patient following an acute illness and hospitalization until the patient is able to return to independent functioning. Home health care can be provided either through a formal system of paid professional health caregivers (e.g., home health care agency) or through an informal system where the care is provided by family, friends, and neighbors[4] (see Chapter 9 for more on caregivers). Medicare is the largest single payer for home health care, accounting for about one-third of the total annual expenditures.[4]

home health care care that is provided in the patient's residence for the purpose of promoting, maintaining, or restoring health

The need for professional health caregivers will continue into the future because of the "increase in the number of older persons and their expressed desire to remain in their homes for care whenever possible."[4] In 2007, there were 9,024 Medicare-certified home health agencies in the United States. That number is almost three times as many as existed in 1980.[23] Even though Medicare and Medicaid are the largest payers for home health care services, the amounts spent are relatively small in comparison to the total dollars spent on the Medicare and Medicaid programs.[38]

accreditation the process by which an agency or organization evaluates and recognizes an institution as meeting certain predetermined standards

Accreditation of Health Care Facilities

One way of determining the quality of a health care facility is to find out if it is accredited by a reputable group. **Accreditation** is the process by which an agency or organization evaluates

Joint Commission
the predominant organization responsible for accrediting health care facilities

and recognizes an institution as meeting certain predetermined standards. The predominant organization responsible for accrediting health care facilities is the **Joint Commission**, formerly known as the Joint Commission on Accreditation of Healthcare Organizations (JCAHO). The Joint Commission is an independent, not-for-profit organization that accredits about 17,000 health care organizations in the United States and in many other countries. The health care facilities/organizations that can be accredited by the Joint Commission include ambulatory care organizations, behavioral health care organizations, critical access hospitals, laboratories, home care organizations, hospitals, long-term care facilities, and office-based surgery practices. To earn and maintain Joint Commission accreditation, a facility or organization must complete an application and undergo an on-site survey (visit) by a Joint Commission survey team. "Organizations receive no notice of the survey date prior to the start of the survey, unless it would not be logical or feasible to conduct an unannounced survey, such as with Department of Defense and Bureau of Prisons facilities and some very small organizations. An organization can have an unannounced survey between 18 and 39 months after its previous full survey (24 months for laboratories, which have their survey (visit) prior to when their accreditation expires)."[39] "Accreditation is awarded to a health care organization that is in compliance with all standards at the time of the on-site survey or has successfully addressed all requirements for improvement (RFI) in an Evidence of Standards Compliance (ESC) submission."[40]

HEALTH CARE SYSTEM: FUNCTION

Like the structure of the health care system, the function of the health care system of the United States is also unique compared to the health care systems of other developed countries of the world. However, at the time this book was being written, some of the structure that had been in place for a number of years was about to change. As noted earlier in this chapter, the Patient Protection and Affordable Health Care Act (PPACA) (Public Law 111-148) and the Health Care and Education Reconciliation Act of 2010 (HCERA) (Public Law 111-152) were signed into law by President Obama in March 2010. (*Note:* Because these two laws were consolidated with each other and some other legislation, we refer to them collectively from here on as the "Affordable Care Act.") The Affordable Care Act is almost 1,000 pages in length and contains many changes that are to be implemented between 2010 and 2020. The bulk of the law goes into effect in 2014, but some became effective in mid-2010. Because of the timing of this new law and the writing of this book the information in the remainder of the chapter includes some of the structure from the past that led to the new law and what can be expected in terms of the change in structure as the new law is implemented.

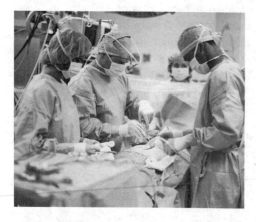

FIGURE 13.10
Health care services offered by U.S. providers are perhaps the best in the world, but at what cost?

Understanding the Structure of the Health Care System

To begin, it must be understood that the health care system of the United States is big and complicated.[41] It is big from the standpoint of cost—it is very expensive (see Figure 13.10)—and because of the many stakeholders that include but are not limited to health care consumers, health care providers, health care administrators, politicians, policymakers, government regulators, insurance companies, and professional and trade associations. It is complicated because health care policy is intertwined with other policies (i.e., the U.S. tax code, for example, credits for employers who provide health insurance for employees and health care consumers who get deductions on their income taxes if their health care spending reaches certain levels in a year) and because of the politics and ideological viewpoints of the decision makers.

The major issues of the health care system in the United States can be represented by the cost containment, access, and quality triangle noted by Kissick[42] (see Figure 13.11). In Kissick's equilateral triangle, the equal 60-degree angles represent equal priorities. That is, access is just as important as quality and cost containment and vice versa. However, an expansion of any one of the angles compromises one or both of the other two. For example, if we were interested in increasing the quality of our already good services, it would also increase the costs and decrease access. Or, some feel, if we increase access, costs will go up, and the quality will decrease. Or, if we concentrate on containing costs, both quality of care and access will decrease. With such dilemmas, the United States continues to struggle to find the right combination of policy and accountability to deal with these shortcomings. Concerns associated with each of the three sides of the cost containment, access, and quality triangle are discussed later in this chapter.

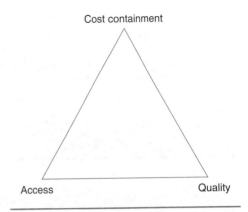

FIGURE 13.11

The cost containment, access, and quality triangle of health care.

Source: Kissick, W. L. (1994). *Medicine's Dilemmas: Infinite Needs versus Finite Resources.* New Haven, CT: Yale University Press. Used with permission.

Access to Health Care

Even with several different means of gaining access to health care services (see Figure 13.12), access has been and continues to be a major health policy issue in the United States. Health insurance coverage and the generosity of coverage are major determinants of access to health care.[43] In 2009, 46.3 million persons of all ages (15.4%) were uninsured, 58.5 million (19.4%) had been uninsured for at least part of the year, and 32.8 million (10.9%) had been uninsured for more than a year[44] (see Box 13.5). Millions more lacked health insurance coverage for shorter periods during that year. The likelihood of being uninsured is greater for younger persons, those with less education, those with lower incomes, nonwhites, those who are not U.S. citizens, and males.[44] It also increases based on where one lives. A greater percentage of those living in the southern (18.6%) and western (17.1%) parts of the United States were uninsured than those living in the Northeast (10.0%) and the Midwest (12.7%)[44] (see Box 13.5). The greatest reason for lack of insurance coverage is cost of insurance followed by lost job or change in employment.[45]

Interestingly enough, the uninsured do not lack emergency or urgent care because no one needing such care and willing to go to a hospital emergency room will be turned away. However, the uninsured usually do not have access to primary care (see Box 13.1), such as checkups, screenings for chronic illnesses, and prenatal care. Without adequate primary care, many patients eventually find themselves in need of more costly and often less effective medical treatment. The primary factors that limit access to this type of care are total lack of health insurance, inadequate insurance, and poverty. Those who are unable to receive medical care because they cannot afford it are referred to as "medically indigent."[46] The medically indigent in America include people and families with income above the poverty level who are thus ineligible for Medicaid, or government health insurance for the poor, but who are unable to afford health care or health insurance. "Eight out of ten uninsured persons are members of working families. In most of these cases, the worker holds a job that does not offer health insurance. In others, subsidized coverage may be offered, but the employee turns it down because of the cost or because they do not perceive the need for coverage."[43] Those who

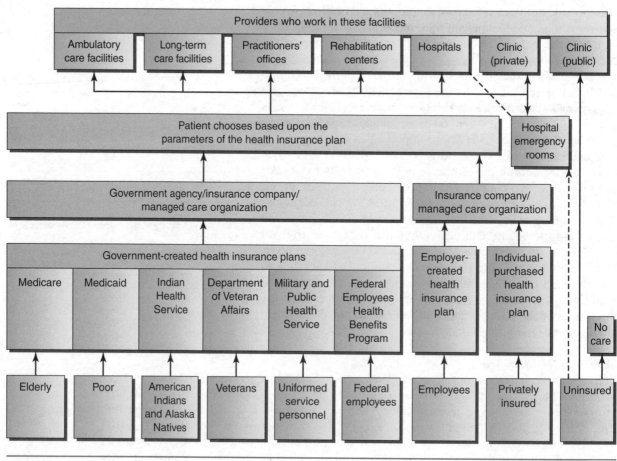

FIGURE 13.12
Means of gaining access to health care.

have a job but are unable to afford health insurance are referred to as the *working poor*. It has been estimated that there are 30 million working poor in the United States.[47] Others may be uninsured because "individual health policies are quite expensive and may be unavailable for those who have a preexisting health problem. Young adults often lose their eligibility under their parent's policy when they turn 19 or graduate from college. Spouses lose coverage under a family policy through separation, divorce, retirement, or upon the death of a policy holder."[43] In summary, in the United States access to a regular source of health care is closely tied to having health insurance.

To deal with the problem of lack of access to health care, a major component of the Affordable Care Act passed in 2010 was aimed at increasing the number of Americans with health insurance. Box 13.6 provides a brief summary of some of the steps that were included in the Affordable Care Act to increase access to care. The Congressional Budget Office has estimated that by taking these steps the number of uninsured will be reduced by 32 million by 2019.[48] If the new law works as planned, the majority of those who will be uninsured in 2019 will be those who have entered the country illegally.

BOX

13.5

HEALTHY PEOPLE 2020: OBJECTIVES

Access to Health Services

Goal: Improve access to comprehensive, quality health care services.

Objective: AHS-1, Increase the proportions of persons with health insurance.

Objective: AHS-1.1, Medical insurance

Target: 100 percent.

Baseline: 83.2 percent of persons had medical insurance in 2008.

Target setting method: Total coverage.

Data source: National Health Interview Survey (NHIS), CDC, NCHS.

Objective: AHS-1.3 (Developmental), Dental insurance

Target: TBD

Baseline: TBD

Target setting method: TBD

Potential data source: National Health Interview Survey (NHIS), CDC, NCHS.

Objective: AHS-1.3 (Developmental), Prescription drug insurance

Target: TBD

Baseline: TBD

Target setting method: TBD

Potential data source: National Health Interview Survey (NHIS), CDC, NCHS.

Objective: AHS-2 (Developmental), Increase the proportion of insured persons with coverage for clinical preventive services

Target: TBD

Baseline: TBD

Target setting method: TBD

Potential data source: Children's Health Insurance Program (CHIP), CMS; AGing Integrated Database (AGID), AoA; CMS claims data and Medicare Current Beneficiary Survey (MCBS), CMS.

TBD = To be determined

For Further Thought

Do you think the Affordable Care Act was the best way to go about reaching these objectives? Defend your response. Do you think the United States should adopt a national health insurance plan like the other developed countries of the world to make sure all persons have health insurance? Why or why not?

Source: U.S. Department of Health and Human Services, Office of Disease Prevention and Health Promotion (2010). *Healthy People 2020.* Available at http://www.healthypeople.gov/2020/default.aspx. Accessed December 2, 2010.

Quality of Health Care

All people are entitled to and should receive quality health care. Yet several different reports, including one completed in 2009 that compared U.S. health care to that of Australia, Canada, Germany, the Netherlands, New Zealand, and the United Kingdom,[49] indicate that people in

BOX 13.6	COMPONENTS OF THE AFFORDABLE CARE ACT TO INCREASE ACCESS TO CARE[*]

1. *Individual mandate.*[†] Beginning in 2014, all individuals will be required to have health insurance or pay a penalty. The penalty will be phased in from 2014–2016. There are some exceptions to this requirement that include financial hardship, religious objections, and for American Indians.

2. *Expansion of public programs.*[‡] Medicaid will be expanded to cover those up to 133% of the federal poverty level. In 2009, that level would have been $14,404 for an individual and $29,327 for a family of four. This expansion will create a national uniform eligibility standard across states. The federal government will pay for much of the expansion.

3. *American Health Benefit Exchanges.* For people who do not receive employer-sponsored insurance and who make more than 133% of the federal poverty level, health insurance will be available through new American Health Benefit Exchanges created by states. Plans in the exchanges must provide benefits that meet a minimum set of standards. Insurers will offer four levels of coverage that vary based on premiums, out-of-pocket costs, and benefits beyond the minimum required plus a catastrophic coverage plan. Various premium subsidies will be available to those with incomes between 100% and 400% of the federal poverty level.

4. *Changes to private insurance.* New health insurance regulations will change the way insurers operate. Insurers will: (1) not be able to deny coverage to people because of health status (i.e., preexisting condition), (2) not be able to charge people more because of health status or gender, (3) for all new health plans, have to provide comprehensive coverage that includes a minimum set of services, caps out-of-pocket spending, does not impose cost-sharing for preventive services, and does not impose annual or lifetime limits on coverage, (4) have to allow young adults to remain on their parents' health insurance up until age 26, and (5) have to limit waiting periods to no longer than 90 days.

5. *Employer requirements.* There is no employer mandate to offer health insurance to employees, but employers with 50+ employees will be assessed a fee of $2,000 per full-time employee (in excess of 30 employees) if they do not offer coverage and if they have at least one employee who receives a premium credit through an exchange. Employers with 50+ employees who do offer health insurance but have at least one employee who receives a premium credit through an exchange will be required to pay the lesser of $3,000 per employee who receives a premium credit or $2,000 per employee (in excess of 30 employees). If employees offer coverage and have workers who do not sign up for the plan or do not opt out of a plan, the employer must automatically enroll employees in the lowest cost premium plan. Also, if employers offer coverage to employees with incomes less than 400% of the federal poverty level and the employees' share of the premium is between 8% and 9.8% of their income, then employers will be required to provide vouchers so that employees can enroll in a plan in an exchange.

[*]Limited to U.S. citizens and legal immigrants.

[†]At the time this book was being written, it appeared that this mandate would be reviewed by the U.S. Supreme Court because in 2010 a federal judge in Virginia ruled it to be unconstitutional.

[‡]At the time this book was being written, approximately 20 states were suing the U.S. government over this component, saying that the Constitution does not allow for such requirements.

Source: Modified from Henry J. Kaiser Family Foundation (2010). *Summary of Coverage Provisions in the Patient Protection and Affordable Care Act* (#8023). Available at http://www.kff.org/healthreform/8023.cfm. Accessed September 29, 2010.

the United States could be receiving better care. *Quality health care* has been defined as doing the right thing, at the right time, in the right way, for the right people, and having the best results.[50] The Institute of Medicine (IOM) has further delineated that quality health care should be:[51]

Effective. Delivering health care based on scientific evidence to all who could benefit based on need

Safe. Delivering health care to patients that avoids injuries to patients from the care that is intended to help them

Timely. Delivering health care in a way that reduces waits and sometimes harmful delays

Patient centered. Providing health care that is respectful of and responsive to individual patient preferences, needs, and values

Equitable. Delivering health care that does not vary in quality because of personal characteristics of patients

Efficient. Delivering health care that maximizes resources and avoids waste

Though the definitions of quality health care are easily understood, operationalizing quality health care is not as easy. Most often health care quality is measured using one or more of the following:[52]

- Clinical performance measures of how well providers deliver specific services needed by specific patients, such as whether children get the immunizations they need

- Assessments by patients of how well providers meet health care needs from the patient's perspective, such as whether providers communicate clearly

- Outcome measures, such as death rates from cancers detectable by screening, which may be affected by the quality of health care received

Based on these variables, a number of groups have created measures for health care quality. Since 2003, the Agency for Healthcare Research and Quality (AHRQ), together with its partners in the Department of Health and Human Services (HHS), has annually reported on progress and opportunities for improving health care quality as mandated by Congress by publishing the *National Healthcare Quality Report* (NHQR)[53] and the *National Healthcare Disparities Report* (NHDR).[52] Both the NHQR and the NHDR are built on the same 200 measures assembled across four dimensions of quality—effectiveness, patient safety, timeliness, and patient centeredness. The themes that came from the 2009 NHQR were: (1) health care quality needs to be improved, particularly for uninsured individuals, who are less likely to get the recommended care; (2) some areas merit urgent attention, including patient safety and health care–associated infections (HAIs); and (3) quality is improving, but the pace is slow, especially for preventive care and chronic disease management.[53] The themes from the 2009 NHDR were: (1) disparities are common, and having no insurance is an important contributor; (2) many disparities are not decreasing; and (3) some disparities merit particular attention, especially care for cancer, heart failure, and pneumonia.[52]

Another group that measures health care quality is the National Committee for Quality Assurance (NCQA).[54] The NCQA is a private, not-for-profit organization that has been assessing and accrediting health care plans (i.e., managed care programs, specifically health maintenance organizations [HMOs] and preferred provider organizations [PPOs]) since 1990. It assesses how well a health plan manages and delivers health care in four different ways: (1) through accreditation (a rigorous on-site review of key clinical and administrative processes); (2) through certification (a rigorous review of certain functions—for example, credentialing or utilization management—that health plans or employers have delegated to another organization); (3) through the Health Plan Effectiveness Data and Information Set (HEDIS—a tool that consists of 71 measures across eight domains that is used to measure performance in key areas such as immunization, mammography screening rates) and members' satisfaction with their care in areas such as claims processing, customer service, and getting needed care quickly; and (4) through physician recognition programs that identify physicians who provide quality care in areas such as diabetes and heart/stroke care. Although participation with NCQA is voluntary, in 2009 NCQA assessed data from 979 health plans.[55] The data available from these assessments are available at NCQA's Web site. Many employers use the data as a way of selecting the best managed care programs for their employees.

Regardless of what method is used to measure the quality of health care delivered in the United States, the results have been similar. The general consensus is that the quality of health care has been getting better at a modest pace but is not as good as it could or should be.

Dealing with the problem of "less than desirable quality in health care" is not easy because it runs through every aspect of care. That is why there are not just a few items in the Affordable Care Act passed in 2010 that deal with quality—there are many. As such, Box 13.7 is presented to provide a sampling of some of the items of the law that address quality.

The Cost of and Paying for Health Care

The cost of health care and paying for health care continue to be burdens on both individuals and the U.S. population as a whole. In 2010, health expenditures were projected to be almost $2.6 trillion and to consume 17.3% of the gross domestic product (GDP), and they are expected to reach $4.5 trillion and $19.3% of the GDP by 2019.[12] America spends more per capita annually on health care (estimated at $8,290 in 2010[12]) than any other nation (see Table 13.4). Under the U.S. system, the actual cost of the service is usually not known until after the service has been provided, unless the consumer is bold enough to inquire ahead of time. Most are not.

BOX 13.7	SOME OF THE COMPONENTS OF THE AFFORDABLE CARE ACT THAT WILL AFFECT QUALITY OF CARE

Wellness and preventive services. New health plans available on or after September 23, 2010, are required to cover recommended preventive services (e.g., screenings, vaccinations, counseling) without charging a copay, co-insurance, or deductible. Similar benefits apply to Medicare. *Effective 01-01-11.*

Center for Medicare & Medicaid Innovation. A new center will begin testing new ways of delivering care to patients. These methods are expected to improve the quality of care and reduce the rate of growth in health care costs for Medicare, Medicaid, and the Children's Health Insurance Program (CHIP). Additionally, by January 1, 2011, HHS will submit a national strategy for quality improvement in health care, including these programs.

Providing better information and accountability for nursing home care. It will be easier to file complaints about the quality of care in a nursing home. Consumers also will have access to more information on nursing home quality and resident rights. *Effective 01-01-11.*

Linking payment to quality outcomes. A hospital Value-Based Purchasing program (VBP) will become a part of traditional Medicare, which will offer financial incentives to hospitals to improve the quality of care. Hospital performance is required to be publicly reported, beginning with measures relating to heart attacks, heart failure, pneumonia, surgical care, health care–associated infections, and patients' perception of care. *Effective after 09-30-12.*

Encouraging integrated health systems. Incentives will be available for physicians to join together to form Accountable Care Organizations (ACOs). These groups allow doctors to better coordinate patient care and improve the quality, help prevent disease and illness, and reduce unnecessary hospital admissions. If ACOs provide high-quality care and reduce costs to the health care system, they can keep some of the money that they have helped save. *Effective 01-01-12.*

Reducing paperwork and administrative costs. A series of changes to be made to standardize billing that requires health plans to begin adopting and implementing rules for the secure, confidential, electronic exchange of health information. Using electronic health records will reduce paperwork and administrative burdens, cut costs, reduce medical errors and, most important, improve the quality of care. *Effective 10-01-12.*

Paying physicians based on value not volume. Physician payments will be tied to the quality of care they provide. Physicians will see their payments modified so that those who provide higher value care will receive higher payments than those who provide lower quality care. *Effective 01-01-15.*

Sources: Data from AARP (2010). *How the Health Care Law Benefits You.* Available at http://assets.aarp.org/www.aarp.org/articles/health/207993_hcr_ed_booklet_6_8_10.pdf; and U.S. Department of Health and Human Services (2010). About the Law. Available at http://www.healthcare.gov/law/about. Accessed September 29, 2010.

Table 13.4
Health Expenditures per Capita and Health Care Rankings: 2007

	Cost per Capita	Overall Health Ranking
Australia	$3,357	3
Canada	$3,895	6
Germany	$3,588	4
Netherlands	$3,837	1
New Zealand	$2,454	5
United Kingdom	$2,992	2
United States	$7,290	7

Source: Adapted from Davis, K., C. Schoen, and K. Stremikis (2010). *Mirror, Mirror on the Wall: How the Performance of the U.S. Health Care System Compares Internationally—2010 Update.* New York, NY: The Commonwealth Fund. Available at http://www.commonwealthfund.org/Content/Publications/Fund-Reports/2010/Jun/Mirror-Mirror-Update.aspx. Accessed September 29, 2010.

Payments for the U.S. health care bill come from four sources. The first is the consumers themselves. In 2010, it was estimated these direct or out-of-pocket payments represented approximately one-tenth (11.4%) of all payments. The remaining portion of health care payments, nine-tenths, comes almost entirely from indirect, or third-party, payments. The first source of third-party payments is private insurance companies. Private insurance companies paid 32.3% of the health care bill in 2010. These payments were made from premiums paid to the insurance company by the employees and/or their employers. The second source of third-party payments is governmental insurance programs (i.e., Medicare, Medicaid, Veterans Administration, Indian Health Service, or military). These government programs are funded by a combination of taxes and premiums from those insured (as in the case of Part B Medicare coverage). In 2010, 37.6% of the health care bill was paid for by federal governmental insurance programs. While state and local governments paid for 11.7%. Finally, a small percentage of health care bills are paid by other private funds. In 2010, it was 7.1% (see Figure 13.13).

It is clear that the cost of health care is going to continue to rise. One of the major selling points of the Affordable Care Act passed in 2010 was to try to slow down the cost of health

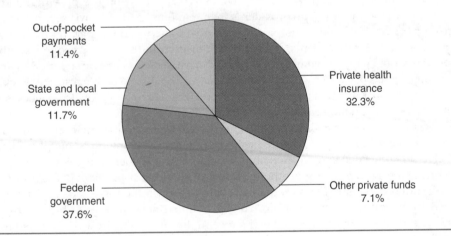

FIGURE 13.13

Health expenditures by source of funds, United States, 2010: projected.

Source: U.S. Department of Health and Human Services, Centers for Medicare and Medicaid Services (2010). "National Health Expenditure Data." Available at http://www.cms.gov/NationalHealthExpenddata/01_Overview.asp#TopofPage. Accessed September 29, 2010.

care, thus the title "Affordable Care." The Congressional Budget Office (CBO) "estimates the cost of the coverage components of the new law to be $938 billion over ten years. These costs are financed through a combination of savings from Medicare and Medicaid and new taxes and fees."[56] Examples of new taxes include taxes on high-cost health insurance and tanning bed use, while examples of new fees include those that have to be paid by pharmaceutical and insurance companies. Many feel that in addition to the cost savings from Medicare and Medicaid, health care costs have the potential to be lower because 32 million people who were uninsured before the law will now be paying premiums, and many of them are young and healthy and will not use a lot of health care.

reimbursement
payments made by the third-party payers to providers

As noted earlier, *third-party payers* (i.e., insurance companies and the federal, state, and local governments) make a majority of the payments for health services. The payments made by the third-party payers to providers are referred to as **reimbursement**.[1] The process for receiving a third-party payment usually begins when a health care provider or his or her staff requests information about the patient's health insurance plan. They normally request the name of the insuring company (e.g., Blue Cross/Blue Shield), the policy number, and a personal identification number (PIN). This information is usually provided to the insured on a wallet-sized card by the insurer. The provider may then ask the patient to sign an insurance claim form in two places. The first signature indicates that the service has been provided and authorizes the provider to submit patient information with the claim for payment. The second signature instructs the insurance company to make the payment directly to the provider. Upon receiving and reviewing the completed and signed form, the insurance company then issues payments to the provider for services based on the provisions of the insurance policy. Depending on the level of reimbursement for the claim, the provider will either consider the bill paid in full or will request payment from the patient in the amount of the difference between the provider's full fee and the portion paid by the insurance company.

fee-for-service
a method of paying for health care in which after the service is rendered, a fee is paid

In recent years, the methods by which the amount of the reimbursement has been determined have changed. Traditionally, providers have favored the **fee-for-service** method, but it is not used much any more because of the cost escalation.[1] The fee-for-service is based on the assumption that services are provided in a set of identifiable and individually distinct units such as a doctor's office visit or a specific medical procedure.[1] Under the fee-for-service format, consumers select a provider, receive care (service) from the provider, and incur expenses (a fee) for the care. The provider is then reimbursed for covered services in part by the insurer (private insurance company or the government) and in part by the consumer, who is responsible for the balance unpaid by the insurer. Initially, the providers set the fees and insurers would pay the claim. But because of increased costs, insurers started to limit the amount they would pay for "usual, customary, and reasonable." The biggest drawback of the fee-for-service format was that providers have a greater incentive to provide services, some of which sometimes are nonessential.[1]

Under the fee-for-service format, consumers are obligated to pay their fee at the time the service is rendered. In the past, before health insurance was common, some physicians provided care when needed and worried about payment later. Others often accepted "in kind" payment, such as farm produce or other products or services, as payment in full for a medical service rendered. Today, for patients to receive care via fee-for-service, they are often required to demonstrate the ability to pay (to assume financial responsibility for the fee) before the service is rendered. A provider's receptionist may ask, "How do you plan to settle your bill?" In other cases, providers have signs placed around the waiting room that state, "Payment is expected when service is rendered, unless other arrangements have been made prior to the appointment."

The more recent methods of paying for health services have included *packaged pricing, resource-based relative value scale, prepaid health care* (i.e., *capitation*), and *prospective reimbursement*. In **packaged pricing**, also referred to as *bundled charges*, several related services are included in one price. For example, optometrists will bundle the cost for an eye exam, frames, and lenses into a single charge.[1]

Resource-based relative value scale was created for Medicare as part of the Omnibus Budget Reconciliation Act of 1989 to reimburse physicians according to the *relative value* of the service provided. The relative values units (RVUs) are derived through a complex formula based on time, skill, and intensity to provide the service. Also, included in the RVU is an overhead charge to run a practice.[21] Each year, Medicare publishes the Medicare Physician Fee Schedule, adjusted for geographic parts of the country, which provides the reimbursement amount for services and procedures under the Current Procedural Terminology (CPT) code.[1]

Managed care organizations (MCOs) (see information about managed care later in this chapter) use a couple different approaches for reimbursement. Preferred provider organizations (PPOs) use a variation of the fee-for-service method. The variation is that the PPOs "establish fee schedules based on discounts negotiated with providers participating in its network."[1] Health maintenance organizations (HMOs), depending on their structure, have either paid providers a salary if they are employed by the HMO or have reimbursed using *prepaid health care* arrangements.

Under **prepaid health care** arrangements, insurers make arrangements with health care providers to provide agreed-upon covered health care services to a given population of consumers for a (usually discounted) set price—the per-person premium fee—over a particular time period. Often the arrangements are set up on a per-member, per-month (PMPM) rate called a *capitated fee*. Thus, this arrangement for reimbursing the providers is referred to as a *capitation system*. The provider receives the capitated fee per enrollee regardless of whether the enrollee uses health care services and regardless of the quality of services provided. The provider is responsible for providing all needed services determined to be medically necessary and covered under the plan.[21] In addition to the capitated fee, consumers may pay additional fees (copayments) for office visits and other services used. The insurer organizes the delivery of care by building an infrastructure of providers and implementing the systems to monitor and influence the cost and quality of care.

Prospective reimbursement has been around since 1983 when it was first used in the form of diagnosis-related groups (DRGs) for hospital stays under Medicare Part A (see discussion of Medicare and DRGs later in the chapter). It replaced *retrospective reimbursement* that was based on the length of stay and services provided. Thus, providers were rewarded for longer stays and more services, which increased costs. **Prospective reimbursement**, referred to as the prospective pricing system (PPS), "uses pre-established criteria to determine in advance the amount of reimbursement."[1] Because of the success of DRGs, the Balanced Budget Act of 1997 mandated implementation of a Medicare PPS for hospital outpatient services and postacute providers such as skilled nursing facilities, home health agencies, and inpatient rehabilitation facilities.[1] Thus, the four primary prospective reimbursement methods used today are DRGs (used for Medicare Part A), ambulatory payment classifications (APCs) (used for payment to hospital outpatient departments), resource utilization groups (RUGs) (used for payment to skilled nursing facilities), and home health resource groups (HHRGs) (used for payment of home health care).[1]

Health Insurance

Health insurance, like all other types of insurance, is a risk- and cost-spreading process. That is, the cost of one person's injury or illness is shared by all in the group. Each person in the group has a different chance (or risk) of having a problem and thus needing health care. Some members of the group, for example, those who suffer from chronic and/or congenital health

---

packaged pricing
several related health services are included in one price

resource-based relative value scale
reimbursement to physicians according to the relative value of the service provided

prepaid health care
a method of paying for covered health care services on a per-person premium basis for a specific time period prior to the service being rendered (also referred to as capitation)

prospective reimbursement
uses preestablished criteria to determine in advance the amount of reimbursement

problems, will probably need more care while others in the group will need less. The concept of insurance has everyone in the group, no matter what their individual risk, helping to pay for the collective risk of the group. The risk of costly ill health is spread in a reasonably equitable fashion among all persons purchasing insurance, and everyone is protected from having to pay an insurmountable bill for a catastrophic injury or illness.

There are some exceptions to the "equitable fashion." If someone in the group knowingly engages in a behavior that increases his or her risk, such as smoking cigarettes or driving in a reckless manner, that person may have to pay more for the increased risk. In short, the greater the risk (or probability of using the insurance), the more the individual or group has to pay for insurance.

The concept of health insurance is not a new one in this country. Group health and life insurance are considered American inventions of the early twentieth century. In 1911, Montgomery Ward and Company sold health insurance policies based on the principles still used today in the business. Currently, hundreds of companies in the United States sell health and life insurance policies.

The Health Insurance Policy

A *policy* is a written agreement between a private insurance company (or the government) and an individual or group of individuals to pay for certain health care costs during a certain time period in return for regular, periodic payments (a set amount of money) called *premiums*. The insurance company benefits in that it anticipates collecting more money in premiums than it has to pay out for services; hence, it anticipates a profit. The insured benefits by not being faced with medical bills he or she cannot pay, because the insurance company is obligated to pay them according to the terms of the contract. The added benefit for those insured as a group is that group premiums are less expensive than premiums for individuals are.

The expectations of both insurers and insured are not always met. An insurer occasionally has to pay out more than it collects in premiums. Alternatively, the insured often purchases insurance that is never used.

Although the language of health insurance policies can be confusing, everyone needs to understand several key terms. One of the most important is **deductible**. The deductible is the amount of expenses (money) that the beneficiary (insured) must incur (pay out of pocket) before the insurance company begins to pay for covered services. A common yearly deductible level is $250 per individual policy holder, or a maximum of $1,000 per family. This means that the insured must pay the first $250/$1,000 of medical costs before the insurance company begins paying. The higher the deductible of a policy, the lower the premiums will be.

Usually, but not always, after the deductible has been met, most insurance companies pay a percentage of what they consider the "usual, customary, and reasonable" charge for covered services. The insurer generally pays 80% of the usual, customary, and reasonable costs, and the insured is responsible for paying the remaining 20%. This 20% is referred to as **co-insurance**. If the health care provider charges more than the usual, customary, and reasonable rates, the insured will have to pay both the co-insurance and the difference. A form of co-insurance, often associated with managed care programs, is **copayment** (or *copay* for short). A copayment is a negotiated set amount a patient pays for certain services—for example, $20 for an office visit and $15 for a prescription. Some insurance policies may have both co-insurance and copayments included. The greater the proportion of co-insurance paid by the insured, the lower the premiums.

A fourth key term, **fixed indemnity**, refers to the maximum amount an insurer will pay for a certain service. For example, a policy may state that the maximum amount of money paid for orthodontia is $2,000. Depending on the language of a policy, the fixed indemnity benefit

deductible
the amount of expenses that the beneficiary must incur before the insurance company begins to pay for covered services

co-insurance
the portion of the insurance company's approved amounts for covered services that a beneficiary is responsible for paying

copayment
a negotiated set amount that a patient pays for certain services

fixed indemnity
the maximum amount an insurer will pay for a certain service

may or may not be subject to the provisions of the deductible or co-insurance clause. Costs above the fixed indemnity amount are the responsibility of the insured.

Another key term related to health insurance is **exclusion**. When an exclusion is written into a policy, it means that a specified health condition is excluded from coverage. That is, the policy does not pay for service to treat the condition. Common exclusions include a pregnancy that began before the health insurance policy went into effect or a chronic disease or condition such as diabetes or hypertension that has been classified as a preexisting condition. A **preexisting condition** is a medical condition that had been diagnosed or treated usually within the 6 months before the date the health insurance policy went into effect. Because of such exclusions, people who have a serious condition or disease are often unable to get health insurance coverage for the condition/disease or in general. Some health insurance policies also exclude a condition/disease for a specified period of time, such as 9 months for pregnancy or 1 year for all other exclusions.

The rule that a preexisting condition could be an exclusion "trapped" many people in jobs, because the employees were afraid of losing their health insurance for the condition if they changed employers. To deal with this issue, Congress passed the Health Insurance Portability and Accountability Act of 1996 (Public Law 104-102, known as HIPAA). This law was created, in part, to ensure that people will not have to wait for health insurance to go into effect when changing jobs. More specifically, a preexisting condition had to be covered without a waiting period when a person joined a new plan if the person had been insured for the previous 12 months. If a person had a preexisting condition and it had not been covered the previous 12 months before joining a new plan, the longest that person had to wait before being covered for that condition is 12 months.

Even with HIPAA many people, mostly older Americans, were unable to get health insurance because of preexisting conditions. Thus, preexisting conditions were addressed in the Affordable Care Act passed in 2010. Beginning 90 days after enactment of the law, older adults with preexisting conditions who had been uninsured for at least 6 months were eligible for subsidized insurance through a national high-risk pool. Then, in 2014, insurance companies will be required to cover all individuals regardless of health status and charge the same premium regardless of preexisting conditions.[57]

Types of Health Insurance Coverage

As has been noted in the previous discussions, there are a number of different types of services that health insurance policies cover. The more common types of coverage are hospitalization, surgical, regular medical, major medical, dental, and disability. Table 13.5 presents a short overview of each of these coverage types.

Though the types of health insurance coverage remain constant, several trends associated with health insurance plans and the products they offer are emerging. The trends that characterize health insurance plans today are (1) the plans are becoming more complex and are concentrated in a fewer number of companies, (2) there is an increase in the diversity of products, so consumers have many more options in the type of plan they select, especially with the passage of the Affordable Care Act in 2010, (3) there is an increased focus on delivering care through a network of providers rather than independent providers, (4) there is a movement of shifting to financial structures and incentives among purchasers, health plans, and providers, and (5) more health insurance plans are developing clinical infrastructures to manage utilization and to improve the quality of care. Such trends will make understanding health insurance plans more challenging for consumers. These trends will require a greater investment in education and information to help consumers understand how insurance products differ, how best to navigate managed care systems, and what differences exist in structure or performance across the plans.

exclusion
a health condition written into the health insurance policy indicating what is not covered by the policy

preexisting condition
a medical condition that had been diagnosed or treated usually within the 6 months before the date a health insurance policy goes into effect

Table 13.5
Types of Health Insurance Coverage

Dental	Dental procedures.
Disability (income protection)	Income when insured is unable to work because of a health problem.
Hospitalization	Inpatient hospital expenses including room, patient care, supplies, and medications.
Long-term care	An umbrella term for an array of supportive services to help people function in their daily lives. Services may include but are not limited to nursing care, home health care, personal care, rehabilitation, adult day care, case management, social services, assistive technology, and assisted living services. Services may be provided at home or in another place of residence like a nursing home.
Major medical	Large medical expenses usually not covered by regular medical or dental coverage.
Optical (vision)	Nonsurgical procedures to improve vision.
Regular medical	Nonsurgical service provided by health care providers. Often has set amounts (fixed indemnity for certain procedures).
Surgical	Surgeons' fees (for inpatient or outpatient surgery).

The Cost of Health Insurance

Over the years, the cost of health insurance has pretty much mirrored the cost of health care. From the early 1970s through the early 1990s, health care costs and the costs of health care insurance were growing in the neighborhood of 10% to 12% per year.[56] But as the cost of health care slowed in the early to mid-1990s, so did the cost of health insurance. This deceleration in premium growth paralleled the dramatic shift in the health insurance marketplace away from traditional fee-for-service indemnity insurance to managed care. However, the managed care revolution created a one-time-only cost savings, and all the underlying cost drivers, such as an aging population, increased use of prescription drugs, and technology, have again increased costs. The burden of the cost of health insurance for those who are working falls primarily on the employer and, to a lesser extent, on the employee. Most Americans younger than 65 years of age receive their health insurance through their employer or the employer of their parent or spouse/partner. Even though the Affordable Care Act passed in 2010 mandates that all citizens and legal immigrants have health insurance, much of the responsibility will continue to fall on employers. Because of the increasing costs of health insurance and its impact on the "bottom line" of companies, employers are shifting more of the cost onto their employees by (1) increasing the workers' share of the premium, (2) raising the deductibles that workers must pay, (3) increasing the copayments for prescription drugs, and (4) increasing the number of items on the exclusion list. A vivid example of the cost of health insurance comes from coffee store giant Starbucks. This company spends more money on health care than it does on coffee beans.[58]

In the end, the actual cost of a policy is determined by two major factors—the risk of those in the group and the amount of coverage provided. An increase in either risk or coverage will result in an increase in the cost of the policy.

Self-Funded Insurance Programs

self-funded insurance programs one that pays the health care costs of its employees with the premiums collected from the employees and the contributions made by the employer

With the high cost of health care today, some employers "(or other group, such as a union or trade association)"[4] that provide health insurance for their employees are deciding to cut their costs by becoming self-insured. With such an arrangement, a **self-funded insurance program** pays the health care costs of its employees with the premiums collected from the employees and the contributions made by the employer instead of using a commercial carrier.[4] Self-funded insurance programs "often use the services of an actuarial firm to set premium rates and a third-party administrator to administer benefits, pay claims, and collect data on utilization. Many third-party administrators also provide case management services for potentially extraordinarily expensive cases to help coordinate care and control employee risk of catastrophic expenses."[4] There are several benefits to being self-funded. First, the organization gets to set most of the parameters of the policy—deductibles, co-insurance, fixed indemnities, and exclusions. If the organization wants to exclude some services and include others, it can. For example, if the organization has an older workforce, it may wish to delete obstetrics from the policy but include a number of preventive health services. Second, the organization holds on to the cash reserves in the benefits account instead of sending them to a commercial carrier, and thus gets to accrue interest on them. Third, the self-funded organizations have been exempt from the *Employee Retirement and Income Security Act of 1974* (ERISA), which mandates minimum benefits under state law.[4] And fourth, generally the administrative costs of self-funded organizations have been less than those of traditional commercial carriers and, in general, health insurance costs to these groups have risen at a slower rate.[4] It appears that these benefits will not be affected by the Affordable Care Act passed in 2010; however, the law did include language that indicates that the Secretary of the U.S. Department of Labor is required to provide an annual report about self-funded insurance programs to the appropriate committees of Congress so that they can study their workings. In addition, the law requires the Secretary of the U.S. Department of Health and Human Services to conduct a study of self-funded insurance programs to determine if there are any adverse effects on the components of health care reform.[59]

For self-funded insurance to work, there must be a sizable group of employees over which to spread the risk. Larger organizations usually find it more useful than smaller ones do. However, if a small workforce is composed primarily of low-health-risk employees, say, for example, younger employees, self-funded programs make sense.

Health Insurance Provided by the Government

Although there are some in the United States who would like to see all health insurance provided by the government—a national health insurance plan—at the present time government health insurance plans are only available to select groups in the United States. The only government health insurance plans—those funded by governments at federal, state, and local levels—that exist today are Medicare, Medicaid, the Children's Health Insurance Program (CHIP) (formerly known as the State Children's Health Insurance Program [SCHIP]), Veterans Administration (VA) benefits (see Figure 13.14), Indian Health Service, and health care benefits for the uniformed services (military and Public Health Service) (TRICARE), federal employees (Federal Employees Health Benefits Program), and prisoners. Our discussion here is limited to Medicare, Medicaid, and CHIP. Medicare and Medicaid were created in 1965 by amendments to the Social Security Act and were implemented for the first time in 1966. CHIP was created in 1997 and codified as Title XXI of the Social Security Act.

Medicare

Medicare, which currently covers more than 46.5 million people,[23] is a federal health insurance program for people 65 years of age or older, people of any age with permanent kidney failure, and certain disabled people under 65. It is administered by the Centers for Medicare and Medicaid Services (CMS) of the U.S. Department of

> **Medicare**
> a national health insurance program for people 65 years of age and older, certain younger disabled people, and people with permanent kidney failure

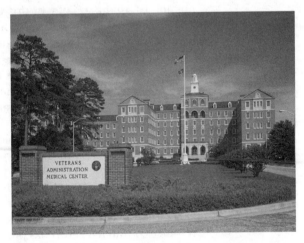

FIGURE 13.14
Insurance provided for veterans is one of several insurance plans paid for by the U.S. government.

Health and Human Services (HHS). The Social Security Administration provides information about the program and handles enrollment. Medicare is considered a contributory program, in that employers and employees are required to contribute a percentage of each employee's wages/salaries through Social Security (FICA) tax to the Medicare fund. Medicare has four parts: hospital insurance (Part A), medical insurance (Part B), managed care plans (Part C), and prescription drug plans (Part D).

The Medicare hospital insurance (Part A) portion is mandatory and is provided for those eligible without further cost. Some seniors who are not eligible for premium-free Part A because they or their spouses did not pay into Social Security at all, or paid only a limited amount, may be able to purchase Part A coverage. In 2010, those premiums were $461 per month.[60] Although Medicare Part A has deductible ($1,100 in 2010) and co-insurance provisions, it helps pay for inpatient care in a hospital and in a skilled nursing facility after a hospital stay, hospice care, and some home health care.[60] Those who are enrolled in Part A of Medicare are automatically enrolled in Part B unless they decline. In 2010, the premium for Part B was $96.40 per month.[60] Most Part A enrollees are also enrolled in Part B and have their premium deducted directly from their Social Security check. Part B of Medicare helps cover physicians' services, outpatient hospital care, and selected other health care services and supplies that are not covered by Part A. Part B also has a deductible ($155 per year in 2010) and co-insurance (80/20 coverage). Whereas most Medicare beneficiaries pay the standard premium rate, a small percentage pay a higher rate based on their income. In 2010, the higher rates ranged from $110.50 to $353.60 per month depending on the extent to which an individual beneficiary's income exceeded $85,000 (or $170,000 for those filing a joint tax return), with the highest rates paid by those whose incomes were more than $214,000 (or $428,000 for those filing a joint tax return).[60]

Part C of Medicare is the managed care plans of Medicare (see the discussion of managed care later in this chapter). Formally, Part C is called Medicare Advantage and was added to Medicare as part of the Balanced Budget Act (BBA) of 1997. It was introduced primarily as a means to try to reduce costs compared with the original fee-for-service Medicare plan. Medicare Advantage plans provide all of the coverage provided in Parts A and B and must cover medically necessary services except for hospice care. They generally offer extra benefits; thus, there is no need to purchase a separate supplemental Medigap policy (see the discussion of Medigap later in this chapter), and many include Part D prescription drug coverage. Part C plans are offered by private insurance companies and are not available in all parts of the country. Because private companies offer them, the specifics of the plans are not consistent from plan to plan. Some are set up on a fee-for-service arrangement while others are offered as managed care plans (i.e., PPOs, HMOs, and medical savings accounts). Most have an annual deductible and require a monthly premium in addition to premiums paid for Part B.[60] In 2010, there were 11.4 million enrolled in Part C plans.[61]

Medicare Part D is the prescription drug program. In 2010, there were 27.7 million enrolled (17.7 million from stand-alone plans and 9.9 million enrolled via Part C plans) in Part D plans.[61] Part D is optional and run by insurance companies and other private companies approved by Medicare. To use it, those eligible must sign up for it and pay a monthly premium (most range from $20 to $40 per month). The premium varies based on the plan selected (most states offer approximately 50 different plans). A special provision in Part D— "Extra Help"—offers drug coverage at low cost for qualified people with limited incomes and resources. Although Part D has provided welcome help with the cost of prescription drugs to those who are eligible, the process of using Part D has been hard for many seniors to understand. It is complicated for several reasons. The first is the large number of plans available.

The plans vary in drugs covered and costs. For example, one drug may be on the list of drugs covered (called the *formulary*) by one plan but not another. Many plans cover only generic drugs, whereas others cover both generic and brand-name drugs. Most plans have copayments or co-insurance. And then there is the coverage gap, or what has become known as the *donut hole*. In 2010, all plans (with the exception of the Extra Help plan) had a $310 deductible. Once the deductible was met, the plans covered the cost of drugs (minus copayment/co-insurance) between $311 and $2,830. Then, at $2,830, the enrollees had to pay out of pocket all costs of drugs while in the coverage gap until they had spent $4,550. (This includes yearly deductible, copayment/co-insurance, and all costs while in the coverage gap. This does not include the plan's premium.) Once enrollees reached the plan's out-of-pocket limit, the donut hole closed and the enrollees had catastrophic coverage. This means that those covered paid a co-insurance amount (e.g., 5% of the drug cost) or a copayment (e.g., $2.15 or $3.15 for each prescription) for the rest of the calendar year.[60] Some of the complexity of Part D will be resolved with the Affordable Care Act passed in 2010. As part of that legislation, the confusing donut hole (i.e., coverage gap) is to be gradually reduced, and by 2020 it will be eliminated.[59]

Finally, it should be noted that when health care providers take assignment (are willing to accept Medicare patients) on a Medicare claim, they agree to accept the Medicare-approved amount as payment in full. These providers are paid directly by the Medicare carrier, except for the deductible and co-insurance amounts, which are the patient's responsibility.

Medicare, like private health insurance programs, is affected by the high costs of health care and, therefore, the government is always looking for ways of cutting the costs of the programs. As noted earlier in the chapter, Medicare has used several types of *prospective reimbursement* to help cut costs. The oldest of these, diagnosis-related groups (DRGs), has been around since 1983. When patients with Medicare coverage are admitted to a hospital they are assigned a DRG and the hospital is reimbursed the predetermined amount of money for the DRG as opposed to the actual cost to render care. "The correct DRG for each patient is decided by considering the patient's major or principal diagnosis; any complications or other problems that might arise; any surgery performed during the hospital stay; and other factors."[62] The amount of money assigned to each DRG is not the same for each hospital. The figure is based on a formula that takes into account the type of service, the type of hospital, the location of the hospital, and the sex and age of the patient. Using this prospective pricing system, hospitals are encouraged to provide services at or below the DRG rate. If the hospital delivers the service below the DRG rate, the hospital can retain the difference. If it is delivered above the DRG rate, the hospital incurs the extra expenses. "However, when a Medicare patient's condition requires an unusually long hospital stay or exceptionally costly care, Medicare makes additional payment to the hospital."[62] Because of DRGs, some have felt that hospitals are quicker to discharge Medicare patients to keep their expenses down. This phenomenon has resulted in an increase in the need for skilled nursing care in homes, in adult day care facilities, and in nursing homes.

In recent years, much discussion has centered around whether there are sufficient funds in Medicare to pay for the health care costs of the 76 million baby boomers when they started to become eligible in 2011. Most projections about the Medicare program indicate that there is enough money to begin to cover the baby boomers, but as they age Medicare will run out of money unless changes are made. To deal in part with this problem, a number of changes were made to Medicare as part of the Affordable Care Act passed in 2010. Box 13.8 presents some of the components of the Affordable Care Act that will affect the way the Medicare program is delivered.

BOX 13.8	IMPLEMENTATION TIMELINE FOR KEY MEDICARE PROVISIONS OF THE 2010 HEALTH CARE REFORM LAW, 2010–2015

2010

Cost containment	• Reduce annual market basket updates for inpatient hospital, home health, skilled nursing facility, hospice and other Medicare providers, and adjust payments for productivity • Ban new physician-owned hospitals in Medicare
Improving quality and health system performance	• Establish a new office within the Centers for Medicare & Medicaid Services (CMS), the Federal Coordinated Health Care Office, to improve care coordination for dual eligibles
Prescription drug benefit	• Provide a $250 rebate for beneficiaries who reach the Part D coverage gap

2011

Cost containment	• Establish a new Center for Medicare and Medicaid Innovation within CMS • Freeze the income threshold for income-related Medicare Part B premiums for 2011 through 2019 at 2010 levels ($85,000/individual and $170,000/couple), and reduce the Medicare Part D premium subsidy for those with incomes above $85,000/individual and $170,000/couple • Provide Medicare payments to qualifying hospitals in counties with the lowest quartile Medicare spending for 2011 and 2012
Medicare Advantage	• Prohibit Medicare Advantage plans from imposing higher cost sharing for some Medicare-covered benefits than is required under the traditional fee-for-service program • Restructure payments to Medicare Advantage (MA) plans by phasing payments to different percentages of Medicare fee-for-service rates; freezes payments for 2011 and 2010 levels
Physician payment	• Provide a 10% Medicare bonus payment to primary care physicians and general surgeons practicing in health professional shortage areas
Prescription drug benefit	• Begin phasing in federal subsidies for generic drugs in the Medicare Part D coverage gap (reducing coinsurance from 100% in 2010 to 25% by 2020) • Require pharmaceutical manufacturers to provide a 50% discount on brand-name prescriptions filled in the coverage gap (reducing coinsurance from 100% in 2010 to 50% in 2011)
Preventive services	• Eliminate Medicare cost sharing for some preventive services • Provide Medicare beneficiaries access to a comprehensive health risk assessment and creation of a personalized prevention plan

2012

Cost containment	• Allow providers organized as accountable care organizations (ACOs) that voluntarily meet quality thresholds to share in the savings they achieve for the Medicare program • Reduce Medicare payments that would otherwise be made to hospitals by specified percentages to account for excess (preventable) hospital readmissions
Improving quality and health system performance	• Create the Medicare Independence at Home demonstration program • Establish a hospital value-based purchasing program and develop plans to implement value-based purchasing for skilled nursing facilities, home health agencies, and ambulatory surgical centers
Medicare Advantage	• Reduce rebates for Medicare Advantage plans • High-quality Medicare Advantage plans begin receiving bonus payments
Prescription drug benefit	• Make Part D cost sharing for dual eligible beneficiaries receiving home and community-based care services equal to the cost sharing for those who receive institutional care

2013

Improving quality and health system performance	• Establish a national Medicare pilot program to develop and evaluate paying a bundled payment for acute, inpatient hospital services, physician services, outpatient hospital services, and post-acute care services for an episode of care
Prescription drug benefit	• Begin phasing in federal subsidies for brand-name drugs in the Part D coverage gap (reducing coinsurance from 100% in 2010 to 25% in 2020, in addition to the 50% manufacturer brand discount)
Tax changes	• Increase the Medicare Part A (hospital insurance) tax rate on wages by 0.9% (from 1.45% to 2.35%) on earnings over $200,000 for individual taxpayers and $250,000 for married couples filing jointly • Eliminate the tax deduction for employers who receive Medicare Part D retiree drug subsidy payments

2014

Cost containment	• Independent Payment Advisory Board comprised of 15 members begins submitting legislative proposals containing recommendations to reduce Medicare spending if spending exceeds a target growth rate • Reduce Disproportionate Share Hospital (DSH) payments initially by 75% and subsequently increase payments based on the percent of the population uninsured and the amount of uncompensated care
Medicare Advantage	• Require Medicare Advantage plans to have medical loss ratios no lower than 85%
Prescription drug benefit	• Reduce the out-of-pocket amount that qualifies for Part D catastrophic coverage (through 2019)

2015

Cost containment	• Reduce Medicare payments to certain hospitals for hospital-acquired conditions by 1%

Source: Reprinted from the Henry J. Kaiser Family Foundation (2010). *Medicare: A Primer (#7615-03).* Available at http://www.kff.org/medicare/7615.cfm. Accessed January 4, 2010.

Medicaid

A second type of government health insurance is **Medicaid**, a health insurance program for low-income Americans. Currently, approximately 46+ million people are covered by Medicaid.[63] Eligibility for enrollment in Medicaid is determined by each state. Many Medicaid recipients are also enrolled in other types of public assistance programs (welfare). Unlike Medicare, there is no age requirement for Medicaid; eligibility requirements are primarily tied to income. Also, unlike Medicare, Medicaid is a noncontributory program jointly paid for and administered through federal and state governments. Both programs cover skilled nursing care but under different conditions.

For many states, one of the more costly items appearing in the annual state budget is the Medicaid program. Thus, like the federal government, state governments are always looking for ways to reshape their programs to become more efficient. Several states have combined their Medicaid program with their Children's Health Insurance Program (CHIP) (see CHIP discussion that follows) to provide better health care for the low-income Americans. In addition, the HHS has provided, on a competitive basis, some states with special grants to develop other plans for extending health care coverage to the uninsured.

The Affordable Care Act passed in 2010 made some significant changes to the Medicaid program. The biggest change deals with eligibility for the program. As noted earlier, eligibility prior to the new law was determined by each state in consultation with the federal government. Under health reform, eligibility will be based solely on income and will be extended to more low-income people, including both parents and adults without dependent children.[63] As a result of these changes, nearly everyone under the age of 65 years with income below 133% of the poverty level (in 2009 that was $29,327 for a family of four) will qualify for Medicaid, significantly reducing the number of uninsured and state variation in coverage.[63] Thus, there will be a degree of standardization in eligibility from state to state that will allow for the coordination between Medicaid and the new health insurance exchanges.[63] It is anticipated that the new eligibility standards will increase the number enrolled in Medicaid and CHIP by 16 million by 2019.[63]

Children's Health Insurance Program

The **Children's Health Insurance Program (CHIP)** was created as part of the Balanced Budget Act of 1997 and funded for 10 years. At some point in 2009, approximately 7.8 million children were enrolled in the program.[64] The program was enacted at the time to extend insurance to a significant portion of the estimated 11.3 million U.S. children without insurance (one in seven, and nearly 25% of all uninsured).[65] On February 4, 2009, President Obama extended CHIP through 2013 by signing the 2009 Children's Health Insurance Program Reauthorization Act (CHIPRA, or Public Law 111-3).[66] Like Medicaid, this is a joint state-federal funded program. To help offset the cost of the reauthorization, the new law included an increase in the federal excise tax rate on tobacco products.[66]

CHIP is specifically targeted at low-income children who are ineligible for other insurance coverage, including Medicaid (almost three-fifths of those covered by Medicaid are children). "Uninsured children pay a heavy price: Study after study shows that they are more likely to report poor health, to see doctors less often (even when they are sick), to go without preventive care, and to turn to emergency rooms when in need of treatment. The result is needless illness, learning problems, disabilities, and sometimes even death."[65] Even with the availability of Medicaid and CHIP, it is estimated that there are still approximately 8.1 million children who are uninsured.[67] Many of these 8+ million are eligible for Medicaid or CHIP, so both CHIPRA and the Affordable Care Act of 2010 have provisions to increase enrollment.

Medicaid
a jointly funded federal-state health insurance program for low-income Americans

Children's Health Insurance Program (CHIP)
a title insurance program under the Social Security Act that provides health insurance to uninsured children

Problems with Medicare and Medicaid

In theory, both the Medicare and Medicaid programs seem to be sound programs that help provide health care to two segments of the society who would otherwise find it difficult or impossible to obtain health insurance. In practice, there are two recurrent problems with these programs. One problem is that some physicians and hospitals do not accept Medicare and Medicaid patients because of the tedious and time-consuming paperwork, lengthy delays in reimbursement, and insufficient reimbursement. As a result, it is difficult if not impossible for many of those eligible for Medicare and Medicaid to receive health care. The second problem occurs when physicians and hospitals file Medicare and Medicaid paperwork for care or services not rendered or rendered incompletely. This is known as *Medicare/Medicaid fraud.*

These problems were known to Congress, so when the Affordable Care Act passed in 2010 it included provisions to both increase payment to physicians and hospitals and crack down on fraud.

Supplemental Health Insurance

Medigap

Medigap
private health insurance that supplements Medicare benefits

As noted earlier, Parts A and B of Medicare have deductibles and co-insurance stipulations. To help cover these out-of-pocket costs and some other services not covered by Medicare, people can purchase supplemental policies from private insurance companies. These policies have come to be known as **Medigap** (also called "Medicare Supplement Insurance") policies because they cover the "gaps" not covered by Medicare. Federal and state laws mandate national standardization of Medigap policies. Since their inception, 14 different standardized Medigap plans (titled A through N) have been used. However, as of June 1, 2010, there are only 10 plans (A–D, F, G, K–N) available[68] (see Box 13.9). All plans are required to have a core set of benefits referred to as *basic benefits*; however, some of the basic benefits of plans K through N are offered at a reduced level. By law, the letters and benefits of the individual plans cannot be changed by the insurance companies. However, they may add names or titles to the letter designations. Companies are not required to offer all the plans. "Insurance companies selling Medigap policies are required to make Plan A available. If they offer any other Medigap plan, they must also offer either Medigap Plan C or Plan F."[68] Three states—Minnesota, Massachusetts, and Wisconsin—have exceptions to the 10-plan setup because they had alternative Medigap standardization programs in effect before the federal legislation was enacted. Individuals should contact the state insurance office in these states if interested in these plans.

Two other variances to these Medigap rules should be noted. The first deals with those individuals enrolled in the Medicare Advantage program. Because Medicare Advantage is more comprehensive in coverage than is the traditional Medicare program, Medigap policies are not needed. In fact, it is illegal for insurance companies to sell a Medigap policy if they know a person is enrolled in Medicare Advantage.[68] Another variance in Medigap policy deals with Medicare SELECT. *Medicare SELECT* is a type of Medigap policy that is available in some states. This type of policy still provides one of the standardized Medigap plans (A–D, F, G, K–N), but requires policy holders to use specific hospitals and, in some cases, doctors (except in emergencies) to receive full Medigap benefits.[68]

Other Supplemental Insurance

Medigap is a supplemental insurance program specifically designed for those on Medicare. However, a number of supplemental insurance policies exist for people regardless of their age. Included are specific-disease insurance, hospital indemnity insurance, and long-term care insurance. Specific-disease insurance, though not available in some states, provides benefits for only a single disease (such as cancer) or a group of specific diseases. Many policies are written as

BOX 13.9 — MEDIGAP POLICIES EFFECTIVE ON OR AFTER JUNE 1, 2010

How to read the chart:

If a checkmark appears in a column of this chart, the Medigap policy covers 100% of the described benefit. If a column lists a percentage, the policy covers that percentage of the described benefit. If a column is blank, the policy doesn't cover that benefit.

Note: The Medigap policy covers coinsurance only after you have paid the deductible (unless the Medigap policy also covers the deductible).

You may buy the following Medigap Plans which became effective June 1, 2010:

Medigap Benefits	A	B	C	D	F*	G	K	L	M	N
Medicare Part A Coinsurance hospital costs up to an additional 365 days after Medicare benefits are used up	✓	✓	✓	✓	✓	✓	✓	✓	✓	✓
Medicare Part B Coinsurance or Copayment	✓	✓	✓	✓	✓	✓	50%	75%	✓	✓***
Blood (First 3 Pints)	✓	✓	✓	✓	✓	✓	50%	75%	✓	✓
Part A Hospice Care Coinsurance or Copayment	✓	✓	✓	✓	✓	✓	50%	75%	✓	✓
Skilled Nursing Facility Care Coinsurance			✓	✓	✓	✓	50%	75%	✓	✓
Medicare Part A Deductible		✓	✓	✓	✓	✓	50%	75%	50%	✓
Medicare Part B Deductible			✓		✓					
Medicare Part B Excess Charges					✓	✓				
Foreign Travel Emergency (Up to Plan Limits)			✓	✓	✓	✓			✓	✓
Medicare Preventive Care Part B Coinsurance	✓	✓	✓	✓	✓	✓	✓	✓	✓	✓

Out-of-Pocket Limit**	
$4,620	$2,310

*Plan F also offers a high-deductible plan. This means you must pay for Medicare-covered costs up to the deductible amount $2,000 in 2010 before your Medigap plan pays anything.

**After you meet your out-of-pocket yearly limit and your yearly Part B deductible ($155 in 2010), the Medigap plan pays 100% of covered services for the rest of the calendar year. Out-of-pocket limit is the maximum amount you would pay for coinsurance and copayments.

***Plan N pays 100% of the Part B coinsurance except up to $20 copayment for office visits and up to $50 for emergency department visits.

Source: Centers for Medicare & Medicaid Services (2010). *2010 Choosing a Medigap Policy: A Guide to Health Insurance for People with Medicare.* Baltimore, MD: Author, 13.

---

fixed-indemnity policies. Hospital indemnity coverage is insurance that pays a fixed amount for each day a person receives inpatient hospital services, and it pays up to a designated number of days. Long-term care insurance, which pays cash amounts for each day of covered nursing home or at-home care, is of great concern to many people, and it is presented next.

Long-Term Care Insurance

With people living longer and the cost of health care on the rise, more and more individuals are considering the purchase of long-term care insurance. It has been estimated that "at least 70 percent of people over age 65 will require some long-term care services at some point in their lives. And, contrary to what many people believe, Medicare and private health insurance programs do not pay for the majority of long-term care services that most people need—help with personal care such as dressing or using the bathroom independently."[69] Women need care for longer than do men (3.7 vs. 2.2 years). Whereas about one-third of today's 65-year-olds may never need long-term care services, 20% of them will need care for more than 5 years.[69] Most—about 80%—of long-term care will be provided in the home by unpaid caregivers,[69] usually family and friends. "The typical caregiver is a 46-year-old woman who is married and employed, and is caring for her widowed mother who does not live with her."[69] Yet, planning for long-term care requires people to think about possible future health care needs and how they will pay for them. Obviously, the cost of long-term care varies based on the level of care, the length of time the care is provided, and where the care is provided. The most costly long-term care is nursing home care. Recent figures show that the average cost of residing in a nursing home was $70,000 per year,[69] while assisted-living facilities averaged $36,000 per year.[70] People who reach age 65 will likely have a 40% chance of entering a nursing home.[71] The costs vary by parts of the country, but such costs for long-term care have many people worried about their financial future. This cost is something that can quickly deplete a lifetime of savings. In fact, the majority of Americans who have to pay for long-term care are impoverished within the first few years of making long-term health care payments. Those caring for a spouse find that they quickly exhaust both their spouse's resources and their own. Though the majority of long-term care is paid for by the government (see Figure 13.15), it is only after patients have exhausted many of their assets that Medicaid will begin to cover the costs.

Though long-term care is expensive, not everyone needs to buy long-term care insurance. Those who do not need it are those with low incomes and few assets who could be covered by Medicaid and the very wealthy who are able to pay the cost of the care out of pocket. Those who are most likely to benefit from long-term care insurance are those in between the poor and wealthy, especially older women. About half of women older than 65 will spend some time in a nursing home. In addition, about 75% of nursing home residents are women and two-thirds of home care consumers are women. However, there are several reasons why all people should consider purchasing long-term insurance. They include the following:

- To preserve financial assets
- To prevent the need for family members or friends to provide the care

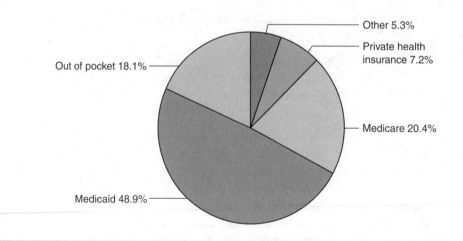

FIGURE 13.15

Who pays for long-term care?

Source: National Clearinghouse for Long-Term Care Information (2010). "National Spending on Long-Term Care." Available at http://www.longtermcare.gov/LTC/main_site/index.aspx. Accessed September 29, 2010.

- To enable people to stay independent in their homes longer
- To make it easier to get into the nursing home or assisted-living home of their choice

As noted in Chapter 9, the Affordable Care Act included the passage of the Community Living Assistance Services and Supports (CLASS) Act. This component adds a great boost to the funding of long-term care. The program will provide individuals with functional limitations a cash benefit to purchase nonmedical services and supports (e.g., housing modification, assistive technologies, personal assistance services, and transportation) necessary to maintain community residence.[69] "The goals of CLASS were to provide workers and future retirees with a financing alternative for long-term services and supports that supports community living and does not require them to become impoverished and turn to Medicaid to access these services"[69] (see Chapter 9 for more information on CLASS).

Managed Care

As noted earlier in this chapter, the failed attempt to adopt universal health care in the United States during the first term of President Clinton led to the movement of managed care. Managed care plans include "a set of techniques used by or on behalf of purchasers of health care benefits to manage health care costs by influencing patient care decision making through case-by-case assessments of the appropriateness of care prior to its provision."[72] The transition to managed care in the United States was largely driven by a desire of employers, insurance companies, and the public to control soaring health care costs. In fact, the goal of managed care is to control costs by controlling health care utilization.[1] Although the exact number of individuals enrolled in managed care programs is constantly changing, it has been estimated that in 2010, more than 135 million Americans[73]—almost one-half of the total population—belonged to some form of a managed health care plan. However, more than 90% of employees insured through employer-sponsored health insurance are enrolled in managed care programs. These numbers cover not only workers who received their health care coverage from employers, but also some individuals who were covered by Medicare, Medicaid, and the military.

Managed health care plans are offered by managed care organizations (MCOs). MCOs function like insurance organizations. They offer policies, collect premiums, and bear financial risk. That is, MCOs take on the financial responsibility if the costs of the services exceed the revenue from the premiums. Approximately 15% to 20% of the premiums are used to manage the risk and to cover administrative expenses, while the remainder is spent on health care services.[1] These organizations have agreements with certain doctors, hospitals, and other health care providers to give a range of services to plan members at reduced cost. MCOs have been structured in a variety of ways and are similar to the other health care organizations with which we are familiar (such as hospitals). Some are structured as nonprofit organizations, while others are for-profit and owned by a group of investors. "Regardless of their structure, their goals, however, are similar: to control costs through improved efficiency and coordination, to reduce unnecessary or inappropriate utilization, to increase access to preventive care, and to maintain or improve quality of care."[74]

The managed health care plans offered by these organizations vary and are always evolving as managed care practices mature. The plans also differ, both in cost and ease of receiving needed services. Although no plan pays for all the costs associated with medical care, some plans cover more than others do. Common features in managed care arrangements include (1) provider panels often referred to as the network—specific physicians and other providers are selected to care for plan members; (2) limited choice—members must use the providers affiliated with the plan or pay an additional amount; (3) gatekeeping—members must obtain a referral from a case manager for specialty care or inpatient services; (4) risk sharing—providers bear some of the health plan's financial risk through capitation and withholds; and (5) **quality management and utilization review**—the plan monitors provider practice patterns and medical outcomes to identify deviations from quality and efficiency standards.[4] The utilization review can take the form of *prospective utilization review* (as precertification), *concurrent utilization review* (i.e., during the course of health care utilization), or *retrospective utilization review* (completed by reviewing medical records after the care has been provided).[1] This latter type of review may involve "analysis of data to examine patterns of excessive utilization or underutilization. *Underutilization* occurs when medically necessary care is not delivered."[1]

Types of Managed Care

As noted earlier, there are several different types of managed care arrangements, and because of the increasing cost of health care and the demands of consumers for better health care service these arrangements continue to be adapted and developed. "Until about 1988, the various types of MCOs were quite distinct. Since then, the differences between traditional forms of health insurance and managed care have narrowed considerably."[1] The following are the most commonly available arrangements.

Preferred Provider Organizations

The **preferred provider organization (PPO)** is a form of managed care closest to a fee-for-service plan. A PPO differs from the traditional fee-for-service plan in that the fee has been fixed (at a discounted rate) through a negotiation process between a health care provider (e.g., physicians, dentists, hospitals) and the PPO, and the provider agrees to accept this discounted rate as payment in full. It works in the following manner: A PPO approaches a provider, such as a group dental practice, and contracts with the dentists to provide dental services to all those covered by the PPO's insurance plan at a fixed (discount) rate. To the extent that the PPO succeeds in obtaining favorable prices, it can offer lower premiums, co-insurance, and copayments, and hence can attract more patients to enroll in its insurance plan. In addition to the PPO doctors making referrals, plan members can refer themselves to other doctors, including ones outside the plan. However, if they do choose to go outside the plan, they will have to meet the deductible and pay higher co-insurance. In addition, they may have to pay the difference between what the provider charges and what the plan pays. PPOs also control costs by requiring (1) preauthorization for hospital admissions (excluding emergencies), and (2) second opinions for major procedures such as surgery.[4] Advantages for the providers are that they (1) do not share in any financial risk as a condition of participation,[4] (2) are reimbursed on a fee-for-service basis to which they are accustomed,[4] (3) are assured a certain volume of patients, and (4) are assured that the patients will pay promptly (via the PPO). Approximately 53 million were enrolled in PPOs in 2010.[73] Much of the increase in enrollment in PPOs was the result of people leaving HMOs (see the discussion of HMOs later in this chapter) because of increased costs and the restrictions in the choice of providers.

Exclusive Provider Organizations

Exclusive provider organizations (EPOs) are like PPOs except that they have stronger financial incentives for enrolled members to use the exclusive (only) provider. Stronger financial incentives usually mean no deductible, co-insurance, or copayments. If the members were to go outside the plan to another provider, they would be responsible for a larger percentage of the bill. Typically, the number of providers (physicians, dentists, hospitals, etc.) is much smaller in an EPO, which strengthens the ability of the organization to receive a greater discount because the providers are guaranteed a larger share of patients. Because of such arrangements, a business or corporation is able to create a more stringent utilization and monitoring program with an EPO.

quality management and utilization review
the analysis of provided health care for its appropriateness by someone other than the patient and provider

preferred provider organization (PPO)
an organization that buys fixed-rate health services from providers and sells them to consumers

exclusive provider organization (EPO)
like a PPO but with fewer providers and stronger financial incentives

Health Maintenance Organizations

Health maintenance organizations (HMOs) are the oldest form of managed care. In 2010, 66+ million people were enrolled in HMOs, but this number was down from a high of about 80 million in 1999.[73] As noted earlier, many of those leaving HMOs switched to PPOs. In an HMO, the insurance coverage and the delivery of medical care are combined into a single organization. The organization hires (through salaries or contracts) an individual doctor or groups of doctors to provide care and either builds its own hospital or contracts for the services of a hospital within the community. The organization then enrolls members, usually, but not always, through the workplace. Members (or their employers or the government [in the case of HMOs for Medicare and Medicaid]) make regular payments in advance on a fixed contract fee to the HMO. This contract may also include a deductible and copayment when service is provided. In return, the HMO is contractually obligated to provide the members with a comprehensive range of outpatient and inpatient services that are spelled out in the contract for a specific time period.

When members enroll in an HMO, they are given a list (network) of specific physicians/providers from which to select their primary care doctor (usually a family physician, internist, obstetrician-gynecologist, or pediatrician) and other health care providers. The primary care doctor (which some have referred to as the gatekeeper) serves as the member's regular doctor and coordinates the member's care, which means the member must contact his or her primary care doctor to be referred to a specialist. In many plans, care by a specialist is only paid for if the member is referred by the primary care doctor, thus the term *gatekeeper*. Also, if patients receive care outside the network, they must pay for all the costs, except in cases of emergency when physically not near a member of the network.

How do HMOs make a profit? An HMO's focus of care is different from that of a traditional fee-for-service provider. In an HMO, ill and injured patients become a "cost." An HMO does not make money on the ill but on keeping people healthy. The less the providers of an HMO see a patient, the lower the costs and the more profitable the organization. Therefore, most HMOs emphasize health promotion activities and primary and secondary care.

There are two main organizational models of HMOs—staff models and individual practice models—and each type has spawned several hybrids. These hybrids are referred to as **mixed model HMOs**.

STAFF MODEL

In **staff model HMOs**, the health care providers are employed (usually salaried) by the HMO and practice in common facilities paid for by the HMO. Staff model HMOs employ providers in all common specialties to provide services to their members. Special contracts are established with subspecialties for infrequently needed services. These providers are expected to follow the practice and procedures determined by the HMO. With the exception of the special contracts, the providers work only for the HMO, and thus do not have their own private practices. In most instances, the HMO contracts with a hospital for inpatient services. Nationwide, the number of staff model HMOs has been declining.

INDEPENDENT PRACTICE ASSOCIATION MODEL

Independent practice associations (IPAs) are the most common type of HMO today. IPAs are legal entities separate from the HMO[1] that are physician organizations composed of community-based independent physicians in solo or group practices who provide services to HMO members.[4] "Instead of establishing contracts with individual physicians or groups, the HMO contracts with the IPA for physician services. Physicians do not have contracts with the HMO, but with the IPA."[1] Thus, the IPA acts as an intermediary and is paid a capitation amount by the HMO.[1]

health maintenance organizations (HMOs) groups that supply prepaid comprehensive health care with an emphasis on prevention

mixed model HMO a hybrid form of health maintenance organization

staff model HMO a health maintenance organization that hires its own staff of health care providers

independent practice associations (IPAs) legal entities separate from the HMO that are physician organizations composed of community-based independent physicians in solo or group practices who provide services to HMO members

group model HMO
one that contracts with a multispecialty group practice

OTHER HMO MODELS

Three other HMO models include the *group model*, the *network model*, and the *direct contract model*. A **group model HMO** contracts with a multispecialty group practice and separately with one or more hospitals to provide services, whereas a **network model HMO** contracts with more than one medical group practice.[1] A **direct contract HMO** contracts with individual physicians as opposed to group practices.[4]

network model HMO
one that contracts with more than one medical group practice

Point-of-Service Option

One of the major objections to HMOs is that the patients cannot freely select their provider. They are restricted to those with whom the HMO has contracted. Some HMOs have solved this problem with the **point-of-service (POS) option**, which allows for a more liberal policy of enabling patients to select providers. With this option, members may choose a provider from within or outside the HMO network. Patients who obtain services outside the network generally must pay a higher deductible and co-insurance.

direct contract HMO
one that contracts with individual physicians as opposed to group practices

Medicare Advantage

As noted earlier, in some parts of the country Medicare recipients may have an HMO option available to them through the Medicare Advantage plan. In such plans, the Medicare recipient receives all Medicare-covered services from the HMO. In addition, the HMO may charge the beneficiary a premium (in addition to the Medicare Part B premium) to cover co-insurance and deductibles of Medicare and may include items and services not covered by Medicare. If this is the case, Medigap coverage cannot be purchased. In other cases, beneficiaries may receive other services not covered by Medicare at no charge or at a much lower cost than might be expected. In 2010, approximately 24.2% of the people in Medicare were covered by managed care plans.[73]

point-of-service (POS) option
an option of an HMO plan that enables enrollees to be at least partially reimbursed for selecting a health care provider outside the plan

Medicaid and Managed Care

As has been noted throughout this chapter, managed care plans are also available for those covered by Medicaid. The rationale for offering such plans is to improve access to care by the establishment of contracted provider networks, as well as by promoting greater accountability for quality and costs. Each state in the United States offers such a plan, and depending on the state requirements, enrollment may or may not be voluntary. If it is mandatory, then the state is required to offer a choice of managed care plans and make efforts to inform beneficiaries about their choices.[4] In 2010, approximately 71% of the people covered by Medicaid were enrolled in managed care plans.[73]

Before leaving our discussion on managed care, we want to remind the reader that, like other aspects of the health care system, there have been efforts to measure the quality of managed care too. Please see our discussion of quality of health care earlier in the chapter where we present information on the National Committee on Quality Assurance (NCQA).

Other Arrangements for Delivering Health Care

Because the majority of people in the United States receive their health care through a managed care plan or a fee-for-service plan, the majority of this chapter focused on those plans. However, there are other ways of delivering health care. A few of the more highly visible arrangements are discussed next.

National Health Insurance

National health insurance, or national health care, suggests a system in which the federal government assumes the responsibility for the health care costs of the entire population. In such a system, the costs are primarily paid for with tax dollars. Presently among all the developed countries of the world, there is only one that does not have a national health care plan for its citizens: the United States.

The national health care systems of the developed countries of the world fall into two basic models. The first is a national health service model with universal coverage and a general tax-financed government ownership of the facilities and doctors as public employees. Countries using this model include the United Kingdom, Spain, Italy, Greece, and Portugal. The second is a social insurance model that provides universal coverage under social security, financed by various ways including taxes or contributions paid by employers and employees. In Canada, contributions are made to a government entity. In France and Germany, contributions go to nonprofit funds with national negotiation on fees. Japan also has a compulsory system that relies heavily on employer-based coverage.

When one considers the level of satisfaction with health care, the better access to health care services, the lower health care costs, and the superior health status indicators in these other countries, one must ask why the United States has not adopted such a program. It is not because the United States has not considered such a plan—in fact, there have been seven failed attempts at addressing the issue over the past 70+ years. The first came when President Roosevelt tried to include it as part of the New Deal. President Harry Truman presented a proposal to Congress on two different occasions, only to have it defeated twice. Other unsuccessful attempts at national health care legislation were made during the Kennedy, Nixon, and Clinton administrations. The most recent talk about a national health insurance program in the United States came during the presidential campaign and debates of 2008. During that campaign, both of the front-running Democratic candidates, Senators Hillary Rodham Clinton and Barack Obama, and the Republican Candidate Senator John McCain pledged to work toward a national program, though all had different plans for getting there. As history has shown us, President Obama was unsuccessful in getting a national health insurance program, but he was successful in getting major health care reform via the Affordable Care Act passed in 2010.

Though the push for national health insurance has not been successful, several states—including Florida, Hawaii, Massachusetts, Minnesota, Oregon, and Vermont—prior to 2010 passed major health care reform packages aimed at providing increased access to health insurance and basic health services to all or most of their residents. It is unclear at this point how the Affordable Care Act will affect the state programs.

HEALTH CARE REFORM IN THE UNITED STATES

Prior to the passage of the Affordable Care Act (ACA) in 2010, the health care reform that has taken place in the United States in recent times has been with specific smaller, but not insignificant, portions of the health care system—for example, President Clinton's creation of the Children's Health Insurance Program (CHIP) in 1997 and the reauthorization of the program by President Obama in 2009. During President George W. Bush's term in office, the reform came in the form of the Medicare Prescription Drug Improvement and Modernization Act (MMA) of 2003 (Public Law 108-173). The portion of MMA that gained the greatest publicity—that dealing with prescription drugs via Medicare Part D—was discussed earlier in the chapter. However another significant component of the MMA was health savings accounts (HSAs). HSAs are one of several different forms of consumer-directed health plans (CDHPs). In the sections that follow, we discuss both CDHPs and the major features of the Affordable Care Act.

Consumer-Directed Health Plans

Consumer-directed health plans (CDHPs) (also called consumer-driven health plans, consumer-directed health arrangements [CDHAs], consumer choice, and self-directed health plans [SDHPs][46]) have been defined several different ways. But whichever definition is used, they are health plan options that combine more consumer responsibility for health care decisions with

Consumer-directed health plans (CDHPs) health plan options that combine more consumer responsibility for decisions with a tax-sheltered account to pay for out-of-pocket costs for health care and a high-deductible health insurance policy

a tax-sheltered account that consumers may use to pay for out-of-pocket health care costs and usually a high-deductible health insurance policy.[75] CDHPs "seek to marshal the power of consumers making cost-conscious choices to constrain rising U.S. health care spending."[76] A critical part of the CDHPs is providing those enrolled in such plans with comparative information to increase their knowledge about health care choices and associated costs.[4] The central idea behind CDHPs is that consumers will still have catastrophic health insurance, but because they are required to use more of their own money to pay for health care they will be more careful about their use of services than they would be under a traditional health plan that provides greater coverage of their initial health care costs.[46,75] Those options usually included in CDHPs are health savings accounts (HSAs) usually coupled with high-deductible health plans (HDHPs), health reimbursement arrangements (HRAs), flexible spending accounts (FSAs), and Archer Medical Savings Accounts (MSAs).

CDHPs are not without critics. There are three major concerns about CDHPs. One, will consumers become educated enough to make good decisions? Health insurance and health care are very complicated, and will consumers take the time to become well educated? Two, is the health care field transparent enough to get enough information to make a good decision? When was the last time that a patient received a health care service and knew in advance what the cost would be? Also, how do consumers know when they are receiving quality care? Who is the best physician in the community? Who is the worst? And three, will consumers seek health care in a timely manner because with CDHPs they have to use more of their own money? For example, on a traditional plan maybe annual influenza vaccinations were covered with a zero deductible, but with a CDHP that has a high deductible it now costs consumers $50 out of pocket. Will they still get the vaccine or will they try to save the $50 and forgo the vaccine?

The most visible of the CDHPs is the *health savings account* (HSA). An HSA is a type of medical savings account that allows people to save money to pay for current and future medical expenses on a tax-free basis. To be eligible for an HSA, people must be covered by a high-deductible plan (in 2010, the deductible was $1,200 for individuals and $2,400 for families), not have any other health insurance (including Medicare), and not be claimed as a dependent on someone else's tax return. Those with HSAs can use this account to pay for qualified health expenses, including expenses that the plan ordinarily does not cover, such as hearing aids.[77] By law, there is a maximum amount that people with HSAs would have to pay out of pocket for health expenses in a year. The amount is adjusted for inflation each year, but in 2010 the amount was $5,950 for individuals and $11,900 for families.

During the year, those with HSAs can make voluntary contributions to the account using before-tax dollars. In 2010, the maximum amount that could be set aside was $3,050 for an individual, $6,150 for families, or the amount of the deductible of the health insurance policy, whichever was lower. People aged 55 and older can make addition "catch-up" contributions (in 2010, $1,000) until they enroll in Medicare. In some cases, employers may set up and help fund HSAs for their employees, but they are not required to do so. An HSA earns interest. If there is a balance in a person's HSA at the end of the year, it will roll over, allowing the person to build up a cushion against future health expenses. In addition, HSAs allow people to accumulate funds and retain them when they change plans or retire.[77] Money can be withdrawn from the account without penalty to pay for care before the deductible is met and for things not covered under the health insurance policy after the deductible is met. Money can be withdrawn and pay for anything (nonhealth expenses) after 65 years of age, but the person must pay income tax on it. The advantages of such a plan are reduced premiums and, it is hoped, more prudent use of health care dollars—which should be good for both employers and employees. In addition, HSAs are portable from one employer to another. The major disadvantage for consumers is that they might have to pay more out of pocket for health care, and therefore might skip needed care. At the present, HSAs seem best suited for the healthy and wealthy. It will be some time before it is known whether this type of reform will have a major impact on health care delivery in the United States.

The Affordable Care Act passed in 2010 made several changes to HSAs. As of January 2011, HSAs could no longer be used tax-free for over-the-counter medications unless the medications were prescribed by a doctor. In addition, if people use their HSA funds for non-medical expenses, they must pay a 20% penalty instead of the former 10% penalty.[56]

Though HSAs must be combined with high-deductible health plans (HDHPs) (usually defined as plans with deductibles of a minimum of $1,000 for individuals and $2,000 for families, but they could be higher; Internal Revenue Service uses $1,200 and $2,200, respectively), HDHPs do not have to be combined with HSAs. In fact, HDHPs are expected to grow in popularity because of their lower premium costs.[1] When these plans are used they are often accompanied by health promotion and wellness, disease management, case management, and health coaching programs to help participants improve and maintain health and keep medical conditions under control.[46]

Another type of CDHP is *health reimbursement arrangements* (HRAs). HRAs may be established by employers to pay employees' medical expenses. Only employers can set up HRAs for employees, and only employers can contribute to them. The employer decides how much money to put in a health reimbursement arrangement, and the employee can withdraw funds from the account to cover allowed expenses. HRAs often are established in conjunction with an HDHP, but they can be paired with any type of health plan or used as a stand-alone account. In addition, federal law allows employers to determine whether employees can carry over all or a portion of unspent funds from year to year. Also, employers can decide whether account balances will be forfeited if an employee leaves the job or changes health plans.[77] The Affordable Care Act passed in 2010 also affected HRAs. Like HSAs, as of January 2011, HRA funds could no longer be used tax-free for over-the-counter medications unless the medications were prescribed by a doctor.[56]

Flexible spending accounts (FSAs) are set up by employers to allow employees to set aside pre-tax money to pay for qualified medical expenses during the year. Only employers may set up an account, and employers may or may not contribute to the account. There may be a limit on the amount that employers and employees can contribute to a health flexible spending arrangement. FSAs can be offered in conjunction with any type of health insurance plan, or they can be offered on a stand-alone basis. In the past, FSAs were subject to a use-it-or-lose-it rule within the year of contributions, but now employers may give employees a $2\frac{1}{2}$-month grace period at the end of the plan year to use up funds in the account. After that time, remaining funds from the previous plan year are forfeited.[77] The tricky part of having an FSA is trying to determine how much money to place in the account in a year to avoid losing any money at year's end. Just like HRAs, as of January 2011, the Affordable Care Act passed in 2010 no longer allowed FSA funds to be used tax-free for over-the-counter medications unless the medications were prescribed by a doctor.[56]

Archer Medical Savings Accounts (MSAs), the oldest of the CDHPs in use today, are individual accounts that may be set up by self-employed individuals and those who work for small businesses (less than 50 employees). To set up an MSA, people must be covered by an HDHP. Either the employee or the employer may contribute to the account, but both cannot contribute to the account in the same year. Individuals control the use of funds in the accounts and can withdraw funds for qualified medical expenses. Funds can be rolled over from year to year, and balances in the accounts are portable when changing jobs or retiring.

The Affordable Care Act passed in 2010 made several changes to MSAs that were much like those made to HSAs. As of January 2011, MSAs could no longer be used tax-free for over-the-counter medications unless the medications were prescribed by a doctor. In addition, if people use their MSA funds for nonmedical expenses, they must pay a 15% penalty instead of the former 10% penality.[56]

Enrollment in CDHPs has been rising in recent years for three major reasons: (1) employers trying to cut health care costs, (2) consumers trying to reduce the cost of health insurance premiums, and (3) the tax advantages of most of the plans. Data from the 2007 National Health Interview Study showed that those more likely to be enrolled in a CDHP were those (1) who directly purchased private health plans, (2) with more education, and (3) with higher incomes.[78] A more recent study,[79] showed that (1) 18% of adults aged 18-64 years with private health insurance were enrolled in an HDHP, including 5% who were enrolled in a CDHP; (2) adults aged 18-64 years enrolled in an HDHP-only or HDHP plus FSA were more likely to report unmet medical or prescription drug needs because of cost than were adults enrolled in a traditional health plan with or without an FSA; (3) adults aged 18-64 years with either an FSA or an HSA were more likely to get an influenza vaccination than were those without an FSA or an HAS; and (4) adults aged 18-64 years with either an FSA or an HSA were more likely to have contact with an eye doctor than were those without an FSA or HSA (see Figure 13.16). In terms of numbers, American Association of Preferred Provider Organizations estimated that 18 million people were enrolled in CDHPs in 2009, up from 14 million in 2008—an increase of more than 28%.[80]

Affordable Care Act

Throughout this chapter, we have made reference to the Affordable Care act (ACA) passed in 2010 when information included in the act applied to a specific topic in the chapter. Here, we would like to provide some background on the ACA and some of its major features. Just as a reminder, one week apart in March 2010 President Obama signed into law two bills—the Patient Protection and Affordable Health Care Act (PPACA) (Public Law 111-148) and the Health Care and Education Reconciliation Act of 2010 (HCERA) (Public Law 111-152). These two acts were consolidated with other approved legislation and are now referred to as the Affordable Care Act. Portions of this ACA went into effect in 2010, and the last portion will go into effect in 2020. Much of the law takes effect in 2014. The process to get the ACA passed was not easy. It took more than a year of discussion, and there was much political wrangling by both Democrats and Republicans. Some called the wrangling an "ideological split." In the end, the Democratic members of the U.S. Senate and House of Representatives were more pleased with the results than were the Republican members. In fact, shortly after the laws were passed, some Republican members were so unhappy with the results that they pledged to do whatever they could to have the law repealed. When this edition of the book went to press, there was still much political posturing going on about the law.

At the heart of the ACA was increasing the number of Americans who had health insurance and providing consumers with some health care/insurance rights that they have not received in the past. As noted throughout this chapter,

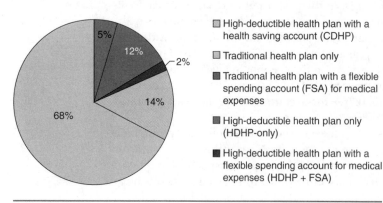

FIGURE 13.16

Percent distribution of type of private health insurance for adults aged 18–64 years: United States, 2007.

Source: Cohen, R. A. (2010). Impact of Type of Insurance Plan on Access and Utilization of Health Care Services for Adults Aged 18–65 with Private Health Insurance: United States, 2007–2008. (NCHS Data Brief, no. 28). Hyattsville, MD: National Center for Health Statistics, 1. Available at http://www.cdc.gov/nchs/data/databriefs/db28.htm. Accessed September 29, 2010.

both the health care that is received and the health of people are better when people are insured. The people helped most by ACA will be "the uninsured and intermittently insured, the underinsured, those who cannot afford their out-of-pocket costs or health insurance premiums, small businesses and their employees, young adults who will be able to stay on their parents' policies until they find a job with health benefits, and those who are denied coverage because they have preexisting conditions or major health problems."[57] Those individuals who are not covered under ACA are undocumented immigrants. Some have estimated this number to be as high as 15 million people.

Earlier in the chapter, we discussed the efforts made during President Clinton's administration to pass a Patient's Bill of Rights at the national level. When those efforts fell short, many states created and passed their own Patient's Bill of Rights. The ACA included several different components that addressed patient's rights "to put American consumers back in charge of their health coverage and care."[81] In June 2010, "the Departments of Health and Human Services (HHS), Labor, and Treasury issued regulations to implement a new Patient's Bill of Rights under the Affordable Care Act—which will help children (and eventually all Americans) with preexisting conditions gain coverage and keep it, protect all Americans' choice of doctors and end lifetime limits on the care consumers may receive. These new protections apply to nearly all health insurance plans."[81] Box 13.10 provides a brief summary of the major components of the ACA that address patient's rights.

As noted throughout this chapter, the ACA is not a simple piece of legislation. It was almost 1,000 pages long and had many items in it that changed the way health insurance is provided in the United States. Some of the changes are very obvious and easy to understand, while others could be skipped over by one not reading closely. Others are complicated and

---

BOX 13.10   THE AFFORDABLE CARE ACT'S NEW PATIENT'S BILL OF RIGHTS

- *No pre-existing condition exclusions for children younger than age 19.* As of September 2010, the ACA prohibited insurance plans from limiting benefits for children and from refusing to sell children coverage at all based on the fact that a child had a pre-existing condition. This policy applies to all types of insurance except for individual market plans that were "grandfathered." This critical policy will be broadened to Americans of all ages in 2014.
- *No unjustified rescissions of insurance coverage.* Prior to passage of ACA, insurance companies were able to retroactively cancel someone's policy when they become sick, or if they or their employers made an unintentional mistake on their paperwork. Under the ACA, insurers are prohibited from rescinding coverage—for individuals or groups of people—except in cases involving fraud or an intentional misrepresentation of material facts. There are no exceptions to this policy.
- *No lifetime limits on coverage.* The ACA prohibited insurance plans from stopping benefits when the cost of care for a patient reached a lifetime limit set by the insurance company. No plan issued or renewed after September 23, 2010, could use such a limit.
- *Restricted annual limits on coverage.* Even more binding than lifetime limits were annual dollar limits on what an insurance company would pay for health care. The ACA is phasing out the use of annual limits over a 3-year period for most health plans before banning such limits entirely in 2014.
- *Protecting choice of doctors.* The ACA made it clear that health plan members were free to designate any available (in the plan network) participating primary care provider as their primary care provider.
- *Removing insurance company barriers to emergency department services.* The ACA made emergency services more accessible for consumers. Health insurers are not able to charge higher cost sharing (copayments or co-insurance) for emergency services obtained outside the health plan's network.

Source: Sebelius, K. (2010). *Health Care Notes: Protecting Patients with Private Insurance.* Available at http://www.healthcare.gov/news/blog/patientprotections.html. Accessed September 29, 2010.

BOX
13.11

BOX 13.11   KEY FEATURES OF THE AFFORDABLE CARE ACT

1. *New federal insurance market rules* that prohibit restricting coverage or varying premiums based on health, set limits on the share of private premiums going for nonmedical costs, and establish essential standard benefit packages that guarantee beneficiaries a comprehensive array of services with limits on levels of cost sharing.

2. *New health insurance exchanges* that will more efficiently pool risk, lower administrative costs, and provide eligible individuals and small businesses a choice of affordable health plans.

3. *Affordability provisions for low- and middle-income families*, including an essential standard benefit package, premium assistance on a sliding scale up to four times poverty income (about $88,000 for a family of four), and expansion of Medicaid eligibility up to 133% of the federal poverty level (almost $30,000 for a family of four).

4. *A commitment to shared responsibility* that preserves employer-sponsored insurance, provides health insurance tax credits to small businesses, assesses a contribution from larger businesses whose employees receive government-financed premium subsidies, and requires that individuals have coverage.

5. *Improvements to Medicare prescription drug benefits*, including $250 rebates for seniors who fell into the "donut hole" in 2010 and elimination of that coverage gap by 2020.

6. *Creation of a new long-term care financing program* to support community living for the disabled.

7. *Investment in a stronger primary care foundation,* one that includes increases in payment for primary care under Medicare and Medicaid, incentives for practices to organize as patient-centered medical homes providing more accessible and coordinated care, and investment in primary care training and expansion of community health centers and the National Health Service Corps.

8. *Establishment of an innovation center* within the Centers for Medicare and Medicaid Services to rapidly test and spread effective payment methods that reward quality of care rather than volume of services. Additional payment and system reform provisions encourage accountability for patient outcomes and use of medical resources and provide incentives for productivity improvement.

9. *Creation of an Independent Payment Advisory Board* with the authority to make recommendations for reducing cost growth and improving quality in both the Medicare program and the health system as a whole.

10. *Investment in the infrastructure required* for a high-performance health system, including publicly reported information on quality, cost, and performance of providers and insurers; use of modern information technology in medical care and health insurance; and national strategies and policies on disease prevention, public health, quality, safety, and the health care workforce.

Source: Davis, K. (2010). *A New Era in American Health Care: Realizing the Potential of Reform.* New York, NY: The Commonwealth Fund, 5–7. Available at http://www.commonwealthfund.org/Content/Publications/Fund=Reports/2010/Jun/A-New-Era-In-American-Health-Care.aspx. Accessed September 29, 2010.

will take many people much time to completely understand and implement. Box 13.11 presents a brief description of 10 key features of ACA as summarized by Davis.[57] Also, to keep consumers up-to-date on the implementation of ACA the U.S. government created an information Web site at www.healthcare.gov.

CHAPTER SUMMARY

- The concept of a health care system has been and continues to be questioned in the United States. Is it really a system or is treatment provided in an informal, cooperative manner?

- Health care in the United States has evolved from home and folk remedies to the modest services of the independent country doctor who often visited the sick in their homes to a highly complex 2 trillion plus industry.

- There are medical specialists and health care facilities for almost every type of illness and health problem.

- The spectrum of health care includes four domains of practice—population-based public health practice, medical practice, long-term practice, and end-of-life practice.

- Within the medical practice domain of health care are the following types of health care providers: independent providers (allopathic, osteopathic, and nonallopathic), limited (restricted) care providers, nurses, nonphysician practitioners, allied health care professionals, and public health professionals.
- Complementary and alternative medicine (CAM) is "a group of diverse medical and health care systems, practices, and products that are not presently considered to be a part of conventional medicine."[4]
- Health care providers perform services in both inpatient and outpatient care facilities.
- Inpatient care facilities include hospitals, nursing homes, and assisted living facilities.
- The types of outpatient care facilities found in communities are health care practitioners' offices, clinics, primary care centers, retail clinics, urgent/emergent care centers, ambulatory surgery centers, and freestanding service facilities.
- Long-term care options include traditional institutional residential care as well as special units within these residential facilities, halfway houses, group homes, assisted-living facilities, transitional (step-down) care in a hospital, day care facilities for patients, and personal home health care.
- The predominant organization responsible for accrediting health care facilities is the Joint Commission.
- The major issues of concern with the health care system in the United States can be summed up by the cost containment, access, and quality triangle.
- Some of the barriers to access to health care in the United States have been the lack of health insurance, inadequate insurance, and poverty.
- There are a number of different methods by which the amount of reimbursement to health care providers is determined. They include fee-for-service, packaged pricing, resource-based relative value scale, prepaid health care, and prospective reimbursement.
- Most health care in the United States is paid for via third-party payment.
- Key health insurance terms include *deductible, coinsurance, copayment, fixed indemnity, exclusion,* and *preexisting condition*.
- The two largest government-administered health insurance programs in the United States are Medicare and Medicaid.
- The government's Children's Health Insurance Program (CHIP) is for many children who were previously uninsured.
- Two major supplemental insurance programs in the United States are Medigap and long-term care insurance.
- A significant portion of Americans today are covered by some form of managed care.

- The more common forms of managed care include health maintenance organizations (HMOs), preferred provider organizations (PPOs), exclusive provider organizations (EPOs), and point-of-service (POS) options.
- The United States is the only developed country in the world without national health insurance.
- Consumer-directed health plans, including health savings accounts (HSAs), high-deductible health plans (HDHPs), health reimbursement arrangements (HRAs), flexible spending accounts (FSAs), and Archer Medical Savings Accounts (MSAs), are becoming more popular health plan options.
- Health care reform in the United States did not come easily, but the Affordable Care Act will significantly increase the number of Americans who have health insurance.

REVIEW QUESTIONS

1. Why have some questioned whether the United States really has a health care system?

2. Describe some of the major changes that have taken place in health care delivery over the years.

3. What is meant by *third-party payment*?

4. Why has the cost of health care in the United States continued to grow faster than the cost of inflation?

5. What is meant by a *spectrum of health care*?

6. What are the domains of practice noted in the spectrum of health care?

7. Is there a demand for health care workers in the United States today? If so, why?

8. In what type of facility are most health care workers employed?

9. What is the difference between independent and limited (restricted) care providers?

10. What are the differences between allopathic and nonallopathic health care providers?

11. Define *complementary* and *alternative medicine* and give a few examples of each.

12. What kind of education do limited (restricted) care providers have?

13. What is the difference between LPNs and RNs?

14. What are advanced practice nurses (APNs)?

15. What are nonphysician practitioners?

16. What role do public health professionals play in health care delivery?

17. What are the advantages of outpatient care facilities?

18. What is meant by a long-term care facility? Give two examples.

SCENARIO: ANALYSIS AND RESPONSE

1. Have you ever experienced a situation similar to the one described in the scenario? If so, briefly describe it.
2. If we truly had a "health care system" in this country, how would this scenario be different?
3. Do you think Chad did the right thing?

4. If you were Chad, what would you have done? If you had zero-deductible health insurance, would it make a difference in what you would do?
5. Which of the options available to Chad do you think was the most expensive? Least expensive? Why?

19. Why has the number of home health care agencies increased in recent years?

20. What is the Joint Commission? What does it do?

21. What are three major problems facing the health care system in the United States?

22. How is the quality of health care services measured?

23. Explain how each of the following types of reimbursement works: fee-for-service, packaged pricing, resource-based relative value scale, prepaid health care, and prospective reimbursement.

24. On what basic concept is insurance based?

25. Explain the following insurance policy provisions: (a) a $200 deductible, (b) 20/80 co-insurance, (c) a $4,500 fixed indemnity for a basic surgical procedure, (d) an exclusion of the preexisting condition of lung cancer, and (e) a $10 copayment.

26. What is the difference between Medicare and Medicaid?

27. What is covered in each of the four parts of Medicare—Parts A, B, C, and D?

28. What relationship does Medigap insurance have to Medicare?

29. What is the Children's Health Insurance Program (CHIP)?

30. Briefly explain the differences among health maintenance organizations (HMOs), preferred provider organizations (PPOs), exclusive provider organizations (EPOs), and a point-of-service option.

31. What are the advantages and disadvantages of managed care?

32. What is meant by the term *consumer-directed health plans*? Give some examples.

33. What is the major result of the Affordable Care Act passed in 2010?

ACTIVITIES

1. Using Table 13.2 from this chapter, identify two different health care facilities in your community for each of the levels of care. Briefly describe each facility and determine whether each one is private, public, or voluntary.

2. Make an appointment to interview three health care workers in your community who have different types of jobs. Ask them what they like and dislike about their work, what kind of education they needed, whether they are happy with their work, and whether they would recommend that others seek this line of work. Summarize your findings in a written paper.

3. Obtain a copy of a local newspaper (the Sunday edition is best) and look through the "want ads" for health care worker jobs. In a one-page paper, briefly describe what you have found and summarize the status of health care position openings in your community.

4. Create a list of all the health care providers from whom your family has sought help in the past 5 years. Group the individuals into the six provider groups outlined in the chapter. When appropriate, identify the providers' specialties and whether they were allopathic, osteopathic, or nonallopathic providers.

5. Make an appointment to interview an administrator in the local (city or county) health department. In the interview, find out what kind of people, by profession, work in the department. Also find out what type(s) of health care services and clinics are offered by the department. Summarize your findings in a two-page paper.

6. Obtain a copy of the student health insurance policy available at your school. After reading the policy, summarize in writing what you have read. In your summary, indicate what type of reimbursement system is used to pay providers, list specifics about the premium costs, deductible, co-insurance, copayment, fixed indemnity, and any exclusions.

7. Visit an HMO in your area and find the answers to the following: (a) What type of HMO is it? (b) How does one enroll? (c) What does it cost? (d) What services are provided? and (e) Why should someone get his or her health care from an HMO instead of the more traditional private-practice physician?

COMMUNITY HEALTH ON THE WEB

The Internet contains a wealth of information about community and public health. Increase your knowledge of some of the topics presented in this chapter by accessing the Jones & Bartlett Learning Web site at **http://health .jbpub.com/book/communityhealth/7e** and follow the links to complete the following Web activities.

- Joint Commission
- Medicare and Medicaid
- Affordable Care Act

REFERENCES

1. Shi, L., and D. A. Singh (2010). *Essentials of the US Health Care System*, 2nd ed. Sudbury, MA: Jones & Bartlett.

2. Institute of Medicine (2003). *The Future of the Public's Health in the 21st Century*. Washington, DC: National Academy Press.

3. Rothstein, W. G. (1972). *American Physicians in the Nineteenth Century: From Sect to Science*. Baltimore, MD: Johns Hopkins University Press.

4. Sultz, H. A., and K. M. Young (2011). *Health Care USA: Understanding Its Organization and Delivery*, 7th ed. Sudbury, MA: Jones & Bartlett.

5. Cambridge Research Institute (1976). *Trends Affecting the U.S. Health Care System* (DHEW pub. no. HRA 75-14503). Washington, DC: U.S. Government Printing Office, 261.

6. U.S. Department of Health, Education and Welfare, Health Resources Administration (September 1974). *Fact Sheet: The Hill-Burton Program*. Washington, DC: U.S. Government Printing Office.

7. Lokkeberg, A. R. (1988). "The Health Care System." In E. T. Anderson and J. M. McFarlane, eds., *Community as Client: Application of the Nursing Process*. Philadelphia: Lippincott, 3-14.

8. Koff, S. Z. (1987). *Health Systems Agencies: A Comprehensive Examination of Planning and Process*. New York: Human Services Press.

9. Stockman, D. A. (1981). "Premises for a Medical Marketplace: A Neoconservative's Vision of How to Transform the Health System." *Health Affairs*, 1(1): 5-18.

10. Wessel, D. (7 September 2006). "In Health Care, Consumer Theory Falls Flat." *Wall Street Journal*, A2.

11. MacKay, A. P., L. A. Fingerhut, and C. R. Duran (2000). *Health, United States, 2000, with Adolescent Health Chartbook*. Hyattsville, MD: National Center for Health Statistics.

12. U.S. Department of Health and Human Services, Centers for Medicare & Medicaid Services (2010). "National Health Expenditure Data." Available at http://www.cms.gov/NationalHealthExpendData/01_ Overview.asp#TopOfPage.

13. Zatkin, S. (1997). "A Health Plan's View of Government Regulation." *Health Affairs*, 16(6): 33-35.

14. Dickerson, J. F. (8 December 1997). "Dr. Clinton Scrubs Up." *Time*, 48.

15. President's Advisory Commission on Consumer Protection and Quality in the Health Care Industry (1998). *Quality First: Better Health Care for All Americans*. Washington, DC: U.S. Government Printing Office.

16. The White House (5 April 2006). "Fact Sheet: Health Savings Accounts: Affordable and Accessible Health Care [Press release]." Available at http://georgewbush-whitehouse.archives.gov/news/releases/ 2006/04/20060405-6.html.

17. Institute of Medicine (2001). *Crossing the Quality Chasm: A New Health System for the 21st Century*. Washington, DC: National Academy Press.

18. World Health Organization (2000). "World Health Organization Assesses the World's Health Systems." Available at: http://www.who .int/whr/2000/media_centre/press_release/en.

19. Turnock, B. J. (2009). *Public Health: What It Is and How It Works*, 4th ed. Sudbury, MA: Jones & Bartlett.

20. U.S. Public Health Service (1994). *For a Healthy Nation: Return on Investments in Public Health*. Washington, DC: U.S. Department of Health and Human Services.

21. Shi, L., and D. A. Singh, (2008). *Delivering Health Care in America: A Systems Approach,* 4th ed. Sudbury, MA: Jones & Bartlett.

22. Bernstein, A. B., E. Hing, A. J. Moss, K. F. Allen, A. B. Siller, and R. B. Tiggle (2004). *Health Care in America: Trends in Utilization*. Hyattsville, MD: National Center for Health Statistics.

23. National Center for Health Statistics (2010). *Health, United States, 2009: With Special Feature on Medical Technology*. Hyattsville, MD: Author.

24. U.S. Department of Labor, Bureau of Labor Statistics (2009). *Spotlight on Statistics: Health Care*. Available at http://www.bls.gov/ spotlight/2009/health_care/.

25. American Osteopathic Association (2010). "What Is a DO?" Available at http://www.osteopathic.org/osteopathic-health/about-dos/what-is-a-do/Pages/default.aspx.

26. National Institutes of Health, National Center for Complementary and Alternative Medicine (2010). *What Is Complementary and Alternative Medicine?* Available at http://nccam.nih.gov/.

27. Barnes, P. M., B. Bloom, and R. L. Nahin (2008). *Complementary and Alternative Medicine Use among Adults and Children: United States, 2007* (National Health Statistics Reports, no. 12). Hyattsville, MD: National Center for Health Statistics.

28. Nahin, R. L., P. M. Barnes, B. J. Stussman, and B. Bloom (2009). *Costs of Complementary and Alternative Medicine (CAM) and Frequency of Visits to CAM Practitioners: United States, 2007* (National Health Statistics Reports, no. 18). Hyattsville, MD: National Center for Health Statistics.

29. National Institutes of Health, National Center for Complementary and Alternative Medicine (2010). *CAM Basics*. Available at http:// nccam.nih.gov/health/whatiscam/.

30. Hassmiller, S. B., and M. Cozine (2006). "Addressing the Nurse Shortage to Improve the Quality of Patient Care." *Health Affairs*, 25(1): 268-274.

31. Stanfield, P. S., N. Cross, and Y. H. Hui (2009). *Introduction to the Health Professions*, 5th ed. Sudbury, MA: Jones & Bartlett.

32. U.S. Department of Labor, Bureau of Labor Statistics (2009). "Licensed Practical and Licensed Vocational Nurses." *Occupational Outlook Handbook, 2010-11 Edition*. Available at http://www.bls.gov/ oco/ocos102.htm.

33. U.S. Department of Labor, Bureau of Labor Statistics (2009). "Registered Nurses." *Occupational Outlook Handbook, 2010-11 Edition*. Available at http://www.bls.gov/oco/ocos083.htm.

34. U.S. Department of Health and Human Services, Health Resources and Services Administration (2010). *The Registered Nurse Population: Initial Findings from the 2008 National Sample Survey of Registered Nurses*. Available at http://bhpr.hrsa.gov/healthworkforce/rnsurvey.

35. Carbonara, P., and J. Caplin (2004). "The Hospital Wars." *Money*, 33(2): 147-148, 151-152.

36. The White House, Council of Economic Advisors (2009). *Recovery Act Investments in Community Health Centers*. Available at http://www.whitehouse.gov/administration/eop/cea/factsheets-reports/economic-impact-arra-4th-quarterly-report/box4-1.

37. Coleman, B. (2000). *Assuring the Quality of Home Care: The Challenge of Involving the Consumer*. Washington, DC: American Association of Retired People.

38. U.S. Department of Health and Human Services, Centers for Medicare & Medicaid Services (2008). *Data Tables.* Available at http://www.cms.gov/NationalHealthExpendData/downloads/tables.pdf.

39. Joint Commission (2010). *Joint Commission Fact Sheets: Facts about the On-Site Survey Process.* Available at http://www.jointcommission.org/AboutUs/Fact_Sheets/onsite_qa.htm.

40. Joint Commission (2009). *Joint Commission Fact Sheets: Facts about Accreditation Decisions for 2010.* Available at http://www.jointcommission.org/AboutUs/Fact_Sheets/10_acc_decisions.htm.

41. Alliance for Health Reform (2010). *Covering Heath Issues,* 5th ed. Available at http://www.allhealth.org/covering-health-issues-5th-edition/toc.asp.

42. Kissick, W. L. (1994). *Medicine's Dilemmas: Infinite Needs versus Finite Resources.* New Haven, CT: Yale University Press.

43. Institute of Medicine (2004). *Insuring America's Health: Principles and Recommendations.* Available at http://www.iom.edu/Reports/2004/Insuring-Americas-Health-Principles-and-Recommendations.aspx.

44. Cohen, R. A., M. E. Martinez, and B. W. Ward (2010). *Health Insurance Coverage: Early Release of Estimates from the National Health Interview Survey, 2009.* Atlanta, GA: Centers for Disease Control and Prevention, National Center for Health Statistics. Available at: http://www.cdc.gov/nchs/data/nhis/earlyrelease/insur201006.htm.

45. Adams, P. F., and P. M. Barnes (2006). "Summary Health Statistics for U.S. Population: National Health Interview Survey, 2004." *Vital and Health Statistics,* 10(229). Available at http://www.cdc.gov/nchs/nhis/nhis_series.htm#04reports.

46. Slee, D. A., V. N. Slee, and H. J. Schmidt (2008). *Slee's Health Care Terms,* 5th ed. Sudbury, MA: Jones & Bartlett.

47. Institute of Medicine (2002). *Care without Coverage: Too Little, Too Late.* Washington, DC: National Academies Press.

48. Kaiser Family Foundation (2010). *Summary of Coverage Provisions in the Patient Protection and Affordable Care Act.* Available at http://www.kff.org/healthreform/8023.cfm.

49. Davis, K., C. Schoen, and K. Stremikis (2010). *Mirror, Mirror on the Wall: How the Performance of the U.S. Health Care System Compares Internationally—2010 Update.* New York: Commonwealth Fund. Available at http://www.commonwealthfund.org/Content/Publications/Fund-Reports/2010/Jun/Mirror-Mirror-Update.aspx.

50. U.S. Department of Health and Human Services, Agency for Healthcare Research and Quality (2005). *Guide to Health Care Quality: How to Know It When You See It* (pub. no. 05-0088). Rockville, MD: Author. Available at http://www.ahrq.gov/consumer/guidetoq/index.html#Contents.

51. Institute of Medicine (1999). *To Err Is Human: Building a Safer Health System.* Washington, DC: Author. Available at http://www.iom.edu/Reports/1999/To-Err-is-Human-Building-A-Safer-Health-System.aspx.

52. U.S. Department of Health and Human Services, Agency for Healthcare Research and Quality (2010). *National Healthcare Disparities Report—2009* (AHRA pub. no. 10-0004). Rockville, MD: Author. Available at http://www.ahrq.gov/qual/nhdr09/nhdr09.pdf.

53. U.S. Department of Health and Human Services, Agency for Healthcare Research and Quality (2010). *National Healthcare Quality Report—2009* (AHRA pub. no. 10-0003). Rockville, MD: Author. Available at http://www.ahrq.gov/qual/nhdr09/nhqr.pdf.

54. National Committee for Quality Assurance (2010). *About NCQA.* Available at http://www.ncqa.org/tabid/675/Default.aspx.

55. National Committee for Quality Assurance (2010). *What Is HEDIS?* Available at http://www.ncqa.org/tabid/187/Default.aspx.

56. Kaiser Family Foundation (2010). *Summary of the New Health Reform Law.* Available at http://www.kff.org/healthreform/8061.cfm.

57. Davis, K. (2010). *A New Era in American Health Care: Realizing the Potential of Reform.* New York: Commonwealth Fund. Available at http://www.commonwealthfund.org/Content/Publications/Fund-Reports/2010/Jun/A-New-Era-in-American-Health-Care.aspx.

58. Jennings, P. (15, December 2005). "Peter Jennings Reporting: Breakdown—America's Health Insurance Crisis." As cited in J. P. Rooney and D. Perrin (2008). *America's Health Care Crisis Solved.* Hoboken, NJ: John Wiley & Sons.

59. The Patient Protection and Affordable Care Act, Public Law Numbers 111-148 and 111-152, Consolidated Print.

60. U.S. Department of Health and Human Services, Centers for Medicare & Medicaid Services (2010). *Medicare and You 2010.* Baltimore, MD: Author.

61. Kaiser Family Foundation (2010). *Medicare: A Primer.* Menlo Park, CA: Author. Available at http://www.kff.org/medicare/7615.cfm.

62. U.S. Department of Health and Human Services (1989). *Your Hospital Stay under Medicare's Prospective Payment System* (DHHS pub. no. HCFA 02163). Washington, DC: U.S. Government Printing Office.

63. Kaiser Family Foundation (2010). *Medicaid: A Primer.* Menlo Park, CA: Author. Available at http://www.kff.org/medicaid/7334.cfm.

64. U.S. Department of Health and Human Services, Centers for Medicare & Medicaid Services (2010). *National CHIP Policy.* Available at http://www.cms.gov/NationalCHIPPolicy/.

65. Dorn, S., M. Teitelbaum, and C. Cortez (1998). *An Advocate's Tool Kit for the State Children's Health Insurance Program.* Washington, DC: Children's Defense Fund.

66. U.S. Department of Health and Human Services, Centers for Medicare & Medicaid Services (2010). *Children's Health Insurance Program Reauthorization Act (CHIPRA) of 2009.* Available at https://www.cms.gov/chipra/.

67. Kaiser Family Foundation (2010). *Health Care Coverage of Children: The Role of Medicaid and CHIP: Fact Sheet.* Menlo Park, CA: Author. Available at http://www.kff.org/uninsured/7698.cfm.

68. Centers for Medicare & Medicaid Services (2010). *2010 Choosing a Medigap Policy: A Guide to Health Insurance for People with Medicare.* Baltimore, MD: Author.

69. Kaiser Family Foundation (2009). *The Sleeper in Health Reform: Long-Term Care and the CLASS Act.* Menlo Park, CA: Author. Available at http://www.kff.org/healthreform/kcmv102009pkg.cfm.

70. Kaiser Family Foundation (2009). *Medicaid and Long-Term Care Services and Supports: Fact Sheet.* Menlo Park, CA: Author. Available at http://www.kff.org/medicaid/2186.cfm.

71. U.S. Department of Health and Human Services (2010). *National Clearinghouse for Long-Term Care Information.* Available at http://www.longtermcare.gov/LTC/Main_Site/index.aspx.

72. Halverson, P. K., A. D. Kaluzny, C. P. McLaughlin, et al., eds. (1998). *Managed Care and Public Health.* Gaithersburg, MD: Aspen Publishers.

73. Managed Care On Line (2010). *Managed Care Fact Sheets.* Available at http://www.mcareol.com/factshts/mcolfact.htm

74. Institute of Medicine (1997). *Managing Managed Care: Quality Improvement in Behavioral Health.* Washington, DC: National Academy Press.

75. Congress of the United States, Congressional Budget Office (2006). *A CBO Study—Consumer-Directed Health Plans: Potential Effects on Health Care Spending and Outcomes.* Washington, DC: Author.

76. Alliance for Health Reform (November 2006). *HSAs and High Deductible Health Plans: A Primer.* Washington, DC: Author.

77. U.S. Department of Health and Human Services, Agency for Healthcare Research and Quality (2007). *What Is Consumer-Directed Coverage?* Available at http://www.ahrq.gov/consumer/insuranceqa/insuranceqa6.htm.

78. Cohen, R. A., and M. E. Martinez (2009). *Consumer-Directed Health Care for Persons under 65 Years of Age with Private Health Insurance: United States, 2007* (NCHS Data Brief, no. 15). Hyattsville, MD: National Center for Health Statistics.

79. Cohen, R. A. (2010). *Impact of Type of Insurance Plan on Access and Utilization of Health Care Services for Adults Aged 18-65 Years of Age with Private Health Insurance: United States, 2007-2008.* (NCHS Data Brief, no. 28). Hyattsville, MD: National Center for Health Statistics.

80. American Association of Preferred Provider Organizations (2010). *2010 Study of Consumer-Directed Health Plan (CDHP) Growth.* Available at http://www.aappo.org/index.cfm?pageid=18.

81. U.S. Department of Health and Human Services (2010). *The Affordable Care Act's New Patient's Bill of Rights.* Available at http://www.healthcare.gov/news/factsheets/aca_new_patients_bill_of_rights.html.

U N I T
T H R E E

ENVIRONMENTAL
HEALTH AND SAFETY

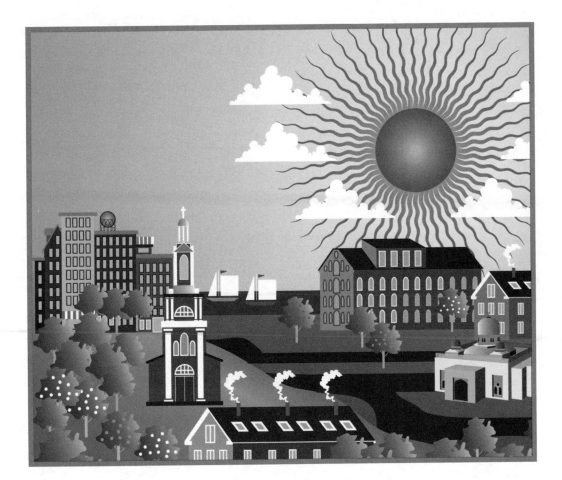

Chapter 14

Community Health and the Environment

Chapter Outline

Chapter Objectives

After studying this chapter, you will be able to:

1 List the sources and types of air pollutants, including the criteria pollutants, and explain the difference between primary and secondary pollutants.

2 Describe the role of the Environmental Protection Agency (EPA) in protecting the environment.

3 Outline the provisions of the Clean Air Act, the National Ambient Air Quality Standards, and the Air Quality Index.

4 List the major types of indoor air pollutants, including radon, and describe ways to reduce exposure to them.

5 Explain the difference between point source and nonpoint source pollution.

6 Define what is meant by the term *waterborne disease outbreak* and list some of the causative agents.

7 Explain why we should not carelessly discard pharmaceuticals and personal care products.

8 Describe the measures communities take to ensure the quality of drinking water and the measures communities take to manage wastewater.

9 Explain the purposes of the Clean Water Act and the Safe Drinking Water Act.

10 Name some of the agents associated with foodborne disease outbreaks and list some of the factors that lead to the occurrence of these outbreaks.

11 List and describe the role of some of the agencies that help protect the safety of our food.

12 Define *pest, pesticides, target organism,* and *nontarget organism.* Explain some of the safety concerns with pesticide use.

13 Describe the composition of our municipal solid waste and outline acceptable municipal solid waste management strategies.

Chapter Objectives (*cont.*)

14 Define *hazardous waste* and give some examples.

15 Explain the purposes of the Resource Conservation and Recovery Act (RCRA) and the Comprehensive Environmental Response, Compensation, and Liability Act (CERCLA).

16 Describe the health hazards associated with lead in our environment.

17 Define the terms *vector* and *vectorborne disease* and explain why these are community concerns.

18 Define *ionizing radiation* and describe the health issues associated with it.

19 List the ways that natural disasters can affect the health of a community.

20 Interpret the relationships among population growth, the environment, and human health.

21 Define *terrorism* and the environmental health repercussions of the World Trade Center attack.

22 Explain the roles of the Federal Emergency Management Agency (FEMA) and the American Red Cross in providing assistance to people and communities after a disaster.

SCENARIO

Juan and Maria had been trying to have a baby for 2 years. Their first child, Elaina, conceived before they moved to their current home and born without a problem, was now 4½ years old. But yesterday, Maria experienced her third miscarriage in the past 14 months. Before they moved into their current home, about 3 years ago, Juan and Maria had taken a sample of the well water and had it tested. At that time, the water was determined to be safe to drink. Six months after that,

however, a large-scale, rural hog farm had been built less than one-half mile away and began operations shortly after that. At first, the smell wasn't noticeable, but now the stench from the huge waste lagoon was evident most days. State inspectors had made several visits to the operation in the past year. Juan wondered whether the water in their well was still safe to drink. He decided to have their well water tested again.

INTRODUCTION

environmental health
the study and management of environmental conditions that affect the health and well-being of humans

Our health is affected by the quality of our environment, including the air we breathe, the water we drink, the food we eat, and the communities in which we live. The activities of our growing population and our demand for ever increasing amounts of energy endanger the quality of our air, the purity of our water, the safety of our food, and the health of our planet. Having recognized implications of environmental degradation on our health and the health of our communities, we have begun to enact regulatory measures to address some of the most egregious environmental assaults and to accept our responsibility for the stewardship of our planet.

environmental hazards
factors or conditions in the environment that increase the risk of human injury, disease, or death

Environmental health is the study and management of environmental conditions that affect our health and well-being. **Environmental hazards** are those factors or conditions in the environment that increase the risk of human injury, disease, or death. The aim of this chapter is to examine common environmental hazards and describe community efforts to protect our health. We begin with a discussion of environmental concerns surrounding our air, water, and food resources. Then, we discuss how communities manage solid and hazardous waste. We conclude with a discussion of natural and sociological environmental hazards.

THE AIR WE BREATHE

Nothing has been more important to the development of life as we know it on earth than the composition of the air we breathe. Yet many of our everyday activities alter the quality of this essential environmental component. By polluting the air, we endanger our health and risk leaving a deteriorating environment to future generations. In some cases, we further endanger our health with unhealthy indoor air.

Outdoor Air Pollution

Air pollution is the contamination of the air by substances—gases, liquids, or solids—in amounts great enough to harm humans, other living organisms, or the ecosystem or that alter climate. These contaminants or pollutants can arise from natural or human sources. Natural sources include dust storms, forest fires, and volcanic eruptions. Human sources can be divided into mobile sources, such as motor vehicles, and stationary sources, such as power plants and factories.

In the United States, major sources are (1) transportation, including privately owned motor vehicles; (2) electric power plants fueled by oil and coal; and (3) industry, primarily mills and refineries. In addition to these major sources, there are many smaller sources, such as wood- and coal-burning stoves, fireplaces, dry-cleaning facilities, and incinerators.

Polluting chemicals are generally divided further into primary and secondary pollutants. **Primary pollutants** include those emanating directly from the sources listed previously. They include carbon monoxide, carbon dioxide, sulfur dioxide, nitrogen oxides, most hydrocarbons, and most suspended particles. **Secondary pollutants** are formed when primary pollutants react with one another or with other atmospheric components to form new harmful chemicals. Secondary pollutants include nitrogen dioxide, nitric acid, nitrate salts, sulfur trioxide, sulfate salts, sulfuric acid, peroxyacyl nitrates, and ozone.[1] Because sunlight promotes the formation of these secondary pollutants, the resulting smog is referred to as **photochemical smog** (brown smog). This term is used to contrast photochemical smog with **industrial smog** (gray smog) formed primarily by sulfur dioxide and suspended solid particles.

Living in communities where air pollution reaches harmful levels can result in both acute and chronic health problems. Acute effects include burning eyes, shortness of breath, and increased incidence of colds, coughs, nose irritation, and other respiratory illness. In severe pollution episodes, deaths have been reported.[2] Chronic effects include chronic bronchitis, emphysema, and increased incidence of bronchial asthma attacks. There is even evidence of increased risk of lung cancer from air pollution (see Figure 14.1).[2]

Ozone, perhaps, represents the single most dangerous air pollutant. Breathing ozone can result in a variety of health problems even at low levels, including chest pain, coughing, throat irritation, congestion, bronchitis, emphysema, asthma, and reduced lung function. Repeated exposure to ground-level ozone may permanently scar lung tissue. Even healthy people can experience breathing problems if exposed to ozone at high enough levels. In many urban and suburban areas throughout the United States concentrations of ground-level ozone exceed air quality standards.

air pollution
contamination of the air that interferes with the comfort, safety, and health of living organisms

primary pollutants
air pollutants emanating directly from transportation, power and industrial plants, and refineries

secondary pollutants
air pollutants formed when primary air pollutants react with sunlight and other atmospheric components to form new harmful compounds

photochemical smog
smog formed when air pollutants interact with sunlight

industrial smog
smog formed primarily by sulfur dioxide and suspended particles from the burning of coal, also known as gray smog

ozone
O_3, an inorganic molecule considered to be a pollutant in the atmosphere because it harms human tissue, but considered beneficial in the stratosphere because it screens out UV radiation

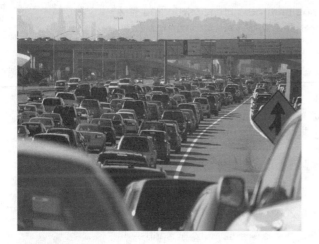

FIGURE 14.1
Air pollution from heavy traffic.

One cause of excessive levels of ground-level ozone is a phenomenon referred to as a **thermal inversion**. This occurs when a layer of warm air settles above cooler air close to the earth's surface, preventing the cooler air from rising. Ozone then accumulates in the cooler air, the air we breathe. The longer a thermal inversion continues, the more likely it is that pollutants will reach dangerously high levels (see Figure 14.2).[2]

Regulation of Outdoor Air Quality

Steady deterioration of air quality in the 1950s and 1960s led to the nation's first serious attempt to regulate air pollution, the **Clean Air Act (CAA)** of 1963. The CAA, which provided the federal government with the authority to address interstate air pollution problems, was amended several times in the late 1960s, but much of the regulation was based on voluntary compliance.

The 1970 amendments to the CAA provided the first comprehensive approach to dealing with air pollution nationwide. Three significant components of these amendments were emission standards for automobiles, emission standards for new industries, and ambient air quality standards for urban areas.[2] The latter are known as the **National Ambient Air Quality Standards (NAAQSs)**.

The **Environmental Protection Agency (EPA)** is the federal agency primarily responsible for setting, maintaining, and enforcing environmental standards. As such, it is empowered to regulate air quality and is authorized to levy fines against those who violate the standards. The EPA sets limits on how much of a pollutant can be in the air anywhere in the United States. The air pollutants of greatest concern in the United States are called **criteria pollutants**. These are sulfur dioxide, carbon monoxide, nitrogen oxides, ground-level ozone, respirable particulate matter, and lead (see Table 14.1). The EPA monitors the levels of each of these six pollutants in the ambient (outdoor) air to determine if and when they exceed the NAAQSs. Between 1990 and 2008, the United States substantially reduced the ambient air concentrations of all six of the criteria pollutants namely, lead by 78%, particulate matter by 31%, ozone by 14%, sulfur dioxide by 59%, carbon monoxide by 68%, and nitrogen oxides by 35%.[3] Nonetheless, in 2008, approximately 127 million people in the United States lived in counties with pollution levels above the NAAQSs.[3] To make it easier for all of us to understand daily air quality and what it means for your health, the EPA calculates the **Air Quality Index (AQI)** for five criteria air pollutants regulated by the Clean Air Act. The index tells you how clean or polluted your air is, and what associated health effects might be of concern for you or sensitive people in your community.

The value of the AQI on a particular day can range from 0 (good air quality) to 500 (hazardous air quality). AQI values below 100 are generally thought of as satisfactory, whereas values above 100 are considered to be unhealthy—at first for certain sensitive groups of people. Weather channels and Web sites might use a color-coded AQI for easier understanding (see Figure 14.3).[4]

The 1990 amendments to the CAA also set deadlines for establishing emission standards for 190 toxic chemicals that had not been previously addressed, established pollution taxes on toxic chemical emissions, and tightened emission standards for automobiles.

thermal inversion
a condition that occurs when warm air traps cooler air at the surface of the earth

Clean Air Act (CAA)
the federal law that provides the government with authority to address interstate air pollution

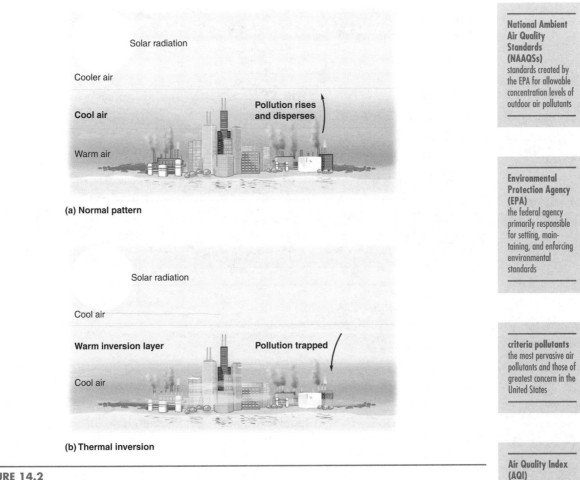

FIGURE 14.2

A thermal inversion.

Source: Chiras, D. D. (2010). *Environmental Science*, 8th ed. Sudbury, MA: Jones & Bartlett Learning.

National Ambient Air Quality Standards (NAAQSs) standards created by the EPA for allowable concentration levels of outdoor air pollutants

Environmental Protection Agency (EPA) the federal agency primarily responsible for setting, maintaining, and enforcing environmental standards

criteria pollutants the most pervasive air pollutants and those of greatest concern in the United States

Air Quality Index (AQI) an index that indicates the level of pollution in the air and the associated health risk

Table 14.1
Criteria Pollutants

Pollutants (Designation)	Form(s)	Major Sources (in order of percentage of contribution)
Carbon monoxide (CO)	Gas	Transportation, industrial processes, other solid waste, stationary fuel combustion
Lead (Pb)	Metal or aerosol	Transportation, industrial processes, stationary fuel combustion, solid waste
Nitrogen dioxide (NO_2)	Gas	Stationary fuel combustion, transportation, industrial processes, solid waste
Ground-level ozone (O_3)	Gas	Transportation, industrial processes, solid waste, stationary fuel combustion
Particulate matter	Solid or liquid	Industrial processes, stationary fuel combustion, transportation, solid waste
Sulfur dioxide (SO_2)	Gas	Stationary fuel combustion, industrial processes, transportation, other wastes

Air Quality Index Levels of Health Concern	Numerical Value	Meaning
Good (green)	0–50	Air quality is considered satisfactory, and air pollution poses little or no risk.
Moderate (yellow)	51–100	Air quality is acceptable; however, for some pollutants there may be a moderate health concern for a very small number of people who are unusually sensitive to air pollution.
Unhealthy for Sensitive Groups (orange)	101–150	Members of sensitive groups may experience health effects. The general public is not likely to be affected.
Unhealthy (red)	151–200	Everyone may begin to experience health effects; members of sensitive groups may experience more serious health effects.
Very Unhealthy (purple)	201–300	Health alert: everyone may experience more serious health effects.
Hazardous (maroon)	> 300	Health warnings of emergency conditions. The entire population is more likely to be affected.

FIGURE 14.3

Color codes for various Air Quality Indices.

Source: Environmental Protection Agency (2009). Air Quality Index (AQI): A Guide to Air Quality and Your Health. Available at http://www.epa.gov/airnow/aqi_brochure_08-09.pdf. Accessed November 18, 2010.

greenhouse gases
atmosphere gases, principally carbon dioxide, chlorofluorocarbons, ozone, methane, water vapor, and nitrous oxide, that are transparent to visible light but absorb infrared radiation

asbestos
a naturally occurring mineral fiber that has been identified as a Class A carcinogen by the Environmental Protection Agency

biogenic pollutants
airborne biological organisms or their particles or gases or other toxic materials that can produce illness

Auto industry lobbyists have successfully influenced Congress not to increase corporate average fuel efficiency (CAFE) standards. But finally, market competition, primarily from other countries and higher fuel prices, has forced American automakers to begin to produce more fuel-efficient models. Still, for the most part, the United States "continues to rely mostly on pollution cleanup rather than prevention."[2] Carpooling, increased reliance on mass transit systems, and further development of hybrid, electric, and solar-powered motor vehicles will all reduce air pollution.

Although our primary focus has been on the health benefits of air quality regulation, some mention should be made of the role of air pollution on climate change. In this regard, it should be noted that reducing the level of **greenhouse gases**, such as carbon dioxide, chlorofluorocarbons, ozone, methane, water vapor, and nitrous oxide, will reduce heat retention in the atmosphere and slow global climate change.

Indoor Air Pollutants

Sources of indoor air pollution include building and insulation materials, biogenic pollutants, combustion by-products, home furnishings and cleaning agents, radon gas, and tobacco smoke. These pollutants can arise from a number of sources (see Figure 14.4). **Asbestos** is a naturally occurring mineral fiber that was commonly used as insulation and fireproofing material. It was often used in older buildings to insulate pipes, walls, and ceilings; as a component of floor and ceiling tiles; and was sprayed in structures for fireproofing. It is harmless if intact and left alone, but, when disturbed, the airborne fibers can cause serious health problems. **Biogenic pollutants** are airborne materials of biological origin such as living and nonliving fungi and their toxins, bacteria, viruses, molds, pollens, insect parts and wastes, and animal dander. They normally enter the human body by being inhaled. These contaminants can trigger allergic

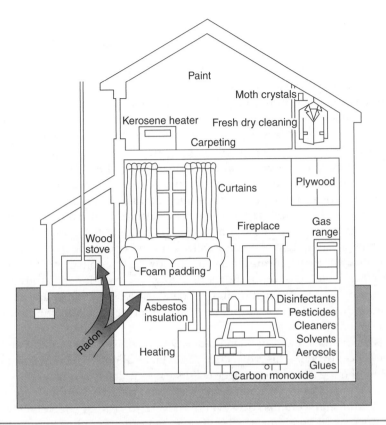

FIGURE 14.4

Air pollution sources in the home.

Source: Environmental Protection Agency (1988). *The Inside Story: A Guide to Indoor Air Quality.* Washington, D.C.: Author, 2.

reactions, including asthma; cause infectious illnesses, such as influenza and measles; or release disease-producing toxins. Symptoms of health problems include sneezing, watery eyes, coughing, shortness of breath, dizziness, lethargy, fever, and even digestive problems. Children, elderly people, and people with breathing problems, allergies, or lung diseases are particularly susceptible to airborne biogenic pollutants. People can minimize exposure to these pollutants by controlling the relative humidity level in a home or office; a relative humidity of 30% to 50% is generally recommended for homes. To reduce airborne biogenic pollutants in their homes, people should clean up standing water, remove any wet or water-damaged materials from around the home, and, if they suspect a problem, have the home inspected by someone knowledgeable about indoor air pollution problems.

Combustion by-products include gases (e.g., carbon monoxide [CO], nitrous dioxide [NO_2], and sulfur dioxide [SO_2]) and particulates (e.g., ash and soot). The major sources of these items are fireplaces, wood stoves, kerosene heaters, gas ranges and engines, candles, incense, secondhand tobacco smoke, and improperly maintained gas furnaces. Prolonged exposure to these substances can cause serious illness and possibly death.

Volatile organic compounds (VOCs) are compounds that exist as vapors over the normal range of air pressures and temperatures. The health effects of these chemicals vary

combustion by-products gases and particulates generated by burning

volatile organic compounds (VOCs) compounds that exist as vapors over the normal range of air pressures and temperatures

formaldehyde (CH$_2$O)
a water-soluble gas used in aqueous solutions in hundreds of consumer products

carcinogens
agents, usually chemicals, that cause cancer

radon
a naturally occurring colorless, tasteless, odorless, radioactive gas formed during the radioactive decay of uranium-238

environmental tobacco smoke
tobacco smoke in the environment that can be inhaled by nonsmokers

secondhand smoke
environmental tobacco smoke

mainstream smoke
tobacco smoke inhaled and exhaled by the smoker

sidestream tobacco smoke
tobacco smoke that comes off the end of burning tobacco products

with their concentration and the length of exposure. Acute symptoms include irritation of the eyes and respiratory tract, headaches, dizziness, and memory impairment. Some of these chemicals are either known or suspected carcinogens. In any one building, one might find hundreds of different VOCs. Sources of VOCs include construction materials (e.g., insulation and paint), structural components (e.g., vinyl tile and sheet rock), furnishings (e.g., drapes and upholstery fabric), cleansers and solvents (e.g., liquid detergent and furniture polish), personal care products (e.g., deodorant and eyeliner pencils), insecticides/pesticides, electrical equipment (e.g., computers and VCRs), and combustion of wood and kerosene.[5] **Formaldehyde**, a pungent water-soluble gas, is one of the most ubiquitous VOCs. It is a widely used chemical that can be found in hundreds of products. Exposure occurs when it evaporates from wood products such as plywood and particle board, in which it is a component of the glue that binds these products together. Formaldehyde can also be found in products such as grocery bags, wallpaper, carpet, insulation, wall paneling, and wallboard.[5] Exposure to formaldehyde can cause watery eyes, burning in the eyes and throat, and difficulty in breathing. It can precipitate asthma attacks in susceptible people. Formaldehyde may also be a **carcinogen**, a cancer-causing agent. So, how can people protect their families and themselves? When building or renovating a residence, use exterior-grade products that emit less formaldehyde. Increase ventilation in the home, use a dehumidifier and air conditioning to control humidity, and keep temperature at moderate levels in the home to reduce formaldehyde emissions.

Radon is the number 1 cause of lung cancer among nonsmokers and the second leading cause of lung cancer overall. This radioactive gas, which cannot be seen, smelled, or tasted, is responsible for about 21,000 lung cancer deaths every year.[6] It is a naturally occurring gas that seeps into a home from surrounding soil, rocks, and water and through openings such as cracks, drains, and sump pumps. However, exposure to radon is preventable, and homeowners can do something about it. Every home and office building should be tested for radon, and homeowners can administer this inexpensive and easy test. More homes with operating radon mitigation systems is one of the *Healthy People 2020* objectives (see Box 14.1).

Environmental tobacco smoke (ETS), also known as **secondhand smoke**, includes both **mainstream smoke** (the smoke inhaled and exhaled by the smoker) and **sidestream tobacco smoke** (the smoke that comes off the end of a burning tobacco product). The involuntary inhalation of ETS by nonsmokers is referred to as **passive smoking**. Hundreds of toxic agents and more than 40 carcinogens are in secondhand smoke. A few of these harmful agents are CO, NO$_2$, carbon dioxide (CO$_2$), hydrogen cyanide, formaldehyde, nicotine, and suspended particles.[7]

Approximately 23.9% (59.8 million) of adult Americans 12 years of age or older were current cigarette smokers in 2008.[8] As a result, many nonsmokers are exposed to environmental tobacco smoke. ETS is classified as a known human (group A) carcinogen and causes approximately 3,000 lung cancer deaths annually in U.S. nonsmokers.[9]

The association between ETS and adverse health effects including cancer and heart disease has been demonstrated in a number of different epidemiological studies.[9-11] In addition, the studies show that about 50% of all American children 5 years of age and younger have been exposed to ETS from prenatal maternal smoking and/or sidestream smoke from household members after their birth. Such exposure has been shown to increase the risk of adverse prenatal consequences and postnatal health conditions in infants. Specifically, this exposure has been associated with intrauterine growth retardation, low birth weight, preterm delivery, respiratory tract infections, and behavioral and cognitive abnormalities.[11] Furthermore, young children are especially susceptible to secondhand smoke and are likely to suffer from coughing, wheezing, phlegm production, breathlessness, and an increased risk of developing asthma.

BOX
14.1

HEALTHY PEOPLE 2020: OBJECTIVES

Objective EH-14   Increase the number of homes with an operating radon mitigation system for persons in homes at risk for radon exposure.

Target setting method: Consistency with national programs/regulations/policies/laws

Data sources: Annual Report to EPA by radon vent fan manufacturers, EPA, Indoor Environments Division

Target and baseline:

Objective	2007 Baseline	2020 Target
EH-14 Increase the number of homes at risk (radon level of 4 Pico curies per liter of air (pCi/L or more) with an operating radon mitigation system	788,000 of 7.7 million homes (10.2%)	3.1 million of 9.2 million homes (30%)

For Further Thought

Have you tested your house for radon? What was the reading? What is the potential radon level in your area? Go to the EPA map of radon zones and search for the map of your state, where you can identify the potential by county.

Source: U.S. Department of Health and Human Services, Office of Disease Prevention and Health Promotion (2010). *Healthy People 2020.* Available at http://www.healthypeople.gov/2020/default.aspx. Accessed December 2, 2010.

Protecting Indoor Air

Because we spend 50% to 90% of our time indoors,[2] we need to take measures to protect the quality of our indoor air. The energy crisis of the 1970s led to a conservation movement that included reducing the ventilation rate. The accepted rate was reduced from 20 cubic feet per minute to 5 cubic feet per minute as a cost savings and energy savings measure. This reduced ventilation resulted in the creation of "tight buildings," known as "sick buildings," as reports of illness traced to such buildings increased.[12] **Sick building syndrome** refers to a situation in which the air quality in a building produces nonspecific signs and symptoms of ill health in the building occupants. Electronic controls and more efficient filtration, heating, and cooling systems have enabled the ventilation rate of 20 cubic feet per minute to be reinstated.

Even though indoor air pollution may be more harmful to human health than outdoor air pollution is, measures to monitor and correct indoor air pollution have been limited. The U.S. government has not yet established a framework for the development of indoor air policies as it has for outdoor air. It has, however, usually supported voluntary industry standards. For example, there are safety codes for kerosene space heaters, an "action guideline" for radon, and smoking restrictions for commercial airlines and an increasing number of public buildings. There also has been federal guidance on the handling of asbestos in schools and a prohibition on new uses of asbestos.

In the absence of a federal indoor clean air act, some states, counties, and municipalities have developed their own. In an attempt to protect workers and citizens from heart disease, cancer, and respiratory illness and to reduce forced inhalation through passive smoking, many U.S. counties and states, as well as countries around the world, have banned or are in the process of outlawing smoking in workplaces, sometimes including bars, restaurants, and casinos. In some areas, even outdoor smoking has been banned within a certain distance of exits and air intakes of public and state-owned building entrances. As of January 2010, 26 states and the District of Columbia have met the American Lung Association's "Smokefree Challenge" to pass comprehensive legislation prohibiting smoking in all public places and workplaces. Still,

passive smoking
the inhalation of environmental tobacco smoke by nonsmokers

sick building syndrome
a term to describe a situation in which the air quality in a building produces generalized signs and symptoms of ill health in the building's occupants

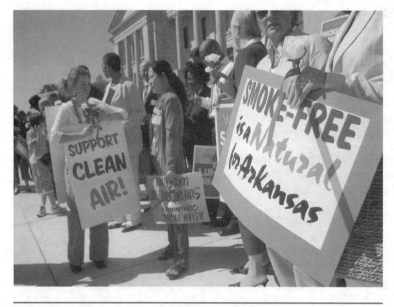

FIGURE 14.5

Nonsmokers' rights advocates sometimes take their campaign to their statehouse.

none of the states or the federal government receive an "A" grade for enacting strong and effective tobacco control laws.[13] The Web site of the American Lung Association includes a summary of the state of tobacco control in each state.

Efforts to pass comprehensive smoking ordinances often originate at the local level. However, some states still have preemptive laws that impede the passage and enforcement of stronger local tobacco control laws. One of the *Healthy People 2010* objectives was to eliminate state laws that preempt stronger local legislation. During the period of 2005–2009, preemptive smoking legislation was rescinded by legislation, ballot initiative, or court ruling in 7 more states, leaving 12 states ("the dirty dozen") with preemptive smoking legislation (see Figure 14.5).[14]

THE WATER WE USE

Clean, uncontaminated water is essential for life and health. In many regions of the world, such as parts of Asia and Africa, the scarcity of potable water limits development and challenges health. Furthermore, lack of basic **sanitation**, including the inability to properly treat wastewater, has immediate and dire health consequences. Consumption of polluted water can result in outbreaks of such waterborne diseases as cholera, typhoid fever, dysentery, and other gastrointestinal diseases. Worldwide, such diseases are responsible for 1.5 million deaths every year. Most of those affected are children in developing countries. In 2006, about two-fifths of the world's population had no access to improved sanitation and 1 billion people had no access to any sanitary facilities at all. One-seventh of the world's population had no access to a supply of clean drinking water.[15]

Here in the United States, virtually 100% of the population has access to both a clean water supply and sanitation; it is the highest reported rate for any world region.[16] Nonetheless, 28 waterborne disease outbreaks (WBDOs) linked to drinking water and 78 WBDOs associated with recreational use were reported in the most recent biennial Centers for Disease Control and Prevention (CDC) report.[17] A major source of drinking water contamination is wastes produced by humans through their daily activities. Thus, both the prevention of water pollution and treatment of polluted water are essential community activities.

Sources of Water

We acquire water for our domestic, industrial, and agricultural needs either from surface water or groundwater. Water in streams, rivers, lakes, and reservoirs is called **surface water**. The water that infiltrates into the soil is referred to as subsurface water or **groundwater**. Groundwater that is not absorbed by the roots of vegetation moves slowly downward until it reaches the zone of soil completely saturated with water, referred to as an aquifer. **Aquifers** are porous, water-saturated layers of underground bedrock, sand, and gravel that can yield economically significant amounts of water.[1]

sanitation
the practice of establishing and maintaining healthy or hygienic conditions in the environment

surface water
precipitation that does not infiltrate the ground or return to the atmosphere by evaporation; the water in streams, rivers, and lakes

groundwater
water located under the surface of the ground

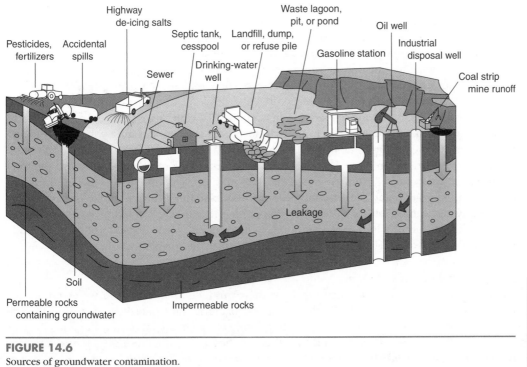

FIGURE 14.6
Sources of groundwater contamination.
Source: U.S. Environmental Protection Agency.

The earth's supply of freshwater available for our use is limited. Only 0.003% of the earth's water is available for use by humans, and much of this is hard to reach and too costly to be of practical value.[2] Thus, the continual contamination of our groundwater through the improper disposal of human waste, trash, and solid and hazardous waste should be of paramount concern to everyone.

Sources of Water Pollution

Water pollution includes any physical or chemical change in water that can harm living organisms or make it unfit for other uses, such as drinking, domestic use, recreation, fishing, industry, agriculture, or transportation.[1] The sources of water pollution fall into two categories—point sources and nonpoint sources (see Figure 14.6).[3] **Point source pollution** refers to a single identifiable source that discharges pollutants into the water, such as a pipe, ditch, or culvert. Examples of such pollutants might include release of pollutants from a factory or sewage treatment plant. Point sources of pollution are relatively easy to identify, control, and treat.

   Nonpoint source pollution includes all pollution that occurs through the runoff, seepage, or falling of pollutants into the water. Examples include the runoff of water from cities, highways, and farms resulting from rain events (called stormwater runoff), seepage of leachates from landfills, and acid rain. Nonpoint source pollution is a greater problem than point source pollution is because it is often difficult to track the actual source of pollution and, therefore, to control it.

Types of Water Pollutants

Water pollutants can be classified as biological or nonbiological. Biological pollutants include pathogens such as parasites, bacteria, viruses, and other undesirable living microorganisms. These pathogens enter the water mainly through human and other animal wastes that were

aquifers
porous, water-saturated layers of underground bedrock, sand, and gravel that can yield economically significant amounts of water

water pollution
any physical or chemical change in water that can harm living organisms or make the water unfit for other uses

point source pollution
pollution that can be traced to a single identifiable source

nonpoint source pollution
all pollution that occurs through the runoff, seepage, or falling of pollutants into the water

runoff
water that flows over land surfaces (including paved surfaces), typically from precipitation

disposed of improperly or without being treated before their disposal. Sources of such contamination include **runoff** from animal farms that contain manure; failed septic systems that leach untreated or only partially treated human fecal waste to groundwater and surface water; combined sewer overflow that discharges a mix of untreated stormwater and human sewage to rivers or streams; and stormwater runoff from our cities, highways, and towns that carries animal and human fecal waste left on land surfaces. These biological wastes spread viruses, bacteria, and parasites into rivers, lakes, reservoirs, and drinking water supplies, where they can cause human illness. For example, people can become ill by drinking water from a groundwater well contaminated with fecal waste from a septic system or from ingesting water while swimming in a lake or reservoir contaminated by runoff from surrounding cities or farms. Although many sanitary districts across the United States are implementing new plans to capture and treat urban stormwater runoff from their streets, it is not yet a common practice. Because of increased urbanization and the growing proportion of land that is covered by impervious concrete, rainwater cannot infiltrate the land surface and is therefore collected by storm and sewer lines and often dumped into rivers without any treatment. Nonbiological pollutants include chemicals, radioactive materials, and heat especially from energy plant cooling towers.

Biological Pollutants of Water

Biological pollutants are living organisms or their products that make the water unsafe for human consumption. Examples include viruses, bacteria, and parasites. Waterborne viral agents and the diseases they cause include poliomyelitis virus (polio) and hepatitis A virus (hepatitis). Waterborne bacteria and the diseases they cause include *Escherichia coli* (gastroenteritis), *Legionella* spp. (legionellosis), *Salmonella typhi* (typhoid fever), *Shigella* spp. (shigellosis or bacillary dysentery), and *Vibrio cholerae* (cholera). Waterborne parasites include *Entamoeba histolytica* (amebiasis or amebic dysentery), *Giardia lamblia* (giardiasis), and *Cryptosporidium parvum* (cryptosporidiosis) (see Table 14.2). Each of these diseases can be serious, and two in particular—typhoid fever and cholera—have killed thousands of people in single epidemics.

waterborne disease outbreak (WBDO)
a disease in which at least two persons experience a similar illness after the ingestion of drinking water or after exposure to water used for recreational purposes and epidemiological evidence implicates water as the probable source of the illness

A **waterborne disease outbreak (WBDO)** is a water exposure in which at least two persons have been epidemiologically linked to recreational or drinking water by location, time, and illness. In the case of a recreational exposure, two or more persons must experience a similar illness after ingestion of drinking water or after exposure to water used for recreational purposes and epidemiological evidence must implicate water as the probable source of the illness.[17]

In recent years, the number of WBDOs associated with drinking water has declined, while the number of those associated with recreational exposure has increased (see Figure 14.7). The Centers for Disease Control and Prevention issues biennial surveillance summaries based on WBDOs reported to the Waterborne Disease and Outbreak Surveillance System (WBDOSS). In the most recent biennial report, 78 WBDOs associated with recreational water were reported from 31 states. These resulted in 4,412 illnesses, 116 hospitalizations, and 5 deaths.[17] Three-fourths of these outbreaks were traced to exposure to treated water venues (swimming pools, wading pools, spas, etc.); one-fourth were associated with untreated water (springs, rivers, reservoirs). In about 60% of the outbreaks, the illnesses were described as acute gastroenteritis illnesses (AGIs), 14% as skin disorders, and 14% as acute respiratory illnesses (ARIs). The remaining outbreaks were described as mixed. The WBDOs associated with gastroenteritis accounted for 4,015 (91%) of the cases of illness. The leading cause WBDO associated with recreational water was parasites (43.6%), followed by bacteria (28.2%), viruses (5.1%), and chemicals/toxins (2.6%) (see Table 14.2).[17]

The 28 WBDOs associated with drinking water were reported from 14 states. Of these, 20 were associated with drinking water, 6 were associated with water not intended for

Table 14.2
Leading Causes of Waterborne Disease Outbreaks—United States, 2005–2006

Predominant Cause of Illness	No. of Outbreaks (%)	No. of Cases (%)
Bacteria	22 (28.2)	255 (5.8)
Legionella sp.	8	124
Shigella sonnei	4	41
Pseudomonas aeruginosa	4	28
Escherichia coli	3	10
Leptospira spp.	2	46
Parasites	34 (43.6)	3,819 (86.6)
Cryptosporidium spp.	31	3,751
Giardia intestinalis	1	11
Naegleria fowleri	1	2
Cryptosporidium/Giardia spp.	1	55
Viruses	4 (5.1)	86 (1.9)
Norovirus	4	86
Chemicals/Toxins	2 (2.6)	22 (0.5)
Copper sulfate	1	3
Chlorine gas	1	19
Suspected/Unidentified	16 (20.5)	230 (5.2)
Total	78 (100)	4,412 (100)

Source: Centers for Disease Control and Prevention (2008). "Surveillance for Waterborne Disease and Outbreaks Associated with Recreational Water Use and other Aquatic Facility-Associated Health Events—United States, 2005–2006" and "Surveillance for Waterborne Disease and Outbreaks Associated with Drinking Water and Water Not Intended for Drinking—United States, 2005–2006." *Surveillance Summaries, Morbidity and Mortality Weekly Report,* 57(No. SS-9).

drinking, and 2 were associated with water of unknown intent. The 20 WBDOs associated with water intended for drinking caused illness in at least 612 people and resulted in 4 deaths. About half of the outbreaks resulted in ARI, slightly less than half resulted in AGI, and one outbreak resulted in hepatitis. In those outbreaks where the etiological agent was determined, the leading cause was bacteria (67%), followed by viruses (17%), parasites (11%), and mixed (6%). In all of the ARI outbreaks, the disease agent was the bacteria *Legionella*. This was the first time since record keeping began that ARI outbreaks outnumbered AGI outbreaks in drinking water-associated outbreaks.

Waterborne disease outbreaks can usually be traced to a source either within or outside of the jurisdiction of a water utility. During 2005–2006, 43.5% of WBDOs associated with drinking water were traced to water utilities, while 52.2% were determined not to be under jurisdiction of a utility. The source of one outbreak was undetermined. Outbreaks associated with municipal water systems can become quite large. The largest WBDO ever reported in the United States occurred in Milwaukee, Wisconsin, in 1993. In that outbreak, 403,000 people became ill and 4,400 were hospitalized. The disease agent was identified as the parasite *Cryptosporidium parvum*. This outbreak occurred because of a breakdown in the city's water treatment plant.[18] Public health laws that set standards for drinking water and for treated recreational water are a community's first line of defense against WBDOs. Although WBDOs occur from time to time in the United States, they occur much less frequently than they do in countries with developing economies, where access to safe drinking water and sanitation is limited or nonexistent.

Nonbiological Pollutants of Water

Nonbiological pollutants include heat; inorganic chemicals such as lead, copper, and arsenic; organic chemicals; and radioactive pollutants. Among the organic chemicals are industrial solvents such as trichloroethylene (TCE); pesticides such as dichlorodiphenyltrichloroethane (DDT) and Atrazine, a commonly used herbicide applied to crops in the spring; and

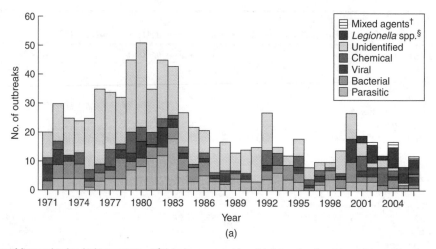

*Single cases of disease related to drinking water (*n* = 16) have been removed from this figure; therefore, it is not comparable to figures in previous *Surveillance Summaries*.
†Beginning in 2003, mixed agents of more than one etiologic agent type were included in the surveillance system. However, the first observation is a previously unreported outbreak in 2002.
§Beginning in 2001, Legionnaires' disesase was added to the survelliance system, and *Legionella* species were classified separately in this figure.

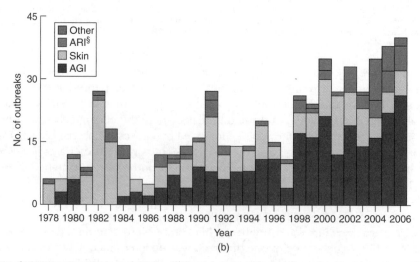

*Single cases of primary amegic meningoencephalitis (*n* = 16) have been removed from this figure; therefore, it is not comparable to figures in previous *Surveillance Summaries*.
†AGI: acute gastrointestinal illness; Skin: illness, condition, or symptom related to skin; ARI: acture respiratory illness; Other: includes keratitis, conjunctivitis, otitis, bronchitis, menigitis, meningoencephalitis, hepatitis, leptospirosis, and combined illnesses.
§All outbreaks of legionellosis (i.e., Legionnaires' diesease and Pontiac fever) are classified as ARI.

FIGURE 14.7

(a) Number of waterborne-disease outbreaks associated with drinking water (n = 814), by year and etiologic agent—United States, 1971–2006. (b) Number of recreational water-associated outbreaks (n = 557), by year and illness—United States, 1978–2006.

Source: Centers for Disease Control and Prevention (2008). "Surveillance for Waterborne Disease and Outbreaks Associated with Recreational Water Use and Other Aquatic Facility–Associated Health Events—United States, 2005–2006" and "Surveillance for Waterborne Disease and Outbreaks Associated with Drinking Water and Water Not Intended for Drinking—United States, 2005–2006." *Surveillance Summaries, Morbidity and Mortality Weekly Report*, 57 (No. SS-9).

---

the insulating chemicals used in transformers and electrical capacitors, such as the polychlorinated biphenyls (PCBs); and dioxin (TCDD), a substance that is a by-product of the incineration of paper products and chlorinated plastics.

Historically, governmental regulation of chemical pollutants has targeted those chemicals discharged by industries and municipal sewage treatment facilities. These pollutants, present in high concentrations and known to be detrimental to human health, are relatively easy to identify. Within the past decade, however, two new types of pollutants have been detected in our waterways and are raising health concerns. These are **endocrine-disrupting chemicals (EDCs)** and **pharmaceuticals and personal care products (PPCPs)**. Endocrine disruptors include pesticides, commercial chemicals, and environmental contaminants that can disrupt, imitate, or block the body's normal hormonal activity, causing developmental or reproductive problems. Evidence for this has been found in certain species of fish and wildlife. Thus far, the relationship between EDCs and human diseases of the endocrine system is poorly understood and remains scientifically controversial.[19] Currently, the EPA Endocrine Disruption Screening Program is evaluating about 87,000 chemicals to try to determine whether they pose a risk to the human endocrine system.

PPCPs are synthetic chemicals found in everyday consumer health care products and cosmetics. These products include prescription and over-the-counter drugs; cosmetics, including soaps and shampoos; fragrances; sunscreens; diagnostic agents; biopharmaceuticals; and many others. PPCPs have been detected in water supplies around the world, and their effects on human health are the subject of scientific investigations. How do PPCPs get into our water sources? They are flushed down our toilets and washed down our drains and transported to our wastewater treatment plants, where they are discharged, mostly unchanged, into our rivers and streams. The risks posed by PPCPs to humans, aquatic life, and wildlife are essentially unknown. The exception is the increase in resistance of some pathogenic bacteria to antibiotics.[20]

While the EPA and other researchers are working to assess the effects of EDCs and PPCPs, there are no governmental regulations or guidance for the disposal of pharmaceuticals meant for personal use. Because it is important to take some personal action to reduce their presence in our environment, we should dispose of unused or unwanted medication in an environmentally sound manner. Disposal into the domestic sewage system is the least desirable option. Two better alternatives are (1) contacting a local pharmacy to see if it takes expired or unwanted medicines, or (2) turning them in to a local hazardous waste collector. If neither of these options is available, disposal in household trash is a better alternative than disposal in the sewage system.[20]

Water quality in the United States has deteriorated in many communities. This deterioration can be attributed to four causes: (1) population growth, (2) chemical manufacturing, (3) reckless land use practices, and (4) mismanagement and irresponsible disposal of hazardous wastes.[21] As the public's knowledge of the endangerment of water quality in the United States grows, it is hoped that greater efforts will be made to protect our water.

endocrine-disrupting chemical (EDC) a chemical that interferes in some way with the body's endocrine (hormone) system

pharmaceuticals and personal care products (PPCPs) synthetic chemicals found in everyday consumer health care products and cosmetics

Ensuring the Safety of Our Water

Ensuring the safety of our water in the United States involves the proper treatment of water intended for drinking and a properly maintained distribution system for that water. It also requires proper construction and maintenance of water-associated recreation facilities. Safe water also depends on the enactment and enforcement of well-conceived water quality regulations. Finally, wastewater treatment and sanitation are required.

Treatment of Water for Domestic Use

Water in the United States is used for many purposes, including agriculture, industry, energy generation, and domestic use. Domestic water use in the United States includes water for drinking, cooking, washing dishes and laundry, bathing, flushing toilets, and outdoor use (such as watering lawns and gardens and washing cars). While domestic use makes up only 6% of the total water usage in the United States, each U.S. resident uses an average of 80–100 gallons of water each day, just by flushing the toilet, showering, washing laundry, and other domestic uses.[22,23]

Whereas many rural residents in the United States obtain their water from untreated private wells (groundwater), urban residents usually obtain their water from municipal water treatment plants. About two-thirds of the municipalities use surface water, while one-third uses groundwater.

Virtually all surface water is polluted and needs to be treated before it can be safely consumed. The steps in the treatment of water for domestic use vary, but usually include removing solids through coagulation, flocculation, and filtration. This is followed by disinfection, during which chlorine (or sometimes ozone) is added to the water to kill remaining viruses, bacteria, algae, and fungi. Disinfection is sometimes accompanied by fluoridation, which helps prevent dental decay.

Fluoridation of community drinking water is a major factor responsible for the decline in dental caries (tooth decay) in the United States since 1950 (see Box 14.2). At first, caries reduction rates of 50% to 70% were reported. More recently, the reduction among adolescents has averaged 25%. Because fluoride has appeared in other products, such as toothpaste and mouthwashes, the difference in rates of caries between those who receive fluoridated water and those who do not has declined. By 1992, 144 million people were receiving fluoridated water, at an average cost of 31 cents per person per year. The savings from prevention of dental caries attributable to fluoridation was estimated for the period 1979–1989 at $39 billion (1990 dollars), a savings per person that in some communities reached $53 per person per year.[24]

The responsibility of municipal water treatment plants is to provide water that is chemically and bacteriologically safe for human consumption. It is also desirable that the water be aesthetically pleasing in regard to taste, odor, color, and clarity. Above all, the municipal

---

BOX 14.2   TEN GREAT PUBLIC HEALTH ACHIEVEMENTS, 1900–1999: FLUORIDATION OF DRINKING WATER

From Toothless Grins to Pearly Whites

At the beginning of the twentieth century, tooth decay was rampant, and because no effective preventive measures existed, tooth extraction was routine. Now, thanks to water fluoridation, combined with other dental health advances, adults in the United States are retaining most of their teeth throughout their lifetime.

In 1901, soon after establishing his dental practice in Colorado Springs, Colorado, Dr. Frederick S. McKay noted an unusual permanent brown stain on the teeth of many of his patients. He concluded that something in the public water supply was probably responsible. McKay also observed that teeth affected by this condition seemed to be less susceptible to dental caries.

In 1931, Dr. H. Trendley Dean, a U.S. Public Health Service Dental Officer, conducted pioneering research into the relationship between fluoride and dental caries. His research laid the groundwork for community water fluoridation in the United States.

In 1945, Grand Rapids, Michigan, became the first city in the world to fluoridate its drinking water. The caries rate among Grand Rapids children born after fluoride was added to the water supply dropped 60%. This finding revolutionized dental care and resulted in tooth decay being preventable for most people.

Water fluoridation is relatively inexpensive in the United States. The benefits of fluoridation are available, on average, for little more than $0.50 per person per year, and even less in large communities.

The documented effectiveness of community water fluoridation in preventing dental caries prompted rapid adoption of this public health measure in cities throughout the United States. In the 1960s, the U.S. Public Health Service provided funding, technical expertise, and leadership to promote and establish fluoridation programs throughout the nation. The federal government continues to promote water fluoridation worldwide.

Source: Centers for Disease Control and Prevention (1999). "Ten Great Public Health Achievements—United States, 1900-1999." *Morbidity and Mortality Weekly Report* 48(12): 241–242. Available at www.cdc.gov/mmwr/PDF/wk/mm4812.pdf. Accessed October 26, 2010.

water supply must be reliable. Reliability in regard to both quantity and quality has always been regarded as nonnegotiable in planning a treatment facility.

Wastewater Treatment

Wastewater is the substance that remains after humans have used water for domestic or commercial purposes. Such water, also referred to as liquid waste or sewage, consists of about 99.9% water and 0.1% suspended and dissolved solids. The solids consist of human feces, soap, paper, garbage grindings (food parts), and a variety of other items that are put into wastewater systems from homes, schools, commercial buildings, hotels/motels, hospitals, industrial plants, and other facilities connected to the sanitary sewer system. The primary purpose of **wastewater treatment** is to improve the quality of wastewater to the point that it might be released into a body of water without seriously disrupting the aquatic environment, causing health problems in humans in the form of waterborne disease, or causing nuisance conditions. Most municipalities and many large companies have wastewater treatment plants that incorporate at least primary and secondary treatment processes (see Figure 14.8).

Primary Wastewater Treatment

Primary wastewater treatment occurs in a sedimentation tank, also called a clarifier, where wastewater remains in a quiescent condition for about 2 to 4 hours. Here, heavier solid particles settle to the bottom, forming a layer referred to as **sludge**. Sludge is a gooey, semisolid mixture that includes bacteria, viruses, organic matter, toxic metals, synthetic organic chemicals, and solids.[1] Above the sludge remains most of the wastewater, including many bacteria and chemicals. On top of this aqueous layer is a layer of oils and fats, also called scum. The layers of sludge and scum are removed, and the clarified wastewater enters the secondary stage of treatment.

Secondary Wastewater Treatment

During secondary treatment, aerobic bacteria are added and mixed with clarified wastewater to break down the organic waste; this mixture then flows to aeration tanks. Here, oxygen is continuously added to support aerobic decomposition of organic waste into carbon dioxide, water, and minerals. When this biological process is completed (after about 6 to 10 hours), the wastewater is sent to sedimentation tanks, where solids and flocks of bacteria are separated from the treated liquid portion of wastewater in quiescent conditions. After this process, many treatment plants disinfect and discharge the treated wastewater to surface water bodies while other wastewater plants perform tertiary treatment.

Tertiary Wastewater Treatment

Tertiary wastewater treatment involves filtration through sand and carbon filters. During this process, many remaining dissolved pollutants are removed. The treated water is finally disinfected and discharged. The least expensive way of disinfecting wastewater is to chlorinate it. After chlorination is completed, chlorine is removed from the water through a process called dechlorination to prevent poisoning of aquatic life in streams or rivers downstream of the discharge point. Discharges of treated wastewater are regulated by the EPA.

wastewater
the aqueous mixture that remains after water has been used or contaminated by humans

wastewater treatment
the process of improving the quality of wastewater (sewage) to the point that it can be released into a body of water without seriously disrupting the aquatic environment, causing health problems in humans, or causing nuisance conditions

sludge
a semiliquid mixture of solid waste that includes bacteria, viruses, organic matter, toxic metals, synthetic organic chemicals, and solid chemicals

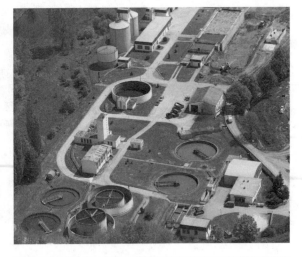

FIGURE 14.8
A wastewater treatment facility.

Septic Systems

Those who live in unsewered areas (25% of Americans) dispose of their wastewater using a septic system. A septic system consists of two major components—a septic tank and a buried sand filter or absorption field (see Figure 14.9). The **septic tank**, which is a watertight concrete or fiberglass tank, is buried in the ground some distance from the house and is connected to it by a pipe. Sewage leaves the home via the toilets or drains and goes through the pipe to the septic tank. The wastewater is retained in quiescent conditions for 1 to 2 days, during which separation of heavier solids and lighter scum from liquid wastewater occurs in the process called sedimentation. The liquid portion of wastewater is then carried by a pipe to an **absorption field**, a system of trenches (dugout channels) where perforated pipes are surrounded by gravel. As wastewater trickles through the gravel, films of aerobic microorganisms develop and feed on this liquid wastewater, causing decomposition of organic waste. This treated wastewater then infiltrates through the soil profile into the groundwater.

Clearly, proper installation and regular maintenance of the septic system are absolutely crucial for its optimal performance. Septic systems cannot be legally installed in most communities without a permit. Local health departments are responsible for issuing permits,

septic tank
a watertight concrete or fiberglass tank that holds sewage; one of two main parts of a septic system

absorption field
the element of a septic system in which the liquid portion of waste is distributed

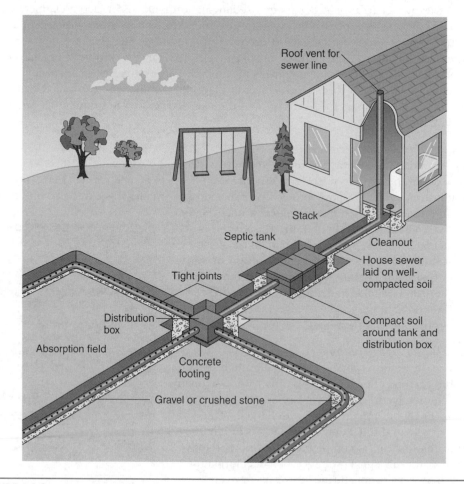

FIGURE 14.9

A septic system consists of a septic tank and an absorption field. This system is commonly used to treat domestic wastewater in suburban and rural areas.

inspecting the systems, and enforcing state and local regulations regarding them. The system must be (1) located in appropriate soil, (2) properly constructed and inspected prior to being buried, and (3) maintained regularly. Septic tanks need to be pumped out every 3 to 5 years to remove sludge and thus prevent overflow, sewage backup to the house, or failure of the absorption field. Failure to properly maintain the system can result in fecal contamination of both land and water sources. Improperly functioning or overflowing septic systems also provide optimal breeding sites for disease-transmitting mosquitoes such as the northern house mosquito, *Culex pipiens* (see Figure 14.10).

Regulating Water Quality

Surface water and drinking water are regulated by two important laws, the Clean Water Act and the Safe Drinking Water Act. Growing public concern over the pollution of surface water sources, such as rivers, lakes, estuaries, coastal waters, and wetlands, led to enactment of the Federal Water Pollution Control Act Amendments of 1972 and 1977, when this law became commonly known as the **Clean Water Act (CWA)**. The goal of the CWA is to restore and maintain the chemical, physical, and biological integrity of the waters in the United States so that they can support "the protection and propagation of fish, shellfish, and wildlife and recreation in and on the water."[25] In other words, the goal is to return the quality of surface waters to swimmable and fishable status. To achieve this goal, the EPA employs various regulatory and nonregulatory programs to reduce direct pollutant discharges into waterways by industrial and wastewater treatment facilities. In addition, the agency attempts to manage polluted runoff by implementing nonregulatory programs.

In the early years of the CWA's implementation, the agency's efforts focused on regulating discharges from traditional point source facilities, such as municipal sewage plants and industrial facilities. The CWA made it unlawful for any person to discharge any pollutant from a point source into navigable waters without a permit. Not much attention was paid to nonpoint source pollution from urban, agricultural, and stormwater runoff. However, since the late 1980s, the EPA has significantly increased its efforts to address polluted nonpoint source runoff and implemented either voluntary or regulatory programs to curb this problem. In its efforts to reduce and manage water pollution, the EPA considers land use and sources of pollution within the entire **watershed** rather than controlling and regulating only individual pollution sources or contaminants. The watershed approach emphasizes protecting healthy waters and restoring impaired ones to protect not only human but also environmental health.

The quality of drinking water is regulated by the **Safe Drinking Water Act (SDWA)** and its amendments. The SDWA implements many actions to protect drinking water and its sources (rivers, lakes, reservoirs, springs, and groundwater). Under the SDWA, the EPA sets national standards to limit the levels of contaminants in drinking water and oversees the states, localities, and water suppliers who implement those standards. The national standard for each contaminant is set at the level allowed in drinking water to protect public health; this standard is known as the maximum contaminant level (MCL). Currently, 87 MCLs are implemented and enforced. The list of contaminants includes organic and inorganic chemicals, microbiological agents, disinfectants, and radionuclides.[26] The SDWA requires the EPA to go through a long and intensive process to identify new contaminants that may require regulation in the future. The EPA must periodically release a list of unregulated contaminants—the Contaminant Candidate List—to prioritize research and data collection that would

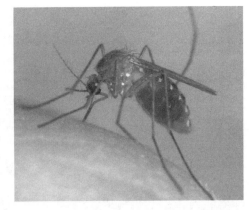

FIGURE 14.10
The northern house mosquito (*Culex pipiens*) is the most important vector of St. Louis encephalitis and West Nile viruses in the eastern United States.

Clean Water Act (CWA) the federal law aimed at ensuring that all rivers are swimmable and fishable and that limits the discharge of pollutants in U.S. waters to zero

watershed the area of land from which all of the water that is under it or drains from it goes into the same place and drains in one point; for example, the Mississippi River watershed drains and collects all the water from the land extending from east of the Rocky Mountains to the Appalachian Mountains and from the upper Midwest all the way south to the Gulf of Mexico

Safe Drinking Water Act (SDWA) the federal law that regulates the safety of public drinking water

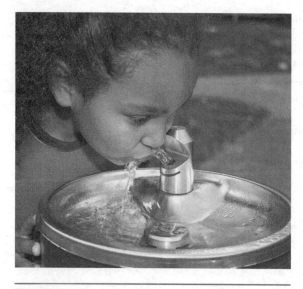

FIGURE 14.11

In the United States, virtually 100% of the population has access to clean, safe drinking water.

help determine whether it should regulate a specific contaminant. The 2009 list included 104 chemicals and 12 microbiological agents.[27]

Environmentalists and others would like to see the provisions of the SDWA strengthened and more vigorously enforced, but others point to the high administrative and enforcement costs of this act and the cost burden it places on municipal and privately owned water supply systems as reasons not to strengthen the provisions. Meanwhile, the quality and safety of our drinking water remain the envy of the world (see Figure 14.11).

THE FOOD WE EAT

One way in which humans interact with their environment is by ingesting bits of it, which we call food. In a worldwide comparison, the U.S. food supply probably ranks as one of the safest. The safety of our food supply is a result of public health efforts and regulatory actions during the past century. In fact, safer and healthier foods in the United States have been designated one of the 10 greatest achievements in public health in the twentieth century (see Box 14.3).[28]

Unfortunately, additional progress must be made before we completely eliminate foodborne disease. "More than 200 known diseases are transmitted through food. In these cases, food is the vehicle; and the agents can be viruses, bacteria, parasites toxins, metals, and prions."[28] Healthy food can become contaminated at several points between the farm or factory and the consumer. When this happens a foodborne disease outbreak can occur.

Foodborne Disease Outbreaks

Symptoms of foodborne illness range from mild to severe, and organs involved can include stomach and intestines, liver, kidneys, and brain and nervous system. Foodborne diseases cause between 6 million and 81 million cases of illness and up to 9,000 deaths each year in the United States.[29] A majority of these cases are never reported to the CDC. A recent report estimated the annual economic cost of foodborne illness in the United States at $152 billion.[30]

The CDC defines a **foodborne disease outbreak (FBDO)** as the occurrence of two or more cases of a similar illness resulting from the ingestion of a common food.[31] During the most recent year for which data are available, 1,270 FBDOs were reported from 48 states, resulting in 27,634 cases and 11 deaths. The cause was confirmed in 624 (49%) of the outbreaks. The leading causes of foodborne illness, including the number of outbreaks and cases, appear in Table 14.3. Of these, norovirus was the most common cause, accounting for 54% of the outbreaks and 11,879 cases, followed by *Salmonella* (18% of outbreaks and 3,252 cases). Among the 11 reported deaths, 10 were attributed to bacterial agents (six *Escherichia coli* O157:H7, two *Listeria monocytogenes*, one *Salmonella* serotype Enteritidis, and one *Clostridium botulinum*) and 1 to mushroom toxin. Common food vehicles were poultry (21%), leafy vegetables (17%), and fruits/nuts (16%).[31]

Leading factors that contributed to FBDOs were inadequate cooking temperatures or improper holding temperatures for foods (especially for bacterial outbreaks); unsanitary conditions or practices at the point of service, such as failure to wash hands (norovirus outbreaks); or drinking raw milk (bacterial outbreaks).[31] Other factors that often contribute to

foodborne disease outbreak (FBDO) the occurrence of two or more cases of a similar illness resulting from the ingestion of food

---

BOX 14.3   TEN GREAT PUBLIC HEALTH ACHIEVEMENTS, 1900–1999: SAFER AND HEALTHIER FOODS

Food for Thought

Early in the twentieth century, contaminated food, milk, and water were responsible for many foodborne diseases, including typhoid fever, tuberculosis, botulism, and scarlet fever. In the first half of the century, scientific discoveries and public health policies, such as food fortification programs, led to large reductions in diseases caused by nutritional deficiency. More recently, the focus of many public health nutrition programs shifted to the prevention and control of chronic disease, such as cardiovascular disease and obesity, through nutrition.

After the characteristics and sources of foodborne diseases were identified, public health professionals began advocating control of those diseases through technology and safer food-handling procedures, including:

- Hand washing
- Better sanitation
- Refrigeration
- Pasteurization
- Pesticide application
- Reduction of foodborne pathogens

- Better animal care and feeding
- Safer food processing

Prompt refrigeration inhibits bacterial growth, thus reducing the risk for disease.

One notable discovery that reduced disease was the process invented by Louis Pasteur—pasteurization.

New foodborne pathogens have emerged in the United States during the past 20 years as a result of changes in agricultural practices and in food-processing operations and the globalization of the food supply. Seemingly healthy food animals can be reservoirs for human pathogens.

Pesticides have played an important role in increasing crop yields, decreasing food costs, and enhancing the appearance of food. However, without proper controls, the residues of some pesticides remaining on foods also create potential health risks.

Source: Centers for Disease Control and Prevention (1999). "Ten Great Public Health Achievements—United States, 1900-1999." *Morbidity and Mortality Weekly Report,* 48(12): 241-242. Available at www.cdc.gov/mmwr/PDF/wk/mm4812.pdf. Accessed October 26, 2010.

FBDOs are contaminated equipment or obtaining food from an unsafe source (such as shellfish from polluted waters).

To protect the public from foodborne diseases requires the coordinated efforts of federal, state, and local health agencies. At the federal level, the CDC, under its Emerging Infections Program, has established the Foodborne Diseases Active Surveillance Network (FoodNet) to provide better data on foodborne diseases. FoodNet tracks diseases caused by enteric pathogens transmitted through foods. The CDC coordinates these surveillance activities with officials from the U.S. Department of Agriculture's Food Safety and Inspection Service, the Food and Drug Administration's Center for Food Safety and Applied Nutrition, and respective state epidemiologists. Data were collected from a combined surveillance population of 44.9 million people (15% of the U.S. population) in 10 states.[32] Among the vehicles associated with outbreaks were bagged fresh spinach, lettuce, and tomatoes. Ground beef was also a source of infection, particularly of *E. coli* O157:H7 bacteria. One set of the *Healthy People 2020* objectives aims to reduce the number of outbreak-associated infections due to foodborne disease agents (see Box 14.4).

Growing, Processing, and Distributing Our Food Safely

In spite of the surveillance efforts described earlier, much remains to be done to ensure the safety of our food supply. Greater efforts need to be made to make sure our plants and animals are free from harmful biological and chemical agents during growing, harvesting, and processing of food products before they reach retail outlets and food service establishments.

Historically, our food was supplied by independent farmers whose field crops or livestock reached the marketplace relatively free from modern chemicals. Over the past century,

Table 14.3
Leading Causes of Reported Foodborne Disease Outbreaks—United States, 2006

Predominant Cause of Illness (Confirmed and Suspected)	No. of Outbreaks (%)		No. of Cases (%)	
Bacteria	**295**	**(23)**	**7,241**	**(26)**
Salmonella sp.	117		3,296	
Clostridium perfingens	34		1,880	
Staphylococcus enterotoxin	29		428	
Escherichia coli, shiga toxin	29		592	
Campylobacter	25		301	
Bacillus cereus	13		72	
Shigella	10		185	
Other bacteria	38		137	
Chemical	**66**	**(5)**	**267**	**(1)**
Scombroid toxin/histamine	32		113	
Ciguatoxin	10		45	
Mushroom toxins	4		16	
Cleaning agents	2		4	
Neurotoxic shellfish poison	2		15	
Plant toxins (herbal toxins)	1		15	
Other chemicals	15		59	
Parasites	**12**	**(1)**	**147**	**(1)**
Cryptosporidium spp.	4		30	
Cyclospora	3		37	
Giardia	2		60	
Trichinella	1		2	
Other parasites	1		18	
Viruses	**511**	**(40)**	**14,855**	**(54)**
Calicivirus (Norovirus)	505		14,753	
Hepatitis A	5		50	
Other viruses	1		52	
Unknown	**363**	**(29)**	**4,330**	**(16)**
Multiple causes	**23**	**(2)**	**794**	**(3)**
Total	**1,270**	**(100)**	**27,634**	**(100)**

Source: Centers for Disease Control and Prevention (2009). Surveillance for Foodborne Disease Outbreaks—United States, 2006. Morbidity and Mortality Weekly Report 58(22): 609–615.

farming has increasingly become "big business" with more and more farmland owned by large corporations. Modern agriculture in the United States has been characterized as the process of converting petroleum into food. Although this seems like an extreme statement, it contains elements of truth. On the modern industrial farm, significant amounts of fuel are required to run the tractors, combines, and other equipment. Tractors are used to apply petroleum-based chemical fertilizers, herbicides, and insecticides, usually from plastic tanks made from petroleum. It is hard to imagine a modern farm operation without these petroleum-based materials.

Two health concerns with the ubiquitous nature of agricultural chemicals, especially pesticides, are (1) the risk of unintentional poisonings where these chemicals are stored and used, and (2) the residues reaching food workers and consumers.

Pesticides

The term **pest** refers to any organism (plant, animal, or microbe) that has an adverse effect on human interests. Some common examples are weeds in the vegetable garden, termites in the house, and mold on the shower curtain. **Pesticides** are natural or synthetic chemicals that have been developed and manufactured for the purpose of killing pests. There are currently

pest
any organism—a multicelled animal or plant, or a microbe—that has an adverse effect on human interests

pesticides
synthetic chemicals developed and manufactured for the purpose of killing pests

---

BOX 14.4	HEALTHY PEOPLE 2020: OBJECTIVES

Objective FS-2   Reduce the number of outbreak-associated infections due to Shiga toxin-producing *E. coli* O157, or *Campylobacter*, *Listeria*, or *Salmonella* species associated with food commodity groups

Target setting method: 10% improvement

Data sources: National Outbreak Reporting System (NORS), CDC, and States

Target and baseline:

Objective		2005–2007 Baseline	2020 Target
FS-2.1	Beef	200	180
FS-2.2	Dairy	786	707
FS-2.3	Fruits and nuts	311	280
FS-2.4	Leafy vegetables	205	185
FS-2.5	Poultry	258	232

For Further Thought

Are you aware of any foodborne outbreaks in your area? Outbreaks of *E. coli* O157:H7 have been associated with undercooked beef. How do you make sure that you are protecting yourself and your guests when you cook hamburgers at home? How do you make sure you do not contaminate fresh leafy vegetables with raw meat or poultry?

Source: U.S. Department of Health and Human Services, Office of Disease Prevention and Health Promotion (2010). *Healthy People 2020.* Available at http://www.healthypeople.gov/2020/default.aspx. Accessed December 2, 2010.

19,140 products containing a total of 1,080 active ingredients that have a current registration. These products are marketed by 1,723 companies.[33] Many of these pesticides are used in agriculture, where it is estimated that pests destroy about 40% of the food crop before it reaches the marketplace. Without the use of agricultural chemicals, farm production could decrease by as much as 30%.[1] Because of this, it seems certain that pesticides will be present in our environment for the foreseeable future.

Although chemical companies market pesticides to control a particular pest, most of them in fact kill a wide range of organisms; that is, they are broad spectrum pesticides. The pest organism against which the pesticide is applied is referred to as the target pest or **target organism** (see Table 14.4). All other organisms in the environment that may also be affected are called **nontarget organisms**. For example, most weed killers will not only kill the weeds

target organism (target pest)
the organism (or pest) for which a pesticide is applied

nontarget organisms
all other susceptible organisms in the environment, for which a pesticide was not intended

---

Table 14.4
Types of Pesticides

Type of Agent	Target Pest to Be Destroyed
Acaricides/miticides	Ticks/mites
Bactericides	Bacteria
Fungicides	Fungi, molds
Herbicides	Weeds, plants
Insecticides	Insects
Larvicides/grubicides	Insect larvae
Molluscicides	Snails, slugs
Nematocides	Worms
Rodenticides	Rats, mice

but also (nontarget) flowers and ornamental plants. Similarly, it is not uncommon for domestic animals to be poisoned and killed by rodenticides (rat poison).

The two most widely used types of pesticides are herbicides (pesticides that kill plants) and insecticides (pesticides that kill insects). These account for 46% and 10% of the pesticides applied for agriculture, respectively.[2] It is also from these two types of pesticides that most human pesticide poisonings occur. The two groups at highest risk for pesticide poisoning are young children and the workers who apply the pesticides. Many of these persons live on farms or are engaged in farm work. Poisonings occur when the pesticides are consumed orally, inhaled, or when they come in contact with the skin. The majority of children poisoned by pesticides consume them orally when the pesticides are left within their reach. Most adult poisonings occur because of careless practice. Examples include eating food without washing hands after handling pesticides, mouth-siphoning to transfer pesticides from one container to another, applying pesticides while one's skin is exposed, or spilling the pesticide on one's body. In agricultural settings, poisonings often occur when agricultural workers fail to follow directions on the pesticide label. For example, workers (who may not be able to read English) may enter sprayed fields too soon after a pesticide application, even a field with posted warning signs, or employers may even tell farm workers to enter the field too soon after a pesticide application. If the workers' children are with them, the children would be at higher risk of becoming poisoned. In addition to occupational exposure of farm workers, consumers may be exposed to low concentrations of pesticides daily through their handling and ingestion of food.

The effects of exposure to pesticides depend on the pesticide type, dose, route and duration of exposure, and the characteristics of the person exposed. Exposures may be acute (single, high-level exposure) or chronic (repeated exposure over an extended period of time). Some signals of poisoning are headaches, weakness, rashes, fatigue, and dizziness. More serious effects include respiratory problems, convulsions, coma, and death. Chronic effects can include cancer, mutations, and birth defects.

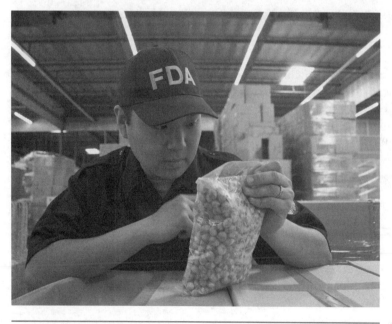

FIGURE 14.12

The Food and Drug Administration (FDA) is charged with ensuring the safety of our foods, except for meat and dairy products.

Regulating Food Safety

Because of the poisonous nature of pesticides, their unregulated manufacture and sale and indiscriminant use are unthinkable. Therefore, they are regulated by a combination of federal and state authorities. The EPA regulates the registration and labeling of pesticides. Individual state agencies license those who can buy, sell, or apply pesticides within their state. The safety of our food supply at the national level is further insured by the United States Department of Agriculture (USDA), which inspects meat and dairy products, and the Food and Drug Administration (FDA), charged with ensuring the safety of the remainder of our foods (see Figure 14.12). In recent years, several instances have occurred that call into question the quality of food processing and its inspection process. These include scares associated with fresh spinach, tomatoes, and peanut butter products.

The task of enforcing state regulations at the local level falls on **registered environmental health specialists (REHSs)**, more commonly known as **sanitarians**. Hired by local health departments, REHSs inspect restaurants and other food-serving establishments (such as hospitals, nursing homes, churches, and schools), retail food outlets (grocery stores and supermarkets), temporary and seasonal points of food service (such as those at fairs and festivals), and food vending machines to ensure that environmental conditions favorable to the growth and development of pathogens do not exist. When unsafe or unhealthy conditions are found, establishments are cited or, in cases of eminent danger to the public, closed. By enforcing food safety laws, public health officials protect the health of the community by reducing the incidence of FBDOs.

Finally, it is important to recognize that consumers, themselves, can further reduce their risk for foodborne illness by following safe food-handling practices and by avoiding consumption of certain unsafe foods. Examples of foods that are often unsafe include unpasteurized milk and milk products, raw or undercooked oysters, raw or undercooked eggs, raw or

> **registered environmental health specialists (REHSs) (sanitarians)** environmental workers responsible for the inspection of restaurants, retail food outlets, public housing, and other sites to ensure compliance with public health codes

---

BOX 14.5 — GUIDELINES FOR PREVENTING FOODBORNE ILLNESSES

To prevent foodborne illness, use the following strategy.

Clean: Wash Hands and Surfaces Often

- Wash your hands with warm water and soap for at least 20 seconds before and after handling food and after using the bathroom, changing diapers, and handling pets.
- Wash your cutting boards, dishes, utensils, and countertops with hot soapy water after preparing each food item and before you go on to the next food.
- Use paper towels to clean up kitchen surfaces. If you use cloth towels, wash them often in the hot cycle of your washing machine.
- Rinse fresh fruits and vegetables under running tap water, including those with skins and rinds that are not eaten.
- Rub firm-skin fruits and vegetables under running tap water or scrub with a clean vegetable brush while rinsing with running tap water.

Separate: Don't Cross-Contaminate!

- Separate raw meat, poultry, seafood, and eggs from other foods in your grocery shopping cart, grocery bags, and in your refrigerator.
- Use one cutting board for fresh produce and a separate one for raw meat, poultry, and seafood.
- Never place cooked food on a plate that previously held raw meat, poultry, seafood, or eggs.

Cook to Proper Temperature

- Use a food thermometer to measure the internal temperature and make sure that the food is cooked to a safe internal temperature (e.g., roasts and steaks to a minimum of 145°F, poultry to a minimum of 165°F in the innermost part of the thigh and wing and the thickest part of the breast). Cook ground meat to at least 160°F.
- Cook eggs until the yolk and white are firm, not runny. Don't use recipes in which eggs remain raw or only partially cooked.
- Cook fish to 145°F or until the flesh is opaque and separates easily with a fork.
- When cooking in a microwave oven, make sure there are no cold spots in food where bacteria can survive. For best results, cover food, stir, and rotate for even cooking.
- Bring sauces, soups, and gravy to a boil when reheating. Heat leftovers thoroughly to 165°F.

Chill: Refrigerate Promptly

- Refrigerate foods quickly and as soon as you get them home from the store because cold temperatures slow the growth of harmful bacteria. Keeping a constant refrigerator temperature of 40°F or below is one of the most effective ways to reduce the risk of foodborne illness.
- Never let raw meat, poultry, eggs, cooked food, or cut fresh fruits or vegetables sit at room temperature more than 2 hours before putting them in the refrigerator or freezer.
- Never defrost food at room temperature. Food must be kept at a safe temperature during thawing, which you can achieve by defrosting your food in the refrigerator, in cold water, and in the microwave.
- Always marinate food in the refrigerator.
- Divide large amounts of leftovers into shallow containers for quicker cooling in the refrigerator.
- Use or discard refrigerated food on a regular basis.

Source: Partnership for Food Safety Education (2010). "Safe Food Handling." Available at http://www.fightbac.org/safe-food-handling. Accessed September 29, 2010.

undercooked ground beef, pork, fish, and poultry. Guidelines for preventing foodborne disease transmission at home are simple and straightforward (see Box 14.5).

THE PLACE WE LIVE

Environmental hazards occur where we live because of our household and land management practices, including the production and mismanagement of our solid waste. The result can be environmental degradation, increased exposure to unsanitary and hazardous materials, and the amplification and transmission of vectorborne diseases.

Solid and Hazardous Waste

Solid waste is the garbage, refuse, sludge, and other discarded solid materials. Most solid waste, 95% to 98%, can be traced to agriculture, mining and gas and oil production, and industry.[1,2] The remaining 2% to 5%, termed **municipal solid waste (MSW)**, comprises the waste generated by households, businesses, and institutions (e.g., universities, schools, and colleges) located within municipalities. In 2008, we produced a daily average of 4.5 pounds of MSW per person, up from the 2.6 pounds of waste produced per person in 1960, but down slightly from the 4.65 pounds per person we generated in 2000 (see Figure 14.13). There are nine major categories—paper, yard waste, food scraps, rubber and textiles, wood, metals, glass, plastics, and other. Paper makes up the largest percentage (31.0%), followed by yard trimmings (13.2%), food scraps (12.7%), and plastics (12.0%) (see Figure 14.14).[34]

Hazardous waste is solid waste with properties that make it dangerous or potentially harmful to human health or the environment and, therefore, requires special management

solid waste
solid refuse from households, agriculture, and businesses

municipal solid waste (MSW)
waste generated by individual households, businesses, and institutions located within municipalities

hazardous waste
a solid waste or combination of solid wastes that is dangerous to human health or the environment

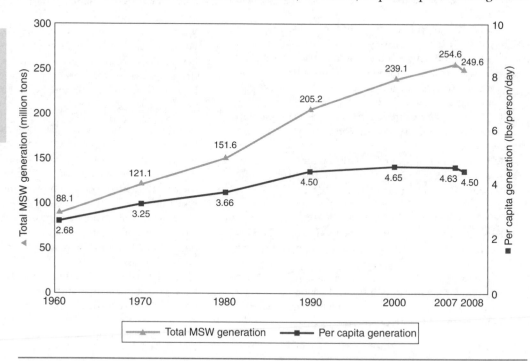

FIGURE 14.13

Municipal solid waste generation rates, 1960–2008.

Source: U.S. Environmental Protection Agency (2009). Municipal Solid Waste Generation, Recycling, and Disposal in the United States: Facts and Figures for 2008. (EPA-530-F-009-021). Washington, DC: Author. Available at http://www.epa.gov/wastes. Accessed November 29, 2010.

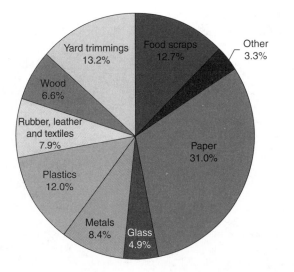

FIGURE 14.14

Total municipal solid waste generation (by material), 2008: 250 million tons (before recycling).

Source: U.S. Environmental Protection Agency (2009). Municipal Solid Waste Generation, Recycling, and Disposal in the United States: Facts and Figures for 2008. (EPA-530-F-009-021). Washington, DC: Author. Available at http://www.epa.gov/epawaste/nonhaz/municipal/pubs/msw2008rpt.pdf. Accessed November 29, 2010.

and disposal. To be classified and regulated as hazardous, the waste must be specifically designated (listed) as hazardous by the U.S. Environmental Protection Agency (EPA), or it must be waste that is ignitable, corrosive, reactive, or toxic. Also, certain wastes, including batteries, mercury-containing instruments, and fluorescent lightbulbs, fall into the category universal (hazardous) wastes. The total amount of hazardous waste created each year in the United States is difficult to estimate, but reliable data are available for large quantity generators that are closely monitored by the EPA. Recent estimates indicate that this group generated approximately 40 million tons of hazardous waste.[35] This figure does not include any wastes that are discarded improperly or illegally. Designated hazardous wastes can be found among the by-products of manufacturing and industrial processes (e.g., solvents that have been used in cleaning or degreasing operations), discarded commercial products (e.g., cleaning fluids), and the by-products of petroleum refining operations and pesticide manufacturing. Electronic waste (e-waste), not included in the preceding total, often contains hazardous components. Each year we discard an estimated 250 million personal computers, 155 million cell phones, and untold millions of television sets[1] (see Box 14.6).

Managing Our Solid Waste

Imagine what would happen if our local garbage and other refuse were not removed for just 2 or 3 weeks. The resulting accumulation of solid waste would produce undesirable odors and attract vermin such as rats, flies, and other disease reservoirs and vectors; it would constitute a community-wide environmental health hazard. Although the necessity of the timely removal of municipal solid waste (MSW) from community neighborhoods is evident to all, its heterogeneous makeup precludes its efficient disposal.

The **Resource Conservation and Recovery Act of 1976 (RCRA)** (pronounced *rick-rah*) was the first comprehensive law to address the collection and disposal of both solid and hazardous wastes. **Solid waste management** encompasses all of approaches to managing all of the constantly accumulating solid waste. These approaches include source reduction,

Resource Conservation and Recovery Act of 1976 (RCRA) the federal law that sets forth guidelines for the proper handling and disposal of hazardous wastes

solid waste management (integrated waste management) the collection, transportation, and disposal of solid waste

BOX
14.6

ELECTRONIC WASTE

As we become more dependent on electronic products to make our lives more convenient, we also generate a vast amount of electronic waste (e-waste) as we dispose of used and obsolete products. In 1998, over 20 million computers became obsolete, and only 13% were reused or recycled. Electronic waste makes up about 1% to 4% of total municipal solid waste production. The European Union estimates that electronic and electrical equipment waste is growing three times faster than municipal solid waste.

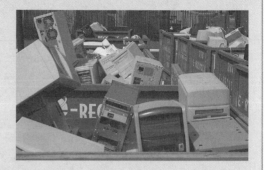

Why Is e-Waste Hazardous?

Color computer monitors and televisions have cathode ray tubes that contain, on average, 4 pounds of lead, as well as other toxic heavy metals, such as chromium, cadmium, mercury, beryllium, nickel, and zinc, and brominated flame retardants used in plastic. These toxic substances require special handling at the end of their lives. When electronics are not properly disposed of or recycled, these toxic materials can be released into the environment through landfill leachate or incinerator ash—both potential pathways to pollution that can negatively affect nearby communities and the health of community members.

What Should I Do with Used and Obsolete Electronic Products?

Individual users of computer monitors and televisions should check with the local municipal solid waste facility to dispose of these wastes properly. Local facilities may recycle these products, thus promoting the safe management of hazardous components and supporting the recovery and reuse of recyclable materials. Another option is recycling used electronic products by donating them for reuse by others. This extends the life of the products, keeps them out of the waste stream for a longer period of time, and prevents unnecessary e-waste pollution. Donating your used electronics for reuse can benefit schools, nonprofit organizations, and lower-income families who would otherwise be unable to obtain such equipment.

Can I Find Environmentally Friendly Products?

When purchasing new equipment, ask your retailer or supplier about electronics that have environmentally preferable attributes and determine whether the manufacturer offers take-back options. *Buying green* involves purchasing new equipment that has been designed with environmentally preferable attributes. Look for electronics that

- Contain fewer toxic constituents
- Use recycled materials in the new product
- Are energy efficient (look for the Energy Star label)
- Are designed for easy upgrading or disassembly
- Use minimal packaging
- Offer leasing or take-back options
- Have been recognized by independent certification groups (such as TCO or Blue Angel) as environmentally preferable

Where Can I Donate Electronic Products?

- Your municipal solids waste disposal facility may have information
- Reuse Development Organization: www.redo.org
- Students Recycling Used Technology: www.strut.org
- Goodwill Industries: www.goodwill.org

Where Can I Recycle Electronic Products?

- Electronic Industries Alliance (Consumer Education Initiative): www.eiae.org
- International Association of Electronic Recyclers: www.iaer.org/search

Source: U.S. Environmental Protection Agency (2010). "Municipal Solid Waste: eCycling." Available at http://www.epa.gov/epaoswer/hazwaste/recycle/ecycling/index.htm. Accessed September 29, 2010.

product reuse and recycling, and disposal. Another term for this combination of approaches is integrated waste management.[1] Of these approaches, the most desirable is **source reduction**. Examples of solid waste source reduction include not buying or using such throwaway products as paper towels and disposable diapers and minimizing packaging associated with groceries and carryout foods. The second best approach to solid waste management is to reuse or recycle the waste. **Recycling** is the collecting, sorting, and processing of materials that would otherwise be considered waste into raw materials that can be used to manufacture new products (see Figure 14.15). Recycling diverts items, such as paper, glass, plastic, and metals, from the waste stream and conserves sanitary landfill

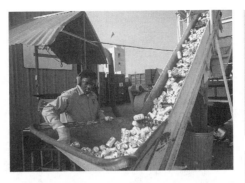

FIGURE 14.15

Recycling involves collecting, sorting, and processing materials to manufacture new products that prevent waste, pollution, and use of virgin natural resources.

space. The United States currently recycles about 33% of its MSW.[34] Only about 59% of our population is served by a curbside recycling program.[36] Although progress has been made, the recycling rate in the United States is far below the rates of some European countries. Austria, for example, recycles or composts 60% of its household solid waste.[37] **Composting** is a form of recycling that can be done easily at home because it doesn't require special knowledge or equipment. In composting, yard waste and food wastes are recycled through a natural process of aerobic biodegradation during which microorganisms convert organic plant and animal matter into compost that can be used as a mulch or fertilizer. Composting conserves precious landfill space.

Once created, MSW that cannot be reused or recycled must be disposed. The currently acceptable methods of disposal are sanitary landfills or combustion (incineration). Currently, 54.2% of municipal solid waste is placed in **sanitary landfills**, sites judged suitable for in-ground disposal of solid waste.[34] RCRA permits only state-of-the-art landfills to operate. At the end of 2008, there were 1,812 approved landfills.[36] These must be located and constructed so that **leachates**, that is, liquids created when water mixes with wastes and drains from beneath a landfill, do not contaminate the groundwater beneath them (see Figure 14.16). Despite these precautions, according to the EPA, all landfills will eventually leak.[1]

Another concern with landfills is the accumulation of dangerous amounts of methane gas (a greenhouse gas) created by the anaerobic decomposition of refuse. In some cases, explosions have occurred when the methane gas was ignited. Although some communities have systems in place to harness the methane gas and use it as an energy source, only a small minority of landfills operating today collect gases. It has been estimated that landfills are responsible for 36% of all methane emissions in the United States.[38]

Nobody wants to live next to a sanitary landfill, even a properly operating one. For this reason, it is exceedingly difficult to establish new landfills in areas where they are needed most. As existing landfill space becomes more restricted, demand will drive up the cost of MSW disposal. This has led to an increased interest in combustion as an alternative to MSW waste disposal.

Combustion (incineration), or the burning of wastes, is the second major method of refuse disposal. The passage of the Clean Air Act of 1970 severely restricted the rights of individuals and municipalities to burn refuse because most could not comply with the strict emission standards. About 13% of all municipal waste was combusted.[36] Some of these incinerators are *waste-to-energy incinerators* or energy recovery plants; that is, they are able

source reduction
a waste management approach involving the reduction or elimination of the use of materials that produce an accumulation of solid waste

recycling
the collecting, sorting, and processing of materials that would otherwise be considered waste into raw materials for manufacturing new products, and the subsequent use of those new products

composting
the natural, aerobic biodegradation of organic plant and animal matter to compost

sanitary landfills
waste disposal sites on land suited for this purpose and on which waste is spread in thin layers, compacted, and covered with a fresh layer of clay or plastic foam each day

leachates
liquids created when water mixes with wastes and removes soluble constituents from them by percolation

combustion (incineration)
the burning of solid wastes

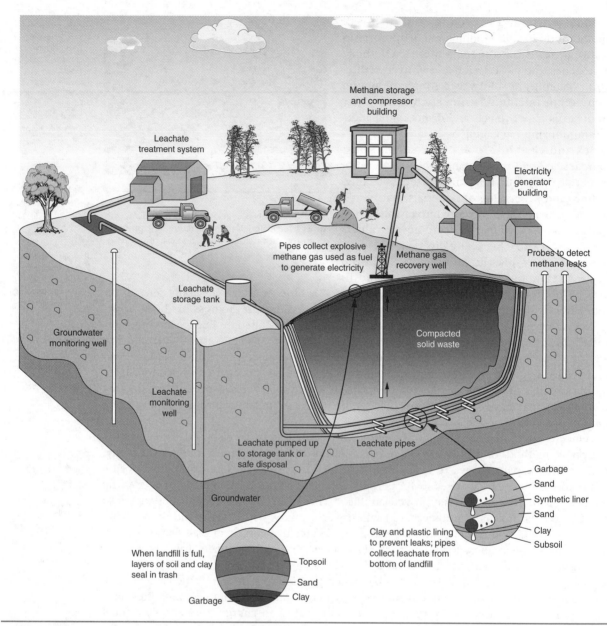

FIGURE 14.16

A state-of-the-art sanitary landfill.

Adapted from Miller, G. T. (2008). *Living in the Environment: Principles, Connections, and Solutions*,16th ed. Pacific Grove, CA: Brooks/Cole; and SWACO Sanitary Landfill Poster, Solid Waste Authority of Central Ohio. Available at http://www.swaco.org/SmartKids/Presentations.aspx. Accessed November 5, 2010.

to convert some of the heat generated from the incineration process into steam and electricity.[36] Combustion reduces the weight of solid waste by 75% and the volume of solid waste by as much as 90%. The resulting waste, if nontoxic, will take up less sanitary landfill space, and because an incinerator can be located closer to the source of the solid waste, transportation costs may be less than for landfills. But there are disadvantages: (1) startup costs are high because large commercial incinerators are expensive, (2) nitrogen oxides, sulfur dioxide, and other toxic air pollutants are produced, and (3) the ash may be too toxic to place in a sanitary landfill. Regular testing is required to ensure that residual ash is nonhazardous before it is placed in a landfill.

Managing Our Hazardous Waste

RCRA also established a system for controlling hazardous waste from the time it is generated until its disposal (called cradle-to-grave regulation) and mandated strict controls over the treatment, storage, and disposal of hazardous waste. It is the responsibility of the EPA to implement the legislation created by RCRA. More than 400 substances are now listed on the EPA's hazardous waste list. The EPA list includes neither radioactive wastes, which are controlled by the Nuclear Regulatory Commission, nor biomedical wastes, which are regulated by the individual states. The EPA Office of Solid Waste has the responsibility to oversee the management of hazardous waste, including its treatment, storage, and disposal. The EPA publishes a report on the hazardous waste generated and managed by the largest waste generators. More than 40 million tons of hazardous waste are generated by these generators in United States in each year.[35] There are about 15 methods of hazardous waste management overseen and regulated by the EPA. The most commonly used method is deep well or underground injection, which is used for disposal of about 50% of hazardous waste.[34] Most of these wells are found in the states of Texas and Florida. The remaining 50% of hazardous waste is managed by various methods, such as special landfills, impoundment, recycling, and incineration.

Managing present and future hazardous wastes is one issue; dealing with the inappropriate past disposal of hazardous wastes is another. Leaking underground storage tanks, abandoned mine lands, and abandoned hazardous chemical waste sites all present serious threats to human health and the environment (see Box 14.7). An underground storage tank (UST) system includes the tank, underground connected piping, and any containment system that stores either petroleum or certain hazardous substances. As of March 31, 2002, 422,573 releases of hazardous substances caused by leaks, spills, and overfills from UST systems had been reported.[39] Gasoline leaking from service stations is one of the most common sources of groundwater pollution. Just 1.5 cups of leaking hazardous chemicals can contaminate more than 1 million gallons of groundwater. Because 40% to 45% of the population of the United States relies on groundwater as its source of drinking water, groundwater pollution is a serious concern.[40] Many municipal and private wells have had to be shut down as a result of contamination caused by leaky UST systems. Additionally, fumes and vapors can travel beneath the ground and collect in areas such as basements, utility vaults, and parking garages,

---

BOX 14.7   BROWNFIELDS, SUPERFUND SITES, AND UNDERGROUND STORAGE TANKS IN YOUR AREA

Search the EPA Web site (www.epa.gov) for brownfields, Superfund sites, USTs, and abandoned mine lands and find the following maps.

- EnviroMapper for Superfund
- EnviroMapper for brownfields
- Abandoned mine lands
- Underground storage tanks

Based on the maps you found, answer the following questions:

1. What types of sites and how many have you found in your area of residence?
2. What specific contaminants of concern are at these sites?
3. Have they been cleaned up?
4. Reflect on your findings and evaluate what this means for the health of your community.

Comprehensive Environmental Response, Compensation, and Liability Act (CERCLA)
the federal law (known as the Superfund) created to clean up abandoned hazardous waste sites

where they can pose a serious threat of explosion, fire, asphyxiation, or other adverse health effects. Cleaning up petroleum releases in the subsurface is difficult and expensive; therefore, the best prevention of groundwater contamination is appropriate management and maintenance of the UST systems to prevent releases.

The primary participant in the cleanup of hazardous waste in the United States has been the federal government. In 1980, Congress passed the **Comprehensive Environmental Response, Compensation, and Liability Act (CERCLA)** in response to the public's demand to clean up leaking dump sites. This law, known as Superfund, created a tax on the chemical and petrochemical industries to clean up abandoned hazardous waste sites that might endanger human health and the environment. CERCLA established a national priority list (NPL) of hazardous waste sites in consultation with various states and provided funds to clean them up. The guiding principle was that the government would make responsible parties pay for those cleanups whenever possible. These sites were placed on the list in order of priority based on the threat to public health or the environment. Once on the NPL, sites were eligible for Superfund dollars that could be used for removing and destroying wastes and for the temporary or permanent relocation of residents affected by the hazardous waste dumps. The Superfund did not provide compensation to victims for health-related problems.

Since the inception of this program, 45,826 contaminated sites have been placed in the database from which the individual states and the U.S. EPA select the sites for the NPL and cleanup. The first NPL in 1983 contained 406 sites. Through the end of 2004, the EPA had listed a total of 1,529 sites and deleted 292 sites from the NPL because of the completion of the cleanup process.[39] The Superfund has provided more than $15,219,000,000 for cleanup of the NPL sites, an average of more than $1 billion per year.[41]

brownfields
property where reuse is complicated by the presence of hazardous substances from prior use

Brownfields

Another problem is the more than 450,000 abandoned industrial plants, factories, commercial worksites, junkyards, and gas stations. These so-called **brownfields** are contaminated properties where expansion, redevelopment, or reuse may be complicated by the presence or potential presence of a hazardous substance, pollutant, or contaminant that can pose a threat to human health.[1] Cleaning up and reinvesting in these properties take development pressures off undeveloped open land, increase local tax bases, facilitate job growth, and improve and protect both the environment and human health.

lead
a naturally occurring mineral element found throughout the environment and used in large quantities for industrial products, including batteries, pipes, solder, paints, and pigments

Lead and Other Heavy Metals

Among the more ubiquitous and harmful environmental hazards are heavy metals, such as lead, mercury, cadmium, chromium, and arsenic. They often contaminate well water and are ingested by unsuspecting people. Heavy metals occur naturally throughout the environment and many are also used in industrial processes or products. For example, lead is used in electric batteries, pipe, solder, paint and plastic pigments, and, until recently, in leaded gasoline.

Because of its past widespread use, **lead** can be found in soil, household dust, air, paint, old painted toys and furniture, and foods and liquids stored in lead crystal or lead-based porcelain. Those who are at greatest risk of lead poisoning are young children, who may inadvertently ingest lead paint, but adults can be poisoned too. It is estimated that as much as 50% of the lead ingested by young children is absorbed, compared with only 10% in adults.

The health problems from exposure to lead include anemia, birth defects, bone damage, depression of neurological and psychological functions, kidney damage, learning disabilities, miscarriages, and sterility.[2] Lead poisoning is the most significant and prevalent disease of environmental origin among American children.[42] A recent study has confirmed that the prevalence of elevated blood lead levels among U.S. children aged 1–5 years has declined significantly since widespread testing began in 1976.[43] Unfortunately, disparities remain among racial and ethnic groups. The children with the highest blood lead levels were non-Hispanic African American children.[43] The major source of lead exposure for these children is dust and chips of lead paint in their homes (see Figure 14.17). In 2000, it was estimated that there were approximately 24 million housing units in the United States that still contain dangerous levels of lead-based paint, and that more than 4 million of these dwellings are homes to children.[44]

The major source of lead intake for adults is occupational exposure. In this case, the method of exposure is usually inhalation. Adults may also be exposed in their homes if they have lead water pipes or have used lead to solder water pipes. The exposed lead dissolves in the flowing water and is delivered to the tap. The EPA has estimated that about 40 million Americans who live in homes built before 1930 (when copper began to replace lead in pipes) are drinking water containing more than the legally permissible level of lead (15 parts per billion). Well water can also become contaminated with lead by the inappropriate disposal of lead-containing materials such as old automobile batteries or solvents containing lead.

The solution to preventing lead poisoning includes several strategies—education, regulation, and prudent behavior. Educational efforts to inform people of the dangers of lead in paint have been in effect for a number of years, and for the most part they seem to have been well received, although an unacceptably high number of children are still being poisoned. Heavy metals are also regulated by the EPA through CERCLA. Those living in older homes with children should have their homes tested for lead paint. Most local health departments provide this service.

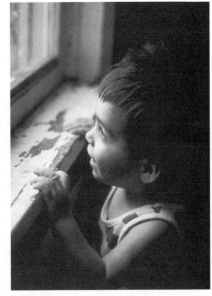

FIGURE 14.17
Lead poisoning from paint dust continues to be a problem in the United States.

Controlling Vectorborne Diseases

Standing water, including runoff water from overflowing septic systems or overloaded sewer systems, and improperly handled solid waste are more than unsavory sights. They provide a habitat for, and support the proliferation of, disease vectors. As discussed in Chapter 4, a **vector** is a living organism, usually an insect or other arthropod, that transmits microscopic disease agents to susceptible hosts. Examples of vectors and the diseases they transmit include mosquitoes (malaria, filariasis, and arthropodborne viruses—arboviruses), fleas (murine typhus and plague), lice (epidemic typhus), and ticks (Rocky Mountain spotted fever and Lyme disease) (see Table 14.5).

vector
a living organism, usually an insect or other arthropod, that can transmit a communicable disease agent to a susceptible host (e.g., a mosquito or tick)

Table 14.5
Vectorborne Biological Hazards

Hazard	Agent	Vector	Disease
Virus	SLE virus	Mosquito	St. Louis encephalitis
	LaCrosse	Mosquito	LaCrosse encephalitis
Rickettsiae	*Rickettsia typhi*	Flea	Murine typhus
	Rickettsia rickettsii	Tick	Rocky Mountain spotted fever
	Ehrlichia chaffeensis	Tick	Ehrlichiosis
Bacteria	*Yersinia pestis*	Flea	Bubonic plague
	Borrelia burgdorferi	Tick	Lyme disease
Protozoa	*Plasmodium* spp.	Mosquito	Malaria
Nematodes	*Wuchereria bancrofti*	Mosquito	Filariasis (elephantiasis)

Source: Heymann, D. L., ed. (2008). *Control of Communicable Diseases Manual*, 19th ed. Washington, DC: American Public Health Association.

vectorborne disease outbreak (VBDO) an occurrence of an unexpectedly large number of cases of disease caused by an agent transmitted by insects or other arthropods

Mosquito larvae require standing water in which to complete their development. The improper handling of wastewater or inadequate drainage of rainwater provides an ideal habitat for mosquitoes and increases the risk for a **vectorborne disease outbreak (VBDO).** Of particular concern in this regard is the northern house mosquito, *Culex pipiens* (see Figure 14.10). *Culex pipiens* is the most important vector of St. Louis encephalitis (SLE) in the eastern United States. In California, SLE virus is transmitted by another mosquito species, *Culex tarsalis,* which proliferates in mismanaged irrigation water. SLE is a disease to which the elderly are particularly susceptible. Those at greatest risk live in unscreened houses without air conditioning.

Culex pipiens also transmits West Nile virus (WNV), which causes West Nile fever, West Nile encephalitis, and West Nile meningitis. The latter two are severe forms of the disease that affect the nervous system. *Encephalitis* refers to an inflammation of the brain; meningitis is an inflammation of the membrane surrounding the brain and spinal cord. West Nile virus first appeared in New York in 1999, where it caused 62 human cases of disease, including 7 deaths.[45] The virus quickly spread westward until it became established throughout the country. In 2009, a relatively mild year for WNV, 663 cases were reported from 34 states. However, as recently as 2006, 4,269 cases were reported from 44 states.[46]

Another species of mosquito that thrives on environmental mismanagement in the north-central and eastern United States is the eastern tree-hole mosquito, *Aedes triseriatus*. Whereas the natural habitat for this mosquito is tree holes, it flourishes in water held in discarded automobile and truck tires. It is estimated that there are 2 billion used tires discarded in various places in the United States today, and 2 million more discarded tires are added to the environment each year. In the eastern United States, *A. triseriatus* transmits LaCrosse encephalitis, an arbovirus that produces a serious and sometimes fatal disease in children.

C. pipiens and *A. triseriatus* are only two of several hundred species of mosquitoes that occur in the United States. Because we have become a global economy, new exotic pest species are constantly being introduced into our country. Two of these are the Asian tiger mosquito, *Aedes albopictus,* first discovered in Texas in 1985,[47] and *Aedes japonicus,* first detected in 1998.[48] Although no human cases of disease have been traced directly to either of these vectors in the United States, laboratory studies indicate that both of them can transmit pathogenic viruses.

Federal, state, and local governments all have units whose primary responsibility is the prevention and control of vectorborne diseases. At the federal level, the lead agency is the CDC's National Center for Zoonotic, Vector-Borne, and Enteric Diseases (NCZVED), located in Ft. Collins, Colorado. They conduct and fund research on vectorborne diseases, maintain surveillance of vectorborne diseases, assist states in investigating vectorborne disease outbreaks, and, in some cases, assist other countries with vectorborne problems. Most state departments of health have offices or labs that maintain vectorborne disease surveillance programs and provide expertise to local health departments, which have the primary task of reducing mosquito populations and preventing disease transmission. Most of us have seen county or mosquito abatement district workers inspecting or treating standing water or driving through our neighborhood with a mosquito sprayer or fogger. Although most of us appreciate these efforts to protect our health and our comfort, it is discouraging to think that despite the millions upon millions of dollars spent on mosquito control in communities across the country, many cases of mosquito-borne diseases are reported annually. Proper land, solid waste, and wastewater management, mosquito control efforts, the promotion of personal protection against mosquito bites, and active surveillance for vectorborne diseases are all important defenses against mosquito-borne disease outbreaks.

The number 1 vectorborne disease in the United States is not a mosquito-borne disease, but a tick-borne disease, Lyme disease. In 2008, more than 35,000 confirmed and probable

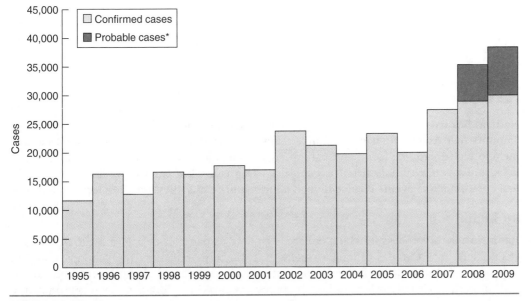

FIGURE 14.18

Number of reported cases of Lyme disease in the United States from 1994 to 2009.

Source: Centers for Disease Control and Prevention (2004). "Lyme Disease—United States 2001–2002." MMWR, 53(17): 365–369; and Centers for Disease Control and Prevention (2006). "Vector-borne Infectious Diseases—Lyme Disease." Available at http://www.cdc.gov/ncidod/dvbid/lyme/ld_UpClimbLymeDis.htm. Accessed November 29, 2010.

cases of Lyme disease were reported to the CDC (see Figure 14.18).[49] Lyme disease is transmitted by the blacklegged tick, *Ixodes scapularis,* a species of tick that flourishes when deer are abundant. During the latter half of the twentieth century, deer populations rapidly increased in the United States through conservation efforts. This resulted in an explosion of populations of the blacklegged tick, sometimes called "the deer tick." The tick transmits the bacterial spirochete *Borrelia burgdorferi*, the cause of Lyme disease. It is important to note that Lyme disease is a bigger problem in some regions of the country. For example, the 10 states reporting the highest incidences of Lyme disease in 2008 were all in the east. Listed in order beginning with the highest incidence they were: New Hampshire, Delaware, Connecticut, Massachusetts, Maine, Vermont, New Jersey, Maryland, Pennsylvania, and New York.[49]

Because there is no vaccine for Lyme disease, and community tick control is virtually nonexistent, personal protection is the best defense. Health departments often remind citizens to take the following precautions: (1) avoid entering tick-infested areas when possible; these are usually wooded and bushy areas with high grass and a lot of leaf litter; (2) if entering an area possibly infested with ticks, dress appropriately—wear long pants and tuck them into your socks and wear a long-sleeved shirt, tucked into your pants; (3) apply a tick repellent; (4) examine oneself and family members for ticks after leaving the area; and (5) carefully remove any ticks found with a pair of tweezers. Finally, support any community efforts at tick control. At home, employ landscaping techniques that discourage ticks—reduce leaf litter and tall grass, and establish a litter-free (and tick-free) border around the perimeter of the yard. Keep the lawn short and, if using acaricides, do so in accordance with instructions on the label.

Improper management of solid waste—such as occurs at open dumps, ill-managed landfills, and urban slums—fosters the expansion of rat and mouse populations. These rodents are hosts for fleas that transmit murine typhus, a rickettsial disease characterized by headache, fever, and rash. The closing of most of the open dumps has relegated murine typhus to the status of an uncommon disease in the United States, but improper MSW management could provide an environment conducive to murine typhus transmission.

NATURAL HAZARDS

natural hazard
naturally occurring phenomenon or event that produces or releases energy in amounts that exceed human endurance, causing injury, disease, or death (such as radiation, earthquakes, tsunamis, volcanic eruptions, hurricanes, tornados, and floods)

Natural hazards are naturally occurring phenomena or events that produce/release energy in amounts that exceed human endurance, causing injury, disease, or death. Natural hazards include high-energy radiation and natural environmental events such as earthquakes, volcanoes, and severe weather related–events such as tornados, hurricanes, and floods. When natural environmental events involve human injuries and deaths, they are often termed disasters.

Radiation

radiation
a process in which energy is emitted as particles or waves

Radiation is the process in which energy is emitted as particles or waves. Heat, sound, and visible light are examples of long-wavelength, low-energy radiation. High-energy (ionizing) radiation is radiation with shorter wavelengths, such as ultraviolet light, X-rays, and gamma rays, or particles, such as alpha or beta particles (see Box 14.8). High-energy **ionizing radiation** is released when atoms are split or naturally decay from a less stable to a more stable form. This type of radiation has enough energy to knock electrons out of orbit and break chemical bonds among molecules in living cells and tissues. Mild tissue damage may be able to be repaired, but if the damage is too severe or widespread, it cannot be repaired and is manifest in radiation burns or radiation sickness or both. Radiation sickness includes nausea, weakness, hair loss, skin burns, diminished organ function, premature aging, cancer, or even death. The amount of radiation and the duration of exposure affect the severity of the injury or illness.

Radiation from Natural Sources

ionizing radiation
high-energy radiation that can knock an electron out of orbit, creating an ion, and can thereby damage living cells and tissues (UV radiation, gamma rays, X-rays, alpha and beta particles)

Radiation arises from both natural and humanmade sources. Sources of natural radiation are extraterrestrial (outer space and the sun) or terrestrial (radioactive minerals emanating from the earth). The radiation we receive originating from outside our solar system can be considered negligible from a health point of view, but the radiation we receive from the sun is considerable. Sunshine comprises energy in many wavelengths, including visible light, heat, and ultraviolet (UV) radiation. UV radiation includes energy at wavelengths between 0 and 400 nanometers (nm). **UV radiation** between 290 and 330 nanometers, called UV-B, causes most of the harm to humans.

ultraviolet (UV) radiation
radiation energy with wavelengths 0–400 nanometers

Much of the UV radiation emanating from the sun is screened out by the layer of ozone in the stratosphere. In recent years, with the erosion of the ozone layer, the quantity of UV-B radiation reaching the earth has been increasing.[1,2] Each year, more than 1 million new cases of skin cancer are reported in the United States, and, in recent years, the incidence rate of skin cancer has been increasing about 3% per year.[50] The vast majority of these cases are the highly curable basal cell and squamous cell carcinomas, the most common forms of cancer. The most serious and least common skin cancer is malignant melanoma. More than 65,000 new cases of melanoma are diagnosed and about 8,600 patients die from this disease each year. This type of skin cancer is the most dangerous because of its ability to grow and spread quickly. However, like the other skin cancers, melanoma is curable if discovered and treated early.[50]

Skin cancer morbidity and mortality rates can be lowered by reducing one's exposure to UV radiation and by early detection and treatment. One can reduce the risk of exposure by staying out of the sun or by covering the skin with clothing or commercial sunscreens.

ABOUT THE ELECTROMAGNETIC SPECTRUM

BOX 14.8

Electromagnetic radiation emitted from different sources has characteristic wavelengths. Taken together, these types of radiation make up the *electromagnetic spectrum*, which ranges from the very-long-wavelength radiation of power lines (thousands of meters) to the very-short-wavelength cosmic radiation that originates in outer space (less than one-trillionth of a meter).

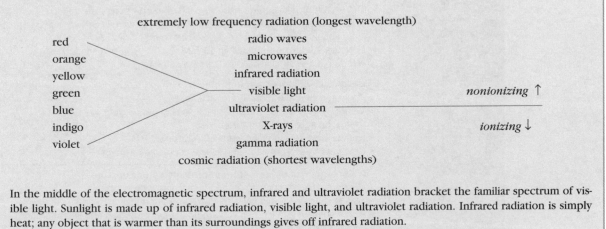

In the middle of the electromagnetic spectrum, infrared and ultraviolet radiation bracket the familiar spectrum of visible light. Sunlight is made up of infrared radiation, visible light, and ultraviolet radiation. Infrared radiation is simply heat; any object that is warmer than its surroundings gives off infrared radiation.

Sunscreens work by absorbing, reflecting, or scattering ultraviolet light, thereby reducing the amount that reaches the skin. To reduce exposure to UV radiation, individuals can also find out the UV index for a specific day through the weather forecast on the Internet, or visit the EPA Web site called Sunwise.[51] The UV index is reported on a scale of 1 (low danger) to 11 (extreme danger) (see Figure 14.19). The EPA also issues UV Alerts, which are warnings when the level of solar radiation in a particular area is predicted to be unusually high. Obtaining information about the strength of UV radiation is the most important step people can take in protecting their health.

The second way people can protect their health is through early diagnosis and prompt treatment. The key to discovering whether treatment is warranted is to practice monthly skin self-examination. Basal and squamous cell carcinomas often appear as a pale, waxlike, peely nodule or a red, scaly, sharply outlined patch. A physician should check either of these abnormalities or the sudden change in a mole's appearance. Melanomas often appear first as small mole-like growths. A new mole that wasn't apparent during a previous month's self-examination should raise concern. The simple ABCD rule from the American Cancer Society outlines warning signs of melanoma.[50]

A is for asymmetry (half of the mole does not match the other half).

B is for border irregularity (the edges are ragged, notched, or blurred).

C is for color (the pigmentation is not uniform).

D is for diameter greater than 6 millimeters (any sudden or progressive change in size should be of concern).

Fortunately, most of us can reduce our exposure to solar radiation through wise behavioral choices. These include avoiding excess direct sun exposure and avoiding tanning beds.

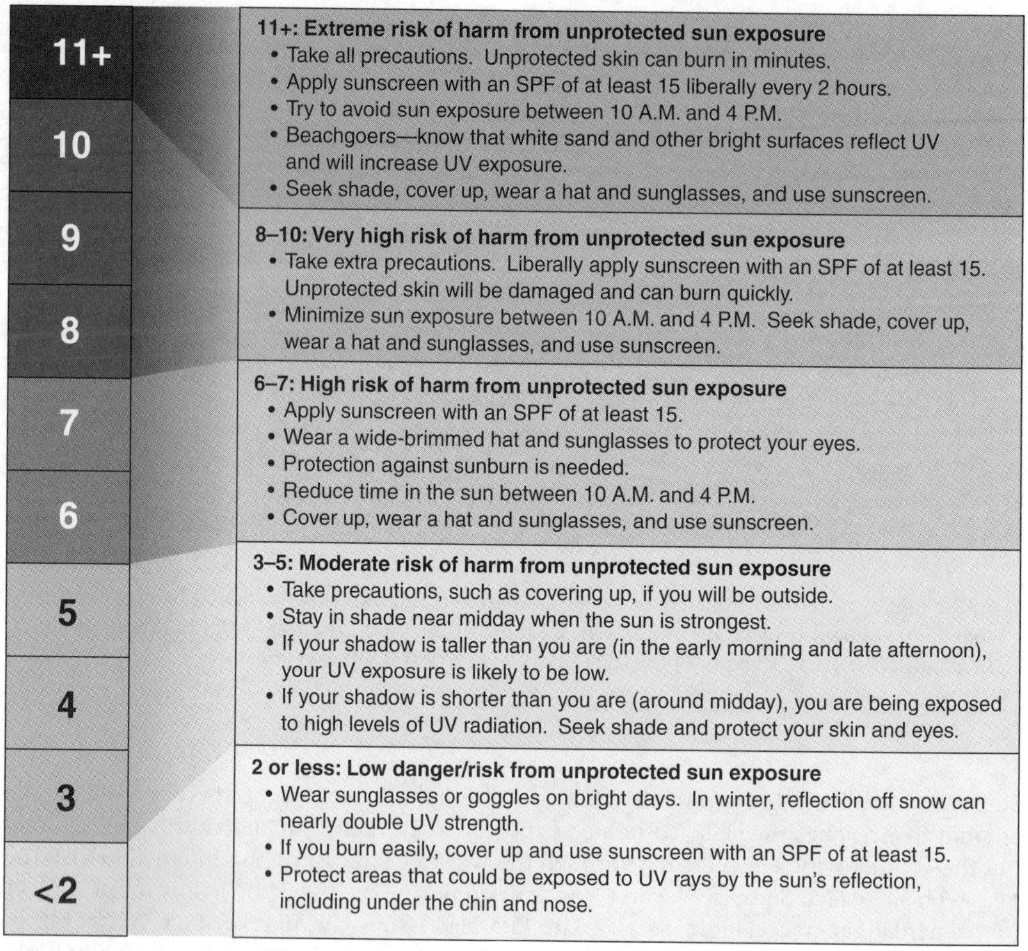

11+	**11+: Extreme risk of harm from unprotected sun exposure** • Take all precautions. Unprotected skin can burn in minutes. • Apply sunscreen with an SPF of at least 15 liberally every 2 hours. • Try to avoid sun exposure between 10 A.M. and 4 P.M. • Beachgoers—know that white sand and other bright surfaces reflect UV and will increase UV exposure. • Seek shade, cover up, wear a hat and sunglasses, and use sunscreen.
10	
9	**8–10: Very high risk of harm from unprotected sun exposure** • Take extra precautions. Liberally apply sunscreen with an SPF of at least 15. Unprotected skin will be damaged and can burn quickly. • Minimize sun exposure between 10 A.M. and 4 P.M. Seek shade, cover up, wear a hat and sunglasses, and use sunscreen.
8	
7	**6–7: High risk of harm from unprotected sun exposure** • Apply sunscreen with an SPF of at least 15. • Wear a wide-brimmed hat and sunglasses to protect your eyes. • Protection against sunburn is needed. • Reduce time in the sun between 10 A.M. and 4 P.M. • Cover up, wear a hat and sunglasses, and use sunscreen.
6	
5	**3–5: Moderate risk of harm from unprotected sun exposure** • Take precautions, such as covering up, if you will be outside. • Stay in shade near midday when the sun is strongest. • If your shadow is taller than you are (in the early morning and late afternoon), your UV exposure is likely to be low. • If your shadow is shorter than you are (around midday), you are being exposed to high levels of UV radiation. Seek shade and protect your skin and eyes.
4	
3	**2 or less: Low danger/risk from unprotected sun exposure** • Wear sunglasses or goggles on bright days. In winter, reflection off snow can nearly double UV strength. • If you burn easily, cover up and use sunscreen with an SPF of at least 15. • Protect areas that could be exposed to UV rays by the sun's reflection, including under the chin and nose.
<2	

FIGURE 14.19

UV index scale.

Source: U.S. Environmental Protection Agency (2006). "Sunwise Program." Available at http://www.epa.gov/sunwise/uviscale.html. Accessed September 29, 2010.

Communities can support healthy behavior by passing and enforcing legislation that bars youths from tanning facilities.

Avoiding terrestrial radiation may be more difficult for some people, those who live near the source of this radiation (uranium ore, for example), or those who live or work in buildings made of brick and stone that contain radioactive materials. Similarly, miners and bricklayers are at greater risk for terrestrial exposure as are those who drink from contaminated wells.

Radiation from Humanmade Sources

Sources of humanmade radiation are those associated with medical and dental procedures, such as X-rays, nuclear medicine diagnoses, and radiation therapy; consumer products, such as smoke detectors, television and computer screens; and nuclear energy and weaponry. Do the benefits derived from the use of radiation outweigh the risks? Most would agree that most of radiation used for medical and dental purposes is justified.

However, there is less agreement about the cost/benefit question in the case of nuclear power plants. The advantages and disadvantages of nuclear power are often discussed. The 103 operating nuclear power stations currently generate about 20% of our nation's total electricity and fit comfortably into the nation's electricity grid.[2] They do this while producing very little air pollution (carbon dioxide, sulfur oxides, nitrogen oxides) and reducing our dependence on foreign oil. However, these facilities produce large volumes of radioactive waste, pose significant environmental and human health risks should failure occur, and are costly to build, run, and decommission at the end of their expected life. The contamination of the environment caused by any accident during shipment or use of nuclear materials is long lasting because the half-life of uranium is measured in the billions of years.

The health effects that have resulted from the 1986 meltdown of the nuclear facility at Chernobyl, in the Ukraine, are staggering. Hundreds of thousands of people, including may children, were exposed to high levels of radiation. A large increase in the incidence of thyroid cancer has occurred among people who were young children or adolescents at the time of the disaster. The incidence of leukemia has doubled in those who experienced high doses of radiation, and there have been an estimated 4,000 additional cancer deaths in the highest exposed groups. Other concerns are cataracts, cardiovascular disease, mental health effects, and reproductive and hereditary effects.[52] It has been more than 20 years since there has been a serious nuclear accident in this country, and there is growing interest in maintaining these nuclear power plants and in building new ones. Many analysts feel nuclear power is a technology whose time has passed because nuclear plants would be too vulnerable to terrorist attacks. However, both the Bush and Obama administrations support the view that nuclear power is an option that should be kept open. Unfortunately, no permanent storage solution for the radioactive wastes generated by nuclear power plants has been identified. The proposed Yucca Mountain site located 90 miles northwest of Las Vegas, Nevada, has become highly controversial, as has the interstate transportation of radioactive waste. States do not want trucks hauling nuclear waste passing through. In March 2010, the Department of Energy under President Obama filed a motion with the Nuclear Regulatory Commission to withdraw the license application for the Yucca Mountain repository.[53] Thus, it would seem that, for the foreseeable future, any new nuclear power plants would have to include on-site storage capacity for newly created nuclear waste materials.

Natural Environmental Events

Natural environmental events include geologic activity such as volcanic eruptions and earthquakes (and resulting tsunamis) and weather-driven events such as tornados, cyclones, hurricanes, and floods. Natural environmental hazards can result in serious physical and psychological health consequences for humans. When these events result in substantial loss of human life and property they are termed **natural disasters** or catastrophic events. Examples of recent natural disasters are Hurricane Katrina, which flooded New Orleans and other Gulf Coast communities in 2005, the tsunami that struck Southeast Asia including Thailand and Indonesia in 2004, and the earthquakes that struck Haiti and Chile in 2010 (see Figure 14.20).

In each of the natural disasters mentioned, health concerns included not only the immediate loss of life and destruction of homes and businesses, but also the unavailability of clean water, food, and sanitation. Also, the loss of loved ones left many survivors feeling sad, depressed, and in need of social services.

Longer-term environmental hazards usually follow for days or months after these natural events. For example, homes flooded because of Hurricane Katrina were contaminated with high levels of mold that lead to respiratory problems. Similarly, volcanic eruptions that release large quantities of ash into the atmosphere are responsible for the acute respiratory

natural disaster
a natural hazard that results in substantial loss of life or property

symptoms commonly reported by people during and after ash falls, including nasal irritation and discharge (runny noses), throat irritation and sore throat, coughing, and uncomfortable breathing. People with preexisting conditions can develop severe bronchitis, shortness of breath, wheezing, and coughing.[54] Flooding from hurricanes or other causes can produce prodigious numbers of mosquitoes, resulting in outbreaks of vectorborne diseases, including encephalitis and malaria.

After a natural disaster, because of the remaining physical, biological, sociological, and psychological conditions, a variety of needs may exist, including clean water, food, shelter, health care, and clothing. Failure of a community, state, or nation to provide for these needs in an efficient and effective manner can exacerbate the extent of human suffering (see Box 14.9).

PSYCHOLOGICAL AND SOCIOLOGICAL HAZARDS

Living around other people exposes us to psychological and sociological hazards that can affect our health. Among these are overpopulation and crowding, hate crimes, wars, and acts of terrorism. Many of these hazards can be related directly or indirectly to population growth.

Population Growth

carrying capacity
the maximum population of a particular species that a given habitat can support over a given period of time

Population growth can be attributed to three factors—birth rate, death rate, and migration. In considering world population growth, migration is not a factor so that when the birth rate and death rate are equal, population growth is zero. When the birth rate exceeds the death rate, the population size increases. As the population grows, more and more environmental resources are needed to support it. The maximum population size that can be supported by available resources (air, water, shelter, etc.) is referred to as the **carrying capacity** of the environment.[1]

The world's six-billionth human inhabitant was born during the first half of 1999; the world's seven-billionth human will be born in 2012[57] (see Figure 14.21). During the past

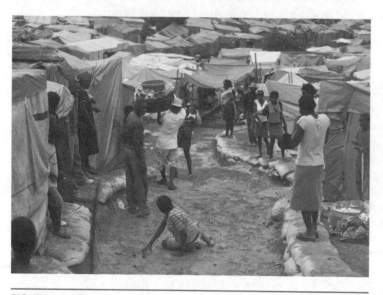

three decades, the rate of world population growth began to decline because of worldwide efforts to curb the growth and avoid disaster caused by exceeding the earth's carrying capacity. Although the *growth rate* of the world's population will continue to decline (see Figure 14.22), the world *population* will continue to grow during the twenty-first century, but at only half the rate it grew in the recent past. At this rate, the U.S. Census Bureau projects that world population will reach 9 billion by the year 2045.[57]

About 80% of the world's population lives in the world's less developed countries (LDCs), and virtually all of the world's population increase between now and 2050 will occur in these countries.[58] The largest percentage of growth during the next 40 years (2010–2050) is expected to occur in sub-Saharan Africa. Only one-third the population size of China in 1950, sub-Saharan Africa was one-half the population

FIGURE 14.20

The 2010 Haiti Earthquake was a natural disaster that resulted in more than 200,000 deaths and 300,000 injuries. The physical disaster was followed by a biological one, as cholera spread among survivors.

HURRICANE KATRINA: A NATURAL DISASTER

Hurricane Katrina ravaged the city of New Orleans and coastal and inland areas of Louisiana and Mississippi in August 2005. The sixth-strongest Atlantic hurricane ever recorded, Katrina was also one of the deadliest, and certainly the costliest. It forced the evacuation of more than 1.5 million people.[55] Storm surges, violent winds, heavy rains, and flooding are to be expected with any hurricane. But with Katrina, the disaster was magnified because most of New Orleans lies below the level of the surrounding bodies of water. The storm surge damaged the levies that protect the city; once these were breached, 80% of New Orleans was flooded, some areas by as much as 3 meters of water. There was extensive damage to buildings, roads, and bridges. Utilities, including communication systems, food distribution, and health care were disrupted. Power outages prevented the operation of 200 sewage treatment plants throughout the disaster area, causing untreated sewage to overflow into streets and houses. Damage to oil and gas platforms meant that floodwaters were contaminated with oil as well as sewage.[56] These environmental conditions increased the risk of waterborne and vector-borne disease outbreaks.

Three weeks after Katrina made landfall, about 1,000 cases of gastrointestinal (diarrheal) disease and 160 cases of dermatological diseases related to arthropod bites and wound infections were reported among evacuees.[51] Those who were evacuated found shelters crowded, unsanitary, and unsafe. Many of the shelters had insufficient food, drinking water, and medicine.

Finally, when floodwaters were pumped out of the inundated areas, a hazardous sludge remained on the land and in buildings and homes. This sludge, and the mold that grew inside damp buildings, caused respiratory problems for people returning to their homes and for recovery workers. Furthermore, 51 cases of carbon monoxide poisoning occurred in the area because some residents used portable generators and other gasoline-powered appliances for electrical power and cleanup. Finally, mental health issues, although not fully known at this time, may well be among the most serious long-term consequences of Katrina.

Sources: Manuel, J. (2006). "News Focus: In Katrina's Wake." *Environmental Health Perspectives*, 114(1): A32-A39; and Centers for Disease Control and Prevention (2005). "Infectious Disease and Dermatological Conditions in Evacuees and Rescue Workers after Hurricane Katrina—Multiple States, August-September, 2005." *Morbidity and Mortality Weekly Report* 54(Dispatch): 1-4.

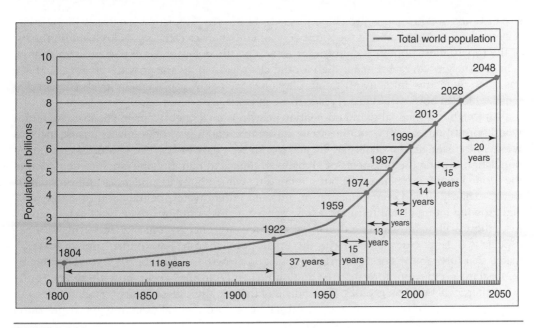

FIGURE 14.21

World population growth in historical perspective between 1750 and 2050, a typical J-shaped curve.

Sources: United Nations (1995) and the U.S. Census Bureau, International Data Base.

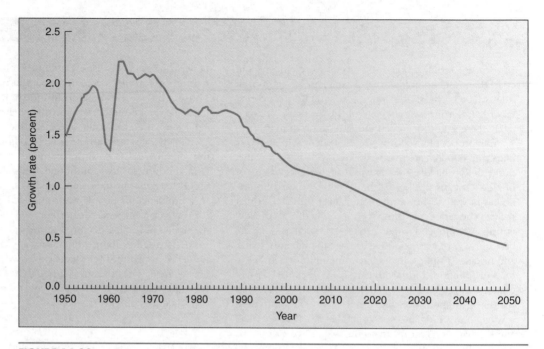

FIGURE 14.22

World population growth rate between 1950 and 2050.

Source: U.S. Census Bureau (2008). *International Data Base, December 2008 Update*. Available at www.census.gov/ipc/www
/img/worldgr.gif. Accessed September 29, 2010.

size of China in 2002 and is projected to surpass China in population size by 2050. By 2050, only the United States, among the more developed countries (MDCs), will remain on the list of the top 10 most populous countries; this will be the result, in large part, of immigration. Whereas the growth rate remains high for the LDCs as a whole, the growth rate for the MDCs has fallen quite low. In many MDCs, fertility rates are below replacement levels (the level at which children born would just replace those persons lost to mortality).[53]

Although exponential world population growth is no longer occurring in absolute terms, world population growth continues to be substantial, and it is at a rate that is unsustainable if we wish to maintain the quality of life and health we enjoy today. The ramifications of over-population include the prospects of global warming, acid rain, bulging landfills, depletion of the ozone layer, increasing crime rates, increasing vulnerability to epidemics and pandemics, smog, exhaustion and contamination of soils and groundwater, degradation of arable land, and growing international tensions. Each year we degrade millions of acres of arable land.[59] Also, there will be a dwindling of natural resources for energy, housing, and living space—especially in large cities. Since 1950, the urban population has more than tripled. It is esti-mated that three-fourths of the current population growth is urban. In 1975, there were only 5 megacities (cities of more than 10 million residents) in the world; now there are 19. By 2015, there will be 23 megacities, with only 2 of them in the United States.[59] Such fast growth and large density of humans in one area results in environmental pollution and degradation that negatively affects the health of every one of us.

Most experts agree that the world population is approaching the maximum sustainable limit. However, no one knows what the ultimate population size will be, what the ultimate carrying capacity of the earth is, and how many people it can support. There are some encouraging signs. The world population growth rate was over 2% just 30 years ago; it is now just 1.2%.[58] Although there are still great concerns with the population growth rates in parts of the Middle East and Africa, some developing countries have succeeded in slowing growth. For example, the average number of children born to a Mexican woman has plunged from 7 to just 2.5 in the past 30 years.[60]

The so-called humane means of limiting population growth include (1) various methods of conception control such as the oral contraceptive pill, physical or chemical barrier methods, or sterilization (tubal ligation and vasectomy); (2) birth control methods such as intrauterine devices, legalized abortion, and morning-after pills; and (3) social policies such as financial incentives and societal disincentives for having children, as is the practice in China's one-child family program. Although some of these methods are unacceptable to certain people, all are proactive solutions to the mounting population problem. The alternative is to allow exponential population growth to continue until it declines naturally, by way of famine, epidemic diseases, and perhaps warfare. Nature's way will require a good deal more environmental deterioration, social disintegration, poverty, and human suffering. The choice is still ours.

The world is more of a global community than ever. The terms *global economy* and *global health* illustrate the notion that we are "all in it together," that we are one big community. Yet ethnic, racial, tribal, and religious differences remain. Whereas some celebrate this diversity, others are unable to shed their prejudices, suspicions, and hatred of peoples unlike themselves. **Bias and hate crimes** are crimes that occur "when offenders choose a victim because of some characteristic—for example, race, ethnicity, or religion—and provide evidence that the hate prompted them to commit the crime."[61] In the United States, race is the leading characteristic associated with bias and hate crimes. Internationally, however, the leading characteristics seem to be religion and ethnicity. One only needs to look to the Middle East to find examples. When these acts are committed not against individuals but against populations, they fall into the realm of terrorism.

bias and hate crimes crimes that occur when offenders choose a victim because of some characteristic— for example, race, ethnicity, or religion— and provide evidence that the hate prompted them to commit the crime

Terrorism

Terrorism is the calculated use of violence (or the threat of violence) against civilians to attain goals that are political or religious or ideological in nature; this is done through intimidation or coercion or instilling fear.[62] Terrorism is a sociological hazard because it affects entire societies, but it is also a psychological hazard because it produces fear, stress, and hysteria and endangers mental health.

terrorism calculated use of violence (or threat of violence) against civilians to attain goals that are political or religious in nature

One or more of these psychological conditions may have been experienced by New Yorkers in the aftermath of the World Trade Center (WTC) attack on September 11, 2001 (see Figure 14.23). Not only did this terrorist attack cause a large number of civilian deaths (2,726), but it was an unprecedented environmental assault on Lower Manhattan that resulted in both physical and mental health problems in survivors.[63] According to the World Trade Center Health Registry survey, the survivors caught in the dust cloud were two to five times more likely to report physical or mental health problems after September 11 than were those who were not. Based on the registry data survey, 64% of building survivors witnessed three or more potentially psychological traumatizing events on September 11, and 11% screened positive for probable serious psychological distress. Also, 15% of adults directly affected by the attacks—such as persons who were in the complex and who were injured; those who lost possessions, a job, a friend, or a relative in this event; or those who were part of the rescue effort—had probable post-traumatic stress disorder (PTSD), compared with only 7.4% of all New York City residents.[63]

A study of Manhattan residents found that 20% of those living near the WTC had symptoms consistent with PTSD 5 to 8 weeks after the attack. Clearly, psychological hazards are an

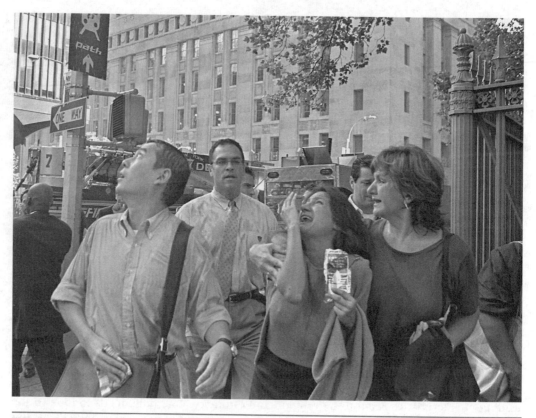

FIGURE 14.23

The September 11, 2001, terrorist attacks on the World Trade Center resulted in fear, stress, and hysteria among some of those who witnessed these events at close range. Others developed post-traumatic stress disorder 1 or 2 months after the attack.

important community health concern, especially during a disaster. In the case of the September 11 terrorist attacks, the full psychological impact on survivors and witnesses of this event is not completely known and continues to be investigated.

RESPONDING TO ENVIRONMENTAL HAZARDS

Federal Emergency Management Agency (FEMA)
the nation's official emergency response agency

Whether to a terrorist attack, such as the World Trade Center attack, or a natural disaster such as Hurricane Katrina, the community must be prepared to respond to minimize the loss of lives, help the injured, and perhaps prevent further catastrophe. In 2005, the response to and recovery of the communities affected by Hurricane Katrina was led by the **Federal Emergency Management Agency (FEMA)**. FEMA, currently an agency within the U.S. Department of Homeland Security, leads efforts to prepare communities around the United States for all hazards and manages federal response and recovery efforts following any national incident, such as earthquake, fire, floods, tornado, landslide, tsunami, wildfires, and winter storms, as well as terrorism. FEMA also initiates proactive mitigation activities, trains first responders, and manages the National Flood Insurance Program.[64]

Although the origins of FEMA can be traced back nearly 200 years, it was then President Jimmy Carter who signed the executive order in 1979 merging many of the separate disaster-related responsibilities into one agency. In March 2003, FEMA was placed in the Department of Homeland Security, where it is part of the Emergency Preparedness and Response Directorate. Today, FEMA has 2,600 regular employees supplemented by nearly 4,000 stand-by disaster assistant employees (see Figure 14.24).[64] The FEMA Web site (www.fema.gov) provides links to a vast array of information, reports, and publications that can help individuals and communities prepare for emergencies. Often FEMA works in partnership with other organizations that are part of the nation's emergency management system, including state and local emergency management agencies, 27 other federal agencies, and the American Red Cross.

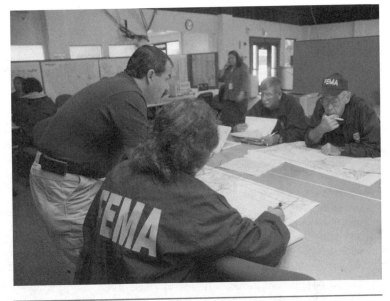

FIGURE 14.24

The Federal Emergency Management Agency (FEMA) helps communities prepare for disasters and manages federal response and recovery efforts following a national incident.

In the United States, the **American Red Cross (ARC)**, a humanitarian organization led by volunteers and guided by its Congressional Charter and the Fundamental Principles of the International Red Cross Movement, provides relief to victims of disaster and helps people prevent, prepare for, and respond to emergencies"[65] (see Chapter 2 for further discussion of the ARC).

American Red Cross
a nonprofit, humanitarian organization led by volunteers and guided by its Congressional Charter that provides relief to victims of disasters

The ARC works to prevent and alleviate human suffering wherever it may be found, with the purpose of protecting life and health while ensuring respect for human beings. The organization is responsible for giving aid to members of the U.S. Armed Forces and to disaster victims in the United States and abroad while staying neutral and impartial. In the history of the ARC, the natural disaster with the highest death toll in the United States was the hurricane that struck Galveston, Texas, in 1900; 6,000 people were killed. Hurricane Katrina was the most expensive single natural disaster in the organization's history and required the largest mobilization of Red Cross workers.[65]

Each year, the ARC responds to more than 70,000 emergencies—from small emergencies such as apartment fires to large ones such as earthquakes and floods. The ARC has 35,000 employees, more than one-half million ARC volunteers, and 700 local chapters throughout the United States.[65]

Natural disasters can occur at any place and at any time. Although a variety of federal and state agencies and organizations have as all or part of their mission to respond to such disasters, recent experiences with disasters should have taught us that local communities, especially those located in high-risk areas, need to prepare too. Only through careful planning and preparation can communities hope to minimize loss of human health and life if a disaster should occur.

CHAPTER SUMMARY

- Environmental health is the study and management of environmental conditions that affect our health and well-being. Environmental hazards increase our risk of injury, disease, or death.

- Air pollution is contamination of the air by gases, liquids, or solids in amounts that harm humans, other living organisms, or the ecosystem or that change the climate. Sources of primary air pollutants are stationary or mobile. Secondary air pollutants arise from the interaction of primary air pollutants and sunlight.

- Efforts to regulate air quality include the Clean Air Act of 1963 and its amendments, which resulted in the establishment of the National Ambient Air Quality Standards. The Environmental Protection Agency calculates the Air Quality Index to help people relate air quality to their health.

- Indoor air pollutants include asbestos, biogenic materials, combustion by-products, and volatile organic compounds. Radon gas and environmental tobacco smoke pose additional indoor air threats to our health.

- The United States has the safest water in the world. Nonetheless, point source and increasingly nonpoint source pollution threaten the safety of our water supply.

- Waterborne disease outbreaks caused by biological and nonbiological pollutants are reported each year, with an increasing proportion of outbreaks being associated with recreational water use.

- Population growth, chemical manufacturing, and reckless land use practices contribute to the deterioration of our water quality.

- Municipal water treatment plants provide water for domestic use, and wastewater treatment plants remove much of the waste before used water is returned to the environment.

- Water quality is regulated by two important laws: the Clean Water Act and the Safe Drinking Water Act.

- More than 200 known diseases are transmitted through the food we eat. Foodborne disease outbreaks occur each year and are reported to the Centers for Disease Control and Prevention.

- The U.S. Department of Agriculture and the Food and Drug Administration inspect food processing plants and enforce health and safety standards. Registered environmental health specialists inspect local restaurants and retail food outlets to enforce food preparation and food handling laws, thereby protecting consumers.

- Solid and hazardous waste management is another environmental concern. The Resource Conservation and Recovery Act governs the management of both municipal and hazardous solid waste, and the Comprehensive Environmental Response, Compensation, and Liability Act governs the cleanup of existing hazardous waste sites.

- Of special concern are the many toxic chemicals and heavy metals, such as lead, that can leach into sources of our drinking water.

- Vectorborne diseases such as West Nile fever, St. Louis encephalitis, LaCrosse encephalitis, Lyme disease, and murine typhus represent another group of environmental health concerns. These diseases affect thousands of people each year and are difficult to predict or control.

- Natural hazards include high-energy radiation and natural environmental events such as earthquakes, tsunamis, volcanic eruptions, and weather-related events such as tornados, hurricanes, and floods.

- Avoiding exposure to ionizing radiation can reduce one's risk for skin cancer and other health problems.

- Natural environmental events, such as earthquakes, volcanoes, floods, and severe weather-related events, that cause extensive loss of human life are called natural disasters.

- Uncontrolled population growth can contribute to psychological and sociological hazards.

- FEMA and the American Red Cross are two agencies that prepare for and respond to natural disasters.

REVIEW QUESTIONS

1. What are the major sources of air pollutants? What are criteria pollutants? What is the difference between primary and secondary pollutants?

2. What role does the Environmental Protection Agency (EPA) play in protecting the environment?

3. What is the Clean Air Act? What are the National Ambient Air Quality Standards? What is the Air Quality Index?

4. What are some major kinds of indoor air pollutants? How can we reduce our exposure to them? What is radon and why is it dangerous?

5. What is the difference between point source and nonpoint source pollution? Which is the bigger problem?

6. What are waterborne disease outbreaks? Name some waterborne disease agents.

7. What are endocrine disruptors and why are they an environmental concern? What are pharmaceuticals and personal care products and why should we be concerned with them?

SCENARIO: ANALYSIS AND RESPONSE

Please take a moment to reread the scenario at the beginning of this chapter. Then, reflect on the questions that follow.

1. Many people like Juan and Maria live where industrial poultry or livestock operations have become established. What additional precautions could Juan and Maria have taken before moving into their current home to protect their health?

2. Suppose the well water is found to contain high levels of nitrates. Assuming that Juan and Maria cannot move, what steps could they take to improve their chances of a successful pregnancy? What might they do to restore the safety of their well water? What local, state, or federal agencies might be able to help them? *Environmental injustice* is a term used to describe situations in which undesirable industries or waste disposal sites are preferentially located in minority areas. Is there anything about this situation that might suggest that this is a case of environmental injustice?

3. Are industrial hog farms a problem in the county or state where you live? What about cattle feedlots? What are your state's regulations regarding the establishment of huge factory farms?

8. How do communities ensure the quality of drinking water, and what steps do communities take to reduce the likelihood that their wastewater harms the environment?

9. What are the purposes of the Clean Water Act and the Safe Drinking Water Act?

10. What is a foodborne disease outbreak? What factors contribute to foodborne disease outbreaks? Name some common foodborne disease causative agents.

11. What are some of the local, state, and federal agencies that help protect our food?

12. What is a pest? What is a pesticide? Explain the difference between target organisms and nontarget organisms and give examples. Explain some safety concerns with pesticides.

13. What types of refuse make up our municipal solid waste? How much MSW do we generate per person per year? What options do communities have for managing MSW?

14. What is hazardous waste? Can you give some examples?

15. What are the purposes of the Resource Conservation and Recovery Act (RCRA) and the Comprehensive Environmental Response, Compensation, and Liability Act (CERCLA)?

16. How do excessive amounts of lead get into our environment? Why is lead detrimental to our health? Which segment of our population is at highest risk for lead poisoning?

17. What is a vector? What is a vectorborne disease? Can you give some examples of each?

18. What is ionizing radiation? Why is it a health issue? How can individuals lower their health risk?

19. What is a natural disaster? How do natural disasters affect the health of a community?

20. How would you interpret the relationships among population growth, the environment, and human health?

21. How would you define *terrorism*? How did the World Trade Center attack result in environmental health repercussions?

22. What role does the Federal Emergency Management Agency (FEMA) play in preparing for and responding to catastrophic events? What is the role of the American Red Cross in providing assistance to people and communities after a natural disaster?

ACTIVITIES

1. For 2 weeks, watch a television weather program that mentions the Air Quality Index (AQI). During that 2-week period, chart the AQI in a graph form and identify the major pollutant for each day.

2. During the next week, create a list of at least 10 things you could have done to conserve the water you use.

3. Write a one-page paper describing either your support for or opposition to (a) nuclear power plants or (b) strengthening the Safe Drinking Water Act.

4. In a one-page paper, identify what you feel to be the number 1 waste or pollution problem faced by the United States, and then detail your rationale for feeling this way.

5. Call your local health department and find out what kind of efforts have been made to eliminate lead poisoning. Ask about education programs and possible state or local laws. Also, find out if the health department will test for lead in the water and paint. If they will, ask about the procedures they use to do so. Write the results of your findings in a two-page paper.

6. For all of us to be better stewards of our environment, we need to be aware of how our community handles various important environmental issues. Find the answers to the following questions about your community and state:

   a. How does your community dispose of solid waste?

   b. How far do you live from a secured landfill? What is the closest community to it?

   c. Where does your community get its water? If you personally get your water from a well, when was the last time the water was evaluated?

   d. Where is the closest nuclear power plant to your home? What are you supposed to do in case of an accident?

   e. Does your state have legislation to protect communities and individuals from factory farm operations that might pollute aquifers or surface water?

7. Make arrangements to interview a director of environmental health in a local health department. Find answers to the following questions and summarize these answers in a two-page paper.

   a. What are all the tasks this division of the health department carries out?

   b. What is the primary environmental health problem of your community? Why is it a problem? How is it being dealt with?

   c. If they inspect restaurants, which ones have the best sanitation practices?

   d. What is an average day like for a health department sanitarian?

COMMUNITY HEALTH ON THE WEB

The Internet contains a wealth of information about community and public health. Increase your knowledge of some of the topics presented in this chapter by accessing the Jones & Bartlett Learning Web site at **http://health .jbpub.com/book/communityhealth/7e** and follow the links to complete the following Web activities:

- Environmental Protection Agency

- National Center for Environmental Health

- FoodNet—Foodborne Diseases Active Surveillance Network

REFERENCES

1. Miller, G. T., Jr., and S. Spoolman (2008). *Environment Science: Principles, Concepts, and Solutions*, 12th ed. Belmont, CA: Brooks/Cole-Thomson Learning.

2. Chiras, D. D. (2010). *Environmental Science*, 8th ed. Sudbury, MA: Jones and Bartlett, Publishers.

3. U.S. Environmental Protection Agency (2009). "Air Trends: Basic Information." Available at http://www.epa.gov/air/airtrends/sixpoll.html.

4. Environmental Protection Agency (2009). *Air Quality Index (AQI): A Guide to Air Quality and Your Health*. Available at http://www .epa.gov/airnow/aqi_brochure_08-09.pdf.

5. Spengler, J. D. (1991). "Sources and Concentration of Indoor Air Pollution." In J. M. Samet and J. D. Spengler, eds., *Indoor Air Pollution: A Health Perspective*. Baltimore, MD: Johns Hopkins University Press, 33-67.

6. U.S. Environmental Protection Agency (2006). "Radon: Health Risks." Available at http://www.epa.gov/radon/healthrisks.html.

7. U.S. Department of Health and Human Services (1991). *Environmental Tobacco Smoke in the Workplace* (DHHS [NIOSH] pub. no. 91-108). Washington, DC: U.S. Government Printing Office.

8. Substance Abuse and Mental Health Services Administration. (2009). *Results from the 2008 National Survey on Drug Use and Health: National Findings* (Office of Applied Studies, NSDUH Series H-36, DHHS pub. no. SMA 09-4434). Rockville, MD. Available at www.oas .samhsa.gov/nsduh/2k8nsduh/2k8Results.cfm.

9. U.S. Environmental Protection Agency (1993). *Respiratory Health Effects of Passive Smoking: Lung Cancer and Other Disorders* (EPA/600/6-90/006f). Washington, DC: U.S. Government Printing Office.

10. U.S. Department of Health and Human Services (1991). *Environmental Tobacco Smoke in the Workplace* (DHHS [NIOSH] pub. no. 91-108). Washington, DC: U.S. Government Printing Office.

11. Overpeck, M. D., and A. J. Moss (1991). *Children's Exposure to Environmental Cigarette Smoke Before and After Birth* (DHHS pub. no. PHS-91-1250). Washington, DC: U.S. Government Printing Office.

12. Moeller, D. W. (1997). *Environmental Health*. Cambridge, MA: Harvard University Press, 93.

13. American Lung Association (2006). *State of Tobacco Control: 2009*. New York: Author. Available at http://www.stateoftobaccocontrol.org/.

14. Centers for Disease Control and Prevention (2010). "State Preemption of Local Smoke-Free Laws in Government Worksites, Private Worksites, and Restaurants—United States, 2005-2009. *Morbidity and Mortality Weekly Report*, 59(4): 105-108.

15. World Health Organization and United Nations Children's Fund Joint Monitoring Programme for Water Supply and Sanitation (JMP) (2008). *Progress on Drinking Water and Sanitation*. New York and Geneva: UNICEF and WHO.

16. World Health Organization and UNICEF (2000). *Global Water Supply and Sanitation Assessment 2000 Report*. Geneva: WHO/UNICEF Joint Monitoring Programme for Water Supply and Sanitation. Available at http://www.who.int/water_sanitation_health/monitoring/globalassess/en/index.html.

17. Centers for Disease Control and Prevention (12 September 2008). "Surveillance for Waterborne Disease and Outbreaks Associated with Recreational Water Use and Other Aquatic Facility-Associated Health Events—United States, 2005-2006 and Surveillance for Waterborne Disease and Outbreaks Associated with Drinking Water and Water Not Intended for Drinking—United States, 2005-2006." *Surveillance Summaries, Morbidity and Mortality Weekly Report*, 57(No. SS-9).

18. Centers for Disease Control and Prevention (1996). "Surveillance for Waterborne-Disease Outbreaks—United States, 1993-1994." *Morbidity and Mortality Weekly Report*, 45(SS-1): 1-33.

19. U.S. Environmental Protection Agency (2006). "The Endocrine Disruption Screening Program." Available at http://www.epa.gov/scipoly/oscpendo/pubs/edspoverview/primer.htm#3.

20. U.S. Environmental Protection Agency (2006). "Pharmaceuticals and Personal Care Products as Environmental Pollutants." Available at http://www.epa.gov/esd/chemistry/pharma/.

21. Steward, J. C. (1990). *Drinking Water Hazards: How to Know If There Are Toxic Chemicals in Your Water and What to Do If There Are*. Hiram, OH: Envirographics.

22. Barber, N. L. 2009. *Summary of Estimated Water Use in the United States in 2005*. U.S. Geological Survey Fact Sheet 2009-3098. Available at: http://pubs.usgs.gov/fs/2009/3098/.

23. U.S. Geological Survey (2009). "Water Q & A: Water at Home Use." Available at http://ga.water.usgs.gov/edu/qahome.html.

24. Centers for Disease Control and Prevention (1999). "Achievements in Public Health, 1900–1999: Fluoridation of Drinking Water to Prevent Dental Caries." *Morbidity and Mortality Weekly Report, 48*(41): 933–940.

25. Federal Water Pollution Control Act (33 U.S.C. 1251 ed seq.) [As Amended Through P.L. 107-303, November 27, 2002]. Available at http://epw.senate.gov/water.pdf.

26. Environmental Protection Agency (2009). *National Primary Drinking Water Regulations*. Available at: http://www.epa.gov/safewater/consumer/pdf/mcl.pdf

27. Environmental Protection Agency (2009). "CCL and Regulatory Determinations at Home." Available at http://www.epa.gov/safewater/ccl/index.html.

28. Centers for Disease Control and Prevention (1999). "Achievements in Public Health, 1900–1999: Safer and Healthier Foods." *Morbidity and Mortality Weekly Report, 48*(4): 905–913.

29. Mead, P. S., L. Slutsker, V. Dietz, L. F. McCaig, J. S. Bresee, C. Shapiro, P. M. Griffin, and R. V. Tauxe (1999). "Food-Related Illness and Death in the United States." *Emerging Infectious Diseases, 5*(5): 607–621.

30. Scharff, R. L., for the Produce Safety Project at Georgetown University. (2010). *Health-Related Costs from Foodborne Illness in the United States*. Available at http://www.producesafetyproject.org/admin/assets/files/Health-Related-Foodborne-Illness-Costs-Report.pdf-1.pdf.

31. Centers for Disease Control and Prevention (2009). "Surveillance for Foodborne Disease Outbreaks—United States, 2006." *Morbidity and Mortality Weekly Report, 58*(22): 609–615.

32. Centers for Disease Control and Prevention (2007). "Preliminary FoodNet Data on the Incidence of Infection with Pathogens Transmitted Commonly Through Food—10 States, 2006. *Morbidity and Mortality Weekly Report, 56*(14): 336–339.

33. National Pesticide Information Retrieval Systems (n.d.). "PPIS." Purdue University. Available at http://ppis.ceris.purdue.edu/.

34. Environmental Protection Agency (n.d.). "Municipal Solid Waste Generation, Recycling, and Disposal in the United States: Facts and Figures for 2008." Available at http://www.epa.gov/osw/nonhaz/municipal/msw99.htm.

35. Environmental Protection Agency (2006). *National Analysis: The National Biennial RCRA Hazardous Waste Report (Based on 2005 Data)* (EPA530-R-06-006). Available at http://www.epa.gov/osw/inforesources/data/br05/national05.pdf.

36. Environmental Protection Agency, Office of Resource Conservation and Recovery (2009). *Municipal Solid Waste Generation, Recycling, and Disposal in the United States Detailed Tables and Figures for 2008*. Available at http://www.epa.gov/epawaste/nonhaz/municipal/pubs/msw2008data.pdf.

37. BBC News (2005). "Recycling around the World." Available at http://news.bbc.co.uk/2/hi/europe/4620041.stm.

38. U.S. Environmental Protection Agency (12 March 1996). "Standards of Performance for New Stationary Sources and Guidelines for Control of Existing Sources: Municipal Solid Waste Landfills." Final rule and guideline, *Federal Register*.

39. U.S. Environmental Protection Agency (September 2005). *FY 2004 Superfund Annual Report* (EPA-540-R-05-001). Washington, DC: Author. Available at http://www.epa.gov/superfund/accomp/fy2004.htm.

40. Centers for Disease Control and Prevention (2008). "Notice to Readers: Ground Water Awareness Week—March 9-15, 2008." *Morbidity and Mortality Weekly Report*, 57(09): 236-237.

41. U.S. Environmental Protection Agency (2006). "Superfund: Superfund Appropriation History." Available at http://www.epa.gov/superfund/accomp/budgethistory.htm

42. Silbergeld, E. K. (1997). "Preventing Lead Poisoning in Children." *Annual Review of Public Health*, 18: 187-210.

43. Jones, R. L., D. M. Homa, P. A. Meyer, D. J. Brody, K. L. Caldwell, J. L. Pirkle, and M. J. Brown. (2009). "Trends in Blood Lead Levels and Blood Lead Testing Among US Children Aged 1 to 5 Years, 1988-2004." *Pediatrics*, 123: e376-e385. Available at http://www.pediatrics.org/cgi/content/full/123/3/e376.

44. Centers for Disease Control and Prevention, National Center for Environmental Health (2000). Eliminating childhood lead poisoning: A federal strategy targeting lead paint hazards. President's task force on environment health risks and safety risks to children. Available at http://www.cdc.gov/nceh/lead/about/fedstrategy2000.pdf.

45. Centers for Disease Control and Prevention. (1999). "Outbreak of West Nile-like Viral Encephalitis—New York, 1999." *Morbidity and Mortality Weekly Report*, 48(38): 845-849.

46. Centers for Disease Control and Prevention, Division of Vector-Borne Infectious Diseases (n.d.). "West Nile Virus." Available at http://www.cdc.gov/ncidod/dvbid/westnile/index.htm.

47. Centers for Disease Control and Prevention, Division of Vector-Borne Infectious Diseases (2005). "Information on *Aedes albopictus*." Available at http://www.cdc.gov/ncidod/dvbid/arbor/albopic_new.htm.

48. Centers for Disease Control and Prevention, Division of Vector-Borne Infectious Diseases (2005). "Information on *Aedes japonicus*." Available at http://www.cdc.gov/ncidod/dvbid/arbor/japonicus.htm.

49. Centers for Disease Control and Prevention (2010). "Lyme Disease: Statistics." Available at http://www.cdc.gov/ncidod/dvbid/lyme/ld_statistics.htm .

50. American Cancer Society (2009). *Cancer Facts & Figures 2009*. Atlanta, GA: Author.

51. U.S. Environmental Protection Agency (2009). "SunWise Program." Available at http://www.epa.gov/sunwise/uviscale.html.

52. World Health Organization (n.d.). "Health Effects of the Chernobyl Accident: An Overview." Available at http://www.who.int/mediacentre/factsheets/fs303/en/index.html.

53. U.S. Department of Energy (2010). "Office of Civilian Radioactive Waste Management." Available at http://www.ocrwm.doe.gov/.

54. Blong, R. J. (1985). *Volcanic Hazards: A sourcebook on the effects of eruptions*. Sydney, Australia: Academic Press, 83–91.

55. Manuel, J. (2006). "News Focus: In Katrina's Wake." *Environmental Health Perspectives*, 114(1): A32–A39.

56. Centers for Disease Control and Prevention (2005). "Infectious Disease and Dermatological Conditions in Evacuees and Rescue Workers after Hurricane Katrina—Multiple States, August-September, 2005." *Morbidity and Mortality Weekly Report*, 54(Dispatch): 1–4.

57. U.S. Census Bureau News (2008). "World Population Approaches 7 Billion." Available at http://www.census.gov/newsroom/releases/archives/population/cb08-95.html.

58. U.S. Census Bureau (2004). *Global Population Profile: 2002* (International Population Reports WP/02). Washington, DC: U.S. Government Printing Office.

59. Hinrichsen, D., and B. Robey (Fall 2000). *Population and the Environment: The Global Challenge* (Population Reports, Series M, no. 15). Baltimore, MD: Johns Hopkins University School of Public Health, Population Information Program.

60. Kluger, J. (2000). "The Big Crunch." *Time* (Special Edition), Earth Day 2000: 44–47.

61. Harlow, C. S. (2005). "Hate Crimes Reported by Victims and Police." *Bureau of Justice Special Report, National Criminal Victimization Survey and Uniform Crime Reporting*. U.S. Department of Justice, Office of Justice Programs, NCH 209911.

62. WordNetWeb (n.d.). "Terrorism." Available at http://wordnetweb .princeton.edu/perl/webwn?s=terrorism.

63. New York City Department of Health and Mental Hygiene (7 April 2006). "Substantial Physical and Mental Health Effects Reported by WTC Building Survivors [Press release]." Available at http://www.nyc.gov/ html/doh/html/pr2006/pr021-06.shtml.

64. Federal Emergency Management Agency (2010). "About FEMA." Available at http://www.fema.gov/about/history.shtm.

65. American Red Cross (2010). "Disaster Services." Available at http://www.redcross.org/portal/site/en/menuitem.d8aaecf214c576bf97 1e4cfe43181aa0/?vgnextoid=477859f392ce8110VgnVCM10000030f387 0aRCRD&vgnextfmt=default.

Chapter 15

Injuries as a Community Health Problem

Chapter Outline

Chapter Objectives

After studying this chapter, you will be able to:

1 Describe the importance of injuries as a community health problem.

2 Explain why the terms *accidents* and *safety* have been replaced by the currently more acceptable terms *unintentional injuries, injury prevention,* and *injury control* when dealing with such occurrences.

3 Briefly explain the difference between intentional and unintentional injuries and provide examples of each.

4 List the four elements usually included in the definition of the term *unintentional injury*.

5 Summarize the epidemiology of unintentional injuries.

6 List strategies for the prevention and control of unintentional injuries.

7 Explain how education, regulation, automatic protection, and litigation can reduce the number and seriousness of unintentional injuries.

8 Define the term *intentional injuries* and provide examples of behavior that results in intentional injuries.

9 Describe the scope of intentional injuries as a community health problem in the United States.

10 List some contributing factors to domestic violence and some strategies for reducing it.

11 List some of the contributing factors to the increase in violence related to youth gangs and explain what communities can do to reduce this level of violence.

12 Discuss local, state, and national resources for preventing or controlling intentional injuries.

SCENARIO

Peter decided to mow the lawn before his ball game. He felt he could complete the task in less than an hour. He checked and filled the gas tank, started the mower, and began mowing. In one corner of the yard, he found it easier to pull the lawnmower backward rather than to push it forward. Peter had done this many times, without incident. This time, he tripped over a stump and lost his balance. In attempting to regain his balance, he pulled harder on the mower, causing it to run over his foot. Instantly he experienced a severe sharp pain and automatically jerked his foot back, but it was too late; the mower blade had cut through Peter's shoe and big toe! Peter quickly turned off the mower and hobbled to the house. As he prepared to go to the emergency room at the local hospital, he was angry with himself as he thought about how his carelessness had caused his injury and might eventually lead to losing his toe.

INTRODUCTION

This chapter first defines and then examines the scope, causes, and effects on the community of both unintentional and intentional injuries. It also reviews approaches to the prevention and control of injuries and injury deaths.

Definitions

The word **injury** is derived from the Latin word for "not right."[1] Injuries result from "acute exposure to physical agents such as mechanical energy, heat, electricity, chemicals, and ionizing radiation interacting with the body in amounts or at rates that exceed the threshold of human tolerance."[2] In this chapter we discuss both **unintentional injuries**, injuries judged to have occurred without anyone intending that harm be done (such as those that result from car crashes, falls, drownings, and fires), and **intentional injuries**, injuries judged to have been purposely inflicted, either by another or oneself (such as assaults, intentional shootings and stabbings, and suicides).

The term *accident* has fallen into disfavor and disuse with many public health officials whose goal it is to reduce the number and seriousness of all injuries. The very word *accident* suggests a chance occurrence or an unpreventable mishap. Yet, we know that many, if not most, accidents are preventable. The term *unintentional injury* is now used in its place. Similarly, the rather vague term *safety* has largely been replaced by **injury prevention** or **injury control**. These terms are inclusive of all measures to prevent injuries, both unintentional and intentional, or to minimize their severity.

There are four significant characteristics of unintentional injuries: (1) they are unplanned events, (2) they usually are preceded by an unsafe act or condition (hazard), (3) they often are accompanied by economic loss, and (4) they interrupt the efficient completion of tasks.

An **unsafe act** is any *behavior* that would increase the probability of an unintentional injury. For example, driving an automobile while being impaired by alcohol or operating a power saw without eye protection is an unsafe act (see Figure 15.1). An **unsafe condition** is any *environmental factor* (physical or social) that would increase the probability of an unintentional injury. Icy streets are an example of an unsafe condition. Unsafe acts and unsafe conditions are **hazards**. Whereas hazards do not actually *cause* unintentional injuries (an alcohol-impaired person may reach home uninjured, even over icy streets), they do increase the probability that an unintentional injury will occur.

---

injury
physical damage to the body resulting from mechanical, chemical, thermal, or other environmental energy

unintentional injury
an injury that occurred without anyone intending that harm be done

intentional injury
an injury that is purposely inflicted, either by the victim or by another

injury prevention (control)
an organized effort to prevent injuries or to minimize their severity

unsafe act
any behavior that would increase the probability of an injury occurring

Cost of Injuries to Society

Injuries are costly to society in terms of both human suffering and economic loss. Injuries are a leading cause of death and disability in the world. An estimated 5.2 million people died from injuries in 2001.[3] This means that more than 14,000 people die each day in the world from injuries. Each year in the United States, more than 150,000 people die from **fatal injuries**, making this the fifth leading cause of death in this country. Specifically, in 2007, there were 182,479 injury deaths, which accounted for 7.5% of all deaths among residents of the United States.[4] Of these deaths, 123,706 (68%) were classified as unintentional injury deaths, 34,598 (19%) as suicides, and 18,316 (10%) as homicides. The remaining 5,793 (3%) deaths were either of undetermined intent or the result of legal intervention (see Figure 15.2).[4]

Deaths are only a small part of the total cost of injuries. Worldwide, 10.9% of the human burden of disease can be attributed to injuries.[3] Here in the United States, each year, there are approximately 33 million medically consulted injuries or poisonings, 25 million of which are considered **disabling injuries** (person was disabled beyond the day of the injury), including some 3 million people who are admitted to hospitals (see Figure 15.3).[5-7]

In addition to the physical and emotional harm caused by these injuries and poisonings, there are significant associated economic costs. For example, in 2008 these costs were estimated at more than $700 billion, including $354.9 billion in wage and productivity losses, $145.1 billion in medical expenses, $122.4 billion in administrative costs, $41.7 billion in motor vehicle damage, $22.3 billion in employer uninsured costs, and $15.5 billion in fire losses.[5] This amounted to about $2,300 per person in the United States.[6] The true economic burden of injuries is much greater than this estimate

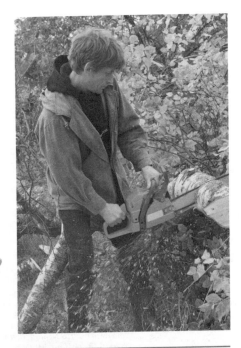

FIGURE 15.1

An unsafe act is a behavior that increases the probability of an injury. Should this person be wearing eye protection?

unsafe condition
any environmental factor or set of factors (physical or social) that would increase the probability of an injury occurring

hazard
an unsafe act or condition

fatal injury
an injury that results in one or more deaths

disabling injury
an injury causing any restriction of normal activity beyond the day of the injury's occurrence

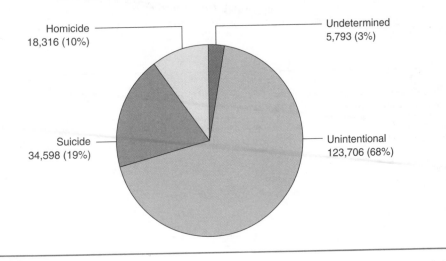

FIGURE 15.2

Injury deaths: United States, 2007.

Source: Xu, J., K. D. Kochanek, S. L. Murphy, and B. Tejada-Vera (2010). "Deaths: Final Data for 2007." *National Vital Statistics Reports,* 59(19):1–73. Available at http://www.cdc.gov/nchs/data/nvsr/nvsr58/nvsr58_19.pdf. Accessed January 5, 2011.

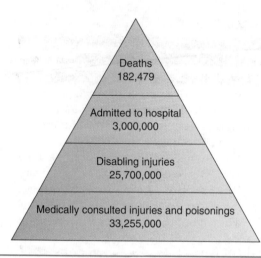

FIGURE 15.3

Burden of injury: United States, 2007.

Sources: Xu, J., K. D. Kochanek, S. L. Murphy, and B. Tejada-Vera (2010). "Deaths: Final Data for 2007." *National Vital Statistics Reports*, 59(19):1-73. Available at http://www.cdc.gov/nchs/data/nvsr/nvsr58/nvsr58_19.pdf; Adams, P. F., K. M. Hayman, and J. L. Vickerie (2009). "Summary Health Statistics for the U.S. Population: National Health Interview Survey, 2008." *Vital and Health Statistics*, 10(243): 1-105. Available at http://www.cdc.gov/nchs/data/series/sr_10/sr10_243.pdf; National Safety Council (2010). *Injury Facts 2010 Edition*. Itasca, IL: Author; and DeFrances, C. J., C. A. Lucas, V. C. Buie, and A. Golosinskiy (30 July 2008). "2006 National Hospital Discharge Survey." *National Health Statistics Reports*, 5. Available at http://www.cdc.gov/nchs/data/nhsr/nhsr005.pdf. Accessed January 5, 2011.

because it does not include value of life lost to premature mortality, loss of patient and caregiver time, and nonmedical expenditures such as insurance costs, property damage, litigation, decreased quality of life, and disability.

Injuries contribute to premature deaths (deaths that occur before reaching the age of one's life expectancy) in the United States. In terms of years of potential life lost before 75 years of age (YPLL-75), unintentional injuries rank third. However, when one considers all injuries, both intentional and unintentional, then injuries are the leading cause of YPLL-75. Leading causes of YPLL-75 and number of deaths for various causes of death are shown in Table 15.1.[8,9]

Table 15.1

Leading Causes of Years of Potential Life Lost (YPLL) and Number of Deaths for Leading Causes of Death: United States, 2006

Disease or Condition	Age-Adjusted YPLL Before Age 75 (per 100,000 population)	Number of Deaths
Injury	1,796	173,472
Cancer	1,586	559,888
Heart disease	1,138	631,636
Stroke	199	137,119
Diabetes mellitus	187	72,449
Chronic lower respiratory diseases	181	124,583
Chronic liver disease and cirrhosis	157	27,555
Human immunodeficiency virus disease	125	12,113
Influenza and pneumonia	79	56,326

Sources: National Center for Health Statistics (2009). *Health, United States, 2009 with Special Feature on Medical Technology*. Hyattsville, MD: Author. Available at http://www.cdc.gov/nchs/hus.htm (accessed January 6, 2011); and Heron, M., D. L. Hoyert, S. L. Murphy, J. Xu, K. D. Kochanek, and B. Tejada-Vera (2009). "Deaths: Final Data for 2006." *National Vital Statistics Reports*, 57(14): 1-136.

Injuries place a special burden on our emergency departments because they are the leading cause of such visits, making up more than one-third of the total visits. There were an estimated 42.4 million injury-related emergency department (ED) visits during 2006, or 14.4 visits per 100 persons per year. This made up 35.5% of all ED visits in 2004. Included in this total were visits for injury, poisoning, or adverse effects of medical treatment.[10]

UNINTENTIONAL INJURIES

Unintentional injuries are the cause of nearly two-thirds of all injury-related deaths in the United States and rank fifth as a leading cause of death (see Table 3.8). There were 112,012 unintentional injury deaths in 2007.[4] Accounting for those deaths were motor vehicle crashes (36%), followed by unintentional poisonings (24%) and falls (18%), along with other causes.[4] In addition to the human death toll were the economic costs, mentioned earlier. Clearly, unintentional injuries constitute one of America's major community health problems. One of the unmet *Healthy People 2010* objectives was to reduce the rate of unintentional injury deaths to below 35.0 per 100,000 population.[11] The Healthy People 2020 objective is less ambitious, namely, to reduce the rate of unintentional injury deaths from 40.0 per 100,000 to 36.0 per 100,000 population. Another Healthy People 2020 objective is to reduce the rate of nonfatal injuries that result in emergency department visits from 9,219.3 per 100,000 to 8,297.4 per 100,000 population.[12]

Types of Unintentional Injuries

There are many types of unintentional injuries. The majority occur as a result of motor vehicle crashes, poisonings, falls, drownings, suffocation, fires and burns, and firearms. These are discussed briefly here.

Motor Vehicle Crashes

Road traffic crash victims can be found throughout the world. Worldwide, 1.26 million people were killed (3,000 each day) and 50 million were injured in road traffic crashes in 2000. An estimated 90% of deaths occurred in middle- or low-income countries as compared with just 10% in developed countries.[13]

In the United States, more people die from unintentional injuries associated with motor vehicle crashes than any other type of injury. In 2007, nearly 6 million police-reported motor vehicle crashes occurred, including more than one and one-half million crashes resulting in injuries. An estimated 1.9 million people were injured and 43,945 people were killed. Fatal injury rates per 100 million vehicle miles traveled (VMT), which had declined almost every year since 1995, reached a record low of 1.25 in 2008. A majority of those killed were drivers (64%), followed by passengers (27%), motorcycle riders (4%), pedestrians (3%), and pedalcyclists (2%).[14] One of the nation's *Healthy People 2020* objectives is to reduce the number of motor vehicle deaths per 100,000 population from the 2007 baseline of 13.8 to 12.4 by 2020. A second objective is to reduce the number of motor vehicle deaths per 100 million vehicle miles traveled from the 2008 baseline of 1.3 to 1.2 by 2020 (see Box 15.1).[12]

Poisonings

Poisonings were the second leading cause of unintentional deaths in 2007, when unintentional poisoning deaths numbered 29,846.[4] These deaths resulted from unintentional ingestion of fatal doses of medicines and drugs, consumption of toxic foods such as mushrooms and shellfish, and from exposure to toxic substances in the workplace or elsewhere. Four-fifths of these poisonings occurred in homes, where poisonings are the leading cause of injury deaths.[6]

Falls

The third leading cause of unintentional fatal injuries is falls, which resulted in 22,631 deaths in 2007.[4] Falls were the leading cause of injury-related ED visits in 2007, with 8.6 million

BOX
15.1   **HEALTHY PEOPLE 2020 OBJECTIVE**

Objective IVP-13   Reduce motor vehicle crash-related deaths
Target-setting method: 10% improvement
Data Sources: National Vital Statistics System–Mortality (NVSS–M), CDC, NCHS, Analysis Reporting System (FARS), U.S. Department of Transportation (DOT), National Highway Transportation Safety Administration (NHTSA)

Target and baseline:

Objective	2007 Baseline	2020 Target
IVP-13.1 Reduce deaths per 100,000 population	13.8	12.4

Objective	2008 Baseline	2020 Target
IVP-13.2 Reduce deaths per 100 million vehicle miles traveled	1.3	1.2

For Further Thought

In 2008, drivers between 16 and 20 years of age experienced the highest rates of involvement in crashes resulting in fatal injuries (44 per 100,000 licensed drivers). This was nearly twice the injury involvement rate for all drivers (24 per 100,000 licensed drivers). Do you think that issuing graduated driver's licenses to new drivers is a solution? If not, how would you suggest states respond to this problem?

Source: U.S. Department of Health and Human Services, Office of Disease Prevention and Health Promotion (2010). *Healthy People 2020.* Available at http://www.healthypeople.gov/2020/default.aspx. Accessed December 2, 2010.

visits.[10] Falls can occur from one surface level to another—stairs or ladders, for example—or on the same level. More than half of the 22,000 or more deaths resulting from falls each year are from falls that occur at home, where falls account for one-third of all deaths from unintentional injuries.[6]

Falls disproportionately affect elders. Each year in the United States, falls affect approximately 30% of elders (adults 65 years of age and older).[15] Falls are the leading cause of both nonfatal and fatal injury among elders, and the Number 1 reason for ED visits among this population. Sixty-two percent of all nonfatal-injury ED visits by elders were attributed to falls.[16]

Other Types of Unintentional Injuries

Other leading causes of unintentional injury deaths in 2007 were fires and burns (3,286), drowning (3,443), all other transport deaths (2,899), and firearms (613). All other types of unintentional injury deaths numbered about 17,043 in 2007.[4]

Epidemiology of Unintentional Injuries

Unintentional injuries are a major community health concern because they account for a disproportionately large number of *early* deaths in our society. However, deaths are only a part of the human toll; incapacitation is another significant aspect of the problem. One in six hospital days can be attributed to unintentional injuries. As mentioned earlier, medical costs from unintentional injuries run into the billions of dollars annually. Many of these injuries, such as head and spinal cord injuries, result in long-term or permanent disabilities that can affect individuals and their families for years.

Some of the factors that describe where, when, and to whom unintentional injuries occur are discussed in the following sections. In addition to describing the occurrence of injuries by person, place, and time, we include a discussion of alcohol and other drugs as risk factors in unintentional injuries.

Person

Unintentional injuries resulting in death and disability occur in all age groups, genders, races, and socioeconomic groupings. However, certain groups are at greater risk for injury than others.

Age

After the first year of life, unintentional injuries become the leading cause of death in children. They are the leading cause of death in the following age groups: 1-4, 5-14, 15-24, 25-34, and 35-44 years of age. They are the third leading cause of death in the 45- to 54-year age group (after cancer and heart disease). Unintentional injuries account for 38% of the deaths in the 5- to 14-year age group; the percentage is higher for males (40%) than for females (32%).[17]

Nearly half of all deaths among older teenagers (15–19 years of age) are caused by unintentional injuries,[17] and the highest rate of injury-related visits to EDs for all types of injuries (19.2 visits per 100,000 persons per year) is by 15- to 24-year-old males (see Figure 15.4).[10]

Children and teenagers are at a higher than average risk of dying as a result of unintentional firearm injury. Unintentional nonfatal firearm-related injury rates are highest among persons aged 15 to 24 years, and these rates decrease with age[18] (see Figure 15.5). Nearly 10% of high school males carried a gun to school at least once in 2009.[19] Some people believe that childhood firearm deaths are a national tragedy in the United States. A child under 15 years of age is nine times more likely to die of an unintentional firearm injury in the United States than in the other 25 industrialized nations (see Figure 15.6).[20] Unintentional firearm injuries constitute an important public health problem. Two states, California and Florida, have enacted legislation making adults legally responsible for the inappropriate storage of firearms.

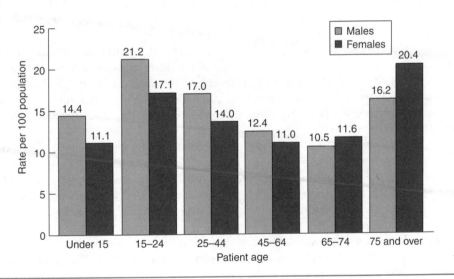

FIGURE 15.4

Rates of injury-related visits to emergency departments by age and sex, 2006.

Source: Pitts, S. R., R. W. Niska, J. Xu, and C. W. Burt (2008). "National Hospital Ambulatory Medical Care Survey: 2006 Emergency Department Summary." *National Health Statistics Reports*, 7.

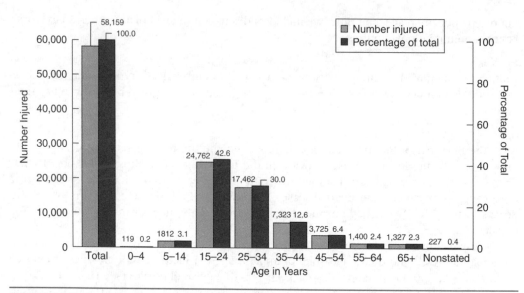

FIGURE 15.5

National estimates of the number and percentage of persons with nonfatal firearm injuries treated in hospital emergency departments, United States, 2004.

Source: U.S. Department of Health and Human Services, Centers for Disease Control and Prevention, National Center for Injury Prevention and Control (2006). *Firearm Injury Surveillance Study, 1993-2004* [Computer file] (ICPSR04595-V1). Atlanta, GA: Author. Available at http://webapp.icpsr.umich.edu/cocoon/ICPSR-STUDY/04595.xml. Accessed January 21, 2011.

For all age groups except persons 75 years and older, motor vehicle crashes are the leading cause of unintentional injury deaths.[4] However, rates of involvement in crashes resulting in fatal injuries in 2008 were the highest for drivers aged 16 to 20 (44 per 100,000 licensed drivers). This was almost twice the fatal injury involvement rate for all drivers (24 per 100,000 licensed drivers).[14]

Among elders (those 65 years and older), injuries are the eighth leading cause of death.[17] Injury deaths would rank higher, but many elders die of other causes resulting from the aging process, such as heart disease, cancer, and stroke. An examination of the rates of death per 100,000 among elders reveals that elders have the highest unintentional injury death rate of any age group (100 per 100,000). For those 85 years and older, the injury death rate climbs to 279 per 100,000.[17]

Falls are the leading cause of unintentional injury deaths for those 80 years and older. At age 80, the death rate from falls surpasses that for motor vehicle crashes and accounts for more than half of the unintentional injury–related deaths of this age group.

Elders are at age-increased risk of dying in car crashes, too. A report published by the AAA Foundation revealed that drivers 65 years and over are almost twice as likely to die in car crashes as drivers aged 55 to 64. Drivers 75 and older were two and one-half times as likely to die, and drivers 85 and older were almost four times as likely to die in car crashes compared with drivers aged 55 to 64.[21] Since this article appeared, more attention has been paid to the topic of safe mobility of elders.

Elders also experience high rates of nonfatal injuries. In 2006, elders made 3.2 million injury-related visits to emergency departments.[10] Elders are three times more likely to be hospitalized following an injury than are those younger than 65.[16]

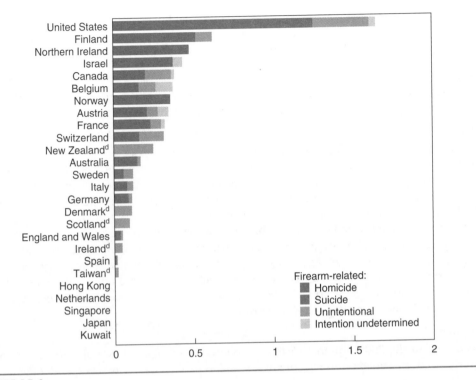

FIGURE 15.6

Rates[a] of firearm-related death[b] among children younger than 15 years in 26 industrialized countries.[c]

[a]Per 100,000 children aged < 15 years and for 1 year during 1990–1995.
[b]Homicides by firearm (*International Classification of Diseases,* 9th Rev., codes E965.0–E965.4), suicides by firearm (E955.0–E955.4), unintentional deaths caused by firearm (E922.0–E922.9), and firearm-related deaths for which intention was undetermined (E985.0–E985.4).
[c]All countries classified in the high-income group with population = 1 million (5) that provided complete data. In this analysis, Hong Kong, Northern Ireland, and Taiwan are considered as countries.
[d]Reported only unintentional firearm-related deaths.

Source: Centers for Disease Control and Prevention (1997). "Rates of Homicide, Suicide and Firearm-Related Deaths among Children—26 Industrial Countries." *Morbidity and Mortality Weekly Report,* 46(5): 101–105.

Gender

Statistics indicate that, at every age level, males are much more likely to become involved in a fatal unintentional injury than are females. Overall, the ratio of male deaths to female deaths is nearly 2:1. In the 15- to 24-year and 25- to 64-year age groups, males die from unintentional injuries at greater than three times the rate of their female counterparts. Although differences in unintentional injury death rates between the sexes decline with age, men retain a marginally higher rate even in the over-75-year age group. One type of unintentional fatality with a wide disparity in rates per 100,000 is motor vehicle crashes (20.9 in males vs. 8.4 in females); the type with the narrowest is falls (7.8 in males vs. 7.2 in females).[4]

Minority Status

In 2005, unintentional injuries and adverse effects were the leading cause of death for all ages through the 25- to 34-year age group in all racial and ethnic groups except for blacks. In this racial group, assault (homicide) and legal intervention replaced unintentional injuries as the leading causes of injury deaths for the 15- to 24-year and 25- to 34-year age groups.[17] Age-adjusted death rates for unintentional injuries in 2005 were highest for the American

Indian/Alaska Native population (51.4 per 100,000) and lowest for the Asian/Pacific Islander population (15.1 per 100,000). The white, non-Hispanic population had a rate of 41.8, while the Hispanic population had a lower rate of 26.9 per 100,000 population.[17]

Place

Unintentional injuries occur wherever people are—at home, at work, or on the road. Although more injuries occur at home, more injury deaths occur on the road.

Home

People spend more time at home than any other place, so it is not surprising that 47.6% of all unintentional injuries and poisonings reported in the 2008 National Health Interview Survey were injuries that occurred in the home (see Figure 15.7).[5] Unintentional injuries in the home result from falls, burns, poisonings, accidental shootings and stabbings, and suffocation. Within the home, some areas are more dangerous than others. The presence of appliances (including stoves, toasters, mixers, and so on) and sharp knives in the kitchen makes this room one of the more dangerous in the house. Another location where many unintentional injuries occur, particularly to the very young and old, is on stairways. For children, the bathroom, garage, and basement are hazardous areas because of the drugs, cleaning agents, and other poisonous materials that are often stored in these areas. In the home, more people die in bedrooms, where they may be sleeping during a fire, than in any other room.

Highway

According to the 2008 National Health Interview Survey of the U.S. population, 14% of all injuries were sustained on streets, highways, and in parking lots.[5] However, with regard to all *fatal* injuries, 33.1% were sustained at these venues. Interestingly, it can no longer be said that more fatal injuries occur on streets, highways, and in parking lots; more injury deaths now occur in or around the home (see Figure 15.8). Two reasons explain this change. First, signif-

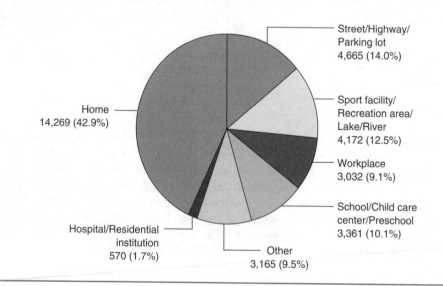

FIGURE 15.7

Number (in thousands) and percentage of injury episodes by place of occurrence: United States, 2008.

Source: Adams, P. F., K. M. Hayman, and J. L. Vickerie (2009). "Summary Health Statistics for the U.S. Population: National Health Interview Survey, 2008." *Vital and Health Statistics,* 10(243): 1–105. Available at http://www.cdc.gov/nchs/data/series/sr_10/sr10_243.pdf. Accessed January 5, 2011.

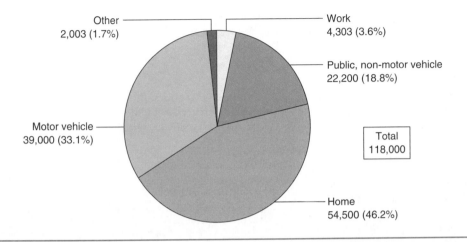

FIGURE 15.8

Unintentional injury deaths by class: United States, 2004. Note: Deaths for sections of chart add to more than the total because some deaths are included in more than one section.

Source: Reprinted with permission of the National Safety Council (2010). National Safety Council (2010). *Injury Facts 2010 Edition.* Itasca, IL: Author.

icant progress has been made in reducing motor vehicle–related deaths, from a rate of 22.5 per 100,000 people in 1980 to 12.25 per 100,000 people in 2008.[14] This has been achieved through effective interventions, including increasing public awareness, education, legal proscriptions (such as child safety seats and safety belts), innovative vehicle and equipment designs, improved roadways, and enhanced medical systems. The second reason why more deaths now occur at home is because of the recent increase in unintentional poison deaths, most of which occur in homes.[4]

One remaining area of concern is the number of unlicensed or improperly licensed drivers on the highways. A 5-year study (1993–1997) revealed that 20% of all fatal crashes— one in five—involve at least one improperly licensed driver. These are drivers with a license that is suspended, revoked, expired, cancelled, or denied. Nearly 4% of drivers involved in fatal crashes had no known license at all.[22]

Recreation/Sports Area

The third most likely place to sustain an injury that results in a visit to an ED is a recreation or sports area, such as a soccer field, baseball diamond, or basketball court. Approximately 12.5% of injuries reported in the 2008 National Health Interview Survey occurred in these settings.[5]

The fourth most common place for injuries to occur is in school, preschool, or child care settings. These settings are not unusually hazardous places, but outside the home, these are places where much of our time is spent.

Workplace

The workplace ranks fifth as a location where unintentional injuries frequently occur. About 9.1% of reported injuries occurred in the workplace.[5] As one might imagine, the risk of injury varies widely among different occupations. Among the most dangerous occupations are mining, farming (including logging), and construction. As America becomes a more service/information-based economy, the typical workplace environment becomes less hazardous. (For more information about workplace injuries, see Chapter 16.)

BOX
15.2

Ten Great Public Health Achievements, 1900–1999: Motor Vehicle Safety

Bumper to Bumper and Curb to Curb . . . Driving Is Safer Now Than in 1900

Although more people are driving automobiles, traveling more miles, and driving at faster speeds than in 1900, driving is much safer now because of safer vehicles, highways, and drivers.

Since 1925, the annual death rate from motor vehicle travel has decreased 90%, despite the increase in miles traveled and the number of vehicles used per capita.

Approximately 85,000 American lives have been saved because of seat belts.

Using child safety seats has reduced the risk of infant death by 69% and of children aged 1 to 4 years by 47%.

Since 1987, community awareness and driving-while-intoxicated regulations have helped reduce alcohol-related traffic fatalities by 32%.

Source: Centers for Disease Control and Prevention (1999). "Ten Great Public Health Achievements—United States, 1900–1999." *Morbidity and Mortality Weekly Report*, 48(12): 241–242. Available at www.cdc.gov/mmwr/PDF/wk/mm4812.pdf. Accessed October 26, 2010.

Time

During the twentieth century, there were declines for some types of unintentional injuries and increases for others. For example, motor vehicle deaths fell from 51,091 in 1980 to 37,261 in 2008. This reduction occurred despite the fact that Americans drove twice as many miles in 2008 as they did in 1980. The fatality rate per 100 million VMT declined from 3.35 to 1.25 during that 28-year period.[14] This reduction in the death rate from motor vehicle crashes in the United States is one of the 10 most significant public health achievements of the twentieth century (see Box 15.2).

Since 1975, unintentional deaths from drowning, fires, and burns have declined by more than half, and from firearms by two-thirds. However, deaths from falls, which declined significantly from 1975 to 1986, have begun to increase in the past few years, as the U.S. population ages. Deaths from poisonings have also increased and now rank second as a leading cause of unintentional injury deaths.[4]

There are seasonal variations in the incidence of some types of unintentional injuries, but these depend on the types of injury. For example, 59% of all drownings occur in four months—May, June, July, and August—when more people take part in water sports. Conversely, 62% of all deaths due to fires and burns are recorded during the six months from November through April, when furnaces, fireplaces, wood-burning stoves, and electric and kerosene space heaters are most often in use.[6]

Motor vehicle crash rates per 100 million VMT in 2008 were highest during November–February. Motor vehicle-related deaths increase markedly at night. Fatalities also occur at a higher rate on weekends (Friday through Sunday). Although more fatal crashes occur on Saturdays, more crashes of all types occur on Fridays. The hours between midnight and 3 A.M. Saturdays and Sundays are the most dangerous 3-hour periods to travel by car (see Figure 15.9).[14]

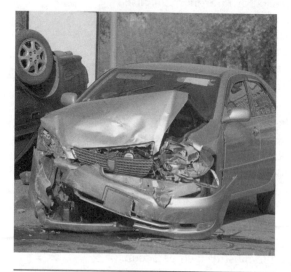

FIGURE 15.9

Motor vehicle fatality rates are higher on weekends.

Much publicity surrounds the number of motor vehicle deaths that occur during the following six major holiday periods: Memorial Day, Fourth of July, Labor Day, Thanksgiving, Christmas, and New Year. However, it has been shown that the number of crash-related deaths for these periods is not significantly different from the number occurring during non-holiday periods. However, the proportion of fatal crashes in which the driver is alcohol impaired is higher during holiday periods (about 41% for New Year's Day, Memorial Day, Fourth of July, and Labor Day; about 36% for Thanksgiving and Christmas) than during non-holiday periods (about 32%).[14]

Alcohol and Other Drugs as Risk Factors

An examination of the factors that contribute to intentional and unintentional injuries reveals that alcohol may be the single most important factor. This is certainly the case with fatal motor vehicle crashes, in which 37% of persons killed in traffic crashes in 2008 died in alcohol-related crashes. Although 37% represents a significant decline from the 55% reported in 1982, it is still too high. There has also been a decline in the percentage of those killed in crashes who were intoxicated—that is, who had blood alcohol concentrations (BACs) that exceeded 0.08% (BAC > 0.08%)—from 48% in 1982 to 37% in 2008.[14]

The percentage of drivers in fatal crashes whose BAC exceeded the legal limit (0.08%) was 22% in 2008, but this percentage was nearly four times higher at night than during the day. Alcohol was involved in 72% of the single-car crashes that occurred on a weekend night in which a 21-year-old or older driver or motorcycle operator was killed (see Figure 15.10). The percentage of drivers or motorcycle operators involved in fatal crashes whose BAC exceeded 0.08% was nearly twice as high for males (25%) as for females (13%).[14] Forty-two

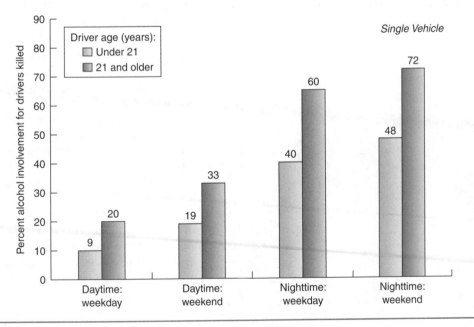

FIGURE 15.10

Alcohol impairment (BAC ≥ 0.08%) for drivers or motorcycle operators killed, by driver age, time of day, and day of week.

Source: U.S. Department of Transportation, National Highway Traffic Safety Administration (2009). *Traffic Safety Facts 2008: A Compilation of Motor Vehicle Crash Data from the Fatality Analysis Reporting System and the General Estimates System* (DOT HS 811 170). Washington, DC: U.S. DOT. Available at http://www-nrd.nhtsa.dot.gov/Pubs/811170.pdf. Accessed January 5, 2011.

percent of drivers and motorcycle operators involved in fatal crashes had a previous record of crashes, license suspension or revocation, DWI conviction, speeding conviction, or other harmful moving violation conviction.[14]

Unfortunately, drivers are not the only persons killed in alcohol-related motor vehicle crashes. Motor vehicle crashes are the leading cause of death among children aged 1 year and older in the United States, and one in four deaths of child passengers aged 14 years and older involves alcohol use. Of the 2,355 children who died in alcohol-related crashes during the period 1997 to 2002, 1,588 (68%) were riding with drinking drivers.[23]

Alcohol use often contributes to motor vehicle injuries and deaths in another way. Safety belt use by drinking drivers is lower than for their nondrinking counterparts, thus increasing the likelihood of a fatal outcome if there is a crash. In 1999, safety belts were used by only 19% of fatally injured *intoxicated* drivers, compared with 30% of fatally injured impaired drivers (with BAC levels between 0.01% and 0.09%) and 48% of fatally injured sober drivers. Child passenger restraint use also decreases as the BAC of the driver increases. Of 1,409 child passengers with known restraint information who died while riding with drinking drivers (1997–2002), only 466 (32%) were restrained at the time of the crash. The likelihood that a child passenger restraint was used decreased with increases in drivers' BAC.[23] Passage of primary enforcement safety belt laws (laws that allow police to stop and ticket a driver solely because an occupant is unbelted) and stricter enforcement of these laws in all states could reduce child passenger deaths. Excessive drinking can also increase a pedestrian's chances of being killed by a motor vehicle. In 2008, 36% of pedestrians 14 years or older killed by motor vehicles were intoxicated.[14]

Alcohol has also been determined to be an important factor in other types of unintentional injuries and deaths, including aquatic-related deaths. Nearly half of those who drown have evidence of alcohol in their blood. Alcohol was the leading contributing factor in 17% of boating fatalities in 2008.[24] A U.S. Coast Guard study estimates that boat operators with a BAC above 0.10% are more than 10 times as likely to be killed in a boating accident than are boat operators with zero BACs.[25] In another study, it was found that nearly half of all boating fatalities occurred when vessels were not under way. This implies that although it is dangerous when the person who is operating the boat is drinking, it is also dangerous when passengers have been drinking (see Figure 15.11). Last, alcohol consumption lowers a person's chance of survival should that person end up in the water. In a study conducted in Louisiana, alcohol and/or metabolites of an illicit drug were found in 60% of drowning victims aged 13 years or older.[26] Clearly, alcohol consumption and aquatic recreation are a dangerous combination.

Alcohol has also been shown to be a risk factor for bicyclists. Nearly 7% of pedalcyclists killed in traffic crashes were under the influence of alcohol or other drugs.[14]

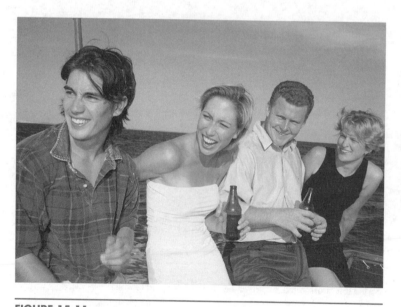

FIGURE 15.11

Alcohol consumption while boating lowers your chances of survival should you end up in the water.

Prevention through Epidemiology

Sometimes it has been society's nature to wait until after a tragedy before correcting an existing hazard or dangerous situation. Most implementation of prevention activities related to injuries occurs only after costly disasters.

Early Contributors to Injury Prevention and Control

The first important efforts toward injury prevention and control began early in the twentieth century. Four of the most important contributors to early efforts at injury control were Hugh DeHaven, John E. Gordon, James Gibson, and William Haddon, Jr. Hugh DeHaven was a World War I combat pilot, who, after surviving a plane crash, dedicated his professional life to studying victims of falls in an effort to design ways to reduce the force of impact on a body. Many of his ideas have led to better design concepts, including structural adaptations to protect drivers and other occupants of moving vehicles. For example, today we have at our disposal the protection of safety belts, air bags, collapsible steering assemblies, and padded dashboards. Many of these safety devices built on the early work of Hugh DeHaven.[27]

In 1949, John E. Gordon proposed that the tools of epidemiology be used to analyze injuries. Because of Gordon's work, a great deal was learned about risk factors, susceptible populations, and the distribution of injuries in populations.

In 1961, James Gibson proposed the idea that injury harm was caused by "energy interchange." Although this definition didn't fit well with certain injury deaths such as drowning and freezing, William Haddon, Jr., realized that in these cases, injury occurred because of the lack of necessary energy elements. Thus, the definition of injury supported by the National Center for Injury Prevention and Control (NCIPC) is "any intentional or unintentional damage to the body resulting from acute exposure to thermal, mechanical, electrical, or chemical energy or from the absence of such essentials as heat or oxygen."[27]

William Haddon, Jr., was both an engineer and a physician and is often considered the founding father of modern injury prevention research.[27] He was an unrelenting proponent of the epidemiological approach to injury control and insisted that the results of this work be used in the development of public policy. He was the foremost expert on highway safety in the 1960s and developed many successful countermeasures to reduce the number of unintentional highway injuries.

A Model for Unintentional Injuries

Until the 1950s, little progress occurred in the reduction of unintentional injuries and deaths. One reason for this was the failure to identify the causative agent associated with unintentional injuries. Chapter 4 discussed the public health model that describes communicable diseases in terms of the host, agent, and environment, arranged in a triangle. A similar **model for unintentional injuries** has been proposed. In this model, the injury-producing agent is *energy* (see Figure 15.12).

Examples of injury-producing energy are plentiful. A moving car, a falling object (or person), and a speeding bullet all have kinetic energy. When one of these moving objects strikes another object, energy is released, often resulting in injury or trauma. Similarly, a hot stove or pan contains energy in the form of heat. Contact with one of these objects results in the rapid transfer of heat. If the skin is unprotected, tissue damage (a burn) occurs. Electrical energy is all around us and represents a potential source of unintentional injuries. Even accidental poisonings fit nicely into

model for unintentional injuries the public health triangle (host, agent, and environment) modified to indicate energy as the causative agent of injuries

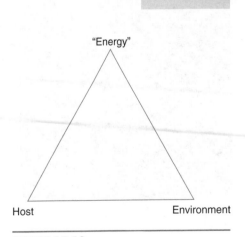

FIGURE 15.12
The public health model for unintentional injuries.

the model that incorporates energy as the causative agent of injury. Cleansers, drugs, and medicines represent stored chemical energy which, when released inappropriately, can cause serious injury or death.

Prevention and Control Tactics Based on the Model

Based on the epidemiological model just described, four types of actions can be taken to prevent or reduce the number and seriousness of unintentional injuries and deaths.[27] These four tactics are modified from those of Haddon. The first is to prevent the accumulation of the injury-producing agent, energy. Examples of implementing this principle include reducing speed limits to decrease motor vehicle injuries, lowering the height of children's high chairs and of diving boards to reduce fall injuries, and lowering the settings on hot water heaters to reduce the number and seriousness of burns. In our electrical example, circuit breakers in the home prevent the accumulation of excess electrical energy.

The second type of action is to prevent the inappropriate release of excess energy or to modify its release in some way. Flame-retardant fabric that will not ignite is an example of such a prevention. Currently, there is a law that requires that such a fabric be used in the manufacture of children's pajamas. The use of automobile safety belts is another example. In this case, excess energy (movement of a human body) is released into the safety belt instead of into the car's windshield (see Figure 15.13). In the prevention of fall injuries, hand rails, walkers, and nonslip surfaces in bathtubs prevent the inappropriate release of kinetic energy resulting from falls.

The third tactic involves placing a barrier between the host and agent. The insulation around electrical wires and the use of potholders and non–heat-transferring handles on cookware are examples of this preventive strategy. The use of sunscreen lotion and the wearing of a hat in the summer place a barrier between the sun's energy and a person's skin. Another example is the cable barriers being installed between opposing traffic lanes on many interstate highways. These installations not only serve as a barrier to protect oncoming traffic but also modify the release of energy and provide drivers and occupants with a relatively soft landing.

Finally, it is sometimes necessary or useful to completely separate the host from potentially dangerous sources of energy. Examples include the locked gates and high fences around electrical substations and swimming pools. At home, locking up guns and poisons provides protection against the likelihood of unintentional injury of young children.

Other Tactics

By viewing energy as the cause of unintentional injuries and deaths, it is possible to take positive steps in their prevention and control. There are still other actions that a community can take. First, injury-control education in the schools and in other public forums can be helpful. Second, improvements in the community's ability to respond to emergencies, such as encouraging the public to enroll in first aid and cardiopulmonary resuscitation (CPR) classes and expanding 911 telephone services, can limit disability and save lives. Third, communities can ensure that they have superior emergency and paramedic personnel by instituting the best possible training programs. The result will be improved emergency medical care and rehabilitation for the injured. Finally, communities can strengthen ordinances against high-risk behaviors, such as driving while impaired by alcohol, and then support their enforcement.

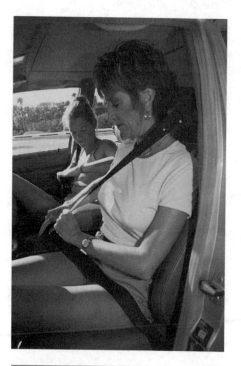

FIGURE 15.13

Safety belts reduce injuries caused by motor vehicle crashes and save lives.

Community Approaches to the Prevention of Unintentional Injuries

There are four broad strategies for the prevention of unintentional injuries—education, regulation, automatic protection, and litigation.

Education

Injury prevention education is the process of changing people's health-directed behavior in such a way as to reduce unintentional injuries. Education certainly has a place in injury prevention. Many of us remember the school fire drill, lessons on bicycle safety, and the school crossing guard. Undoubtedly, millions of injuries were prevented in these ways. However, injury prevention education has its limitations. Figure 15.14 illustrates both the inefficiency of public education and the difficulties of measuring a successful outcome.

injury prevention education
the process of changing people's health-directed behavior so as to reduce unintentional injuries

Regulation

The former 55-mile-per-hour national speed limit is an example of the power of **regulation**—the enactment and enforcement of laws to control conduct—as a means of reducing the number and seriousness of unintentional injuries. For years, motorists were advised to drive more responsibly. Public service announcements in the 1960s and 1970s informed audiences that "speed kills," and advised motorists not to "drink and drive." However, the highway

regulation
the enactment and enforcement of laws to control conduct

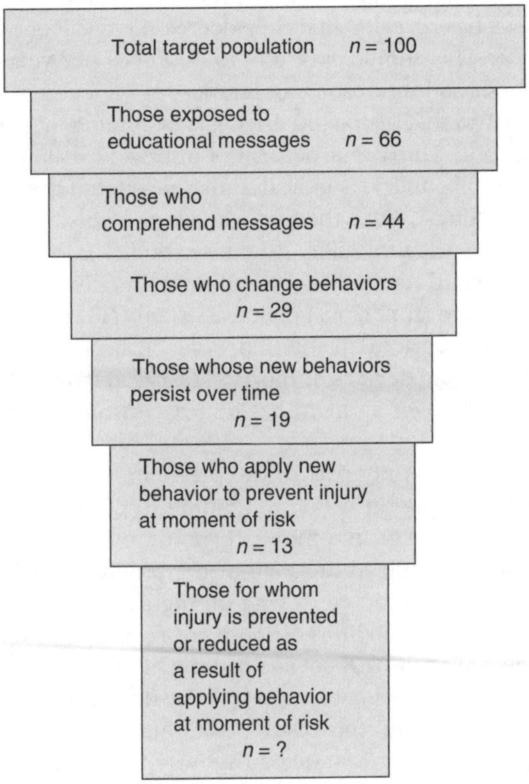

FIGURE 15.14
Attenuation of the effect of a public health education program.

Source: Adapted from McLoughlin, E., C. J. Vince, A. M. Lee et al. (1982). "Project Burn Prevention: Outcome and Implications," *American Journal of Public Health,* 72(3): 241–247. As presented in U.S. Congress, Office of Technology Assessment (February 1988). *Healthy Children: Investing in the Future* (pub. no. OTA-H-345). Washington, DC: U.S. Government Printing Office.

death toll continued to mount until 1974, when then President Gerald Ford issued the national 55-mile-per-hour speed limit. Although the primary purpose of the slower speed limit was to conserve gasoline during the Arab oil embargo, more than 9,000 lives were saved as the number of motor vehicle deaths dropped from 55,511 in 1973 to 46,200 in 1974 because of the slower speeds.

State laws requiring child safety seats and safety belt use are another example of regulation to reduce injuries. Beginning in the 1980s, automobile child restraint and safety belt legislation spread across the United States. All states now have child passenger safety seat or restraint requirements for children, and all states except for New Hampshire have safety belt use laws for adults.[14] There is quite a bit of variation in the provisions of these laws from state to state with regard to enforcement, level of fines, seats of the vehicle covered (front seat or all seats), and type of vehicle covered. To check state seat belt laws, visit http://health.jbpub.com/book/communityhealth/7e. Passage and vigorous enforcement of safety belt regulations are one reason why motor vehicle fatalities have declined in recent years. Regulation is often aimed not at the consumer, but at the industry. For example, beginning with the 1990 models, car makers were required to equip all passenger cars with safety belts or air bags.

Another regulatory change that has helped reduce motor vehicle–related injuries is the lowering of the blood alcohol concentration at which a person is legally intoxicated to 0.08%. In 2004, Delaware became the final state to adopt this standard, which has now been adopted by all 50 states, Puerto Rico, and the District of Columbia. A systematic review of the effectiveness of such laws has revealed that they decrease fatal alcohol-related motor vehicle crashes an average of 7%. This should save 400 to 600 lives per year nationally and significantly decrease the number and seriousness of injuries.[28]

A recent survey indicates that distracted driving is becoming increasingly recognized as a roadway hazard for everyone. Thirty-four percent of interviewees indicated they felt less safe on the road today than before, and 31% indicated that distracted driving was the single most common reason for this feeling.[29] Since the first workshop on distracted driving research was held by the National Highway Traffic Safety Administration (NHTSA) in 2000, the number of personal electronic devices in use has increased dramatically. Examples are cell phones (including iPhones), Blackberries, personal digital assistants (PDAs), laptops, electronic notebooks, and global positioning devices. In addition, availability of in-car entertainment devices, such as DVD players and gaming devices, is more widespread than in the past. "Drivers using handheld cell phones at any given moment has increased from 4% in 2002 to 6% in 2008," according to the NHTSA.[30]

Use of electronic devices is only part of the problem. Drivers also become distracted when eating or drinking, putting on makeup, tending to children, talking to a passenger, looking for something in the car or in a purse, fidgeting with controls, singing along with music, and reading a map. But add to these all of the technological devices now in widespread use, and the impact of distracted driving on highway safety becomes significant. In 2008, 5,870 of the 37,261 traffic fatalities (16%) were recorded as distracted-related traffic fatalities.[30] Drivers younger than 20 years of age had the highest proportion of fatal crashes in which the driver was reported as being distracted at the time of the crash (16%).

Twenty-seven states, Guam, and the District of Columbia have indicated that distracted driving has become a priority in their Strategic Highway Safety Plans. Eight states have indicated that the governor or legislature has set up a task force or summit on distracted driving. In 2010, 34 states collected data on crashes in which distraction was a factor. Collecting such data may soon become a federal requirement.[30]

Texting and e-mailing while driving are the latest distracted driving issues. The American Automobile Association's Foundation for Traffic Safety reports that 21% of drivers admit to having read or sent a text message or e-mail while driving in the past 30 days. This figure increases to 40% of drivers younger than 35 and 51% of drivers 16–19 years of age.[29] States are taking a comprehensive approach to reducing text messaging and e-mailing while driving, including education, legislation, and enforcement. Forty-one states indicate that they have initiated public education/information campaigns on this topic using either traditional methods or new media/social networking, and eight states indicate that they have begun efforts to educate judges on the issue of distracted driving. Text messaging has been banned for all drivers in 30 states and Guam and for novice drivers in an additional 8 states. Efforts to regulate cell phone usage and texting are ongoing; to see the laws in a particular state, visit the Governors' Highway Safety Association Web site: www.ghsa.org.[31]

In a "free society," such as the one in which Americans live, there is a limit to how much can be accomplished through legislation. For example, it has been very difficult to reduce the number of firearm injuries in the United States through legislation because the National Rifle Association (NRA) has been able to lobby successfully against restrictions on gun ownership.

Another example of the difficulty of achieving a balance between personal freedoms and society's legitimate health interests is motorcycle helmet legislation. Studies show that helmet laws are associated with a 29% to 33% decrease in annual per capita motorcycle fatalities.[32] In 1975, all but two states required motorcyclists to use helmets. Beginning in 1976, states began to repeal these laws. By the end of 2008, only 20 states, Puerto Rico, and the District of Columbia required a helmet for all motorcyclists. To check the motorcycle helmet laws in a particular state, visit the textbook's Web site at http://health.jbpub.com/book/communityhealth/7e.[14]

automatic (passive) protection the modification of a product or environment so as to reduce unintentional injuries

The strategy of prevention through regulation can be difficult to implement. The idea of regulating health behavior grates against the individual freedom that Americans have come to expect. Why should someone be required to wear a safety belt? The answer to that is: For the good of the total public, to protect the resources, including human life, of the greater public. Others say, "It's my life, and if I choose to take the risk of dying by not wearing a safety belt, who should care?" That response is all well and good; but when life is lost, it affects many others, such as family members, friends, and coworkers, not just the deceased. This scenario would become worse if the person not wearing a safety belt does not die but becomes a paraplegic and a ward of the state. Many public resources then would have to be used.

At what point is some legislation enough? It is known that safety belts and air bags are good and effective, but so are helmets—at least they think so at the Indianapolis 500. So, should people now work to pass a law that requires all automobile and truck drivers to wear helmets? How much legislated health behavior is enough?

Automatic Protection

When engineered changes are combined with regulatory efforts, remarkable results can sometimes be achieved. The technique of improving product or environmental design to reduce unintentional injuries is termed **automatic (or passive) protection**.[27] A good example is child-proof safety caps (see Figure 15.15). Child-proof safety caps on aspirin and other medicine were introduced in 1972. By 1977, deaths attributed to ingestion of analgesics and antipyretics

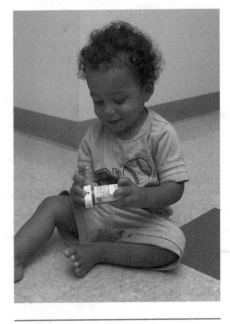

FIGURE 15.15

Child safety caps are an example of automatic or passive protection.

had decreased 41%.[33] We are all familiar with automatic protection devices. Common examples include automatic shut-off mechanisms on power tools (such as lawn mowers), safety caps on toxic products, and the warning lights and sounds that remind us to buckle our safety belts in motor vehicles.

Litigation

litigation
the process of seeking justice for injury through courts

When other methods fail, behavioral changes can sometimes come about through the courts. **Litigation**—lawsuits filed by injured victims or their families—has been successful in removing dangerous products from store shelves or otherwise influencing changes in dangerous behavior. Litigation against a manufacturer of unsafe automobile tires, for example, might result in safer tires. Lawsuits against bartenders and bar owners for serving alcohol to drunken customers, who have later injured other people, have produced more responsible server behavior at public bars. Alcohol-related deaths and injuries on college campuses have caused insurance companies to re-examine their liability insurance policies with fraternities and sororities. This has forced some of these organizations and the universities themselves to restrict the way alcohol is used. The outcome may be a drop in unintentional injuries on these campuses.

INTENTIONAL INJURIES

Intentional injuries, the outcome of self-directed and interpersonal violence, are a staggering community health problem in the United States. More than 50,000 people die, and millions of others receive nonfatal injuries each year, as a result of self-directed or interpersonal violence.[4,9] In 2006, an estimated 1.8 million persons were treated for nonfatal physical assault–related injuries in EDs.[10] Although the physical assault rate is higher for males than for females, the rate of ED visits for sexual assault–related injuries can be five times higher for females. The highest injury rates for both males and females was for the 15- to 24-year age group.[10] The injury rate for black males was about 2.6–3.5 times higher than the rate for non-Hispanic white males.[34]

Types of Intentional Injuries

The spectrum of violence includes assaults, rapes, suicides, and homicides. These acts of violence can be perpetrated against family members (children, elders, and intimate partners), community members, or complete strangers. In 2008, residents of the United States 12 years of age or older reported being victims of an estimated 4.9 million violent crimes. Violent and property crimes were at or near their lowest levels in more than three decades.[35]

Interpersonal violence is a costly community health problem, not only because of the loss of life and productivity but also because of the economic cost to the community. Consider the community resources expended for each violent act. There are those of the police, the legal system, the penal system, emergency health care services, medical services, social workers, and many others. Clearly, this is a problem for which prevention is the most economic approach.

Epidemiology of Intentional Injuries

To better understand the problem of intentional injuries, it is instructive to look more closely at both the victims and the perpetrators of violence. Interpersonal violence disproportionately affects those who are frustrated and hopeless, those who are jobless and live in poverty, and those with low self-esteem. More violent acts, whether self-directed or directed at others, are committed by males. Firearms are increasingly involved in violent acts, with ever-increasing fatal consequences. Abuse of drugs, especially alcohol, also contributes to the number of intentional injuries. Additionally, perpetrators of violent acts are more likely to have been abused or neglected as children or exposed to violence and aggression earlier in their lives.

Homicide, Assault, Rape, and Property Crimes

Between 1991 and 2005, the homicide rate declined from 9.8 to 5.6 per 100,000 people.[36] In 2008, 14,180 murders were reported to the FBI.[37] Both the upswing in the homicide rate prior to 1991 and the subsequent decline afterward resulted from large swings in the victimization rates of those less than 25 years of age. During that same period, the homicide victimization rate for blacks was six times higher than for whites during some years.[38] Much of the increase in homicides could be traced to the use of handguns by juveniles involved in the distribution of crack cocaine.[38] While the U.S. homicide rate has declined in recent years and has leveled off at about 6 per 100,000 people, it remains higher than the rates of most other industrialized nations. Homicide and legal intervention ranked as the fifteenth leading cause of death in the United States in 2007. In the 15- to 24-year age group, homicide ranked as the second leading cause of death.[34] Most of the homicides in the United States (69%) are committed with firearms, which are abundant and easy to acquire.

Research indicates an inverse relationship between income level and risk for becoming a victim of violence. In 2008, persons in households with annual incomes less than $7,500 were about 1.5 times as likely as persons in households with incomes of $75,000 or more to become victim of a property crime.[35]

Males and blacks as well as the poor are more vulnerable to violence. Except for rape and sexual assault, every violent crime victimization rate is higher for males than for females. Males experienced violent crime at higher rates than females, and they account for about three-fourths of all murder victims. However, females were victims of rape and sexual assault four times more often than males. In 2008, 26 blacks, 18 whites, and 15 persons of other races per 1,000 were victimized. Individuals of more than one race experienced violent crimes at rates two to three times higher than whites, blacks, or people of other races. In 2008, there were 5.2 aggravated assaults per 1,000 black persons, 3.0 per 1,000 white persons, 2.8 per 1,000 persons of other races, and 6.8 per 1,000 persons of more than one race.[35]

Overall, it is estimated that less than half of all violent crimes committed in 2008 were reported to police. Furthermore, only 41% of rapes or sexual assaults were reported to police. This makes the acquisition of accurate statistics on rape and attempted rape difficult. Although reported offenders are usually strangers, 63% of all rapes and sexual assaults against females are committed by someone acquainted with, known to, or related to the victim and 18% by an intimate partner (current or former boyfriend or spouse).[35]

Suicide and Attempted Suicide

As previously indicated, more than 30,000 suicides are reported each year in the United States, accounting for one-fifth of all injury mortality. In 2008, 34,598 suicide deaths were reported.[33] The suicide rate for men (18.3 per 100,000) was four times that for women (4.8 per 100,000) in 2007.[4] The rates of suicide in young people (15 to 24 years of age) nearly tripled between 1950 and 1995 but have since declined to 9.7 per 100,000.[4] Those for the elderly have also declined in recent years. Suicide rates in older men, however, remain quite high. Senior men (65 years old and older) are eight times more likely to commit suicide than are senior women.[4]

Firearm Injuries and Injury Deaths

Statistics on fatal and nonfatal firearm injuries include data covering both intentional and unintentional incidents. When one considers all firearm deaths—those that result from both intentional and unintentional acts—firearms were the third leading cause of injury deaths after motor vehicles and poisoning in 2006 (see Figure 15.16).[39] In 2007, there were 31,285 firearm injury deaths. Of these, 17,352 (56%) were classified as suicides, 12,632 (41%) as homicides, 412 (1%) as resulting from legal intervention, and 276 (<1%) were of undetermined intent. Only 613 (<2%) were classified as unintentional deaths. In 2007, firearms were used in 69% of all homicides, 50% of all suicides, and less than 1% of all unintentional injury deaths.[4] Males were six times more likely to die or be treated in an emergency department for a gunshot wound than were females.

At highest risk for homicide and suicide involving firearms are teenage boys and young men, aged 15 to 24 years. A national survey found that in 2008, nearly 10% of high school males had carried a handgun to school at least once in the past year.[19] The gun-toting behavior continues even in college. In a random sample of 10,000 undergraduate students, 4.3% reported that they had a working firearm at college, and 1.6% said they had been threatened with a gun while at college.[40] The banning of firearms on college and university campuses was successfully challenged in Utah where, in 2006, the Utah Supreme Court ruled that the University of Utah cannot bar guns from campus.[41] This decision has raised concern among educators and administrators in institutions of higher education, where campus safety is an ever-present concern. Although there have been heinous and well-publicized violent crimes on campuses, statistics reveal that college and university campuses are much safer than other busy venues. The average homicide rate on American campuses is one homicide per 1 million students. By comparison, the homicide rate in New York City is 70 times greater.[42]

But guns on campus could change this. About 40% of college students binge drink regularly and 85% of campus arrests involve alcohol.[42] Allowing students to possess/carry guns would virtually guarantee that violence on college campuses would become more deadly. Also, college students are under considerable stress, often citing relationship problems, financial matters, or academic or career concerns. The reported suicide ideation rate among college students is estimated at about 10%. More than 50% of suicides involve firearms. Firearms on campus would probably increase the suicide completion rate among college students.

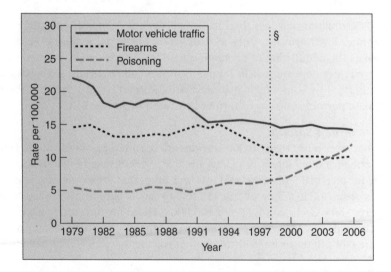

FIGURE 15.16

Firearms were the third leading cause of injury deaths after motor vehicle accidents and poisonings in 2006.

Source: Centers for Disease Control and Prevention (2009). QuickStats: Age-Adjusted Death Rates Per 100,000 Population* for the Three Leading Causes of Injury Death—United States, 1979–2006. *Morbidity and Mortality Weekly Report,* 58(24); 675.

When one compares the ratios of firearm-related fatalities to nonfatal injuries, the lethality of firearms becomes clear. When one looks at injuries from all causes, for each death, nine others are hospitalizations and 189 more are treated and released. When one looks at firearm-related injuries, for each death, only 1.2 people are hospitalized and one person is treated and released (Figure 15.17).

One barrier to preventing firearm injuries and deaths is the absence of a detailed, federally supported reporting system. Unlike the highly developed reporting system for motor vehicle crashes and crash injuries, there is no such system for firearm-related injuries. Until a more comprehensive, national reporting system is in place, the Firearm Injury Surveillance Study, 1993–2004, is the single best source for nonfatal firearm injury data in the United States.[18]

Violence in Our Society and Resources for Prevention

A sixth-grade student brings a gun to school and kills a teacher and three students, a man is killed for "cutting" in line, and a child dies from punishment for breaking a rule at home. These are signs of the violent society in which Americans now find themselves living. Over the past few years, violence in America has increased. Many young people do not have the interest or skills to work out a solution to a conflict through verbal negotiation, and they resort to physical violence to resolve it. Some of these confrontations are gang-related, while

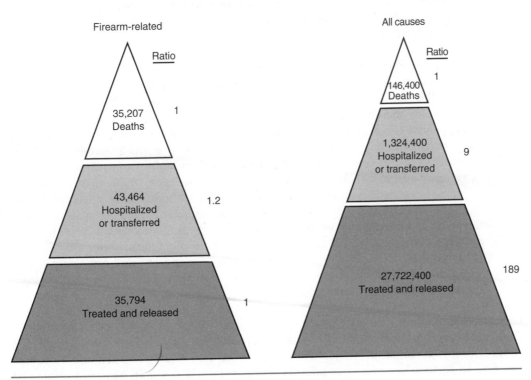

FIGURE 15.17
Injury pyramids for firearm-related injury versus all causes of injury: Firearm injuries are more deadly than other types of injuries.

Source: U.S. Department of Health and Human Services, Centers for Disease Control and Prevention, National Center for Injury Prevention and Control (2006). "Firearm Injury Surveillance Study, 1993–2004 [United States] [Computer File]" (ICPSR04595-V1). Atlanta, GA: Author. Ann Arbor, MI: Inter-university Consortium for Political and Social Research, Distributor. Available at http://webapp.icpsr.umich.edu/cocoon/ICPSR-STUDY/04595.xml. Accessed January 21, 2011.

others are simply individual actions. The availability of firearms in America makes violence all the more deadly, both for those in conflict and for innocent bystanders. In the next sections, we discuss individual, family, and gang violence.

Individuals and Violence

A significant number of violent acts committed in the United States each year are committed by individuals who lack basic communication and problem-solving skills. Many of these people are not interested in resolving an argument through discussion or compromise. Instead, they are intent on "winning" their argument, by physical force if necessary. (After all, isn't that the way arguments are won in the movies?)

The availability and proliferation of firearms makes this approach particularly deadly. In 2001, homicide and legal intervention were the Number 1 cause of death for black Americans aged 15 to 24.[34] Unfortunately, violent confrontations often result in injuries and deaths not only for the victim, but also to others not directly involved in the confrontation.

Because of the level of violence, many schools and community organizations offer conflict resolution programs that teach youth alternative ways to resolve disagreements. These programs are designed for various grade levels and teach about the nature of conflicts, the harmful effects of violence, alternatives to violent behavior, and how to make safe decisions. Some of these programs, aimed specifically at reducing handgun-related violence, are listed in a report by the Office of Juvenile Justice and Delinquency Programs, United States Department of Justice. This report, *Promising Strategies to Reduce Gun Violence*, lists 60 of the more than 400 programs examined that were judged to be successful or "promising" at reducing gun violence.[43]

Family Violence and Abuse

One in every six homicides is the result of family violence. **Family violence** includes the maltreatment of children, intimate partner violence, sibling violence, and violence directed toward elder family members. Because children are our most important resources, and because being abused or neglected as a child increases one's risk for violent behavior as an adult, it is of paramount importance that society increase its efforts to intervene in cases of family violence. In recent years there has been increased attention paid to family violence, including violence against children and intimate partners. Between 1993 and 2001, the victimization rates for intimate partners and children declined. Whereas some might credit this decline to improved efforts by the governmental and nongovernmental agencies involved with intervening and preventing violence among these groups, others would credit it to the strong economy during this period. Lower rates of unemployment mean better financial situations for families, lower levels of stress among family members, and fewer reports of domestic violence. Some social workers may be concerned about how the "Great Recession of 2008–2009" will influence family violence rates.

Child Maltreatment

Child maltreatment is an act or failure to act by a parent, caretaker, or other person as defined under state law that results in physical abuse, neglect, medical neglect, sexual abuse, emotional abuse, or an act or failure to act that presents an imminent risk of serious harm to a child. Also included are other forms of child maltreatment, such as child abandonment and congenital drug addiction. **Child abuse** can be physical, emotional, verbal, or sexual. Physical abuse is the intentional (nonaccidental) inflicting of injury on another person by shaking, throwing, beating, burning, or other means. Emotional abuse can take many forms, including showing no emotion and the failure to provide warmth, attention, supervision, or normal living experiences. Verbal abuse is the demeaning or teasing of another verbally. Sexual abuse includes the physical acts of

family violence the use of physical force by one family member against another, with the intent to hurt, injure, or cause death

child maltreatment an act or failure to act by a parent, caretaker, or other person as defined under state law that results in physical abuse, neglect, medical neglect, sexual abuse, emotional abuse, or an act or failure to act that presents an imminent risk of serious harm to a child

child abuse the intentional physical, emotional, verbal, or sexual mistreatment of a minor

fondling or intercourse, nonphysical acts such as indecent exposure or obscene phone calls, or violent physical acts such as rape and battery. **Child neglect** is a type of maltreatment that refers to the failure by the parent or legal caretaker to provide necessary, age-appropriate care when financially able to do so, or when offered financial or other means to do so. Neglect may be physical, such as the failure to provide food, clothing, medical care, shelter, or cleanliness. It also may be emotional, such as the failure to provide attention, supervision, or other support necessary for a child's well-being (see Figure 15.18). Or, it may be educational, such as the failure to ensure that a child attends school regularly. Educational neglect is one of the most common categories of neglect, followed by physical, and then emotional neglect.

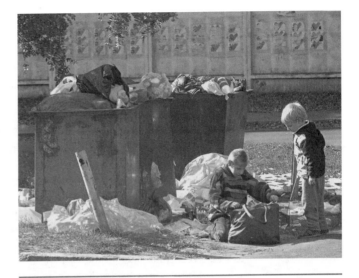

FIGURE 15.18

Child neglect is the failure to provide care or other necessary subsistence for a child.

In 2008, 772,000 children under the age of 18 years were victims of abuse or neglect nationwide at a rate of 10.3 per 1,000 children. Eighty-one percent of the perpetrators were parents. There has been a steady decline from the rate of reported child maltreatment since 1993, when the rate was 15.3 per 1,000 children (see Figure 15.19). Of the 772,000 children who were maltreated in 2008, 71% suffered

child neglect
the failure of a parent or guardian to care for or otherwise provide the necessary subsistence for a child

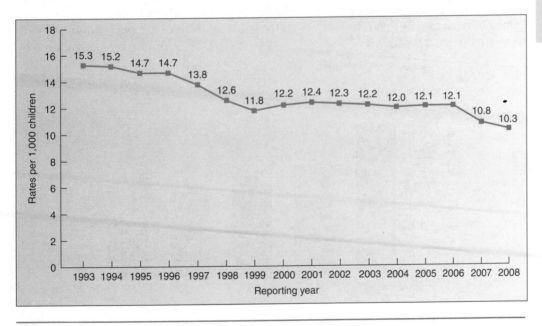

FIGURE 15.19

There has been a fairly steady decline in the child maltreatment rates since 1993 when the rate was 15.3 victims per 1,000 children.

Source: U.S. Department of Health and Human Services, Administration on Children, Youth and Families (2010). *Child Maltreatment 2008.* Available at http://www.acf.hhs.gov/programs/cb/pubs/cm08/cm08.pdf. Accessed January 6, 2011.

neglect, 16% suffered physical abuse, 9% were sexually abused, 7% were psychologically abused, and 2% were medically neglected.[44] In 15% of all cases, other or additional types of maltreatment were reported, including abandonment, threats of harm to the child, and congenital drug addiction. The highest victimization rates were for infants (21.7 maltreatments per 1,000 children under 1 year of age), and these rates decline with age (see Figure 15.20). Rates of many types of maltreatment are the same for males and females, but the sexual abuse rate for female children was higher than the rate for male children. Victimization rates vary by race and ethnicity. In 2008, the lowest rates were for Asian children (2.4 children per 1,000), and the highest rates were for African American children (16.6 children per 1,000), followed by children of multiple races (13.8 per 100,000). Although recurrence of child maltreatment does occur, data reveal that in about 95% of cases, no recurrence occurs in the first 6 months after initial occurrence.[44]

An estimated 1,630 children died of abuse or neglect in 2008, at a rate of approximately 2.36 deaths per 100,000 children. Four-fifths of the fatalities occurred in children under 4 years of age and 45% occurred in infants (see Figure 15.21). Maltreatment deaths were most often associated with neglect.[44]

Children who physically survive maltreatment may be scarred emotionally. "What happens to abused and neglected children after they grow up? Do the victims of violence and neglect later become criminals or violent offenders?"[45] In an attempt to answer these questions, researchers followed 1,575 child victims of abuse and neglect between 1967 and 1971. By the mid-1990s, 49% of the victims had been arrested for some type of nontraffic offense, compared with 38% of the control group (who shared other risk factors such as poverty). Eighteen percent had been arrested for a violent crime, compared with 14% in the control group. These differences were regarded as significant by the researchers. A key finding of the study was that neglected children's rates of arrest for violence were almost as high as physically abused children's. Another key finding was that black individuals who had been abused or neglected as children were being arrested at much higher rates than white individuals with the same background.[45]

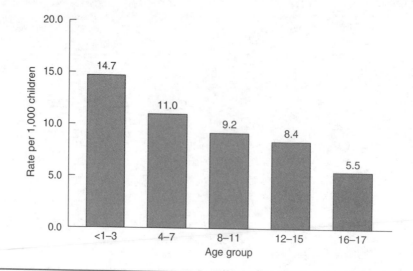

FIGURE 15.20

The highest victimization rates of child maltreatment occur in infants (21.7 per 100,000). Victimization rates decline with increasing age of the victim.

Source: U.S. Department of Health and Human Services, Administration on Children, Youth and Families (2010). *Child Maltreatment 2008.* Available at http://www.acf.hhs.gov/programs/cb/pubs/cm08/cm08.pdf. Accessed January 6, 2011.

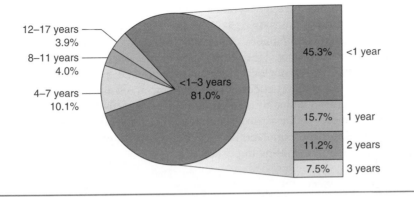

FIGURE 15.21

Percentage of child fatalities resulting from abuse or neglect by age, 2008.

Source: U.S. Department of Health and Human Services, Administration on Children, Youth and Families (2010). *Child Maltreatment 2008.* Available at http://www.acf.hhs.gov/programs/cb/pubs/cm08/cm08.pdf. Accessed January 6, 2011.

Prevention of Child Maltreatment

One of the keys to protecting children from maltreatment is a system of timely reporting and referral to one of the many state and local child protective service (CPS) agencies. Anyone may make such a report (e.g., relative, neighbor, or teacher). In 2008, 58% of child abuse and neglect reports were received from professionals—people who came into contact with the victim through their jobs.[44] Signs of neglect are apparent to the trained professional, such as a teacher, a school nurse, or another community health professional. Signs of neglect include extremes in behavior, an uncared-for appearance, evidence of a lack of supervision at home, or the lack of medical care.

CPS agencies provide services to prevent future instances of child abuse or neglect and to remedy harm that has occurred as a result of child maltreatment.[44] These services are designed to increase the parents' child-rearing competence and knowledge of developmental stages of childhood. There may be an assessment of the family's strengths and weaknesses, the development of a plan based on the family's needs, and post-investigative follow-up services. Services might include respite care, parenting education, housing assistance, substance abuse treatment, day care, home visits, counseling, and other services. The goal is to ensure the safety of the child or children.[44]

There are many useful sources of information and support for those interested in preventing child abuse and neglect. The Child Welfare Information Gateway, sponsored by the Children's Bureau of the U.S. Department of Health and Human Services' Administration for Children and Families provides information, products, and technical assistance services to help professionals locate information related to child abuse and neglect and related child welfare issues (available at www.childwelfare.gov/). Another source of information is the *Committee for Children.* Its mission is to promote the safety, well-being, and social development of children (available at www.cfchildren.org). The *National Foundation for Abused and Neglected Children (NFANC)*, created in 1992, is a nonprofit organization dedicated to the prevention of child abuse and neglect (available at www.gangfreekids.org/).

Elder Maltreatment

There were more than 40 million elders (persons 65 years of age and older) in the United States in 2010.[46] Although elders experience violent crime and thefts at a lower rate than people of other age groups (3.1 per 1,000 population vs. 19.3 per 1,000 for the population as a whole in 2008),[35] between 1 million and 2 million of them have been abused, neglected, exploited, or otherwise mistreated.[47] Women over the age of 75 are particularly vulnerable, and elders over 80 are three times more likely to be abused as are younger elders. More than half of the abusers are family members, either adult children or other relatives.[48]

Abuse can be physical, sexual, psychological or emotional, or financial, or may involve abandonment, neglect, or self-neglect. Elders may be kicked, hit, denied food and medical care, or have their Social Security checks or other financial resources stolen or otherwise misappropriated. Most cases of elder abuse are not reported or only become apparent following other legal or medical proceedings; thus, accurate statistics on the incidence of elder abuse are unavailable. As the American population ages, elder maltreatment is likely to become a community health problem of increasing importance.

Intimate Partner Violence

intimate partner violence (IPV)
rape, physical assault, or stalking perpetrated by current or former dates, spouses, or cohabiting partners

Intimate partner violence (IPV) can be defined as rape, physical assault, and stalking perpetrated by current and former dates, spouses, and cohabiting partners (cohabiting meaning living together at least some of the time as a couple).[49] Each year countless women and men are victimized by their intimate partners. About 552,000 females age 12 or older experienced nonfatal violent victimization (rape/sexual assault, robbery, or aggravated or simple assault) by an intimate partner in 2008.[50] Sometimes intimate partner violence is deadly. In 2008, 1,640 women and 440 men were murdered by an intimate partner.[50] Fifty-seven percent of rapes and sexual assaults against females were committed by an offender whom they knew, 20% by an intimate partner.[50] Injuries to women from intimate partner physical violence are underreported, but more than 500,000 women injured as a result of IPV require medical treatment each year. Women spend more days in bed, miss more work, and suffer more from stress and depression than men. The health care costs of intimate partner rape, physical assault, and stalking exceed $5.8 billion each year.[51]

One in four women residing in the United States has been physically assaulted or raped by an intimate partner; one of 14 men has reported such an experience.[51] Women are also more likely than men to be murdered by an intimate partner. From 2007, 45% of all women who were murdered were killed by an intimate partner, whereas only 5% of male murder victims were killed by an intimate partner.[50] Each year, thousands of American children witness IPV within their families. Witnessing such violence is a risk factor for developing long-term physical and mental health problems, including alcohol and substance abuse, becoming a victim of abuse, and perpetrating IPV.[51]

Despite the grim statistics just presented, the rates of victimization by an intimate partner have declined since 1993, when the rates were 9.8 per 1,000 for females and 1.6 per 1,000 for males. In 2008, these rates were 4.3 per 1,000 for females and 0.8 per 1,000 for males.[50]

Risk factors for women who are likely to experience IPV include having a family income below $10,000, being young (19–29 years of age), and living with an intimate partner who uses alcohol or other drugs. Another risk factor is a previous episode of abuse. In a dysfunctional relationship, the male intimate partner may seek to exert power and control over his female intimate partner, resulting in a cycle in which violence recurs (see Figure 15.22). The *cycle of violence* depicts the progression of steps leading up to an attack or episode of violence and the restoration of calm. A violent episode may result from the loss of a job, a divorce, illness, death of a family member, or misbehavior (actual or perceived) of children or an intimate partner. The likelihood that abuse will occur is greatly increased if alcohol has been consumed. While selected interventions aimed at one factor (for example, the abuser) might mitigate against family violence, community efforts to reduce violence should be both comprehensive, involving a variety of approaches, and coordinated among all agencies involved in order to be effective.

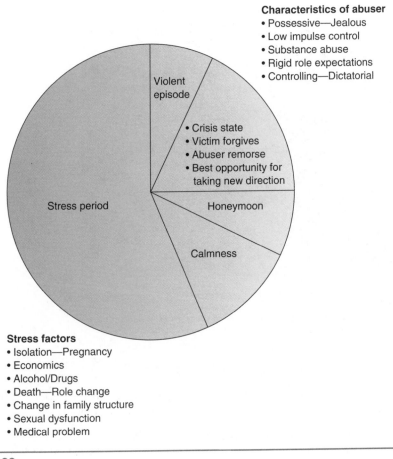

Characteristics of abuser
- Possessive—Jealous
- Low impulse control
- Substance abuse
- Rigid role expectations
- Controlling—Dictatorial

Violent episode

- Crisis state
- Victim forgives
- Abuser remorse
- Best opportunity for taking new direction

Stress period

Honeymoon

Calmness

Stress factors
- Isolation—Pregnancy
- Economics
- Alcohol/Drugs
- Death—Role change
- Change in family structure
- Sexual dysfunction
- Medical problem

FIGURE 15.22

Cycle of violence.

Source: Domestic Abuse Intervention Project in Duluth, Minnesota, as reported in the *AHEC News*, a publication of the Area Health Education Centers of Oklahoma, *AHEC News* (February 1994), 2(1): 9. Used with permission.

Prevention of Intimate Partner Violence

Prevention of IPV involves improvements in identifying and documenting cases of IPV and increasing access to services for victims and perpetrators of IPV and their children. Coordinating community initiatives strengthens the safety networks for high-risk individuals and families. Some communities have established a "Violence Coordinating Council" that holds monthly meetings to set an agenda and action plans for the community and to determine and clarify the roles and responsibilities of agencies and individuals. It is important for communities to develop and implement a coordinated response with strong advocates from criminal justice, victim services, children's services, and allied professions. One of the important groups of allied professionals are health care providers. Educational materials and programs on IPV and sexual assault are available at the National Center for Injury Prevention and Control Web site (www.cdc.gov/injury/).

Violence in Schools

Although schools are one of the safest places for children to spend their time (see Figure 15.23), even rare acts of violence strike terror into parents, teachers, and the children themselves.

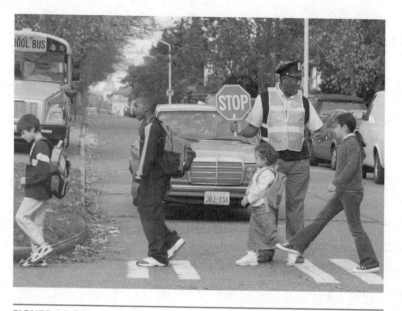

FIGURE 15.23

Despite several highly publicized tragic events, schools are one of the safest places for students to spend time.

Highly publicized incidents of fatal shootings on school grounds have focused the nation's attention on the question of just how safe (or unsafe) our nation's schools are.

> Our nation's schools should be safe havens for teaching and learning, free of crime and violence. Any instance of crime or violence at school not only affects the individuals involved but also may disrupt the educational process and affect bystanders, the school itself, and the surrounding community.[52]

The National Center for Educational Statistics (NCES), Institute of Education Sciences (IES), in the U.S. Department of Education, and the Bureau of Justice Statistics (BJS) in the U.S. Department of Justice jointly collect and publish data annually on the frequency, seriousness, and incidence of violence in elementary and secondary schools.[53] During the 2007–2008 school year, 43 student, staff, and nonstudent, school-associated violent deaths were recorded, including 21 homicides and 5 suicides of youth aged 5–18 years at school. The percentage of homicides of youths at school has remained less that 2% of all youth homicides, and the percentage of youth suicides has remained less than 1% of all youth suicides occurring nationwide. This amounts to about 1 homicide or suicide per 2.1 million students enrolled during the 2007–2008 school year. In 2007, among students aged 12–18 years, there were about 1.5 million victims of nonfatal crimes at school, including 826,800 thefts and 684,100 violent crimes (simple assault and serious violent crime). During 2007–2008, 85% of public schools recorded that one or more incidents of crime had occurred at their school, and 75% reported one or more violent incidents of violent crime.[53]

There has been an overall decline in victimization rates at school for students aged 12–18 years, but most of that decline occurred before 2004; victimization rates have remained steady during the past 3 years at about 4% of students. Theft was reported by 3%, violent victimization by 2%, and serious violent victimization by less than 0.5%. Although student victimization rates remained unchanged in 2004–2007, an increase has been noticed in teachers reporting being threatened. The percentage of teachers who reported being threatened varied by type of school—10% in city schools, 7% in town schools, and 6% in rural schools and suburban schools.[53]

Fighting and weapon carrying are also concerns. In 2007, more than one-third of students in grades 9–12 reported they had been in a fight during the previous year, 12% on school property. Eighteen percent reported having carried a weapon in the past 30 days, 6% on school property. Three times as many males reported carrying a weapon as did females.[53] As stated earlier, 9.8% of males in grades 9–12 reported carrying a gun to school in the past 30 days in 2009.[19]

Most schools try to deal with violence problems by instituting zero tolerance policies toward serious student offenses. These policies, defined as school or district policy mandating predetermined consequences for various student offenses, have recently come under fire because administering such policies sometimes leads to somewhat ridiculous outcomes. In 2007–2008, almost all schools also utilized some type of security measures, such as requiring visitor sign-ins (99%), controlling access to school buildings during school hours (90%), establishing electronic notification systems for school-wide emergencies (43%), and implementing structured anonymous threats systems (31%). Only 1% of schools required students to pass through metal detectors daily. School safety and security practices are becoming more widespread. More schools are requiring student, faculty, and staff identification badges; placing telephones in classrooms; requiring students to wear uniforms; and drug testing more students involved in athletics and other extracurricular activities.[53]

Bullying and being bullied at school are increasingly being recognized as associated with violence-related behavior (such as carrying a weapon to school, fighting, or becoming injured in a fight). Bullying includes being made fun of; being made the subject of rumors; being threatened with harm; being pushed, shoved, tripped, or spat on; being pressured to do something one does not want to do; being excluded, or having one's property destroyed. In 2007, 32% of 12- to 18-year-olds reported having been bullied at school within the past 6 months.[53]

Safe Schools/Healthy Students Initiative

The *Safe Schools/Healthy Students Initiative* is a unique grant program jointly administered by the U.S. Departments of Education, Health and Human Services, and Justice. The program promotes a comprehensive, integrated problem-solving process for use by communities in addressing school violence. "Since 1999, more than 240 urban, rural, suburban, and tribal school districts—in collaboration with local mental health and juvenile justice providers—have received grants using a single application process."[54] Steps in the process are as follows:

1. Establishing school–community partnerships
2. Identifying and measuring the problem
3. Setting measurable goals and objectives
4. Identifying appropriate research-based programs and strategies
5. Implementing programs and strategies in an integrated fashion
6. Evaluating the outcomes of programs and strategies
7. Revising the plan on the basis of evaluation information

The initiative requires comprehensive, integrated community-wide plans to address at least the following six elements:[54]

1. A safe school environment
2. Alcohol and other drugs and violence prevention and early intervention programs
3. School and community mental health preventive and treatment intervention services
4. Early childhood psychosocial and emotional development services

5. Supporting and connecting schools and communities (2004–present grantees); education reform (1999–2003 grantees)
6. Safe school policies

Youth Violence after School

Although violence in schools has grabbed the headlines, the real problem area is violence after school. Fewer and fewer children have a parent waiting for them at home after school. Whereas many youths are able to supervise themselves and their younger siblings responsibly after school or are engaged in sports or other after-school activities, some are not. Statistics show that serious violent crime committed by juveniles peaks in the hours immediately after school (see Figure 15.24). Also, during these after-school hours, juveniles are most likely to become victims of crime, including violent crimes such as robberies and aggravated assaults. This is because at this unsupervised time, youth are more vulnerable to exploitation, injuries, and even death.[55]

For communities that want to become involved in reducing the problem of youth violence, the federal government has a variety of resources. One of these is *Best Practices of Youth Violence Prevention: A Sourcebook for Community Action*.[56] In addition, the federal government has established a Web site, www.afterschool.gov, that provides resources for communities that wish to develop after-school programs for youths.[57] The Web site provides links to successful after-school programs, ideas for after-school activities, and Web sites for youths to visit after school. Additional information and resources are available at the National Center for Injury Prevention and Control's Web site.[58]

Violence in Our Communities

Youth gangs and gang violence contribute to the overall level of violence in the community and are a drain on community resources.

Youth Gang Violence

Whereas most young women and men in the United States grow up subscribing to such American ideals as democracy, individualism, equality, and education, others do not. Many of those who do not are economically disadvantaged and have lost faith in society's capacity to

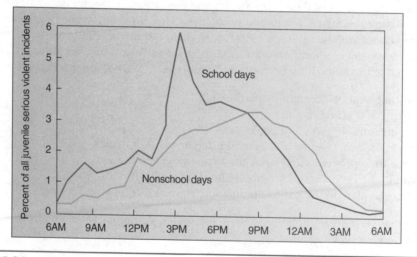

FIGURE 15.24

Serious violent crime committed by juveniles peaks in the hours immediately after school.

Source: U.S. Department of Justice, Office of Justice Programs, Office of Juvenile Justice and Delinquency Prevention (1999). *Violence After School, 1999 National Report Series, November 2000*. Washington, DC: Author.

work on their behalf. Some of these seek refuge and reward in organized subculture groups of youngsters who feel similarly disenfranchised.

One popular subculture structure is the **youth gang**, a self-formed association of peers bound together by mutual interests, with identifiable leadership and well-defined lines of authority. Youth gangs act in concert to achieve a specific purpose, and their acts generally include illegal activities and the control over a particular territory or enterprise. Types of illegal activities in which gang members participate include larceny/theft, aggravated assault, burglary/breaking and entering, and street drug sales.

A recent survey of a representative sample of 3,330 law enforcement agencies revealed youth gang activity in 32% of the districts under their jurisdiction. This is a significant decline since 1996, when 53% of jurisdictions reported youth gang activity. An estimated 27,900 gangs were active in the United States in 2008. Gang activity is more prevalent in cities with a population of 250,000 or greater. There were more than 774,000 active gang members in 2008.[59]

> **youth gang**
> an association of peers, bound by mutual interests and identifiable lines of authority, whose acts generally include illegal activity and control over a territory or an enterprise

Costs to the Community

Youth gangs and youth-gang-related violence present an enormous drain on the law enforcement resources of a community beyond the injuries and injury deaths that result from their activities. Pressured to "do something," field officers may be pulled from other duties and not replaced. If additional police are hired, it can cost the community $50,000 per year per officer. Next, there is the additional need to strengthen the prosecutor's office if the operation is to be effective. In short, the suppression of gangs by law enforcement is costly for communities, often depleting resources for other needed community improvements.

Another problem is vandalism and the defacing of public and private buildings by gang-related graffiti. This money spent repairing damage and erasing graffiti could be used to hire teachers or to support educational activities.

Community Response

Many communities have responded effectively to the increased violence resulting from gang-related activity. Perhaps the best approach is a multifaceted effort involving law enforcement, education, diversion activities, and social services support. Suppression of gang activity by law enforcement is justified because many gang-related activities—such as selling illicit drugs, carrying and discharging weapons, and defacing property—are illegal. Education of children, teachers, parents, and community leaders is another facet of gang-related violence prevention. Just as there are drug abuse prevention curricula in schools, there are now anti-gang awareness programs in some schools. Diversion activities, including job opportunities and after-school activities such as enrichment programs, sports, and recreation, can reduce the attractiveness of less wholesome uses of free time. Sports and recreational activities have long been touted as a healthy outlet for pent-up physical energy. It seems logical to assume that young persons who participate in such activities would be less likely to become involved in destructive, violent behavior (see Figure 15.25).

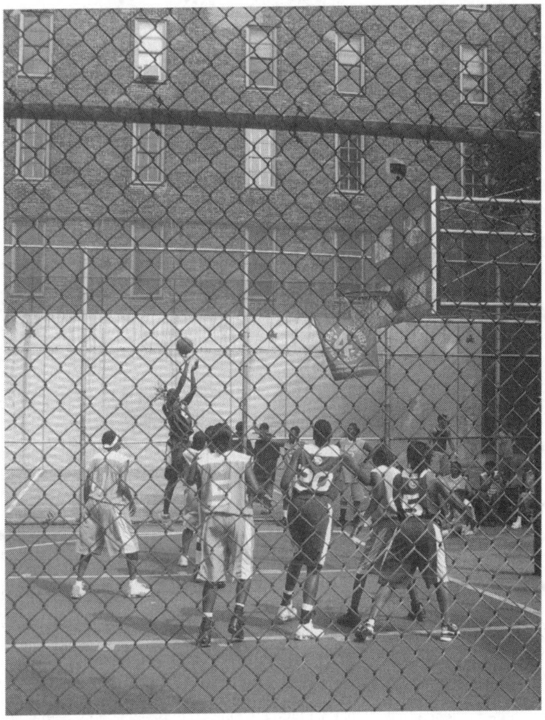

FIGURE 15.25
Adequate recreational opportunities for youth can reduce violence in a community.

State Response

Most, if not all, states have agencies with programs aimed at preventing or reducing the level of injuries caused by intentional violence. By searching the Internet using the words "injury prevention" or "violence prevention," and "state," one can find many of these state-funded agencies and programs. Many of the agencies or programs are concerned with both unintentional and intentional injury prevention. For example, one agency might include programs for child occupant safety, older driver safety, residential fire prevention, domestic violence, or violence against women programs, youth violence prevention, suicide prevention, and so on, with links to other injury prevention and control agency Web sites. Funding sources for these programs are variable. Some are funded as line items on state budgets; other programs are grant driven.

Federal Response

Several federal agencies house programs aimed at preventing or reducing the number and seriousness of intentional and unintentional injuries. The Centers for Disease Control and Prevention, in the Department of Health and Human Services, has a Web site that provides links to a vast array of programs specifically aimed at preventing injury and violence and promoting safety (www.cdc.gov/InjuryViolenceSafety/).[60] Programs and topics are wide-ranging, from child abuse/maltreatment, to dog bites, to falls among older adults, to youth violence, just to name a few.

The Office of Justice Programs is another federal agency whose mission includes improving public safety by supporting law enforcement and the justice system.[61] The agency monitors crime and victimization, gang-related activity, substance abuse and crime, juvenile justice, and the corrections system. The Office of Justice Programs offers a variety of programs to state and local agencies aimed at reducing intentional violence. Included are programs to empower communities (Community Prosecution, Safe Schools Initiative, Safe Start, Weed and Seed, and Offender Reentry). There are also programs aimed at breaking the cycle of drug abuse and crime (the Drug Free Communities Program, the Drug Prevention Demonstration Program, and Enforcing Underage Drinking). Other programs combat family violence, violence against women, and violence on college campuses. Still others address youth violence and protect and support victims of crime. The purpose of these programs is to support communities in their efforts to reduce intentional violence and violence-related injuries.[62]

Injuries, including intentional injuries, are a worldwide problem, but here in the United States, firearm availability is much greater than in most other countries. Legislative attempts aimed at making it more difficult for certain persons to acquire hand guns and/or automatic weapons have failed to reduce the level of firearm injuries and deaths.[63] Some local governments have banned guns in their jurisdictions in an effort to reduce the frequency of firearm injuries. However, many of these bans are now in jeopardy. In June 2010, the Supreme Court ruled 5–4 that the Second Amendment applies to states and city governments in regard to gun laws and ended a nearly 30-year handgun ban in the city of Chicago.

In conclusion, intentional injuries resulting from interpersonal violence remain a national as well as a community concern. Significant resources are available at the federal level (from the Departments of Health and Human Services and Justice) to help states and local communities reduce the number and seriousness of violence-related injuries. It is up to each concerned citizen to make sure that his or her own community is taking advantage of these resources.

CHAPTER SUMMARY

- Injuries are the fifth leading cause of death in the United States.

- Unintentional and intentional injuries represent a major community health problem, not only because of the loss of life but also because of lost productivity, medical costs, and the increase in the number of disabled Americans.

- Unintentional injuries are unplanned events that are usually preceded by an unsafe act or condition. They are often accompanied by economic loss, and they interrupt the efficient completion of a task.

- More fatal and nonfatal unintentional injuries occur in the home than at any other location.

- Unintentional injuries occur across all age groups; however, they are the leading cause of death for younger Americans.

- Motor vehicle accidents are the leading cause of unintentional injury deaths, followed by poisonings, falls, fires and burns, and drownings.

- Males and certain minority groups suffer proportionately more unintentional injuries.

- Prevention and control of unintentional injuries and fatalities can be instituted based on a model in which energy is the causative agent for injuries.

- There are also four broad strategies that can prevent unintentional injuries—education, regulation, automatic protection, and litigation. Together, these strategies may be used to reduce the numbers and seriousness of unintentional injuries in the community.

- Intentional injuries are the outcome of self-directed or interpersonal violence.

- The spectrum of violence includes assaults, rapes, robberies, suicides, homicides, and the maltreatment of children, elders, and intimate partners.

- Minorities and young adults are at highest risk for injury or death from an intentional violent act.

- Family violence, including child and elder maltreatment, and intimate partner violence, is a serious and pervasive community health problem.

- Widely publicized fatal shootings in schools have once again focused national attention on violence in our schools. However, schools remain a relatively safe place for the nation's youth.

- Youth violence, including youth gang violence, grew in the 1990s but has since declined, in part because of federal, state, and local initiatives to address this problem.

- Significant resources are available at the state and federal levels (from the Departments of Health and Human Services and Justice) to assist local communities in reducing the number and seriousness of violence-related injuries.

REVIEW QUESTIONS

1. List the ways in which injuries are costly to society and quantify the costs in terms of the United States.

2. Identify the leading types of unintentional injury deaths and the risk factors associated with each type of death.

3. Why have the terms *accident* and *safety* lost favor with injury prevention professionals?

4. What is a hazard? Do hazards cause accidents? Explain your answer.

5. What types of injuries are most likely to occur in the home, and in which rooms are they most likely to occur?

6. Characterize injuries from the following activities by time—motor vehicle driving, swimming, and heating the home.

7. How does alcohol consumption contribute to unintentional injuries?

8. Summarize the contributions of Hugh DeHaven, John E. Gordon, and William Haddon, Jr., to injury prevention and control.

9. Describe the epidemiological model for injuries and provide three examples of how energy causes injuries.

10. For each of your examples from Question 9, explain how the injury could have been prevented using prevention and control tactics.

11. List four broad strategies for the reduction of unintentional injuries and give an example of each.

12. Identify the different types of violent behavior that result in intentional injuries.

13. Describe the cost of intentional injuries to society.

14. Define *family violence* and give some examples.

15. Explain the difference between child abuse and child neglect. List some contributing factors to these phenomena. What is intimate partner violence?

16. How safe are our schools? How are schools responding to safety concerns?

17. What is a youth gang? Why are they attractive to some youths? How can communities compete for youths' attention?

18. Describe the best ways in which communities can respond to youth gang violence.

SCENARIO: ANALYSIS AND RESPONSE

Please take a moment to reread the scenario at the beginning of this chapter. Then, reflect on the questions that follow.

1. How does the description of the unintentional injury fit the definition provided in the chapter? Can you identify each element of the definition as it pertains to this particular scenario?

2. Think about the four approaches to the prevention of unintentional injuries (education, regulation, automatic protection, and litigation). Provide an example of how each of these four approaches could prevent another similar injury from occurring.

---

19. What resources are available at the state and federal levels to help communities reduce the number and seriousness of injuries?

ACTIVITIES

1. Obtain a copy of a local newspaper and find three stories dealing with unintentional injuries. Provide a two- or three-sentence summary of each article and then provide your best guess of (a) what the unsafe act or condition that preceded the event was, (b) what the resulting economic loss or injury was, and (c) what task was not completed.

2. Make an appointment and interview the director of safety on your campus. Find out what the most prevalent unintentional injuries are on campus, what strategies have been used to deal with them, and what could be done to eliminate them.

3. With guidance from your course instructor, conduct a random survey of safety belt use at your campus. Collect the data in such a manner that you can compare the results between school employees and students. Then, analyze your results and draw some conclusions.

4. Survey your home, apartment, or residence hall and create a room-by-room list of the unsafe conditions that may exist. Then, create a strategy for changing each condition.

5. Using a local newspaper, locate three articles that deal with violence. For each article, (a) provide a two-sentence summary, (b) identify and describe the victim and the perpetrator, (c) identify what you feel was the underlying cause of the violence, and (d) offer a suggestion as to how the violence could have been avoided or prevented.

6. Make an appointment with an officer of the local police department to interview him or her about violent crime

in your hometown. Write a two-page summary of your interview and include answers to the following questions: (a) What is the Number 1 violent crime? (b) What is the law enforcement department doing to control violent crime? (c) Does the city have a comprehensive program against crime? (d) What can the typical citizen do to help reduce violence?

7. Write a two-page paper on what the typical citizen can do about violence.

8. Think about the public health triangle model of disease (agent, host, and environment) and gang violence. Describe in writing who or what represents each of these factors. What steps can be taken to reduce gang-related violence using this public health model? List the steps explaining each one.

COMMUNITY HEALTH ON THE WEB

The Internet contains a wealth of information about community and public health. Increase your knowledge of some of the topics presented in this chapter by accessing the Jones & Bartlett Learning Web site at **http://health .jbpub.com/book/communityhealth/7e** and follow the links to complete the following Web activities.

- National Center for Injury Prevention and Control
- Family Violence Prevention Fund
- Children's Safety Network

REFERENCES

1. Baker, S. P. (1989). "Injury Science Comes of Age." *Journal of the American Medical Association*, 262(16): 2284–2285.

2. Miniño, A. M., and R. N. Anderson (2006). "Deaths: Injuries, 2002." *National Vital Statistics Reports*, 54(10): 1–128.

3. Lopez, A. D., C. D. Mathers, M. Ezzati, D. T. Jamison, and C. Murray (2006). *Global Burden of Disease and Risk Factors*. New York: World Bank and Oxford University Press.

4. Xu, J., K. D. Kochanek, S. L. Murphy, and B. Tejada-Vera (2010). "Deaths: Final Data for 2007." *National Vital Statistics Reports*, 59(19):

1-73. Available at http://www.cdc.gov/nchs/data/nvsr/nvsr58/nvsr58_19.pdf.

5. Adams, P. F., K. M. Hayman, and J. L. Vickerie (2009). "Summary Health Statistics for the U.S. Population: National Health Interview Survey, 2008." *Vital Health Statistics*, 10(243): 1-105. Available at http://www.cdc.gov/nchs/data/series/sr_10/sr10_243.pdf.

6. National Safety Council (2010). *Injury Facts 2010 Edition*. Itasca, IL: Author.

7. DeFrances, C. J., C. A. Lucas, V. C. Buie, and A. Golosinskiy (30 July 2008). "2006 National Hospital Discharge Survey." *National Health Statistics Reports*, 5. Available at http://www.cdc.gov/nchs/data/nhsr/nhsr005.pdf.

8. National Center for Health Statistics (2009). *Health, United States, 2009 with Special Feature on Medical Technology*. Hyattsville, MD: National Center for Health Statistics. Available at http://www.cdc.gov/nchs/hus.htm.

9. Heron, M., D. L. Hoyert, S. L. Murphy, J. Xu, K. D. Kochanek, and B. Tejada-Vera (2009). "Deaths: Final Data for 2006." *National Vital Statistics Reports*, 57(14): 1-136.

10. Pitts, S. R., R. W. Niska, J. Xu, and C. W. Burt (2008). "National Hospital Ambulatory Medical Care Survey: 2006 Emergency Department Summary." *National Health Statistics Reports*, 7.

11. U.S. Department of Health and Human Services, Office of Disease Prevention and Promotion (2010). *Healthy People 2020*. Available at http://www.healthypeople.gov/2020/default.aspx.

12. U.S. Department of Health and Human Services (2009). *Data 2010: The Healthy People 2010 Database*. Available at http://wonder.cdc.gov/data2010/focus.htm.

13. Peden, M., R. Scurfield, D. A. Sleet, D. Hohan, A. A. Hyder, E. Jarawan, and C. Mathers, eds. (2004). *World Report on Road Traffic Injury and Prevention*. Geneva, Switzerland: World Health Organization.

14. U.S. Department of Transportation, National Highway Traffic Safety Administration (2009). *Traffic Safety Facts 2008: A Compilation of Motor Vehicle Crash Data from the Fatality Analysis Reporting System and the General Estimates System* (DOT HS 811 170). Washington, DC: U.S. DOT. Available at http://www-nrd.nhtsa.dot.gov/Pubs/811170.PDF.

15. Centers for Disease Control and Prevention (2006). "Fatalities and Injuries from Falls among Older Adults—United States, 1993-2003 and 2001-2005." *Morbidity and Mortality Weekly Report*, 55(45): 1221-1224.

16. Centers for Disease Control and Prevention (2003). "Public Health and Aging: Nonfatal Injuries among Older Adults Treated in Hospital Emergency Departments—United States, 2001." *Morbidity and Mortality Weekly Report*, 52(42): 1019-1022.

17. Anderson, R. H., and B. L. Smith (2005). "Deaths: Leading Causes for 2002." *National Vital Statistics Reports*, 53(17): 1-92.

18. U.S. Department of Health and Human Services, Centers for Disease Control and Prevention, National Center for Injury Prevention and Control (2006). "Firearm Injury Surveillance Study, 1993-2004 [United States] [Computer file]" (ICPSR04595-V1). Atlanta, GA: Author. Ann Arbor, MI: Inter-university Consortium for Political and Social Research, distributor. Available at http://webapp.icpsr.umich.edu/cocoon/ICPSR-STUDY/04595.xml.

19. Centers for Disease Control and Prevention (2010). "Youth Risk Behavior Surveillance—United States, 2009." *Morbidity and Mortality Weekly Report*, 59(SS-5): 1-146. Available at http://www.cdc.gov/mmwr/pdf/ss/ss5905.pdf.

20. Centers for Disease Control and Prevention (1997). "Rates of Homicide, Suicide and Firearm-Related Deaths among Children—26 Industrial Countries." *Morbidity and Mortality Weekly Report*, 46(5): 101-105.

21. Griffin III, L. I. (2004). *Older Driver Involvement in Injury Crashes in Texas, 1975-1999*. Washington, DC: AAA Foundation for Traffic Safety. Available at http://www.aaafoundation.org/e-news/issue7/seniorcrashes.cfm.

22. Griffin, L. I., and S. DeLaZerda (2000). *Unlicensed to Kill*. Washington, DC: AAA Foundation for Traffic Safety. Available at www.aaafoundation.org/pdf/unlicensed2kill.pdf.

23. Centers for Disease Control and Prevention (2004). "Child Passenger Deaths Involving Drinking Drivers—United States, 1997-2002." *Morbidity and Mortality Weekly Report*, 53(4): 77-79.

24. U.S. Department of Homeland Security, U.S. Coast Guard (2009). *Boating Statistics—2008* (COMDTPUB P16754.19). Available at http://www.uscgboating.org/assets/1/Publications/Boating_Statistics_2008.pdf.

25. U.S. Department of Homeland Security, U.S. Coast Guard (2000). *Boating Statistics—1999* (COMDTPUB P16754.16). Available at http://www.uscgboating.org/assets/1/Publications/Boating_Statistics_1999.pdf.

26. Centers for Disease Control and Prevention (2001). "Drowning—Louisiana, 1998." *Morbidity and Mortality Weekly Report*, 50(20): 413-414.

27. Christoffel, T., and S. S. Gallagher (2006). *Injury Prevention and Public Health: Practical Knowledge, Skills, and Strategies*, 2nd ed. Sudbury, MA: Jones & Bartlett.

28. Centers for Disease Control and Prevention (2010). "Effectiveness of 0.08% Blood Alcohol Concentration (BAC) Laws." *Guide to Community Preventive Services*. Available at http://www.thecommunityguide.org/mvoi/AID/BAC-laws.html.

29. AAA Foundation for Traffic Safety (2009). *2009 Traffic Safety Culture Index*. Washington, DC: Author. Available at http://www.aaafoundation.org/pdf/2009TSCIndexFinalReport.pdf.

30. Vermette, E. (2010). *Curbing Distracted Driving: 2010 Survey of State Safety Programs*. Washington, DC: Governors Highway Safety Association. Available at http://www.ghsa.org/html/publications/survey/index.html.

31. Governors Highway Safety Association (n.d.). Web site. Available at http://www.ghsa.org.

32. Waller, P. F. (2002). "Challenges in Motor Vehicle Safety." *Annual Review of Public Health*, 23: 93-113.

33. Centers for Disease Control and Prevention (1982). "Unintentional and Intentional Injuries—United States." *Morbidity and Mortality Weekly Report*, 31(18): 240-248.

34. Centers for Disease Control and Prevention (2010). "Welcome to WISQARS." Available at http://www.cdc.gov/injury/wisqars/index.html.

35. Rand, M. R. (2009). "Criminal Victimization, 2008." *National Crime Victimization Survey* (NCJ 227777). Washington, DC: U.S. Department of Justice, Bureau of Justice Statistics. Available at http://bjs.ojp.usdoj.gov/content/pub/pdf/cv08.pdf.

36. Fox, J. A., and M. W. Zawitz (2006). *Homicide Trends in the United States*. Washington, DC: U.S. Department of Justice, Bureau of Justice Statistics. Available at http://bjs.ojp.usdoj.gov/content/pub/pdf/htius.pdf.

37. Federal Bureau of Investigation (2009). "2008 Crime in the United States: Expanded Homicide Data." Available at http://www2.fbi.gov/ucr/cius2008/documents/expandedhomicidemain.pdf.

38. Blumstein, A., F. P. Rivara, and R. Rosenfeld (2000). "The Rise and Decline of Homicide—and Why." *Annual Review of Public Health*, 21: 505-541.

39. Centers for Disease Control and Prevention (2009). "QuickStats: Age-Adjusted Death Rates per 100,000 Population for the Three Leading Causes of Injury Death—United States, 1979-2006." *Morbidity and Mortality Weekly Report*, 58(24): 675.

40. Miller, M., D. Hemenway, and H. Wechsler. (2002). "Guns and Gun Threats at College." *Journal of American College Health*, 51(2): 57-65.

41. Jaschik, S. (2006). "Gun Rights vs. College Rights." *Inside Higher Ed*. Available at http://www.insidehighered.com/news/2006/09/11/guns.

42. Schwartz, V., J. Kay, and P. Appelbaum. (12 May 2010). "Keep Guns off College Campuses." *Huffington Post*. Available at http://www.huffingtonpost.com/victor-schwartz/keep-guns-off-college-cam_b_573634.html.

43. Office of Juvenile Justice and Delinquency Programs, U.S. Department of Justice (n. d.). *Promising Strategies to Reduce Gun Violence*. Available at http://ojjdp.ncjrs.org/pubs/gun%5Fviolence/contents.html.

44. U.S. Department of Health and Human Services, Administration on Children, Youth and Families (2010). *Child Maltreatment 2008*. Available at http://www.acf.hhs.gov/programs/cb/pubs/cm08/cm08.pdf.

45. National Institute of Justice (1996). *The Cycle of Violence Revisited.* Washington, DC: U.S. Department of Justice.

46. U.S. Census Bureau (2010). "U.S. Population Projections." Available at http://www.census.gov/population/www/projections/2008projections.html.

47. Bonnie, R. J., and R. B. Wallace (2003). National Research Council. *Elder Mistreatment: Abuse, Neglect, and Exploitation in an Aging America.* Washington, DC: National Academies Press.

48. Teaster, P. B., T. A. Dugar, M. S. Mendiondo, E. L. Abner, and K. A. Cecil (2006). *The 2004 Survey of State Adult Protective Services: Abuse of Adults 60 Years of Age and Older.* National Committee for the Prevention of Elder Abuse and National Adult Protective Services Administration. Available at http://www.ncea.aoa.gov/ncearoot/Main_Site/pdf/APS_2004NCEASurvey.pdf.

49. Catalano, S., E. Smith, H. Snyder, and M. Rand (2009). "Female Victims of Violence." *Bureau of Justice Statistics, Selected Findings*, NCJ 228356. Available at http://bjs.ojp.usdoj.gov/content/pub/pdf/fvv.pdf.

50. Catalano, S. (2006). "Intimate Partner Violence in the United States." Data from the Bureau of Justice Statistics, U.S. Department of Justice, Office of Justice Programs. Available at http://www.ojp.usdoj.gov/content/intimate/ipv.cfm.

51. Centers for Disease Control and Prevention, National Center for Injury Control and Prevention (2009). *Understanding Intimate Partner Violence* [Fact Sheet]. Available at http://www.cdc.gov/violence prevention/pdf/IPV_factsheet-a.pdf.

52. Henry, S. (2000). "What Is School Violence? An Integrated Definition." *Annals of the American Academy of Political and Social Science*, 567: 16–29. As cited in U.S. Department of Education, National Center for Education Statistics (2007) "Indicators of School Crime and Safety: 2006" (NCES 2007-003).

53. Dinkes, R., J. Kemp, and K. Baum (2009). *Indicators of School Crime and Safety: 2009* (NCES 2010–012/NCJ 228478). Washington, DC: National Center for Education Statistics, Institute of Education Sciences, U.S. Department of Education, and Bureau of Justice Statistics, Office of Justice Programs, U.S. Department of Justice. Available at http://nces.ed.gov/programs/crimeindicators/crimeindicators2009/.

54. Substance Abuse and Mental Health Services Administration, Department of Health and Human Services (2006). "About the Safe Schools/Healthy Students (SS/HS) Initiative." Available at http://www.sshs.samhsa.gov/initiative/about.aspx.

55. U.S. Department of Justice, Office of Juvenile Justice and Delinquency Prevention (1999). *Violence After School* (1999 National Report Series). Washington, DC: Author.

56. Thornton, T. N., C. A. Craft, L. L. Dahlberg, B. S. Lynch, and K. Baer (2002). *Youth Violence: Best Practices of Youth Violence Prevention: A Sourcebook for Community Action.* Atlanta, GA: Centers for Disease Control and Prevention, National Center for Injury Prevention and Control. Available at http://www.cdc.gov/violenceprevention/pub/YV_bestpractices.html.

57. U.S. Department of Health and Human Services, Administration for Children and Families (n.d.). Web site. Available at http://www.afterschool.gov.

58. Centers for Disease Control and Prevention, National Center for Injury Prevention and Control (2007). "Youth Violence: Prevention Strategies." Available at http://www.cdc.gov/ncipc/factsheets/yvprevention.htm.

59. Egley, Jr., A., J. C. Howell, and J. P. Moore (March 2010). "Highlights of the 2008 National Youth Gang Survey." *OJJDP Fact Sheet*, NCJ 229249. U.S. Department of Justice, Office of Justice Programs, Office of Juvenile Justice and Delinquency Prevention. Available at http://www.ncjrs.gov/pdffiles1/ojjdp/229249.pdf.

60. Centers for Disease Control and Prevention. *Injury, Violence and Safety.* Available at http://www.cdc.gov/InjuryViolenceSafety/.

61. U.S. Department of Justice, Office of Justice Programs. "Mission and Vision." Available at http://www.ojp.usdoj.gov/about/mission.htm.

62. U.S. Department of Justice, Office of Justice Programs. "Welcome to OJP: Our Mission." Available at http://www.ojp.usdoj.gov/ccdo/welcome_flash.html.

63. Centers for Disease Control and Prevention (2003). "First Reports Evaluating the Effectiveness of Strategies for Preventing Violence: Firearm Laws: Findings from the Task Force on Community Preventive Services." *Morbidity and Mortality Weekly Report*, 52(RR-14): 11–20.

Chapter 16

Safety and Health in the Workplace

Chapter Objectives

After studying this chapter, you will be able to:

1 Describe the scope of the occupational safety and health problem in the United States and its importance to the community.

2 Identify some of the pioneers in the prevention of occupational injuries and disease.

3 Provide a short history of state and federal legislation on occupational safety and health.

4 Explain the difference between occupational injuries and occupational diseases and give several examples of each.

5 Discuss the types of injuries that frequently occur in the workplace and describe their occurrence with regard to person, place, and time.

6 Briefly describe broad strategies for preventing injuries in the workplace.

7 Outline the causes of, and risk factors for, violence in the workplace and describe prevention strategies.

8 Identify the different types of occupational illnesses and disorders and list some of the causative agents.

9 Outline some general strategies for preventing and controlling these disorders and illnesses.

10 List several occupational safety and health professions and describe what the professionals in each of these do.

11 List and briefly describe several occupational safety and health programs for the workplace.

SCENARIO

At first Jen was excited about her new job. Now that she had turned 21, she was permitted to work in the Terrace Lounge and Restaurant, where alcohol was served and the tips were excellent. She politely resigned from her job as a waitress at another restaurant where she had worked for more than 2 years. That restaurant, which enjoyed a clientele primarily of seniors, did not serve alcohol and had a no-smoking policy. She looked forward to working at the Terrace because she believed that she would make as much in tips in two nights as she made all week at her old job. This increase in earnings would help her buy many of the things she wanted for her baby, which was due in 6 months.

That was 2 months ago. Now she was wondering whether she really liked working at the Terrace. The problem was all the cigarette smoke. Her mother was the first to notice that her clothes smelled smoky. But Jen had also noticed the effects of working in the lounge. Her eyes always burned at the end of a night's work and lately her throat burned too. She had started to take her 10-minute breaks outside to enjoy a few breaths of clean air.

Then, she had begun to think about the effects of the inhaled cigarette smoke on the health of her baby. During her first checkup with the doctor after she realized she was pregnant, she had been asked whether she smoked. She had proudly answered, "No." But now she wondered, "Could working in such a smoky environment be harmful to my baby?" She hated the thought of having to quit this job because she was making good money, and her manager was very complimentary of her work.

INTRODUCTION

occupational disease
an abnormal condition, other than an occupational injury, caused by an exposure to environmental factors associated with employment

The global workforce stands at about 3 billion workers and is continuously growing. Approximately 85% of these workers are in less developed countries, where working conditions are more hazardous than in more developed countries. Each year there are as many as 270 million occupational injuries including 360,000 fatalities. Diseases acquired in the workplace result in an estimated 1.95 million deaths annually. The estimated 2.3 million work-related fatalities mean that each day 1 million workers suffer a workplace injury and 5,500 die from a workplace injury or disease. It is estimated that the equivalent of $1.25 trillion are lost from the global gross domestic product by direct and indirect costs of occupational injuries and diseases.[1]

The number of civilian Americans employed in the labor force is approximately 139.1 million.[2] After home, Americans spend the next largest portion of their time at work; thus, safe and healthy workplaces are essential if America is to reach its future health objectives. It is not always easy to distinguish between the terms *occupational injury* and *occupational illness* or *disease*. However, it is generally accepted that an **occupational disease** is any abnormal condition or disorder, other than one resulting from an occupational injury, caused by factors associated with employment. It includes acute or chronic illnesses or disease that may be caused by inhalation, absorption, ingestion, or direct contact. An **occupational injury** is any injury, such as a cut, fracture, sprain, or amputation, that results from a work-related event or from a single, instantaneous exposure in the work environment.[3]

occupational injury
an injury that results from exposure to a single incident in the work environment

Scope of the Problem

Each day in the United States, on average, 14 workers die from an injury sustained at work. Although even one worker death is one too many, it is instructive to note that the work-related fatality rates in America have declined significantly over the past 100 years. In 1912, an estimated 18,000 to 21,000 work-related unintentional injury deaths occurred, a death rate of 21 per 100,000 workers.[4] In 2008, there were 5,214 such deaths, and the death rate for occupational injury deaths had fallen to below 4 per 100,000 workers.[5,6]

A total of 3.7 million nonfatal injuries and illnesses were reported in private industry workplaces during 2008, resulting in a rate of 3.9 cases per 100 equivalent full-time workers. A total of 1.1 million injuries and illnesses in private industry required recuperation away from work beyond the day of the incident in 2008. The vast majority of these events, 3.7 million, were classified as injuries; about 5% were classified as illnesses.[7]

Even though more workplace injuries are reported than workplace illnesses, the estimated number of deaths is higher for workplace illnesses. For example, a 2000 study estimated that for each worker who died from a workplace injury in the United States, eight workers died from work-related diseases.[8] Worldwide, it is estimated that fewer than one in five work-related deaths is the result of an injury.[1]

Although significant progress has been made in reducing morbidity and mortality in the workplace in the United States, the U.S. occupational fatality rate is not the lowest among the highly developed nations. All but two of the reporting members of the European Union—Austria and Portugal—have lower occupational fatality rates than the United States. The average occupational fatality rate for the 15 reporting members in 2007 was 2.1 per 100,000 full-time workers.[9]

Occupational injuries and illnesses are an economic issue, too. It has been estimated that workplace injuries and deaths cost $183 billion in 2008, including $88.4 billion in lost wages and productivity, $38.3 billion in medical expenses, and $37.7 billion in administrative costs and other costs. Thus, each worker in America must produce $1,250 in goods or services just to offset the cost of work-related injuries.[4]

Importance of Occupational Safety and Health to the Community

Because of the grim statistics previously stated, it is important to recognize how occupational and community health problems are linked. The population of those working in industry is a subset of the population of the larger community in which the industry is located. Workers, usually the healthiest people in the community, are exposed in the course of their jobs to specific hazardous materials at the highest concentrations. It is in the factory that the most accurate exposure and health data are available for extrapolation to the general community. Most pollutants for which safe exposure levels have been adopted are workplace materials for which occupational exposures were studied first.

Hazardous agents in the workplace affect not only workers but also those outside the worksite. This can occur through soil and groundwater contamination with solids and liquids or air pollution with industrial gases and dusts. It can also occur through clothing and vehicle contamination, as in the case of asbestos workers whose wives and children became exposed to asbestos from these sources. It is important to note that the general population, which includes children, the elderly, and pregnant women, is more sensitive to exposure to pollutants than the workforce is.

Another way that industries and their communities share health problems is in the instance of an industrial disaster. Examples include the Three Mile Island (Pennsylvania) nuclear reactor near-meltdown in the United States in 1979, the Bhopal tragedy in India in 1984, and the Chernobyl nuclear catastrophe in the Ukraine in 1986. In these cases, the risk of exposure to a chemical or nuclear energy source, which was originally limited to the workplace, became a community-wide risk.

Finally, it is important to recognize the workers themselves as a community, with common social problems and environmental risks. The failure to recognize the community nature of occupational groups and to monitor chronic conditions such as dermatitis, headaches, blood pressure, or blood chemistries has been a major weakness in our conventional approach to occupational health problems.

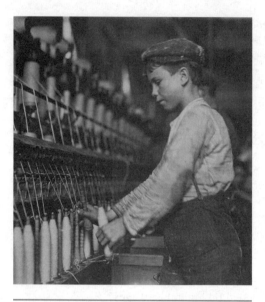

FIGURE 16.1
Cotton mills in the late nineteenth century offered little protection from injuries.

HISTORY OF OCCUPATIONAL SAFETY AND HEALTH PROBLEMS

Occupational risks undoubtedly occurred even in prehistoric times, not only during hunting and warfare, but also in more peaceful activities such as the preparation of flint by knapping. The discovery of flint heaps suggests that even these earliest of workers may have been at risk for silicosis (dust in the lungs).

An extensive historical review of occupational safety and health problems from early Egyptian times to the present day has been published.[10] The first of these milestones occurred in 1561 with George Agricola's treatise on mining, *De Re Metallica,* which emphasized the need for ventilation of mines. In 1567, the work of Philippus Aureolus Theophrastus Bombastus von Hohenheim, also known as Paracelsus, was published under the title *On the Miners' Sickness and Other Miners' Diseases.* These were the first significant works describing specific occupational diseases. The first work on occupational diseases in general was Ramazzini's *Discourse on the Diseases of Workers,* which appeared in 1700.[11,12] In this chapter, we concentrate only on recent events in the United States and make only brief references to earlier milestones.

Occupational Safety and Health in the United States Before 1970

The Industrial Revolution, which began in Britain in the eighteenth century, soon spread to continental Europe and then to the United States. Factors creating and driving the Industrial Revolution were the substitution of steam and coal for animal power, the substitution of machines for human skills, and other advances in industrial technology. These changes resulted in the rise of mass manufacturing, the organization of large work units such as mills and factories, and eventually the exposure of masses of workers to new hazards. Although mining remained the most dangerous form of work, there were soon other unsafe occupations, such as iron smelting and working in cotton mills and textile factories (see Figure 16.1).

The recognition of the need to reduce workplace injuries began long before any attention was paid to workplace diseases. The earliest efforts of those responsible for inspecting workplaces were aimed primarily at the sanitation and cleanliness of workplaces. They soon became concerned with equipment safeguards and tending to those who had become injured or ill at work.[12] These efforts, while much needed and appreciated, did little to improve the overall health of the workforce.

State Legislation

The first official responses to new hazards in the workplace did not occur until 1835, when Massachusetts passed the first Child Labor Law, and later in 1867, when it created a Department of Factory Inspection to enforce it (see Figure 16.2). Under this law, factories were prohibited from hiring children younger than 10 years of

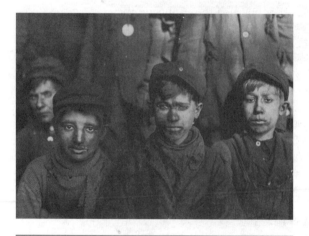

FIGURE 16.2
Before child labor laws were passed, many children worked long hours at dangerous jobs such as mining.

age.[13] At this time the federal government was concerned only with working conditions of federal employees. In 1877, Massachusetts passed the first worker safety law, aimed at protecting textile workers from hazardous spinning machinery.[14]

In 1902, Maryland became the first state to pass any kind of workers' compensation legislation. In 1908, Congress, at the insistence of President Theodore Roosevelt, finally enacted the first of several **workers' compensation laws**; this first law covered certain federal employees. Over the next 40 years, all states and territories eventually enacted some type of workers' compensation legislation, beginning with New York in 1910 and ending with Mississippi in 1948.[10] So ended the first wave of reform in occupational safety and health. With the exception of several other legislative efforts, little progress was achieved during the first half of the century in protecting workers from injuries in the workplace, and almost nothing was done about occupational illnesses.

There was one exception. Alice Hamilton (1869–1970) was a strong proponent of occupational health and a true pioneer in this field (see Figure 16.3). Over her 40-year career in occupational health, she led crusades to reduce poisonings from heavy metals such as lead and mercury. She investigated silicosis in Arizona copper mines, carbon disulfide poisoning in the viscose rayon industry, and many other industrial health problems.[13]

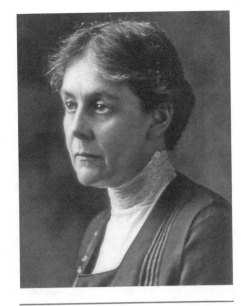

FIGURE 16.3
Alice Hamilton (1869–1970) was a pioneer in occupational safety and health in America.

In spite of Hamilton's efforts, progress in occupational health legislation was slow in the first half of the twentieth century. Occupational diseases were by and large ignored. There was some safety legislation, such as the Coal Mine Safety Act of 1952. Beginning in the 1960s, some people began to take a closer look at the various state workers' safety and workers' compensation laws. It then was discovered that in most states, legislation was a fragmentary patchwork of laws; some states had good laws, but many had inadequate legislation. Many of the laws had failed to keep up with new technology or with inflation. Some groups of workers, including agricultural workers, were not covered at all by legislation. Other problems were the division of authority among various departments within state governments, fragmented record keeping, and inadequate administrative personnel.[15]

workers' compensation laws
a set of federal laws designed to compensate those workers and their families who suffer injuries, disease, or death from workplace exposure

Federal Legislation

In 1884, the federal government created a Bureau of Labor, in 1910 the Federal Bureau of Mines, and in 1914 the Office of Industrial Hygiene and Sanitation in the Public Health Service. In 1916, Congress passed the Federal Employees' Compensation Act, which provided federal employees compensation if injured while on the job.[14] Quite a few important laws were passed between 1908 and 1970 (see Table 16.1), but the two most comprehensive laws were the Coal Mine Health and Safety Act of 1969 and the **Occupational Safety and Health Act of 1970 (OSHAct)**, also known as the Williams-Steiger Act in honor of Senator Harrison A. Williams, Jr., and Congressman William A. Steiger, who worked for passage of the act. At the time the act was passed, 14,000 workers died each year on the job. Since its passage, the act has served to raise the consciousness of both management and labor to the problems of health and safety in the workplace.

Occupational Safety and Health Act of 1970 (OSHAct)
comprehensive federal legislation aimed at ensuring safe and healthful working conditions for working men and women

Occupational Safety and Health Act of 1970

The purpose of the Occupational Safety and Health Act of 1970 is to ensure that employers in the private sector furnish each employee "employment and a place of employment which are

Table 16.1
Highlights of Federal Occupational Safety and Health Legislation

Year	Legislation
1908	Federal Workmen's Compensation Act—limited coverage
1916	Federal Highway Aid Act
1926	Federal Workmen's Compensation Act—amended to include all workers
1927	Federal Longshoremen's and Harbor Workers' Compensation Act
1936	Walsh-Healey Public Contracts Act
1952	Coal Mine Safety Act
1958	Federal Longshoremen's and Harbor Workers' Compensation Act—amended to include rigid safety precautions
1959	Radiation Standards Act
1960	Federal Hazardous Substances Labeling Act
1966	National Traffic and Motor Vehicle Safety Act
1966	Child Protection Act—banned hazardous household substances
1967	National Commission on Product Safety created
1968	Natural Gas Pipeline Safety Act
1969	Construction Safety Act
1969	Child Protection Act—amended to broaden the coverage
1969	**Coal Mine Health and Safety Act**
1970	**Occupational Safety and Health Act**

Occupational Safety and Health Administration (OSHA) the federal agency located within the Department of Labor and created by the OSHAct that is charged with the responsibility of administering the provisions of the OSHAct

free from recognized hazards that are causing or likely to cause death or serious physical harm."[14] Furthermore, employers were henceforth required to comply with all occupational safety and health standards promulgated and enforced under the act by the **Occupational Safety and Health Administration (OSHA)**, which was established by the act.

Also established by the OSHAct was the **National Institute for Occupational Safety and Health (NIOSH)**, a research body now located in the Centers for Disease Control and Prevention of the Department of Health and Human Services. NIOSH is responsible for recommending occupational safety and health standards to OSHA, which is located in the Department of Labor.

The OSHAct contains several noteworthy provisions. Perhaps the most important is the employee's right to request an OSHA inspection. Under this right, any employee or any employee representative may notify OSHA of violations of standards or of the general duty obligation (to provide a safe and healthy workplace) by the employer. Under the act, the employee's name must be withheld if desired, and the employee or a representative may accompany the OSHA inspectors in their inspection. By another provision of the OSHAct, individual states can regain local authority over occupational health and safety by submitting state laws that are and will continue to be as effective as the federal programs.[14]

National Institute for Occupational Safety and Health (NIOSH) a research body within the Department of Health and Human Services that is responsible for developing and recommending occupational safety and health standards

PREVALENCE OF OCCUPATIONAL INJURIES, DISEASES, AND DEATHS

In this section, a brief overview of current trends in workplace injuries and illness is followed by a discussion of the occurrence and prevalence of work-related injuries and work-related diseases.

Overview of Recent Trends in Workplace Injuries and Illnesses

Since 1992, there has been a decline in the number of workplace injuries and illnesses reported in private industry. There were 3.7 million injuries and illnesses reported in 2008, resulting in a rate of 3.9 cases per 100 equivalent full-time workers per year.[7] Approximately 1.1 million of these injuries and illnesses were cases with days away from work.[16] Ninety-five percent of the 3.9 million injuries and illnesses were injuries. About 187,400 new, nonfatal cases of occupational illnesses were reported in private industry in 2008. This figure does not include long-term latent illnesses, which are often difficult to relate to the workplace and therefore are underreported.[7]

In the private sector, the goods-producing industries had a higher rate of nonfatal injuries and illnesses per 100 full-time workers (4.9) than the service-providing industries (3.6). Within the goods-producing industries, agriculture, forestry, fishing, and hunting had the highest rate of nonfatal injuries and illnesses (5.3 per 100 full-time workers), followed by manufacturing (5.0), construction (4.7), and mining (2.9). Within the service-providing industries, education and health care had the highest rate (5.0), followed by trade, transportation, and utilities (4.4); leisure and hospitality (4.2); and other services (3.1). Information (2.0), financial activities (1.5), and professional and business services (1.9) had the lowest rates (see Figure 16.4).[7] Specific industries within industry groups had higher nonfatal injury and illness rates. For example, the animal production industry had a rate of 6.9 per 100 full-time workers, transportation and warehousing 5.7, hospital workers 7.6, and nursing homes and residential facilities workers had a nonfatal injury and illness rate of 8.4 per 100 full-time workers. Workplace injury and illness rates and cases with and without lost workdays have declined steadily since 1992 (see Figure 16.5).[16]

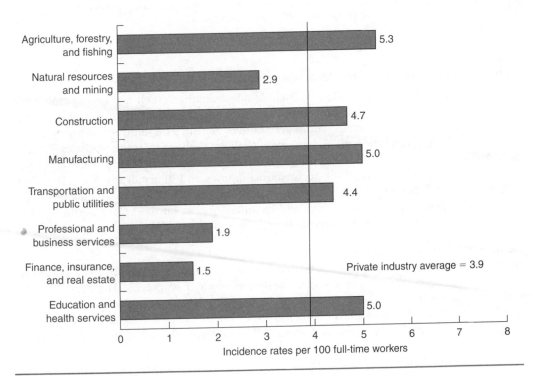

FIGURE 16.4

Nonfatal workplace injury and illness incidence rates by industry division, 2008.

Source: U.S. Department of Labor, Bureau of Labor Statistics (2009). *Workplace Injuries and Illness in 2008.* Available at http://www.bls.gov/news.release/archives/osh_10292009.pdf. Accessed January 6, 2011.

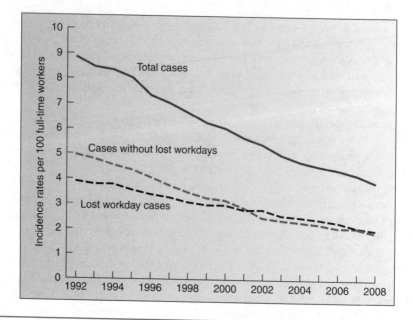

FIGURE 16.5

Workplace injury and illness incidence rates by type of case, 1992 to 2008.

Sources: U.S. Department of Labor, Bureau of Labor Statistics (2009). *Workplace Injuries and Illness in 2008.* Available at http://www.bls.gov/news.release/archives/osh_10292009.pdf; and U.S. Department of Labor, Bureau of Labor Statistics (2009). *Nonfatal Occupational Injuries and Illnesses Requiring Days Away from Work, 2008.* Available at http://www.bls.gov/news.release/archives/osh2_12042009.pdf. Accessed January 6, 2011.

Unintentional Injuries in the Workplace

Unintentional injuries in the workplace include minor injuries (such as bruises, cuts, abrasions, and minor burns), and major injuries (such as amputations, fractures, severe lacerations, eye losses, acute poisonings, and severe burns). Statistics on injuries and injury deaths are available from several sources, including the National Center for Health Statistics (NCHS), the National Safety Council (NSC), the Bureau of Labor Statistics (BLS), and NIOSH. For this reason, estimates of the number of occupational injuries and injury deaths vary. However, beginning in 1992, the NSC adopted the figures published by BLS reports, including its *Census of Fatal Occupational Injuries (CFOI)* and its annual report on workplace injuries and illnesses. The BLS reports are the source of figures used in this text.[5,6]

Fatal Work-Related Injuries

In 2008, there were 5,214 fatal work-related injuries, or about 14.3 per day. The fatal work injury rate for 2008 was 3.7 per 100,000 full-time equivalent workers.[5,6] Highway incidents continued to lead the way, with 1,215 deaths (23% of the total); followed by falls with 700 deaths (13%), being struck by object with 508 (10%), homicides with 526 deaths (10%), exposure to harmful substances or environments with 439 deaths (8%), and fire and explosions with 173 deaths (3%) (see Figure 16.6).[5,6,17]

Overall, the 2008 total of fatal work injuries was the lowest annual total since the fatality census was first conducted in 1992. Several counts were high though; 263 workplace suicides occurred in 2008, the highest number ever reported. Also, the number of fatal work injuries among 16- and 17-year-old workers increased in 2008 as did the number of fatalities in farming, fishing, and forestry. Fatal transportation incidents fell 13% from 2007 levels.[5,6]

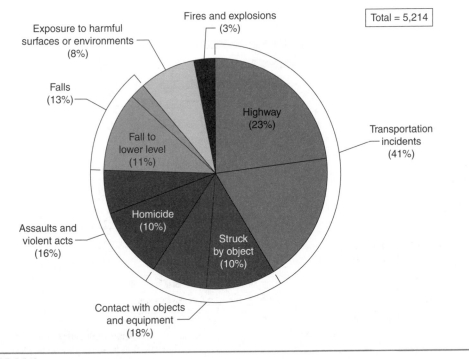

FIGURE 16.6

Manner in which fatal work injuries occurred, 2008.

More fatal work injuries resulted from transportation incidents than from any other event. Highway incidents alone accounted for almost one out of every four fatal work injuries in 2008.

Note: Percentages may not add to totals because of rounding.

Source: U.S. Department of Labor, Bureau of Labor Statistics (2009). "Census of Fatal Occupational Injuries Charts 1992–2008 (Revised Data)." Available at http://www.bls.gov/iif/oshcfoi1.htm#charts. Accessed January 6, 2011.

The industries with the highest rates of fatal occupational injuries per 100,000 employees in 2008 were agriculture, forestry, fishing, and hunting (30.4), mining (18), transportation and warehousing (14.9), and construction (9.7). Industries with the lowest fatality rates were financial activities (1.5), information (1.1), and educational and health services (0.7) (see Figure 16.7).[5,6,17]

Nonfatal Work-Related Injuries

In 2007, an estimated 34 million occupational injury and illness cases were treated in emergency departments; approximately 94,000 (2.7%) of these were hospitalized.[18] A recent study determined that males accounted for 69% of the workers treated, but 85% of those hospitalized. Younger workers (<25 years) had the highest nonfatal workplace injury/illness rates, while workers 45 years of age and older had the lowest rates. More than three-fourths of the nonfatal workplace injuries/illnesses involve contact with objects or equipment (being struck by a falling tool or caught on machinery), bodily exertion or reaction (sprain or strain), and falls. Approximately 57% of all injuries/illnesses were categorized as sprains and strains or lacerations, punctures, amputations, or avulsions.[19]

Disabling injuries or illnesses are those in which the injured worker remains away from work because of injury beyond the day on which the injury occurred. In 2008, sprain or strain injuries accounted for nearly two-fifths of all cases of disabling injuries and illnesses. Within this category, the most common site of injury was the back (40% of all cases).[16] The most disabling type of injury or illness is carpal tunnel syndrome, which results in 25 days

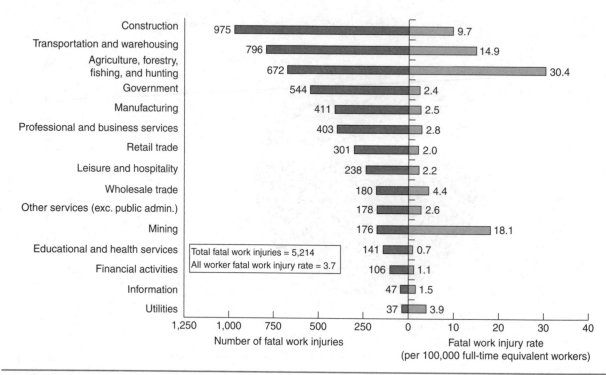

FIGURE 16.7

Number and rate of fatal occupational injuries, by industry sector, 2008.

Although construction had the highest number of fatal injuries in 2008, agriculture, forestry, fishing, and hunting had the highest fatal work injury rate.

Note: In 2008, CFOI implemented a new methodology, using hours worked for fatal work injury rate calculations rather than employment. For additional information on the fatal work injury rate methodology changes please see www.bls.gov/iif/oshnotice10.htm.

Source: U.S. Department of Labor, Bureau of Labor Statistics (2009). "Census of Fatal Occupational Injuries Charts 1992–2008 (Revised Data)." Available at http://www.bls.gov/iif/oshcfoi1.htm#charts. Accessed January 6, 2011.

away from work (see Figure 16.8).[20] The average cost of a disabling workplace injury was calculated at $48,000 in 2008.[4] One set of *Healthy People 2020* objectives is to reduce nonfatal work-related injuries in private sector industries. The first is aimed at injuries resulting in medical treatment, lost time from work, or restricted work activity; a second objective targets nonfatal injuries treated in emergency departments. A third objective aims at reducing nonfatal injuries among adolescent workers (see Box 16.1).

Characteristics of Workers Involved in Work-Related Injuries

Differences in injury and injury death rates are often related to the age and gender of the worker. Injury death rate differences also occur between those of different income levels and races.

Age

Younger workers aged 15–24 years account for 14% of all employed workers and 12.9% of the injuries and illnesses involving days away from work.[16,21] But younger workers spent the fewest days (4–5 days) away from work for each disabling injury or illness of any age group. Days away from work for each disabling injury increase with age; 55- to 66-year-olds average 12 days away from work, and workers 65 years and older average 15 days away from work for each disabling injury or illness.[16] The youngest workers (16–17 years of age) have the lowest

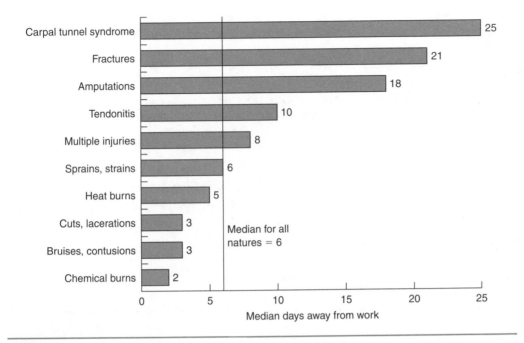

FIGURE 16.8

Characteristics of occupational injuries or illnesses. Median days away from work due to occupational injuries or illnesses in private industry by nature of injury or illness, 2001.

Source: U.S. Department of Health and Human Services, Centers for Disease Control and Prevention, National Institute of Occupational Safety and Health (2004). *Worker Health Chartbook, 2004* (DHHS [NIDSH] pub. no. 2004-146). Available at http://www.cdc.gov/niosh/docs/2004-146. Accessed January 6, 2011.

workplace fatality rates of any age group, 2.4 deaths per 100,000 full-time workers. Workplace fatality rates increase with age; the highest rates are for working elders (65 years of age and older), 12.7 per 100,000 full-time workers (see Figure 16.9).[17] The fewer days away from work per disabling injury or illness and the lower fatality rates being experienced by younger workers may reflect the types of employment today's young people find—fewer are finding manufacturing jobs and more are finding employment in the service-providing industries.[20]

One group of workers that is of special concern is children. An estimated 70% to 80% of teens have worked for pay at some time during their high school years; 50% of employed youths work more than 15 hours during the school week. One in six works more than 25 hours during the school week. Although some level of employment may be desirable, studies show that teens who work more than 20 hours a week do worse academically and are more likely to abuse drugs and alcohol. There are other dangers, too. Every 30 seconds, a teenaged worker is injured in the workplace, and every 4 days a teenager dies because of a workplace injury.[21,22] In 2008, 2.3 million adolescents aged 15–17 years worked in the United States. Many of these youths are employed in jobs that are hazardous even for adult workers; in 2008, 34 workers under the age of 18 died in the workplace.[22]

At particular risk are those youth who are employed in violation of child labor laws. An estimated 148,000 youth are illegally employed during an average week in the United States. This figure does not include the roughly 800,000 youth aged 6 to 17 years who are working as migrant and seasonal farmworkers.[22] A child labor survey found 4,059 child labor violations in the 32 states reporting violations in 2004. The top five child labor violations related to minors

<table>
<tr><td>BOX
16.1</td><td colspan="3">HEALTHY PEOPLE 2020: OBJECTIVES</td></tr>
</table>

OSH-2.1 Reduce nonfatal work-related injuries in private sector industries

Target-setting method: 10% improvement

Data Sources: Survey of Occupational Injuries and Illnesses (SOII), DOL, BLS; National Electronic Injury Surveillance System-Work Supplement (NEISS-Work), CDC, NIOSH; Current Population Survey, U.S. Bureau of the Census.

Target and baseline:

Objective		2008 Baseline	2020 Target
		Injuries per 100 full-time equivalent workers	
OSH-2.1	Reduce nonfatal work-related injuries resulting in medical treatment, lost time from work, or restricted work activity, as reported by employers.	4.2	3.8
OSH-2.2	Reduce nonfatal work-related injuries treated in emergency departments.	2.4	2.2
OSH-2.3	Reduce nonfatal work-related injuries among adolescent workers aged 15 to 19 years.	5.5	4.9

For Further Thought

The target for each of these reductions in nonfatal work-related injuries is 10%. If that seems modest, remember that significant achievements have already been made in worksite safety during the past 100 years. What do you think the effect of a stronger or weaker economy would have on meeting the target level? How does the shift to a "service economy" from a "manufacturing economy" affect the rate of nonfatal injuries in the workplace?

Source: U.S. Department of Health and Human Services, Office of Disease Prevention and Health Promotion (2010). *Healthy People 2020.* Available at http://www.healthypeople.gov/2020/default.aspx. Accessed December 2, 2010.

engaged in prohibited hazardous work in 2004 involved working alone in a cash-based business, cooking, baking, serving alcohol, and working without adult supervision (in retail and restaurants); construction; power-driven machinery; driving on public roads or operating forklifts; and roofing.[23]

Youth employment peaks during summers, when an estimated 5.5 million youths find jobs. Young workers are at particular risk for injury because (1) they may not be trained to perform the assigned task, (2) they may not be adequately supervised, (3) they lack experience and maturity needed to perform assigned tasks and to recognize hazards, and (4) they may be unaware of child labor laws aimed at protecting them. The most dangerous types of work for youth are (1) agriculture, (2) retail trades, especially at night and handling cash, (3) transportation, and (4) construction. Box 16.2 provides recommendations for protecting the safety and health of young workers.[24]

Gender

More than 66 million women are part of the American labor force.[2] Since 1950, the labor force participation rate of women has nearly doubled, so that today more than half of all adult women work. In 2008, females made up 47% of the American workforce.[2] Although males made up 53% of the workforce, they worked 57% of all the hours worked. Because they work more hours and because there are still some dangerous jobs filled predominantly by males, males accounted for nearly two-thirds (64%) of all the injury and illness cases involving days away from

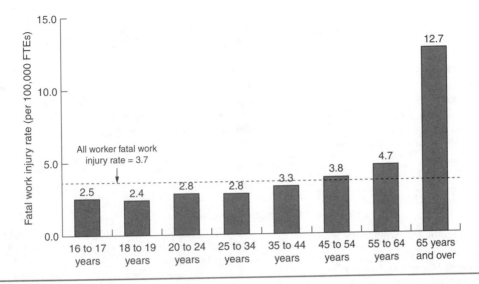

FIGURE 16.9

Fatal work injury rates, by age group, 2008.

Fatal work injury rates for workers 45 years of age and over were higher than the overall U.S. rate, but workers 44 years of age and under had lower rates.

Note: In 2008, CFOI implemented a new methodology, using hours worked for fatal work injury rate calculations rather than employment. Rates are expressed per 100,000 full-time equivalent workers (FTEs). For additional information on the fatal work injury rate methodology changes please see www.bls.gov/iif/oshnotice10.htm.

Source: U.S. Department of Labor, Bureau of Labor Statistics (2009). "Census of Fatal Occupational Injuries Charts 1992–2008 (Revised Data)." Available at http://www.bls.gov/iif/oshcfoi1.htm#charts. Accessed January 6, 2011.

work.[16] Women die of work-related injuries at much lower rates than do men. In 2008, only 7% of those who died of an injury in the workplace were women (see Figure 16.10).[17] When figures are adjusted for the numbers of each sex in the workforce, the overall occupational death rate for men is over 10 times higher than for women (6.1 deaths per 100,000 for men, compared with 0.6 per 100,000 workers for women).[5] A significant portion of the difference results from men being employed in more dangerous jobs. Industries with the highest fatality rates are the same for both men and women—mining, agriculture, construction, and transportation. Although the number of homicides is higher among men, proportionally homicides are greater for women, accounting for one in four of women's job-related fatalities.[17]

Working women are more likely than nonworking women to receive certain health benefits such as workplace prenatal education (offered in 9% of workplaces), weight control programs (24%), and cancer education (23%). Women in the workforce are more likely to be covered by health insurance than nonworking women (73% vs. 46%) and were more likely to have a Pap test within the past 3 years (83% vs. 73%).[25] One group of disorders in which females make up a higher proportion of cases with days away from work is anxiety, stress, and neurotic disorders. In 2001, female workers accounted for 64.9% of these cases.[20]

Poverty and Race

Studies show that those living in counties where income is lower have significantly higher occupational death rates than those living in higher-income counties. In general, since 1998, little difference in workplace fatality rates exists among races.[20] However, machinery injury death rates for whites are twice those of blacks. Hispanics, which make up 10.9% of the workforce, experience 15.2% of all occupational fatalities.[20] Native Americans are at highest risk for

BOX
16.2

HAZARDOUS WORK FOR ADOLESCENTS AND PRACTICAL STEPS FOR PROTECTING THEIR SAFETY AND HEALTH

Work Too Hazardous for Adolescents

- Working in or around motor vehicles
- Operating tractors and other heavy equipment
- Working in retail and service industries where there is a risk of robbery-related homicide
- Working on ladders, scaffolds, roofs, or construction sites
- Continuous manual lifting or lifting of heavy objects

Recommendations

Young Workers

Young workers should take the following steps to protect themselves:

1. *Know about and follow safe work practices.*
   - Recognize the potential for injury at work.
   - Follow safe work practices.
   - Seek information about safe work practices from employers, school counselors, parents, state labor departments, and the Department of Labor (DOL). Visit www.youthrules.dol.gov, or call 1-866-4-USWAGE.
2. *Ask about training:* Participate in training programs offered by your employer, or request training if none is offered.
3. *Ask about hazards:* Don't be afraid to ask questions if you are not sure about the task you are asked to do. Discuss your concerns with your supervisor or employer first.
4. *Know your rights:* Be aware that you have the right to work in a safe and healthful work environment free of recognized hazards. Visit www.osha.gov/sltc/teenworkers/index.html.
   - You have the right to refuse unsafe work tasks and conditions.
   - You have the right to file complaints with DOL when you feel your rights have been violated or your safety has been jeopardized.
   - You are entitled to workers' compensation for a work-related injury or illness.

5. *Know the laws:* Before you start work, learn what jobs young workers are prohibited from doing. State child labor laws may be more restrictive than federal laws, and they vary considerably from state to state. Visit www.youthrules.dol.gov or call 1-866-4-USWAGE.

Employers

Employers should take the following steps to protect young workers:

1. *Recognize the hazards.*
   - Reduce the potential for injury or illness in young workers by assessing and eliminating hazards in the workplace.
   - Make sure equipment used by young workers is safe and legal. Visit www.dol.gov/dol/topic/youthlabor/hazardousjobs.htm or call 1-866-4-USADOL.
2. *Supervise young workers.*
   - Make sure that young workers are appropriately supervised.
   - Make sure that supervisors and adult coworkers are aware of tasks young workers may or may not perform.
   - Label equipment that young workers cannot use, or color-code uniforms of young workers so that others will know they cannot perform certain jobs.
3. *Provide training.*
   - Provide training in hazard recognition and safe work practices.
   - Have young workers demonstrate that they can perform assigned tasks safely and correctly.
   - Ask young workers for feedback about the training.
4. *Know and comply with the laws:* Know and comply with child labor laws and occupational safety and health regulations that apply to your business. State laws may be more restrictive than federal laws, and they vary considerably from state to state. Post these

death from explosions and falling objects. Asians have very low death rates for occupational injuries. Although they make up 4.7% of the workforce, they experience only 2.5% of all occupational fatalities.[20] Occupational injury rates may reflect the types of employment in which workers find themselves.

BOX	(CONTINUED)
16.2	

regulations for workers to read. For information about federal child labor laws, visit www.dol.gov/dol/topic/youthlabor/index.htm or call 1-866-4-USADOL. Links to state labor offices are available at www.youthrules.dol/gov/states.htm (1-866-4-USWAGE). Information about OSHA regulations that apply to workers of all ages is available at www.osha.gov.

5. *Develop an injury and illness prevention program:* Involve supervisors and experienced workers in developing a comprehensive safety program that includes an injury and illness prevention program and a process for identifying and solving safety and health problems. OSHA consultation programs are available in every state to help employers identify hazards and improve their safety and health management programs.

Educators

Educators should take the following steps to protect young workers:

1. *Talk to students about work:* Talk to students about safety and health hazards in the workplace and students' rights and responsibilities as workers.

2. *Ensure the safety of school-based work experience programs:* Ensure that vocational education programs, school-to-work, or Workforce Investment Act partnerships offer students work that is allowed by law and is in safe and healthful environments free of recognized hazards. All such programs should include safety and health training.

3. *Include worker safety and health in the school curriculum:* Incorporate occupational safety and health topics into high school and junior high curricula (e.g., safety and health regulations, how to recognize hazards, how to communicate safety concerns, where to go for help). Information is available from NIOSH at 1-800-35-NIOSH.

4. *Know the laws:* If you are responsible for signing work permits or certificates, know the child labor laws. State laws may be more restrictive than federal

laws, and they vary considerably from state to state. Visit www.dol.gov/gol/topic/youthlabor/ResourcesforEducators.htm (or call 1-866-USADOL), or www.youthrules.dol.gov (or call 1-866-4-USWAGE).

Parents

Parents should take the following steps to protect young workers:

1. *Take an active role in your child's employment.*
   • Know the name of your child's employer and your child's work address and phone number.
   • Ask your child about the types of work involved, work tasks, and equipment he or she uses at work.
   • Ask your child about training and supervision provided by the employer.
   • Be alert for signs of fatigue or stress as your child tries to balance demands of work, school, home, and extracurricular activities.

2. *Know the laws:* Be familiar with child labor laws. State laws may be more restrictive than federal laws, and they vary considerably from state to state. Don't assume that your child's employer knows about these laws. Visit www.dol.gov/dol/topic/youthlabor/ParentsofYoung.htm (or call 1-866-4-USADOL) or www.youthrules.dol.gov (or call 1-866-4-USWAGE).

3. *Be aware of young workers' rights:* Report unsafe working conditions or employment in violation of child labor laws to DOL. Young workers are eligible for workers' compensation benefits if injured on the job.

4. *Share information with other parents:* Studies have shown that most young workers and parents are not aware of the laws and rights of young workers.

Source: U.S. Department of Health and Human Services, Centers for Disease Control and Prevention, National Institute for Occupational Safety and Health (2003). *NIOSH Alert: Preventing Deaths, Injuries, and Illnesses of Young Workers* (DHHS [NIOSH] pub. no. 2003-128). Available at http://www.cdc.gov/niosh/topics/youth. Accessed September 29, 2010.

Geographic Differences in Workplace Injuries

For the 21-year period ending in 2000, occupational injury death rates were highest in Alaska (20.9 per 100,000 workers), followed by Wyoming, Montana, Idaho, Mississippi, and West Virginia (see Figure 16.11).[20] Deaths from nonfarm machinery are higher in the mountain states,

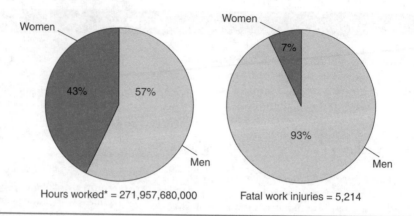

Hours worked* = 271,957,680,000   Fatal work injuries = 5,214

FIGURE 16.10

Hours worked and fatal work injuries, by gender of worker, 2008.

Men recorded a disproportionate share of fatal work injuries relative to their hours worked in 2008.

*Starting with reference year 2008, calculations are based on total hours worked rather than total workers. The figure shown represents the full-time equivalent (working 40 hours a week, 50 weeks a year) of 135,978,840 civilian workers.

Source: U.S. Department of Labor, Bureau of Labor Statistics (2009). "Census of Fatal Occupational Injuries Charts 1992–2008 (Revised Data)." Available at http://www.bls.gov/iif/oshcfoi1.htm#charts. Accessed January 6, 2011.

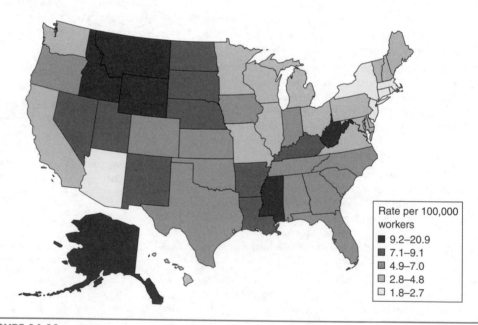

Rate per 100,000 workers

◼ 9.2–20.9
◼ 7.1–9.1
◼ 4.9–7.0
◻ 2.8–4.8
◻ 1.8–2.7

FIGURE 16.11

Average annual rate of fatal occupational injuries per 100,000 workers by state of death, 1980–2000. (All data for 1980–2000 exclude New York City.) The states with the highest fatality rates for occupational injury during 1980–2000 include Alaska (20.9 per 100,000 workers), Wyoming (14.9), Montana (11.1), Idaho (9.7), Mississippi (9.6), and West Virginia (9.6). The greatest number of fatal occupational injuries occurred in California (12,221), Texas (11,635), Florida (7,252), Illinois (5,145), and Pennsylvania (4,420).

Source: U.S. Department of Health and Human Services, Centers for Disease Control and Prevention, National Institute for Occupational Safety and Health (2004). *Worker Health Chartbook, 2004* (HHS [NIOSH] pub. no. 2004-146). Available at http://www.cdc.gov/niosh/docs/2004-146. Accessed January 6, 2011.

but deaths from farm machinery are higher in the north-central states. Work-related death rates from machinery, falling objects, electric current, and explosion are all higher in rural states. Within states, work-related deaths are higher in rural areas than in more urban areas.

Temporal Variations in Workplace Injuries

As mentioned previously, between 1912 and 2008 injury death rates among workers have declined 82% (from 21 per 100,000 workers to 3.7 per 100,000). During this period, the workforce in America has nearly quadrupled in size, and the amount of goods and services produced has increased ninefold.[4] These improvements in workplace safety have been considered one of the 10 greatest achievements in public health during the past century (see Box 16.3).

There is a seasonality to work-related deaths. Injury death rates from machinery, falling objects, electric current, and explosions are highest in the summer, when farming and construction work increase. Deaths from these causes are also more often reported during weekdays than on weekends, when, in general, more injury deaths occur.

Workplace Injuries by Industry and Occupation

Fatal and nonfatal occupational injury rates vary according to type of industry and type of occupation.

Fatal Occupational Injuries by Industry

Some jobs are more dangerous than others. Injury death rates are one indication of the risk associated with employment in an industry or in a particular job within an industry. Although the total number of deaths is highest in the construction industry, workers in agriculture, forestry, fishing, and hunting have the highest workplace fatality rates (32.5 deaths per 100,000 full-time workers) (see Figure 16.7).[17] Within this industry category, commercial fishing is the single most dangerous occupation. During the period 1992–2008, an annual average of 58 deaths were reported (128 deaths per 100,000 workers).[26] (Remember the overall fatality rate for American workers is less than 4 deaths per 100,000 workers.) Loggers and aircraft pilots usually join fishers at the top of the annual list of America's "Top 10 Most Dangerous Jobs" (see Table 16.2).[27]

BOX 16.3   TEN GREAT PUBLIC HEALTH ACHIEVEMENTS, 1900–1999: SAFER WORKPLACES

Saving Lives, Promoting Health, and Protecting Jobs

A Sharp Increase in the Workforce, but an Even Sharper Decline in Work-Related Deaths

At the beginning of the twentieth century, workers in the United States faced remarkably high risks to their health and safety. Today, despite a much larger workforce than ever before, work-related deaths have declined sharply. Identifying and correcting occupational health hazards has greatly reduced the health and safety risks for such occupations as construction workers, miners, and farmers.

From 1933 to 1997, according to the National Safety Council, work-related injuries declined 90%. And, although the workforce tripled during those years, deaths declined from 37 per 100,000 to 4 per 100,000 workers.

If today's workforce of approximately 130 million were at the same risk for dying from injuries as workers in 1933, an additional 40,000 workers would have died in 1997 from preventable events.

In the coal mining industry, for example, improvements in workers' enviromental health and safety have resulted in lower rates of fatal injury, which were once common among miners.

Source: Centers for Disease Control and Prevention (1999). "Achievements in Public Health, 1900–1999: Improvements in Workplace Safety—United States, 1900–1999." *Morbidity and Mortality Weekly Report* 48(22):241–242. Available at www.cdc.gov/mmwr/preview/mmwrhtml/mm4822a1.htm. Accessed October 26, 2010.

Table 16.2
Top Ten Most Dangerous Jobs in 2008

Rank	Occupation	Death Rate/ 100,000	Total Deaths
1	Fishers and fishing workers	111.8	38
2	Logging workers	86.4	76
3	Aircraft pilots	66.7	82
4	Structural iron and steel workers	45.5	40
5	Farmers and ranchers	38.4	285
6	Roofers	29.4	79
7	Electrical power line installers/repairers	32.7	36
8	Driver/sales workers and truck drivers	29.1	993
9	Refuse and recylable material collectors	22.8	18
10	Police sheriffs and patrol officers	21.4	143

Source: Kirdahy, M. (2008). "America's Most Dangerous Jobs." Forbes.com. Available at http://www.forbes.com/2008/08/25/dangerous-jobs-fishing-lead-careers-cx_mk_0825danger.html. Accessed January 7, 2011.

The industry with the second highest workplace fatality rate is mining (25.6 deaths per 100,000 workers). On April 6, 2010, an explosion at the Upper Big Branch mine in West Virginia killed 29 miners. This was the country's worst disaster in four decades,[28] and an unneeded reminder of the hazardous nature of coal mining (see Figure 16.12). One set of *Healthy People 2020* objectives is to reduce deaths from work-related injuries in private sector industries. Mining, construction, transportation and warehousing, and agriculture, forestry, fishing, and hunting offer the best opportunities for improvement (see Box 16.4).

Nonfatal Occupational Injuries and Illnesses by Industry
A total of 3.7 million injuries and illnesses were reported in private industry workplaces during 2008, resulting in a rate of 3.9 cases per 100 equivalent full-time workers.[7] Goods-producing industries had higher rates than service-producing industries. Among goods-producing industries, agriculture, forestry, fishing, and hunting had the highest incidence rate in 2008 (5.3 cases per 100 full-time workers). In the service-producing industries, education and health services has the highest incidence rate (5.0 cases per 1,000 full-time workers) (see Figure 16.4). All 2008 incidence rates showed declines from 1998 levels.[7]

Agricultural Safety and Health
One particularly hazardous occupation is farming. Those working on farms are at considerable risk not just for injuries, but for lung diseases, noise-induced hearing loss, skin diseases, and certain cancers associated with chemical use and sun exposure. About 3 million people are involved in farm operations and, if unpaid farm workers and family members are counted, the number is much higher. In 2008, 307 farm-related deaths were reported.[5] In 2008, agriculture (including forestry, fishing, and hunting) ranked first among major U.S. industries for

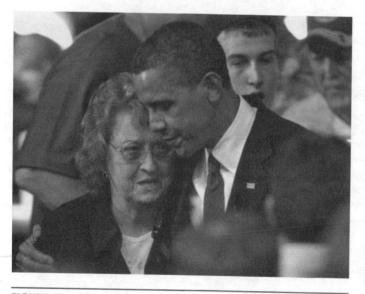

FIGURE 16.12
President Barack Obama attended the memorial service for miners killed in the Upper Big Branch mine disaster in West Virginia, in April, 2010.

BOX
16.4

HEALTHY PEOPLE 2020: OBJECTIVES

Objective OSH-1:   Reduce deaths from work-related injuries

Target-setting method: 10% improvement

Data Source: Census of Fatal Occupational Injuries (CFOI), DOL, BLS; Current Population Survey (CPS), U.S. Bureau of the Census.

Target and baseline:

Objective		2007 Baseline	2020 Target
		Deaths per 100,000 full-time equivalent workers	
OSH-1.1	All industry	4.0	3.6
OSH-1.2	Mining	21.4	19.3
OSH-1.3	Construction	10.8	9.7
OSH-1.4	Transportation and warehousing	16.5	14.8
OSH-1.5	Agriculture, forestry, fishing, and hunting	27.0	24.3

For Further Thought

Targets call for reducing deaths from work-related injuries by 10%. In view of the significant progress made in the past, do you feel this target is attainable? Which industry do you think has the best chance of meeting their target? Why?

Source: U.S. Department of Health and Human Services, Office of Disease Prevention and Health Promotion (2010). *Healthy People 2020*. Available at http://www.healthypeople.gov/2020/default.aspx. Accessed December 2, 2010.

work-related, unintentional injury fatality rates (see Figure 16.7),[17] and farming and ranching alone ranked fifth among the top 10 most dangerous jobs in 2008 (see Table 16.2).[27]

A major contribution to farm-related fatalities is farm machinery, particularly farm tractors. For more than two out of five farm worker deaths, the source of the fatal injury was a tractor, and more than half of these deaths resulted from tractor rollovers. Rollover incidents are those in which the tractor tips sideways or backward (especially when the tractor is improperly hitched), crushing the operator (see Figure 16.13). While all tractors manufactured since 1985 are fitted with seat belts and **rollover protective structures (ROPS)**, many tractors in use in the United States lack this equipment. The effectiveness of ROPS in protecting the tractor operator was demonstrated by statistics collected in Nebraska, where only 1 (2%) of 61 persons operating ROPS-equipped tractors that rolled over died. These data compare favorably with a 40% death rate for the 250 persons involved in unprotected tractor rollover incidents. The single fatality in the ROPS-equipped tractor was not wearing a seat belt and was ejected from the ROPS-protected area.[29]

rollover protective structures (ROPS) factory-installed or retrofitted reinforced framework on a cab to protect the operator of a tractor in case of a rollover

Although today's tractors are the safest ever, they are still a leading cause of farm injuries and deaths.[29] The OSHA standard requiring ROPS be installed on all tractors is not actively enforced on farms with fewer than 11 employees, and family farms without other employees are exempt from OSHA regulations. NIOSH can promote ROPS use but has no authority to require their use.[30]

Another concern about farming is that it is one of the few industries in which the families of workers are also exposed to many of the same risks. In 2006, more than 1 million youths 0 to 19 years of age lived in farm operator households, while an estimated 307,000 children and adolescents were hired to work on farms and 29.3 million youths visited a farm.[31] It is not unusual for farm boys under the age of 12 to be seen driving tractors (see Figure 16.14). Each

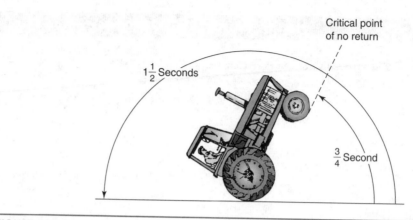

FIGURE 16.13

The timing of events during rear rollovers of farm tractors.

Source: Reproduced with permission from Deere & Company. © 1994 Deere & Company. All rights reserved.

year about 100 children are killed and thousands of children and adolescents are injured in agriculture-related activities.[31] The fatality rate for youths on farms in 2006 was 8.4 per 100,000.[31] Many of those injured belong to the migrant workforce, where children as young as 12, 10, 8, and even 4 years of age can be found working in the fields. Testimony before the U.S. Senate Committee on Labor and Human Resources by Fernando Cuevas, Jr., paints a grim picture of migrant children (see Box 16.5).[32]

Of our 50 states, 48 rely heavily on migrant workers during the peak harvest season. These migrant workers have poor access to health care facilities; infant mortality is about 50 per 1,000 compared with the national average of about 7.2 per 1,000. In many cases, working conditions are hazardous, and water shortages require workers to drink water from irrigation ditches. Not only is such water unpurified, it is usually laden with agricultural chemicals and biological wastes. Migrant workers are also exposed to long hours in the sun, other unsanitary conditions, and numerous harmful pesticides from crop-dusting airplanes.

It is an unfortunate fact that virtually no progress has been made in addressing the plight of migrant farm workers. In 2000, Human Rights Watch (HRW) documented the exploitive and dangerous conditions under which these workers and their children labor in a report titled *Fingers to the Bone: United States Failure to Protect Child Farmworkers*. Nearly 10 years later, when HRW reexamined the situation, they discovered that conditions for child farmworkers were essentially unchanged.[33] Children often work 10 or more hours a day and, during peak harvest times, may work dawn to dusk (see Figure 16.15). They typically earn less than the minimum wage and are often forced to spend their own money on tools, gloves, and even drinking water. They may be exposed to agricultural chemicals that make them sick. Because of missed days at school, farm-working youth drop out of school at a rate four times higher than the national average. "Under current U.S. law, children can do agricultural work that the U.S. Department of Labor deems 'particularly hazardous' for children at age 16 (and at any age on farms owned or operated by their

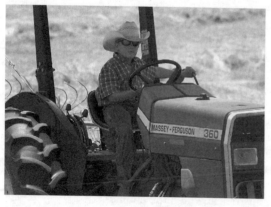

FIGURE 16.14

It is not unusual for farm boys under the age of 12 to be seen driving tractors.

BOX
16.5

COMMENTS OF A YOUNG FARM WORKER

"When I was younger it was all a game to me. But as I started getting older it became a job, and at the age of about 7 and 8, I was competing with my parents and my older sisters. . . . I was able to get out of the fields permanently at the age of 15 to try and get a decent education. I also became an organizer for the Farm Labor Organizing Committee at the age of 16, and I continue to see many, many young children working out in the fields

at the same age that I was—4-, 5-, 6-, 7-, and 8-year-olds. They are still working out in the fields. I see it every year, up in Ohio, I see it down in Texas, I see it in Florida, I see it anywhere that we go and organize."

Source: Committee on Labor and Human Resources (19 March 1991). "Prepared Statement of Fernando Cuevas, Jr." *Childhood Labor Amendments of 1991* (S. HRG. 102-201, S. 600). Washington, DC: U.S. Government Printing Office.

parents). In non-agricultural sectors, no one under age 18 can do such jobs."[33] Even these lax labor laws are not enforced diligently. Between 2001 and 2009, enforcement of child labor laws overall by the U.S. Department of Agriculture declined dramatically. Despite the hazardous conditions and frequent injuries and illnesses suffered by farmworkers, relatively few complain for fear of being fired or even deported. Even though many of the children may be U.S. citizens, the entire family may fear being deported.

"The United States spent more than $26 million in 2009 to eliminate child labor around the world, yet the country's law and practice concerning child farmworkers are in violation of or are inconsistent with international conventions on the rights of children."[33] Legislation aimed at eliminating the double standard in child labor laws is introduced during each session of Congress. So far, none of these bills has reached a vote.

Prevention and Control of Unintentional Injuries in the Workplace

Reducing the number and seriousness of injuries and illnesses in the workplace involves four fundamental tasks: anticipation, recognition, evaluation, and control.[34] *Anticipation* involves the foresight to envision future adverse events and take action to prevent them. A hazard inventory should be conducted to detect and record physical, ergonomic, chemical, biological, and psychological hazards in the workplace. *Recognition* involves surveillance and monitoring of the workforce for injuries and illnesses, including near misses. It includes inspections of the workplace for hazards, monitoring it for toxins, recording injuries, and conducting employee health screenings. All of the aforementioned activities include data collection. *Evaluation* is the assessment of the data that were collected during the recognition and monitoring activities. This includes toxicological, exposure, and clinical assessment as well as risk assessment.

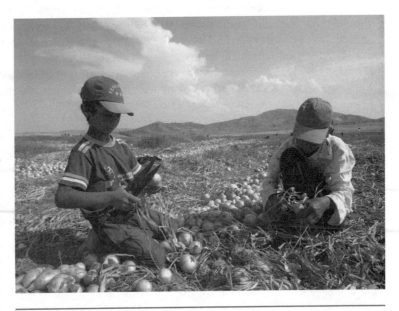

FIGURE 16.15
Children of migrant workers often work ten or more hours a day and tend to drop out of school at a rate four times the national average.

Epidemiology is part of the evaluation process. Risk assessment enables the translation of scientific information about hazards into decisions and policies that can improve workplace safety and health. Upon establishing the need for intervention, a decision concerning *control* can be made. The control may involve changes in the production process to make it safer, changes in the work environment to make it safer, or improvements in the use of personal protective equipment or apparel to protect individual workers. Finally, the education and training of workers can help to reduce workplace injuries and illnesses.[34]

National leadership in reducing the number and seriousness of workplace injuries and illnesses resides with OHSA and NIOSH. In an effort to chart the future course for research on workplace safety and health problems, NIOSH has developed a partnership with more than 500 public and private outside organizations and individuals. In 2006, the National Occupational Research Agenda (NORA), a framework to guide occupational safety and health research into the twenty-first century, marked 10 years of achievement. A review of past accomplishments under NORA and the agenda for the future are available online.[35]

Workplace Violence: Intentional Workplace Injuries

Although only a small number of the incidents of workplace violence that occur each day make the news, some 1.7 million Americans are victims of workplace violence each year.[36] Many of us have heard about a teacher who was attacked by a student, a female worker who was sexually assaulted in the parking lot, a woman shot in her place of work by an irate boyfriend, or a pizza delivery man killed for a few dollars. In 2008, 526 homicides occurred in the workplace, making homicide the third leading cause of workplace fatalities behind highway incidents and falls, and the second leading cause of workplace deaths among women.[20]

In the early 1990s, there was extensive media coverage of work-related homicides at U.S. Postal Service facilities. The phrase "Don't go postal on me," meaning don't become crazy or violent, is still heard occasionally. However, an examination of the occupational injury death rates for postal workers in the 1980s revealed that workplace injury death rates for postal workers were approximately 2.5 times lower than those for all workers combined.[37] A more recent study found that "'going postal' is a myth and a bad rap," and that postal workers are only one-third as likely as those in the national workforce to be victims of homicide at work. Some occupations are significantly more dangerous. For example, taxi drivers are 150 times likelier than letter carriers to be victims of homicide at work (31.54 vs. 0.21 per 100,000).[38]

There are many reasons for workplace homicides and violence. Researchers have divided workplace violence into four categories:[39]

Criminal intent (Type I): The perpetrator has no legitimate relationship to the business or its employees and is usually committing a crime, such as robbery, shoplifting, and trespassing. This category makes up 85% of the work-related homicides.

Customer/Client (Type II): The perpetrator has a legitimate relationship with the business and becomes violent while being served. This category includes customers, clients, patients, students, and inmates. This category represents 3% of the work-related homicides.

Worker-on-worker (Type III): The perpetrator is an employee or past employee of the business who attacks or threatens another employee or past employee of the workplace. Worker-on-worker violence accounts for 7% of workplace homicides.

Personal relationship (Type IV): The perpetrator usually does not have a relationship with the business but has a personal relationship with the intended victim. This category, which includes victims of domestic violence assaulted or threatened at work, makes up just 2% of workplace homicides.

Data on nonfatal workplace violence are more difficult to obtain than data on workplace homicides. One estimate is that about 1.7 million people are victims of nonfatal workplace violence each year.[39] Assaults occur almost equally among men and women. Most of these assaults occur in service settings such as hospitals, nursing homes, and social service agencies. Forty-eight percent of nonfatal assaults in the workplace are committed by health care patients.[39]

Risk Factors

Risk factors for encountering violence at work are listed in Box 16.6. They include working with the public, working around money or valuables, working alone, and working late at night. Additionally, certain industries and occupations put workers at particular risk. For workplace homicides, the taxicab industry has the highest risk at 41.4 per 100,000, nearly 60 times the national average rate of 0.70 per 100,000. Other jobs that carry a higher than average risk for homicide are jobs in liquor stores (7.5), detective and protective services (7.0), gas service stations (4.8), and jewelry stores (4.7). The workplaces that have the highest risk of nonfatal assault (and the highest percentage of all assaults that occurred) are nursing homes (27%), social services (13%), hospitals (11%), grocery stores (6%), and restaurants or bars (5%).[39]

Prevention Strategies

Prevention strategies for workplace violence can be grouped into three categories—environmental designs, administrative controls, and behavior strategies. Before these strategies can be implemented, a workplace violence prevention policy should be in place. Such a policy should clearly indicate a zero tolerance of violence at work. Just as workplaces have mechanisms for reporting and dealing with sexual harassment, they must also have a policy in place to deal with violence. Such a policy must spell out how such incidents are to be reported, to whom, and how they are to be addressed.

Environmental designs to limit the risk of workplace violence might include implementing safer cash handling procedures, physically separating workers from customers, improving lighting, and installing better security systems at entrances and exits. Administrative controls include staffing policies (having more staff is generally safer than having fewer staff), procedures for opening and closing the workplace, and reviewing employee duties (such as handling money) that may be especially risky. Behavior strategies include training employees in nonviolent response and conflict resolution and educating employees about risks associated with specific duties and about the importance of reporting incidents and adhering to administrative controls. Training should also include instruction on the appropriate use and maintenance of any protective equipment that may be provided.[39]

BOX 16.6	FACTORS THAT INCREASE A WORKER'S RISK FOR WORKPLACE ASSAULT

- Contact with the public
- Exchange of money
- Delivery of passengers, goods, or services
- Having a mobile workplace such as a taxicab or police cruiser
- Working with unstable or volatile persons in health care, social services, or criminal justice settings
- Working alone or in small numbers

- Working late at night or during early morning hours
- Working in high-crime areas
- Guarding valuable property or possessions
- Working in community-based settings

Source: Centers for Disease Control and Prevention, National Institute for Occupational Safety and Health (2004). "Violence on the Job" (NIOSH pub. no. 2004-100d). Available at http://www.cdc.gov/niosh/docs/video/violence.html. Accessed January 7, 2011.

Occupational Illnesses and Disorders

Precise data on the number of cases of occupational illnesses are more difficult to acquire than data on injuries. It is more difficult to link illnesses to occupational exposure. Some illnesses that can result from occupational exposure (e.g., tuberculosis, cancer, and asthma) appear no different from those that result from exposure elsewhere. Also, there is usually a lengthy period of time between exposure and the appearance of disease, unlike injuries, which are usually evident immediately. Reported cases of illnesses in the workplace in 2008 accounted for only 5% of the 3.7 million injury and illness cases. In private industry, 187,000 new cases of occupational illness were reported, a rate of 19.7 per 10,000 full-time workers. Skin diseases and disorders had the highest incidence, 3.8 cases per 10,000 full-time workers.[7] The illnesses reported in the figures are only the cases reported during 2008. Some conditions, such as various cancers, are slow to develop and are difficult to associate with the workplace. These diseases and conditions are often unrecognized and underreported in annual reports of injuries and illnesses.[7]

Types of Occupational Illnesses

Occupational diseases can be categorized by cause and by the organ or organ system affected. For example, repeated trauma is the cause, and the musculoskeletal system is the affected organ system. Exposure to asbestos is a cause of illness; the respiratory system, especially the lung, is the system affected.

Musculoskeletal Disorders

Musculoskeletal disorders are the most frequently reported occupational disorders. They include both acute and chronic injury to muscles, tendons, ligaments, nerves, joints, bones, and supporting vasculature. The leading type of musculoskeletal disorder was repeated trauma disorders, which can make up 65% of all cases of nonfatal occupational illness in a given year.[20] Included in this category are carpal tunnel syndrome and noise-induced hearing loss. These disorders are sometimes referred to as repeated trauma disorders.

Skin Diseases and Disorders

Reported skin disorders included allergic and irritant dermatitis, eczema, rash, oil acne, chrome ulcers, and chemical burns. The highest incidences of occupational skin disorders were reported in agriculture, foresty, and fishing.[20] The skin may serve as the target organ for disease, or it may be the route through which toxic chemicals enter the worker's body.

Noise-Induced Hearing Loss

Noise-induced hearing loss is another form of repeated trauma. Approximately 30 million Americans are exposed to hazardous noise on the job, and an additional 9 million are at risk for hearing loss from other agents such as solvents and metals. Cases include workers with a permanent noise-induced hearing loss or with a standard threshold shift. Most of the cases were reported within manufacturing; within the manufacturing sector, 51% of the cases were associated with manufacturing.[20]

Respiratory Disorders

Occupational respiratory disorders are the result of the inhalation of toxic substances present in the workplace. The lungs, like the skin,

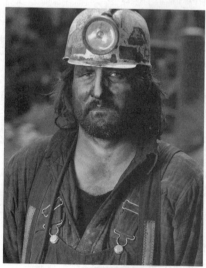

FIGURE 16.16

Mining is a dangerous occupation because of exposure to both injuries and disease.

can be both the target organ of disease and a portal of entry for toxic substances. Characteristic of occupational lung diseases are their chronic nature and the difficulty in early recognition (the latent period for such diseases may be 15 to 30 years). Also, there is the problem of multiple or mixed exposures in the home and the workplace.

Work-related asthma (WRA) is the most commonly reported occupational respiratory disease, even though estimates suggest that most cases are not recognized or reported as being work related. There is no estimate on how many cases of WRA occur nationwide. The highest percentage of cases occur among operators, fabricators, and laborers.[20]

One of the most important categories of lung diseases is **pneumoconiosis**, a fibrotic lung disease caused by the inhalation of dusts, especially mineral dusts. During the period 1968 through 1999, a total of 121,982 pneumoconiosis deaths were reported in U.S. residents.[20]

Types of pneumoconioses include coal workers' pneumoconiosis, asbestosis, silicosis, and byssinosis. The largest number of pneumoconiosis deaths were from coal workers' pneumoconiosis (CWP). **Coal workers' pneumoconiosis** (also called *black lung disease*) is an acute or chronic lung disease that is caused by inhaling coal dust (see Figure 16.16). Historically, deaths from CWP clearly outnumber all other types of pneumoconiosis deaths. During the period from 1987 to 1996, CWP made up 54% of all pneumoconiosis deaths. However, deaths from CWP have declined during the last 30 years, from a high of 2,870 in 1972 to 635 (26%) in 2005.[20,40] The human cost of CWP can be measured another way, through analysis of years of potential life lost (YPLL). During the period 1998–2006, a total of 22,625 YPLL were attributed to CWP, an average of 5.7 years per fatality.[41] This means that workers who developed CWP during this period died, on average, 5.7 years sooner than expected. Most troubling is the finding that, after a period of decline, the number of YPLL has been increasing, from an average of 5.3 during 1968–1972 to 7.8 in 2002–2006. This increase could be caused by increased exposure to coal dust because of inadequate enforcement of standards and unrepresentative dust sample measurements. One-fourth of the coal mine dust samples tested exceeded the NIOSH recommended exposure limit for respirable coal dust. Also, miners worked an average of 25.6% more hours underground during 2003–2007 than they did during 1978–1982, thereby increasing their exposure to coal dust.[41] No effective medical treatment is available for pneumoconiosis; therefore, primary prevention is essential.

Asbestos workers suffer from diseases that include **asbestosis** (an acute or chronic lung disease), lung cancer, and mesothelioma (cancer of the epithelial linings of the heart and other internal organs). In contrast to CWP, asbestosis deaths have increased from 77 in 1968 to nearly 1,423 in 2005. It now accounts for 58% of pneumoconiosis deaths.[20,40]

Workers in mines, stone quarries, sand and gravel operations, foundries, abrasive blasting operations, and glass manufacturing run the risk of **silicosis** (sometimes referred to as dust on the lungs) that is caused from inhaling crystalline silica. Silicosis deaths represent nearly 6% of all pneumoconiosis deaths in the United States Mortality from silicosis has significantly declined in recent years from 1,157 in 1968 to 161 in 2005.[20,40]

Textile factory workers who inhale dusts from cotton, flax, or hemp often acquire **byssinosis** (sometimes called *brown lung disease*), an acute or chronic lung disease. In comparison with the other types of pneumoconiosis, byssinosis deaths are uncommon—10 or fewer cases were reported annually between 1996 and 2005. There were also 216 unspecified pneumoconiosis deaths in 2005.[40]

Other agents that can affect the lungs include metallic dusts, gases and fumes, and aerosols of biological agents (viruses, bacteria, and fungi). Health conditions that can result from exposure to these agents include occupational asthma, asphyxiation, pulmonary edema, histoplasmosis, and lung cancer.

pneumoconiosis fibrotic lung disease caused by the inhalation of dusts, especially mineral dusts

coal workers' pneumoconiosis (CWP) acute and chronic lung disease caused by the inhalation of coal dust (black lung disease)

asbestosis acute or chronic lung disease caused by the deposition of asbestos fibers on lungs

silicosis acute or chronic lung disease caused by the inhalation of free crystalline silica

byssinosis acute or chronic lung disease caused by the inhalation of cotton, flax, or hemp dusts (brown lung disease)

Other Work-Related Diseases and Disorders

Other types of work-related illnesses and disorders are those that arise from poisonings and infections. Poisoning agents include heavy metals (including lead), toxic gases, organic solvents, pesticides, and other substances. Pesticides, when used properly, offer benefits to society, increasing crop production, preserving produce, and combating insect infestations. However, pesticides do represent a health risk, especially for agricultural workers. Approximately 1 billion pounds of pesticide active ingredients are used annually in the United States, where 16,000 separate pesticide products are marketed. Each year, 10,000 to 20,000 physician-diagnosed pesticide poisonings occur among the approximately 3,380,000 agricultural workers.[42] During 1998–2005, 3,271 cases of acute pesticide-related occupational illness were identified in the United States.[43] The vast majority of these cases (71%) occurred in farm workers. Insecticides are responsible for the highest percentage of occupational poisoning cases (49%).[20]

In 2009, 11 million people were employed by hospitals or in the health care industry in the United States, making up 8% of the employed workforce.[2] More than 8 million of these workers are exposed to a variety of hazardous conditions, including infectious disease agents. Among the agents of concern are hepatitis B virus and human immunodeficiency virus (HIV). Health care workers are at risk if they become exposed to the blood or bodily fluids of patients or coworkers. The major route of exposure to these agents (82% of the cases) is percutaneous exposure (injuries through the skin) via contaminated sharp instruments such as needles and scalpels (see Figure 16.17). Exposure also occurs through contact with the mucous membranes of the eyes, nose, or mouth (14%), exposure to broken or abraded skin (3%), and through human bites (1%). Up to 800,000 percutaneous injuries occur annually, with an average risk of infection for HIV of 0.3% (3 per 1,000) and for hepatitis B of from 6% to 30%.[20] Health care workers are also at increased risk for acquiring other infectious diseases such as tuberculosis (TB); the incidence for health care workers is 3.7 cases per 100,000 workers.[20]

Another risk in health care settings is occupational exposure to antineoplastic drugs (drugs used in cancer treatment) and other hazardous drugs. Exposure to these substances can cause skin rashes, infertility, miscarriage, birth defects, and possibly leukemia or other cancers.[44] Exposure can occur while crushing tablets, reconstituting powdered drugs, expelling air from syringes filled with hazardous drugs, administering these drugs, or handling contaminated clothing, dressings, or body fluids. Currently, no statistics are available on the incidence of diseases and disorders resulting from these exposures, but NIOSH has issued an alert and guidelines for preventing exposure.[44]

In 2001, more than 5,000 cases of anxiety, stress, or neurotic disorders with time away from work were reported in the Survey of Occupational Injuries and Illnesses (SOII). This is about 0.6 cases per 10,000 workers. Half of these cases required 25 or more days away from work, and women constituted 65% of the cases.[20]

As stated previously, there are any number of health problems that, although prevalent and serious, could be the result of dual or multiple exposures (workplace and home). Among these

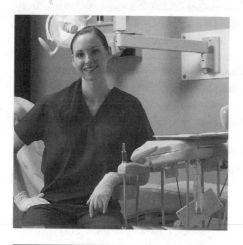

FIGURE 16.17
Health care workers are exposed to a variety of workplace hazards, including infectious diseases.

are cardiovascular diseases, cancers, and reproductive disorders. Perhaps a million or more workers are exposed to agents that can produce cancer, for example. However, there are no reliable estimates on the actual number of cancer deaths that can be traced directly to occupational exposure. Thus, we have discussed here only conditions generally accepted to be solely or predominantly related to work.

Prevention and Control of Occupational Diseases and Disorders

Preventing and controlling occupational diseases requires the vigilance of employer and employee alike and the assistance of governmental agencies. The agent-host-environment disease model discussed earlier in this book is applicable to preventive strategies outlined here. Specific activities that should be employed to control occupational diseases include identification and evaluation of agents, standard setting for the handling of and exposure to causative agents, elimination or substitution of causative factors, engineering controls to provide for a safer work area, environmental monitoring, medical screenings, personal protective devices, health promotion, disease surveillance, therapeutic medical care and rehabilitation, and compliance activities. In this regard, prevention and control of occupational diseases and disorders is similar to the prevention of occupational injuries.[34] Coordinated programs to monitor and reduce occupational hazards require professionally trained personnel. In a well-functioning program, these professionals work together as members of the occupational health and safety team.

RESOURCES FOR THE PREVENTION OF WORKPLACE INJURIES AND DISEASES

Community resources for the prevention of injuries and diseases attributable to the workplace include a variety of professional personnel and programs.

Occupational Safety and Health Professionals

The need for health professionals in the workplace is substantial. Among those with specialized training in their fields are safety engineers and certified safety professionals, health physicists, industrial hygienists, occupational physicians, and occupational health nurses.

Safety Engineers and Certified Safety Professionals

Approximately 400 academic institutions offer accredited programs that train occupational safety professionals. Many of these professionals will join the professional organization called the American Society of Safety Engineers (ASSE). "Founded in 1911, ASSE is the oldest and largest professional safety organization."[45] It has about 32,000 members who are involved in safety, health, and environmental issues in industry, insurance, government, and education. In spite of the name of this society, not all members are engineers. In fact, the background of the group is varied and includes a number of health educators.

Another recognizable group of trained professionals in this field is the Board of Certified Safety Professionals (BCSPs). This group is somewhat smaller; there are about 11,000 CSPs. "The Board of Certified Safety Professionals (BCSP) was organized as a peer certification board with the purpose of certifying practitioners in the safety profession."[46] Certification usually requires a bachelor's degree in engineering or in another scientific curriculum and the passing of two examinations.

Safety engineers and **certified safety professionals (CSPs)** design safety education programs, detect hazards in the workplace, and try to correct them (see Figure 16.18). Increased federal regulations have made the workload heavier for these occupational health professionals.

safety engineer
a safety professional employed by a company for the purpose of reducing unintentional injuries in the workplace

certified safety professional (CSP)
a health and safety professional, trained in industrial and workplace safety, who has met specific requirements for board certification

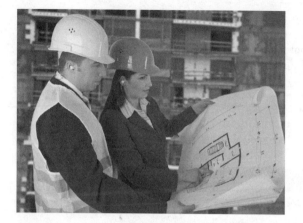

FIGURE 16.18

Safety engineers prevent workplace injuries by detecting hazards.

Health Physicists

Health physicists are concerned with radiation safety in the workplace. They monitor radiation within the work environment and develop plans for decontamination and coping with accidents involving radiation. It is estimated that there are approximately 11,000 health physicists in the United States. Many of these belong to the Health Physics Society, a 6,000-member, international scientific organization of professionals who are dedicated to promoting the practice of radiation safety.[47,48]

Industrial Hygienists

Whereas the safety engineer or certified safety professional is primarily concerned with hazards in the workplace and injury control, the **industrial hygienist** is concerned with environmental factors that might cause illness. Examples of such factors might include poor ventilation, excessive noise, poor lighting, and the presence of hazardous substances.

It is estimated that there are 7,600 industrial hygienists practicing in the United States. Perhaps a third of them hold the title of Certified Industrial Hygienist (CIH), and many belong to the American Industrial Hygiene Association. To be certified requires a two-part written examination; the first part is given following one year of postbaccalaureate experience. The second is given after 5 years of professional activity. Many industrial hygienists belong to the American Conference of Governmental Industrial Hygienists (ACGIH). This 5,000-member organization advances worker health and safety through education and the development and dissemination of scientific and technical knowledge through their publications.[49]

Occupational Physicians

The **occupational physician (OP)** or **occupational medical practitioner (OMP)** is a medical practitioner whose primary concern is preventive medicine in the workplace. Many OPs or OMPs belong to the American College of Occupational and Environmental Medicine (ACOEM), which represents more than 5,000 physicians specializing in the field of occupational and environmental medicine (OEM). "The American Board of Preventive Medicine (ABPM) recognizes and certifies qualified physicians in the medical specialty of occupational medicine. Approximately 2,200 physicians have been 'board certified' in occupational medicine within the United States."[50]

Because physicians are highly skilled and highly salaried occupational health professionals, only the largest companies maintain full-time OPs. Smaller companies may hire OPs on a part-time basis or as consultants.

Occupational Health Nurses

The role of the **occupational health nurse (OHN)** has changed over the years from running the company's medical department and first aid station to one of greater emphasis on health promotion and illness prevention. Because the OHN may be the only health professional employed in smaller plants, it is clear that if injury prevention and health promotion programs are to be offered, the job will fall to this individual.

The OHN must be a registered nurse (RN) in the state in which he or she practices. It is unlikely that these persons will have had much formal training in occupational health nursing prior to receiving their baccalaureate degrees because most nursing curricula do not provide

health physicists safety professionals with responsibility for developing plans for coping with radiation accidents

industrial hygienists health professionals concerned with health hazards in the workplace and with recommending plans for improving the healthiness of workplace environments

occupational physician (OP) or occupational medical practitioner (OMP) a physician whose primary concern is preventive medicine in the workplace

much training in this area. However, the American Board of Occupational Health Nurses, Inc., established in 1972, now offers certifications. Requirements include many hours of continuing-education credits and 5 years' experience in the field of occupational health nursing. ABOHN is the only certifying body for occupational health nurses in the United States. More than 12,000 active, certified occupational health nurses are working today.[51] Many OHNs belong to the American Association of Occupational Health Nurses (AAOHN), which was founded in 1942 and includes about 10,000 members.[52]

Occupational Safety and Health Programs

A number of programs can be put in place in occupational settings to reduce injuries and diseases. These include preplacement examinations, health maintenance programs, safety awareness programs, health promotion programs, investigation of accidents, stress management programs, employee assistance programs, and rehabilitation programs.

Preplacement Examinations

The purpose of **preplacement examinations** is to make sure that the worker fits the job. By selecting the employee who is the best physically and mentally qualified for a specific job, probabilities of job-related injuries or illnesses are minimized. Periodic evaluations are necessary to ensure that the selected individual continues to be physically and mentally qualified to carry out the job assignment. Examinations are also recommended for transferred and return-to-work employees. Sometimes a phasing in of these employees is desirable.

Occupational Disease Prevention Programs and Safety Programs

Occupational health services that facilitate preventive activities in the workplace include disease prevention programs and safety programs.

Disease Prevention Programs

Originally, occupational disease programs focused on controlling occupational diseases that one might succumb to from exposure in the work environment. Agents of concern were chemicals, radiation, and perhaps even psychological and social factors that could lead to sickness or disability. Gradually, these disease prevention efforts broadened into health maintenance programs and included the early detection and treatment of such diseases as hypertension, diabetes, obesity, and heart disease to keep employees healthier and on the job longer.

Safety Programs

Safety programs are those portions of the workplace health and safety program aimed at reducing the number and seriousness of unintentional injuries on the job. Each company needs to have a policy statement, safe operating procedures, a disaster plan, policies for hazard control, and policies for the investigation of injuries in the workplace. Provisions must be made for regular safety inspections of the workplace and for the maintenance of accurate records for each injury and for analysis of such records. Each safety program should include safety orientation and training programs and programs on first aid and cardiopulmonary resuscitation.

Worksite Health Promotion Programs

Worksite health promotion (WHP) programs are workplace-based programs aimed at improving the health of employees through changes in behavior and lifestyle. The goals for the employer include reduction of absenteeism, lowering health insurance premiums, increasing productivity, and improving employee morale. Other reasons why employers might support WHP programs include reducing workers' compensation costs, increasing employee retention, and enhancing the company's image.[53]

occupational health nurse (OHN) a registered nurse (RN) whose primary responsibilities include prevention of illness and promotion of health in the workplace

preplacement examination a physical examination of a newly hired or transferred worker to determine medical suitability for placement in a specific position

safety programs those parts of the workplace safety and health program aimed at reducing unintentional injuries on the job

worksite health promotion (WHP) programs health promotion programs in the workplace that include health education, screening, and/or intervention designed to change employees' health behavior and reduce risks associated with disease or injury

In the United States, historically, health care insurance has come through one's employment. In 1965, the employers' share of the nation's health care bill was 18%; in 2006, it was 40%. In some companies the cost of providing health care for employees is equal to about 50% of the companies' profits.[53] Obviously, this upward trend in the cost of health care for employers cannot continue much longer. Until this system changes, however, employers are making serious efforts to reduce health care costs, and one effective way to do this is worksite health promotion.

Health promotion programs range in size from very modest programs that might include only hypertension screening to more comprehensive programs that offer cancer risk screening, nutrition and weight management, fitness, smoking cessation, stress management programs, and more. Generally, the objectives of these programs are to facilitate changes in behavior or lifestyle to prevent disease and to promote health.[53]

All indications are that WHP programs will continue to grow. Corporations not only see them as a means to control health care costs and show a concern for the employees, but also as a means by which to recruit new employees and to retain the ones currently in the organization. (See Chapter 5 for more information on health promotion programs.)

employee assistance programs (EAPs) workplace-based programs that assist employees who have substance abuse, domestic, psychological, or social problems that interfere with their work performance

Employee Assistance Programs

Employee assistance programs (EAPs) are programs that assist employees who have substance abuse, domestic, psychological, or social problems that interfere with their work performance. These programs, which arrived at many workplaces before WHP programs, originally arose in response to occupational alcohol problems. EAPs provide help to employees with a variety of problems that affect their work performance. Whereas WHP programs are primary prevention efforts, EAPs are secondary prevention or tertiary prevention efforts. They have as their goal the intervention and sometimes rehabilitation of employees with behavioral or other problems before such problems become costly for both the employer and employee.

CHAPTER SUMMARY

- After time spent at home, Americans spend the next largest portion of their time at work; thus, safe and healthy workplaces are essential if America is to reach its health potential.

- Every day approximately 14 people die from work-related injuries and many more people die of work-related diseases.

- Occupational health issues affect the quality of life economically as well as medically in communities in which workers live. Although occupational injuries and illnesses have been a long-standing concern of workers in America, rapid progress in reducing the number and seriousness of workplace injuries and illnesses became possible only after the passage of the Occupational Safety and Health Act (OSHAct) of 1970.

- The OSHAct established the Occupational Safety and Health Administration (OSHA) and the National Institute of Occupational Safety and Health (NIOSH) and required private industry to provide safe jobs and workplaces.

- The number and type of workplace injuries vary by person, place, time, and type of industry. Highway injuries are the leading cause of fatal work-related injuries. Falls and being struck by an object or equipment are the second and third leading causes of unintentional workplace deaths.

- Nonfatal work-related injuries cost both employees and employers in terms of lost wages and lost productivity.

- Workplace violence affects 1.7 million workers in the United States each year, and homicide is the third leading cause of workplace fatalities.

- Work-related injuries can be controlled by applying a variety of injury prevention strategies, including eliminating a dangerous job, improving the work environment, using safer machinery, and improving the selection and training of workers.

- Work-related illnesses and disorders kill thousands of workers and former workers each year.

SCENARIO: ANALYSIS AND RESPONSE

Please take a moment to reread the scenario at the beginning of this chapter. Then, reflect on the questions that follow.

1. If you were Jen, what would you do?

2. In 1998, California passed legislation protecting waitresses like Jen and bartenders by outlawing smoking in not only restaurants but also in bars. Do you support such legislation? How likely is it that your state legislature would pass a similar law?

3. Ambient smoke in a restaurant or bar is an example of situations that occur daily in the workplace. Suppose you suspected that you were being exposed to a toxic agent where you worked. What would you do? Who would you contact? How could OSHA be of assistance?

4. Think about some of the jobs held by your fellow classmates. Do any of those jobs expose them to hazardous substances? Do any of the jobs students have put them at risk for injuries?

- The types of illnesses and disorders that can be attributed to workplace exposure are many, including musculoskeletal conditions, dermatological conditions, lung diseases, and cancers, among many others.

- Repeated trauma is the leading cause of work-related nonfatal illnesses.

- There are numerous resources to aid in the prevention of occupational injuries and diseases, including occupational health professionals and workplace injury and illness prevention programs and worksite health promotion programs.

REVIEW QUESTIONS

1. Provide definitions of the terms *occupational injury* and *occupational disease* and give three examples of each.

2. In what ways are health problems in the workplace related to health problems in the general community?

3. How did the Industrial Revolution contribute to an increase in occupational health problems?

4. Who was Alice Hamilton? What did she do?

5. What were the deficiencies in state occupational safety and health laws in the early 1960s?

6. Discuss briefly the purpose of the Occupational Safety and Health Act of 1970 and outline its provisions.

7. What is OSHA and what does it do? What is NIOSH and what does it do?

8. What are some of the most frequently reported workplace injuries? Which are the leading causes of workplace injury deaths?

9. Which age group and gender of workers suffer the most occupational injuries? Which have the most fatal injuries?

10. Why is farming a particularly hazardous occupation? What are ROPS and how do they prevent deaths? Describe some of the workplace hazards experienced by migrant farmworkers and their children.

11. What are the risk factors for encountering violence in the workplace? Which occupation is at greatest risk for workplace homicides?

12. Outline some general control strategies that can reduce the number and seriousness of workplace injuries.

13. What is the most frequently reported occupational disorder?

14. What determines whether a musculoskeletal condition or skin condition should be considered an injury or a disease?

15. List four well-documented lung conditions that are related to occupational exposure. Name the occupations whose workers are at high risk for each of these conditions.

16. Why is it often difficult to prove that a disease or condition resulted from workplace exposure?

17. Outline some features of a workplace program to prevent or control occupational diseases. For each activity, indicate whether it is aimed at the agent, host, or environment aspect of the disease model.

18. List five health occupations that deal with worker safety and health. Describe their training and job assignments.

19. Name and describe four occupational safety and health programs.

20. What are some of the benefits of worksite health promotion programs for employers and employees?

ACTIVITIES

1. Examine your local newspaper every day for a week for articles dealing with occupational injury or illness. Find three articles and, after reading them, provide the following: a brief summary, the resulting injury or disease, the cause of the injury or disease, and a brief plan for how the organization could eliminate the cause.

2. Interview an individual who works in the profession you wish to enter after graduation. Ask him or her to describe what he or she feels are the most prevalent injuries and illnesses connected with his or her job. Also ask about specific preservice and in-service education the interviewee has had to protect against these problems. Finally, ask him or her to propose measures to limit future problems. Summarize your interview on paper in a two-page report.

3. If you have ever become injured or ill as a result of a job, explain what happened to you. In a two-page paper, identify the causative agent, how the injury could have been prevented, and what kind of training you had to prepare you for a safe working environment.

4. Go to the school library and research the injuries and diseases connected with your future profession. In a two-page paper, identify the major problems and what employers and employees should do about them and express concerns that you have about working in the profession because of these problems.

5. Visit any job site related to your future profession. At that site, find 10 things that employers and employees are doing to make it a safe work environment. List these 10 things briefly and explain the benefit of each one.

COMMUNITY HEALTH ON THE WEB

The Internet contains a wealth of information about community and public health. Increase your knowledge of some of the topics presented in this chapter by accessing the Jones & Bartlett Learning Web site at **http://health .jbpub.com/book/communityhealth/7e** and follow the links to complete the following Web activities.

- National Institute for Occupational Safety and Health
- Occupational Safety and Health Administration
- American Industrial Hygiene Association

REFERENCES

1. International Labour Organization (2009). *World Day for Safety and Health at Work 2009: Facts on Safety and Health at Work*. Geneva: Author. Available at http://www.ilo.org/wcmsp5/groups/public/dgreports/dcomm/documents/publication/wcms_105146.pdf.

2. U.S. Department of Labor, Bureau of Labor Statistics (2010). "Labor Force Statistics from the Current Population Survey." Available at http://www.bls.gov/cps/demographics.htm.

3. U.S. Department of Labor, Bureau of Labor Statistics (2008). *BLS Glossary*. Available at http://www.bls.gov/bls/glossary.htm.

4. National Safety Council (2010). *Injury Facts 2010 Edition*. Itasca, IL: Author.

5. U.S. Department of Labor, Bureau of Labor Statistics (2009). *National Census of Fatal Occupational Injuries in 2008*. Available at http://www.bls.gov/news.release/archives/cfoi_08202009.pdf.

6. U.S. Department of Labor, Bureau of Labor Statistics (2009). "Revisions to the 2008 Census of Fatal Occupational Injuries (CFOI) Counts." Available at http://www.bls.gov/iif/oshcfoi1.htm.

7. U.S. Department of Labor, Bureau of Labor Statistics (2009). *Workplace Injuries and Illnesses in 2008*. Available at http://www.bls.gov/news.release/archives/osh_10292009.pdf.

8. Health and Safety Executive (United Kingdom) (2006). "European Comparisons—Fatal Injuries." Available at http://www.hse.gov.uk/statistics/european/fatal.htm.

9. European Commission (2010). "Fatal Accidents at Work: Incidence Rate." Eurostat, Your Key to European Statistics. Available at http://epp.eurostat.ec.europa.eu/portal/page/portal/health/health_safety_work/data/main_tables.

10. Felton, J. S. (1986). "History of Occupational Health and Safety." In J. LaDou, ed., *Introduction to Occupational Health and Safety*. Chicago: National Safety Council.

11. Rosen, G. (1958). *A History of Public Health*. New York: M.D. Publications.

12. LaDou, J., J. Olishifski, and C. Zenz (1986). "Occupational Health and Safety Today." In J. LaDou, ed., *Introduction to Occupational Health and Safety*. Chicago: National Safety Council.

13. Schilling, R. S. F. (1989). "Developments in Occupational Health." In H. A. Waldron, ed., *Occupational Health Practice*. Boston: Butterworths.

14. Ashford, N. A. (1976). *Crisis in the Workplace: Occupational Disease and Injury—A Report to the Ford Foundation*. Cambridge, MA: MIT Press.

15. Page, J. A., and M. W. O'Brien (1973). *Bitter Wages*. New York: Grossman.

16. U.S. Department of Labor, Bureau of Labor Statistics (2009). *Nonfatal Occupational Injuries and Illnesses Requiring Days Away from Work, 2008* [News release]. Available at http://www.bls.gov/news.release/archives/osh2_12042009.pdf.

17. U.S. Department of Labor, Bureau of Labor Statistics (2009). "Census of Fatal Occupational Injuries Charts 1992-2008 (Revised Data)." Available at http://www.bls.gov/iif/oshcfoi1.htm#charts.

18. Centers for Disease Control and Prevention (2010). "Workers Memorial Day—April 28, 2010." *Morbidity and Mortality Weekly Report*, 59(15): 449. Available at http://www.cdc.gov/mmwr/pdf/wk/mm5915.pdf.

19. Centers for Disease Control and Prevention (2007). "Nonfatal Occupational Injuries and Illnesses—United States, 2004." *Morbidity and Mortality Weekly Report*, 56(16): 393-397. Available at http://www.cdc.gov/mmwr/preview/mmwrhtml/mm5616a3.htm.

20. U.S. Department of Health and Human Services, Centers for Disease Control and Prevention, National Institute for Occupational Safety and Health (2004). *Worker Health Chartbook, 2004* (DHHS [NIOSH] pub. no. 2004-146). Available at http://www.cdc.gov/niosh/docs/2004-146.

21. Centers for Disease Control and Prevention (2010). "Occupational Injuries and Deaths among Younger Workers—United States, 1998-2007." *Morbidity and Mortality Weekly Report*, 59(15): 449-455. Available at http://www.cdc.gov/mmwr/pdf/wk/mm5915.pdf.

22. National Consumers' League (2003). "Teens, Avoid These Jobs in 2010." Available at http://www.nclnet.org/worker-rights/54-teen-jobs/401-teens-avoid-these-jobs-in-2010.

23. Child Labor Coalition (2005). "2004 Child Labor State Survey." Available at http://www.stopchildlabor.org/USchildlabor/2004_survey_results.htm.

24. U.S. Department of Health and Human Services, Centers for Disease Control and Prevention, National Institute for Occupational Safety and Health (2003). *NIOSH Alert: Preventing Deaths, Injuries, and Illnesses of Young Workers* (DHHS [NIOSH] pub. no. 2003-128). Cincinnati, OH: NIOSH Publications. Available at http://www.cdc.gov/niosh/topics/youth/.

25. Wagner, D. K., J. Walstedt, L. Jenkins, et al. (1997). *Women: Work and Health* (DHHS pub. no. PHS 97-1415). Hyattsville, MD: National Center for Health Statistics.

26. Centers for Disease Control and Prevention (2010). "Commercial Fishing Deaths—United States, 2000-2009." *Morbidity and Mortality Weekly Report*, 59(27): 842-845. Available at http://www.cdc.gov/mmwr/preview/mmwrhtml/mm5927a2.htm?s_cid=mm5927a2_w.

27. Kirdahy, M. (2008). "America's Most Dangerous Jobs." Forbes.com. Available at http://www.forbes.com/2008/08/25/dangerous-jobs-fishing-lead-careers-cx_mk_0825danger.html.

28. Urbina, I. (9 April 2010). "No Survivors Found After West Virginia Mine Disaster." *New York Times*. Available at http://www.nytimes.com/2010/04/10/us/10westvirginia.html.

29. Ayers, P. D. (2005). *Safety: General Tractor Safety* (Farm and Ranch Series, no. 5.016). Ft. Collins: Colorado State University Extension. Available at http://www.ext.colostate.edu/pubs/farmmgt/05016.pdf.

30. Centers for Disease Control and Prevention (1997). "Use of Rollover Protective Structures—Iowa, Kentucky, New York, and Ohio, 1992-1997." *Morbidity and Mortality Weekly Report*, 46(36): 842-845.

31. U.S. Department of Health and Human Services, Centers for Disease Control and Prevention, National Institute for Occupational Safety and Health (2009). "Injuries to Youth on Farms and Safety Recommendations, U.S. 2006" (DHHS [NIOSH] pub. no. 2009-117). Available at http://www.cdc.gov/niosh/docs/2009-117/pdfs/2009-117.pdf.

32. Novello, A. C. (1991). "A Charge to the Conference." Presented at the Surgeon General's Conference on Agricultural Safety and Health: Farm Safe 2000, Des Moines, IA.

33. Human Rights Watch (2010). *Fields of Peril: Child Labor in U.S. Agriculture*. New York: Author. Available at http://www.hrw.org/node/90126.

34. Weeks, J. L., G. R. Wagner, K. M. Rest, and B. S. Levy (2005). "A Public Health Approach to Preventing Occupational Diseases and Injuries." In B. S. Levy, G. R. Wagner, K. M. Rest, and J. L. Weeks, eds., *Preventing Occupational Disease and Injury*, 2nd ed. Washington, DC: American Public Health Association.

35. Centers for Disease Control and Prevention, National Institute of Occupational Safety and Health (2006). "The National Occupational Research Agenda (NORA)." Available at http://www.cdc.gov/niosh/nora/default.html.

36. Centers for Disease Control and Prevention, National Institute for Occupational Safety and Health (2004). *Violence on the Job* (NIOSH pub. no. 2004-100d). Available at http://www.cdc.gov/niosh/docs/video/violence.html.

37. Centers for Disease Control and Prevention (1994). "Occupational Injury Deaths of Postal Workers—United States, 1980-1989." *Morbidity and Mortality Weekly Report*, 43(32): 587-595.

38. National Center on Addiction and Substance Abuse at Columbia University (2000). *The United States Postal Service Commission on a Safe and Secure Workplace*. New York: Author.

39. Centers for Disease Control and Prevention, National Institute for Occupational Safety and Health (2004). "Violence on the Job" (NIOSH pub. no. 2004-100d). Available at http://www.cdc.gov/niosh/docs/video/violence.html.

40. Centers for Disease Control and Prevention, National Institute for Occupational Safety and Health (2005). "Work-Related Lung Disease (WoRLD) Surveillance Report: December 2007 Updated Tables and Figures." Available at http://www2a.cdc.gov/drds/WorldReportData/.

41. Centers for Disease Control and Prevention (2009). "Coal Worker's Pneumonoconiosis-Related Years of Potential Life Lost Before Age 65 Years—United States, 1968-2006." *Morbidity and Mortality Weekly Report*, 58(50): 1412-1416. Available at http://www.cdc.gov/mmwr/PDF/wk/mm5850.pdf.

42. Centers for Disease Control and Prevention, National Institute for Occupational Safety and Health (2005). "NIOSH Topic: Pesticide Illness and Injury Surveillance." Available at http://www.cdc.gov/niosh/topics/pesticides/.

43. Calvert, G. M., J. Karnik, L. Meler, J. Beckman, B. Morrissey, J. Sievert, R. Barrett, M. Lackovic, L. Mabee, A. Schwartz, Y. Mitchell, and S. Moraga-McHaley (2008). "Acute Pesticide Poisoning among Agricultural Workers in the United States, 1998-2005." *American Journal of Industrial Medicine*, 51: 883-898. Available at http://www.cdc.gov/niosh/topics/pesticides/ajim2008.html.

44. Centers for Disease Control and Prevention, National Institute for Occupational Safety and Health (2004). "NIOSH Alert: Preventing Occupational Exposures to Antineoplastic and Other Hazardous Drugs in Health Care Settings" (DHHS [NIOSH] pub. no. 2004-165). Cincinnati, OH: Author.

45. American Society of Safety Engineers (2010). Web site. Available at http://www.asse.org.

46. Board of Certified Safety Professionals (2010). Web site. Available at http://www.bcsp.org.

47. Health Physics Society (2010). "About the Health Physics Society." Available at http://hps.org/aboutthesociety/.

48. American Academy of Health Physics (2010). "Welcome to the Home Page of the AAHP." Available at http://hps1.org/aahp/.

49. American Conference of Governmental Industrial Hygienists (2010). Web site. Available at http://www.acgih.org.

50. American College of Occupational and Environmental Medicine (2010). Web site. Available at http://www.acoem.org/.

51. American Board for Occupational Health Nurses, Inc. (2010). "Who We Are and What We Do." Available at http://www.abohn.org.

52. American Association of Occupational Nurses, Inc. (2010). Web site. Available at http://www.aaohn.org.

53. Chenoweth, D. H. (2007). *Worksite Health Promotion*, 2nd ed. Champaign, IL: Human Kinetics.

Appendix I

Case/Control Studies: How to Calculate an Odds Ratio

Let us assume that you selected 100 lung cancer cases and 1,000 controls of the same age, sex, and socioeconomic status as the cases. Suppose 90 of 100 cases of lung cancer had been regular smokers, but only 270 of 1,000 controls smoked. An odds ratio could be calculated by the formula $(A \times D) \div (B \times C)$, where cases and controls are designated as follows:

		Disease Present	
		Yes	No
Risk Factor Present	Yes	A	B
	No	C	D

In our example:

		Disease Present	
		Yes	No
Risk Factor Present	Yes	90	270
	No	10	730

Substituting our data into the formula:

$[(90 \times 730) \div (270 \times 10)] = 65,700 \div 2,700 = 24.33$. Thus, lung cancer victims have 24.33 times greater probability of having been a smoker.

COHORT STUDIES: HOW TO CALCULATE RELATIVE AND ATTRIBUTABLE RISK

Let us assume that in a cohort of 4,000 there were 1,000 smokers and 3,000 nonsmokers. If, after 20 years, cancer develops in 22 smokers (22 per 1,000) and in 6 nonsmokers (6 per 3,000 or 2 per 1,000), *relative risk* is the ratio of the incidence rates, 22 per thousand: 2 per thousand or 22:2 or 11 to 1.

Further, one can calculate an *attributable risk* by subtracting the deaths in the nonsmoking group (2 deaths) from the number of lung cancer deaths in the smoking group (22 deaths). Thus, 20 deaths are attributable to smoking; the attributable risk is 20 per 1,000.

Appendix 2

Operational Definitions for the 1990 Census

American Indian, Eskimo, or Aleut Includes persons who classified themselves as such in one of the specific race categories identified below.

American Indian Includes persons who indicated their race as "American Indian," entered the name of an Indian tribe, or reported such entries as Canadian Indian, French-American Indian, or Spanish-American Indian.

Eskimo Includes persons who indicated their race as "Eskimo" or reported entries such as Arctic Slope, Inupiat, and Yupik.

Aleut Includes persons who indicated their race as "Aleut" or reported entries such as Alutiiq, Egegik, and Pribilovian.

Asian or Pacific Islander Includes persons who reported in one of the Asian or Pacific Islander groups listed on the questionnaire or who provided write-in responses such as Thai, Nepaili, or Tongan.

Asian Includes "Chinese," "Filipino," "Japanese," "Asian Indian," "Korean," "Vietnamese," and "Other Asian."

Chinese Includes persons who indicated their race as "Chinese" or who identified themselves as Cantonese, Tibetan, or Chinese American. In standard census reports, persons who reported as "Taiwanese" or "Formosan" are included here with Chinese. In special reports on the Asian or Pacific Islander population, information on persons who identified themselves as Taiwanese are shown separately.

Filipino Includes persons who indicated their race as "Filipino" or reported entries such as Philipino, Philipine, or Filipino-American.

Japanese Includes persons who indicated their race as "Japanese" and persons who identified themselves as Nipponese or Japanese-American.

Asian Indian Includes persons who indicated their race as "Asian Indian" and persons who identified themselves as Bengalese, Bharat, Dravidian, East Indian, or Goanese.

Korean Includes persons who indicated their race as "Korean" and persons who identified themselves as Korean-American.

Vietnamese Includes persons who indicated their race as "Vietnamese" and persons who identified themselves as Vietnamese-American.

Cambodian Includes persons who provided a write-in response such as Cambodian or Cambodia.

Hmong Includes persons who provided a write-in response such as Hmong, Laohmong, or Mong.

Laotian Includes persons who provided a write-in response such as Laotian, Laos, or Lao.

Thai Includes persons who provided a write-in response such as Thai, Thailand, or Siamese.

Other Asian Includes persons who provided a write-in response of Bangladeshi, Burmese, Indonesian, Pakistani, Sri Lankan, Amerasian, or Eurasian.

Pacific Islander Includes persons who indicated their race as "Pacific Islander" by classifying themselves into one of the following race categories or identifying themselves as one of the Pacific Islander cultural groups of Polynesian, Micronesian, or Melanesian.

Hawaiian Includes persons who indicated their race as "Hawaiian" as well as persons who identified themselves as Part Hawaiian or Native Hawaiian.

Samoan Includes persons who indicated their race as "Samoan" or persons who identified themselves as American-Samoan or Western Samoan.

Guamanian   Includes persons who indicated their race as "Guamanian" or persons who identified themselves as Chamorro or Guam.

Other Pacific Islander   Includes persons who provided a write-in response of a Pacific Islander group such as Tahitian, Northern Mariana Islander, Palauan, Fijiian, or a cultural group such as Polynesian, Micronesian, or Melanesian.

Black   Includes persons who indicated their race as "black or Negro" or reported entries such as African-American, Afro-American, black Puerto Rican, Jamaican, Nigerian, West Indian, or Haitian.

White   Includes persons who indicated their race as "white" or reported entries such as Canadian, German, Italian, Lebanese, Near Easterner, Arab, or Polish.

Other race   Includes all other persons not included in "white," "black," "American Indian, Eskimo, or Aleut," and "Asian or Pacific Islander" race categories described above. Persons reporting in the "Other race" category and providing write-in entries such as multiracial, multiethnic, mixed, interracial, Wesort, or a Spanish/Hispanic origin group (such as Mexican, Cuban, or Puerto Rican) are included here.

Hispanic origin   Of Hispanic origin are those who classified themselves in one of the specific Hispanic origin categories listed on the questionnaire—"Mexican," "Puerto Rican," or "Cuban"—as well as those who indicated that they were of "other Spanish/Hispanic" origin. Persons of "Other Spanish/Hispanic" origin are those whose origins are from Spain, the Spanish-speaking countries of Central or South America or the Dominican Republic, or they are persons of Hispanic origin identifying themselves generally as Spanish, Spanish-American, Hispanic, Hispano, Latino, and so on.

Note: These definitions were taken directly from U.S. Department of Commerce (1990). *Census of Population and Housing, Summary Population and Housing, Characteristics, United States.* Washington, DC: U.S. Government Printing Office.

Appendix 3

Revised Operational Definitions for 1997*

American Indian or Alaska Native A person having origins in any of the original peoples of North and South American (including Central America), and who maintains tribal affiliation or community attachment.

"Alaska Native" should replace the term "Alaskan Native."

Alaska Native should be used instead of Eskimo and Aleut.

Asian A person having origins in any of the original peoples of the Far East, Southeast Asia, or the Indian subcontinent including, for example, Cambodia, China, India, Japan, Korea, Malaysia, Pakistan, the Philippine Islands, Thailand, and Vietnam.

Native Hawaiian or Other Pacific Islander A person having origins in any of the original peoples of Hawaii, Guam, Samoa, or other Pacific Islands.

Hispanic or Latino A person of Cuban, Mexican, Puerto Rican, South or Central American, or other Spanish culture or origin, regardless of race. The term "Spanish origin" can be used in addition to "Hispanic or Latino."

*Federal programs had until January 1, 2003, to adopt these revised standards.

Source: Office of Management and Budget (30 October 1997), *Revisions to the Standards for the Classification of Federal Data on Race and Ethnicity.* Available at http://www.white house.gov/omb/fedreg_1997standards.

Self-Assessment Checklist Promoting Cultural Diversity and Cultural Competency

SELF-ASSESSMENT CHECKLIST FOR PERSONNEL PROVIDING SERVICES TO CHILDREN WITH SPECIAL HEALTH NEEDS AND THEIR FAMILIES

This checklist was developed by HRSA's Maternal and Child Health Bureau/Children with Special Health Needs component of the National Center for Cultural Competence. It is for personnel providing health services and supports to children with special health needs and their families and is intended to heighten the awareness and sensitivity of personnel to the importance of cultural diversity and cultural competence in human service settings. The checklist provides concrete examples of the kinds of values and practices that foster such an environment. ***Directions: Select A, B, or C for each item listed below.***

A = Things I do frequently   B = Things I do occasionally   C = Things I do rarely or never

Physical environment, materials, and resources

____1. I display pictures, posters, and other materials that reflect the cultures and ethnic backgrounds of children and families served by my program or agency.

____2. I ensure that magazines, brochures, and other printed materials in reception areas are of interest to and reflect the different cultures of children and families served by my program or agency.

____3. When using videos, films, or other media resources for health education, treatment, or other interventions, I ensure that they reflect the cultures of children and families served by my program or agency.

____4. When using food during an assessment, I ensure that meals provided include foods that are unique to the cultural and ethnic backgrounds of children and families served by my program or agency.

____5. I ensure that toys and other play accessories in reception areas and those which are used during assessment are representative of the various cultural and ethnic groups within the local community and the society in general.

Communication styles

____6. For children who speak languages or dialects other than English, I attempt to learn and use key words in their language so that I am better able to communicate with them during assessment, treatment, or other interventions.

____7. I attempt to determine any familial colloquialisms used by children and families that may impact on assessment, treatment, or other interventions.

____8. I use visual aids, gestures, and physical prompts in my interactions with children who have limited English proficiency.

____9. I use bilingual staff or trained volunteers to serve as interpreters during assessment, meetings, or other events for parents who would require this level of assistance.

____10. When interacting with parents who have limited English proficiency I always keep in mind that:

   ____* limitations in English proficiency is in no way a reflection of their level of intellectual functioning.

   ____* their limited ability to speak the language of the dominant culture has no bearing on their ability to communicate effectively in their language of origin.

   ____* they may or may not be literate in their language of origin or English.

____11. When possible, I ensure that all notices and communiqués to parents are written in their language of origin.

____12. I understand that it may be necessary to use alternatives to written communications for some families, as word of mouth may be a preferred method of receiving information.

Values and attitudes

____13. I avoid imposing values that may conflict or be inconsistent with those of cultures or ethnic groups other than my own.

____14. In group therapy or treatment situations, I discourage children from using racial and ethnic slurs by helping them understand that certain words can hurt others.

____15. I screen books, movies, and other media resources for negative cultural, ethnic, or racial stereotypes before sharing them with children and their parents served by my program or agency.

____16. I intervene in an appropriate manner when I observe other staff or parents within my program or agency engaging in behaviors that show cultural insensitivity or prejudice.

____17. I understand and accept that family is defined differently by different cultures (e.g., extended family members, fictive kin, godparents).

____18. I recognize and accept that individuals from culturally diverse backgrounds may desire varying degrees of acculturation into the dominant culture.

____19. I accept and respect that male–female roles may vary significantly among different cultures (e.g., who makes major decisions for the family, play and social interactions expected of male and female children).

____20. I understand that age and life cycle factors must be considered in interactions with individuals and families (e.g., high value placed on the decisions of elders or the role of the eldest male in families).

____21. Even though my professional or moral viewpoints may differ, I accept the family/parents as the ultimate decision makers for services and supports for their children.

___22. I recognize that the meaning or value of medical treatment and health education may vary greatly among cultures.

___23. I accept that religion and other beliefs may influence how families respond to illnesses, disease, and death.

___24. I recognize and accept that folk and religious beliefs may influence a family's reaction and approach to a child born with a disability or later diagnosed with a disability or special health care needs.

___25. I understand that traditional approaches to disciplining children are influenced by culture.

___26. I understand that families from different cultures will have different expectations of their children for acquiring toileting, dressing, feeding, and other self-help skills.

___27. I accept and respect that customs and beliefs about food, its value, preparation, and use are different from culture to culture.

___28. Before visiting or providing services in the home setting, I seek information on acceptable behaviors, courtesies, customs, and expectations that are unique to families of specific cultures and ethnic groups served by my program or agency.

___29. I seek information from family members or other key community informants, which will assist in service adaptation to respond to the needs and preferences of culturally and ethnically diverse children and families served by my program or agency.

___30. I advocate for the review of my program's or agency's mission statement, goals, policies, and procedures to ensure that they incorporate principles and practices that promote cultural diversity and cultural competence.

There is no answer key. However, if you frequently responded "C", you may not necessarily demonstrate values and engage in practices that promote a culturally diverse and culturally competent service delivery system for children and families.

For more information contact: Tawara D. Goode, Georgetown University Child Development Center UAP. Adapted from "Promoting Cultural Competence and Cultural Diversity in Early Intervention and Early Childhood Settings" (Revised 1999).

Source: U.S. Department of Health and Human Services (January 2000). "Promoting Cultural Diversity and Culture Competency." Office of Minority Health, *Closing the Gap*, 6–7.

Glossary Terms

absorption field The element of a septic system in which the liquid portion of waste is distributed.

accreditation The process by which an agency or organization evaluates and recognizes an institution as meeting certain predetermined standards.

acculturated The cultural modification of an individual or group by adapting to or borrowing traits from another culture.

activities of daily living (ADLs) Eating, toileting, dressing, bathing, walking, getting in and out of a bed or chair, and getting outside.

acute disease A disease in which the peak severity of symptoms occurs and subsides within 3 months of onset, usually within days or weeks.

Administration on Aging An operating division of the Department of Health and Human Services designated to carry out the provisions of the Older Americans Act of 1965.

Administration for Children and Families An operating division of the Department of Health and Human Services that coordinates programs that promote the economic and social well-being of families, children, individuals, and communities.

adolescents and young adults Individuals between the ages of 15 and 24 years.

adult day care programs Daytime care provided to seniors who are unable to be left alone.

aftercare The continuing care provided to former drug abusers or drug-dependent persons.

age pyramid A conceptual model that illustrates the age distribution of a population.

age-adjusted rates Rates used to make comparisons of relative risks across groups and over time when groups differ by age structure.

aged The state of being old.

ageism Prejudice and discrimination against the aged.

Agency for Healthcare Research and Quality (AHRQ) An operating division of the Department of Health and Human Services that has the responsibility of overseeing health care research.

Agency for Toxic Substances and Disease Registry (ATSDR) An operating division of the Department of Health and Human Services created by Superfund legislation to prevent or mitigate adverse health effects and diminished quality of life resulting from exposure to hazardous substances in the environment.

agent (pathogenic agent) The cause of the disease or health problem; the factor that must be present for the disease to occur.

aging The physiological changes that occur normally in plants and animals as they grow older.

air pollution Contamination of the air that interferes with the comfort, safety, and health of living organisms.

Air Quality Index (AQI) An index (number between 0 and 500) that indicates the level of pollution in the air and associated health risk.

airborne disease A communicable disease that is transmitted through the air (e.g., influenza).

Alcoholics Anonymous (AA) A fellowship of recovering alcoholics who offer support to anyone who desires to stop drinking.

alcoholism   A disease characterized by impaired control over drinking, preoccupation with drinking, and continued use of alcohol despite adverse consequences.

alien   A person born in and owing allegiance to a country other than the one in which he or she lives.

allied health care professionals   Health care workers who provide services that assist, facilitate, and complement the work of physicians and other health care specialists.

allopathic providers   Independent health care providers whose remedies for illnesses produce effects different from those of the disease. These people are doctors of medicine (MDs).

American Cancer Society   A voluntary health agency dedicated to fighting cancer and educating the public about cancer.

American Health Security Act of 1993   The comprehensive health care reform introduced by then President Clinton, but never enacted.

American Red Cross   A nonprofit, humanitarian organization led by volunteers and guided by its Congressional Charter that provides relief to victims of disasters.

amotivational syndrome   A pattern of behavior characterized by apathy, loss of effectiveness, and a more passive, introverted personality.

amphetamines   A group of synthetic drugs that act as stimulants.

anabolic drugs   Compounds, structurally similar to the male hormone testosterone, that increase protein synthesis.

analytic study   A type of epidemiological study aimed at testing hypotheses (e.g., observational, experimental).

anthroponosis   A disease that infects only humans.

aquifers   Porous, water-saturated layers of underground bedrock, sand, and gravel that can yield economically significant amounts of water.

asbestos   A naturally occurring mineral fiber that has been identified as a class A carcinogen by the Environmental Protection Agency.

asbestosis   Acute or chronic lung disease caused by the deposit of asbestos fibers on lungs.

assisted-living facility   "A special combination of housing, personalized supportive services, and health care designed to meet the needs—both scheduled and unscheduled—of those who need help with activities of daily living" (see Chapter 9, reference 37).

attack rate   A special incidence rate calculated for a particular population for a single disease outbreak and expressed as a percentage.

automatic (passive) protection   The modification of a product or the environment in such a way as to reduce unintentional injuries.

bacteriological period   The period in public health history from 1875 to 1900 during which the causes of many bacterial diseases were discovered.

barbiturates   Depressant drugs based on the structure of barbituric acid; for example, phenobarbital.

behavioral health care services   The managed care term for mental health and substance abuse/dependence care services.

benzodiazapines   Nonbarbiturate depressant drugs; examples: Librium, Valium.

best experience   Intervention strategies used in prior or existing programs that have not gone through the critical research and evaluation studies and thus fall short of best practice criteria.

best practices   "Recommendations for interventions based on critical review of multiple research and evaluation studies that substantiate the efficacy of the intervention" (see Chapter 5, reference 31).

best processes   Original intervention strategies that the planners create based on their knowledge and skills of good planning processes including the involvement of those in the priority population and the theories and models.

bias and hate crimes   Crimes that occur when offenders choose a victim because of some characteristic—for example, race, ethnicity, or religion—and provide evidence that the hate prompted them to commit the crime.

binge drinking   Consuming five or more alcoholic drinks in a row for males, four or more for females.

biogenic pollutants   Airborne biological organisms or their particles or gases or other toxic materials that can produce illness.

biological hazards   Living organisms (and viruses), or their products, that increase the risk of disease or death in humans.

bioterrorism   The threatened or intentional release of biological agents for the purpose of influencing the conduct of government or intimidating or coercing a civilian population to further political or social objectives.

bipolar disorder   An affective disorder characterized by distinct periods of elevated mood alternating with periods of depression.

birth rate   See *natality (birth) rate.*

blood alcohol concentration (BAC)   The percentage of concentration of alcohol in the blood; a BAC of 0.08% or greater is regarded as the legal level of intoxication in all states.

Bloodborne Pathogen Standard   A set of regulations promulgated by OSHA that sets forth the responsibilities of employers and employees with regard to precautions to be taken concerning bloodborne pathogens in the workplace.

bloodborne pathogens   Disease agents, such as HIV, that are transmissible in blood and other body fluids.

body mass index (BMI)   The ratio of weight (in kilograms) to height (in meters, squared). To calculate in pounds and inches, divide (weight in pounds)/2.20 by [(height in inches)/32.27]^2.

bottom-up community organization   Organization efforts that begin with those who live within the community affected.

brownfields   Property where reuse is complicated by the presence of hazardous substances from prior use.

Bureau of Alcohol, Tobacco, Firearms, and Explosives (ATF)   The federal agency in the Department of Justice that regulates alcohol, tobacco, firearms, and explosives.

Bureau of Indian Affairs (BIA)   The original federal government agency charged with the responsibility for the welfare of American Indians.

byssinosis   Acute or chronic lung disease caused by the inhalation of cotton, flax, or hemp dusts; those affected include workers in cotton textile plants (sometimes called *brown lung disease*).

capitation   See *prepaid health care*.

carcinogens   Agents, usually chemicals, that cause cancer.

care manager   One who helps identify the health care needs of an individual but does not actually provide the health care services.

care provider   One who helps identify the health care needs of an individual and also personally performs the caregiving service.

carrier   A person or animal that harbors a specific communicable disease agent in the absence of discernible clinical disease and serves as a potential source of infection to others.

carrying capacity   The maximum population of a particular species that a given habitat can support over a given period of time.

case fatality rate (CFR)   The percentage of cases of a particular disease that result in death.

case/control study   An epidemiological study that seeks to compare those diagnosed with a disease (cases) with those who do not have the disease (controls) for prior exposure to specific risk factors.

cases   People afflicted with a disease.

categorical programs   Those programs available only to people who can be categorized into a specific group based on disease, age, family means, geography, or other variables.

cause-specific mortality rate (CSMR)   An expression of the death rate due to a particular disease; the CSMR is calculated by dividing the number of deaths due to a particular disease by the total population and multiplying by 100,000.

census   The enumeration of the population of the United States that is conducted every 10 years; begun in 1790.

Center for Mental Health Services (CMHS)   The federal agency, housed within the Department of Health and Human Service's Substance Abuse and Mental Health Services Administration, whose mission it is to conduct research on the causes and treatments for mental disorders.

Centers for Disease Control and Prevention (CDC)   One of the operating divisions of the Public Health Service; charged with the responsibility for surveillance and control of diseases and other health problems in the United States.

Centers for Medicare and Medicaid Services (CMS)   The federal agency responsible for overseeing Medicare, Medicaid, and the related quality assurance activities.

cerebrovascular disease (stroke)   A disease in which the blood supply to the brain is interrupted.

certified safety professional (CSP)   A health and safety professional, trained in industrial and workplace safety, who has met specific requirements for board certification.

chain of infection   A model to conceptualize the transmission of a communicable disease from its source to a susceptible host.

chemical hazards   Hazards caused by the mismanagement of chemicals.

chemical straitjacket   A drug that subdues a mental patient's behavior.

child abuse   The intentional physical, emotional, verbal, or sexual mistreatment of a minor.

child maltreatment   The act or failure to act by a parent, caretaker, or other person as defined under state law that results in physical abuse, neglect, medical neglect, sexual abuse, or emotional abuse, or an act or failure to act that presents an imminent risk of serious harm to the child.

child neglect   The failure of a parent or guardian to care for or otherwise provide the necessary subsistence for a child.

childhood diseases   Infectious diseases that normally affect people in their childhood (e.g., measles, mumps, rubella, and pertussis).

children   Persons between 1 and 14 years of age.

Children's Health Insurance Program (CHIP) A title insurance program under the Social Security Act that provides health insurance to uninsured children.

chiropractor A nonallopathic, independent health care provider who treats health problems by adjusting the spinal column.

chlorpromazine The first and most famous antipsychotic drug, introduced in 1954 under the brand name Thorazine.

chronic disease A disease or health condition that lasts longer than 3 months, sometimes for the remainder of one's life.

citizen-initiated community organization See *bottom-up community organization*.

Clean Air Act (CAA) The federal law that provides the government with authority to address interstate air pollution.

Clean Water Act (CWA) The federal law aimed at ensuring that all rivers are swimmable and fishable and that limits the discharge of pollutants in U.S. waters to zero.

club drugs A general term for those illicit drugs, primarily synthetic, that are most commonly encountered at night clubs and "raves." Examples include MDMA, LSD, GHB, GBL, PCP, ketamine, Rohypnol, and methamphetamines.

coal workers' pneumoconiosis (CWP) Acute and chronic lung disease caused by the inhalation of coal dust (sometimes called black lung disease).

coalition "A formal alliance of organizations that come together to work for a common goal" (see Chapter 5, reference 14).

cocaine The psychoactive ingredient in the leaves of the coca plant, *Erythoxolyn coca*.

cognitive-behavioral therapy Treatment based on learning new thought patterns and adaptive skills, with regular practice between therapy sessions.

cohort A group of people who share some important demographic characteristic—year of birth, for example.

cohort study An epidemiological study in which a cohort is selected, classified on the basis of exposure to one or more specific risk factors, and observed to determine the rates at which disease develops in each class.

co-insurance Portion of insurance company's approved amounts for covered services that the beneficiary is responsible for paying.

combustion (incineration) The burning of solid wastes.

combustion by-products Gases and other particles generated by burning.

communicable disease (infectious disease) An illness due to a specific communicable agent or its toxic products, which arises through transmission of that agent or its products from an infected person, animal, or inanimate reservoir to a susceptible host.

communicable disease model A visual representation of the interrelationships of agent, host, and environment—the three entities necessary for communicable disease transmission.

community A group of people who have common characteristics; communities can be defined by location, race, ethnicity, age, occupation, interest in particular problems or outcomes, or other common bonds.

community analysis A process by which community needs are identified.

community building "[A]n orientation to community that is strength based rather than need based and stresses the identification, nurturing, and celebration of community assets" (see Chapter 5, reference 20).

community capacity "The characteristics of communities that affect their ability to identify, mobilize, and address social and public health problems" (see Chapter 5, reference 7).

community diagnosis See *community analysis*.

community health The health status of a defined group of people and the actions and conditions to promote, protect and preserve their health.

community mental health center (CMHC) A fully staffed center originally funded by the federal government that provides comprehensive mental health services to local populations.

community organizing "A process through which communities are helped to identify common problems or goals, mobilize resources, and in other ways develop and implement strategies for reaching their goals they have collectively set" (see Chapter 5, reference 5).

Community Support Program A federal program that offers financial incentives to communities to develop a social support system for the mentally ill.

complementary/alternative medicine (CAM) "A group of diverse medical and health care systems, practices, and products that are not presently considered to be a part of conventional medicine" (see Chapter 13, reference 4).

composting The natural, aerobic biodegradation of organic plant and animal matter to compost.

Comprehensive Drug Abuse Control Act of 1970 (Controlled Substances Act) The central piece of legislation that regulates controlled substances (drugs subject to abuse).

Comprehensive Environmental Response, Compensation, and Liability Act (CERCLA) The federal law (known as the Superfund) created to clean up abandoned hazardous waste sites.

congregate meal programs Community-sponsored nutrition programs that provide meals at a central site, such as a senior center.

consumer-directed health plans (CDHPs) Health plan options that combine more consumer responsibility for decisions with a tax-sheltered account to pay for out-of-pocket costs for health care and a high-deductible health insurance policy.

continuing care Long-term care for chronic health problems, usually including personal care.

continuing-care retirement communities (CCRCs) Planned communities for elders that guarantee a lifelong residence and health care.

controlled substances Drugs regulated by the Comprehensive Drug Abuse Control Act of 1970, including all illegal drugs and many legal drugs that can produce dependence.

coordinated school health program "An organized set of policies, procedures, and activities designed to protect and promote the health and well-being of students and staff which has traditionally included health services, healthful school environment, and health education. It should also include, but not be limited to, guidance and counseling, physical education, food service, social work, psychological services, and employee health promotion" (see Chapter 6, reference 4).

copayment A negotiated set amount the insured will pay for a certain service after paying the deductible.

core functions of public health Health assessment, policy development, and health assurance.

coronary heart disease (CHD) A noncommunicable disease characterized by damage to the coronary arteries, which supply blood to the heart.

criteria of causation Aspects of the association between two variables that should be considered before deciding that the association is one of causation.

criteria pollutants The most pervasive air pollutants in the United States.

crude birth rate An expression of the number of live births per unit of population in a given period of time. For example, the crude birth rate in the United States in 1999 was 14.5 births per 1,000 population.

crude death rate (CDR) An expression of the total number of deaths (from all causes) per unit of population in a given period of time. For example, the crude death rate in the United States in 2004 was 800.0 per 100,000 population.

crude rate A rate in which the denominator includes the total population.

cultural competence Service provider's degree of compatibility with the specific culture of the population served, for example, proficiency in language(s) other than English, familiarity with cultural idioms of distress or body language, folk beliefs, and expectations regarding treatment procedures (such as medication or psychotherapy) and likely outcomes.

cultural and linguistic competence A set of congruent behaviors, attitudes, and policies that come together in a system, agency, or among professionals that enables effective work in cross-cultural situations.

culturally sensitive Having respect for cultures other than one's own.

curriculum Written plan for instruction.

cycles per second (cps) A measure of sound frequency.

death rate See *mortality (fatality) rate*.

deductible The amount of expense that the beneficiary must incur before the insurance company begins to pay for covered services.

deinstitutionalization The process of discharging, on a large scale, patients from state mental hospitals to less restrictive community settings.

demography (demographers) The study of a population and those variables bringing about change in that population.

Department of Health and Human Services (HHS) The largest federal department in the United States government, formed in 1980 and headed by a secretary who is a member of the president's cabinet.

dependency ratio A ratio that compares the number of individuals whom society considers economically productive (the working population) to the number of those it considers economically unproductive (the nonworking or dependent population).

depressant A psychoactive drug that slows down the central nervous system.

descriptive study An epidemiological study that describes an epidemic with respect to person, place, and time.

designer drugs Mind-altering drugs, synthesized in clandestine laboratories, that are similar to but structurally different from known controlled substances.

diagnosis-related groups (DRGs) A procedure used to classify the health problems of all Medicare patients when they are admitted to a hospital.

direct contract HMO Contracts with individual physicians as opposed to group practices.

direct transmission The immediate transfer of an infectious agent by direct contact between infected and susceptible individuals.

disability-adjusted life years (DALYs) A measure for the burden of disease that takes into account premature death and years lived with disability of specified severity and duration. One DALY is one lost year of healthy life.

disabling injury An injury causing any restriction of normal activity beyond the day of the injury's occurrence.

diseases of adaptation Diseases that result from chronic exposure to excess levels of stressors which elicit the General Adaptation Syndrome.

disinfection The killing of communicable disease agents outside the host, on countertops, for example.

dose The number of program units as part of the intervention.

drug A substance other than food or vitamins that, upon entering the body in small amounts, alters one's physical, mental, or emotional state.

drug abuse Use of a drug despite the knowledge that continued use is detrimental to one's health or well-being.

drug abuse education Providing information about the dangers of drug abuse, changing attitudes and beliefs about drugs, providing skills necessary to abstain from drugs, and ultimately changing drug abuse behavior.

drug (chemical) dependence A psychological and sometimes physical state characterized by a craving for a drug.

Drug Enforcement Administration (DEA) The federal government's lead agency with the primary responsibility for enforcing the nation's drug laws, including the Controlled Substances Act of 1970.

drug misuse Inappropriate use of prescription or non-prescription drugs.

drug use A non-evaluative term referring to drug-taking behavior in general; any drug-taking behavior.

Earth Day Annual public observance for concerns about the environment; the first was held April 22, 1970.

elderly (or elder) Individuals older than 65 years of age.

electroconvulsive therapy (ECT) A method of treatment for mental disorders involving the administration of electric current to induce a coma or convulsions.

employee assistance programs (EAPs) Worksite-based, employer-sponsored programs that assist employees whose work performance suffers because of substance abuse or domestic, psychological, or social problems.

encore careers Those when individuals transition out of their work careers and into jobs and volunteer opportunities in nonprofit and public sectors.

endocrine-disrupting chemical (EDC) A chemical that interferes in some way with the body's endocrine (hormone) system.

end-of-life practice Health care services provided to individuals shortly before death.

endemic disease A disease that occurs regularly in a population as a matter of course.

environmental hazards Factors or conditions in the environment that increase the risk of human injury, disease, or death.

environmental health The study and management of environmental conditions that affect the health and well-being of humans.

Environmental Protection Agency (EPA) The federal agency primarily responsible for setting, maintaining, and enforcing environmental standards.

environmental sanitation The practice of establishing and maintaining healthy or hygienic conditions in the environment.

environmental tobacco smoke (ETS) Tobacco smoke in the environment that can be inhaled.

epidemic An unexpectedly large number of cases of an illness, specific health-related behavior, or other health-related event.

epidemic curve A graphic display of the cases of disease according to the time or date of onset of symptoms.

epidemiologist An investigator who studies the occurrence of disease or other health-related conditions or events in defined populations.

epidemiology The study of the distribution and determinants of health-related states or events in specific populations, and the application of this study to control health problems.

equilibrium phase Last phase of the population growth S-curve, when the birth and death rates are equal.

eradication The complete elimination or uprooting of a disease (e.g., smallpox eradication).

etiology The cause of a disease (e.g., the etiology of mumps is the mumps virus).

evaluation Determining the value or worth of the objective of interest.

evidence-based practices Ways of delivering services to people using scientific evidence that shows that the services actually work.

exclusion A condition that is written into a health insurance policy indicating what is not covered by the policy.

exclusive provider organization (EPO) Similar to a preferred provider organization but with fewer providers and stronger financial incentives. See *preferred provider organization (PPO)*.

experimental study An analytic, epidemiological study in which investigators allocate exposure to the risk factor(s) and follow the subjects to observe disease development.

exploritas Educational programs specifically for elders held on college campuses or at a variety of sites around the world.

exponential phase Middle phase of the population growth S-curve, when the birth rate is greater than the death rate.

Family and Medical Leave Act (FMLA) Federal legislation that provides up to a 12-week unpaid leave to men and women after the birth of a child, an adoption, or an event of illness in the immediate family.

family planning The process of determining the preferred number and spacing of children in one's family and choosing the appropriate means to achieve this preference.

family violence The use of physical force by one family member against another, with the intent to hurt, injure, or cause death.

fatal injury An injury that results in one or more deaths.

fatality rate See *mortality (fatality) rate.*

Federal Emergency Management Agency (FEMA) The nation's official emergency response agency.

Federal Water Pollution Control Act Amendments See *Clean Water Act (CWA).*

fee-for-service A method of paying for health care in which a bill (fee) is paid after the care (service) is rendered.

fertility rate The number of live births per 1,000 women of childbearing age (15–44 years).

fetal alcohol syndrome (FAS) A group of abnormalities that may include growth retardation, abnormal appearance of face and head, and deficits of central nervous system function including mental retardation in babies born to mothers who have consumed heavy amounts of alcohol during their pregnancies.

fetal deaths Deaths in utero with a gestational age of at least 20 weeks.

fight or flight reaction An alarm reaction that prepares one physiologically for sudden action.

fixed indemnity The maximum amount an insurer will pay for a certain service.

Food and Drug Administration (FDA) An operating division of the Department of Health and Human Services that regulates all food, over-the-counter and prescription drugs, medical devices, and cosmetics.

foodborne disease A disease transmitted through the contamination of food.

foodborne disease outbreak (FBDO) The occurrence of two or more cases of a similar illness resulting from the ingestion of food.

formaldehyde (CH_2O) A water-soluble gas used in aqueous solutions in hundreds of consumer products.

formative evaluation The evaluation that is conducted during the planning and implementing processes to improve or refine a program.

full-service hospitals Hospitals that offer services in all or most of the levels of care defined by the spectrum of health care.

functional limitations Difficulty in performing personal care and home management tasks.

gag rule Regulations that bar physicians and nurses in clinics receiving federal funds from counseling clients about abortions.

gatekeepers Those who control, both formally and informally, the political climate of the community.

General Adaptation Syndrome (GAS) The complex physiological responses resulting from exposure to stressors.

geriatrician "A physician specializing in the care of patients with multiple chronic diseases who may not be able to be cured but whose care can be managed" (see Chapter 9, reference 3).

geriatrics "The branch of medicine concerned with medical problems and care of the elderly" (see Chapter 9, reference 3).

gerontology "The multidisciplinary study of the biological, psychological, and social processes of aging and the elderly" (see Chapter 9, reference 3).

government hospital A hospital that is supported and managed by governmental jurisdictions.

governmental health agency (or official health agencies) Health agencies that are part of the governmental structure (federal, state, or local) and that are funded primarily by tax dollars.

grass-roots community organizing A process that begins with those affected by the problem/concern.

greenhouse gases Atmospheric gases, principally carbon dioxide, chlorofluorocarbons, ozone, methane, water vapor, and nitrous oxide, that are transparent to visible light but absorb infrared radiation.

groundwater Water located under the surface of the ground.

group model HMO An HMO that contracts with a multispecialty group practice.

hallucinogens Drugs that produce profound distortions of the senses.

hard-to-reach population Those in a priority population that are not easily reached by normal programming efforts.

hate crimes See *bias and hate crimes*.

hazard An unsafe act or condition.

hazardous waste A solid waste or combination of solid wastes that is dangerous to human health or the environment.

health A dynamic state or condition of the human organism that is multidimensional in nature, a resource for living, and results from a person's interactions with and adaptations to his or her environment; therefore, it can exist in varying degrees and is specific to each individual and his or her situation.

health disparities The difference in health between different populations.

health education "Any combination of planned learning experiences based on sound theories that provide individuals, groups, and communities the opportunity to acquire information and the skills to make quality health decisions" (see Chapter 5, reference 30).

health maintenance organizations (HMOs) Groups that supply prepaid comprehensive health care with an emphasis on prevention.

health physicist A safety professional with responsibility for monitoring radiation within a plant environment, developing instrumentation for that purpose, and developing plans for coping with radiation accidents.

health promotion "Any planned combination of educational, political, environmental, regulatory, or organizational mechanisms that support actions and conditions of living conducive to the health of individuals, groups, and communities" (see Chapter 5, reference 30).

health resources development period The period in public health history from 1900 to 1960; a time of great growth in health care facilities.

Health Resources and Services Administration (HRSA) An operating division of the Department of Health and Human Services established in 1982 to improve the nation's health resources and services and their distribution to underserved populations.

health-adjusted life expectancy (HALE) The number of years of healthy life expected, on average, in a given population.

healthy school environment "The promotion, maintenance, and utilization of safe and wholesome surroundings, organization of day-by-day experiences and planned learning procedures to influence favorable emotional, physical and social health" (see Chapter 6, reference 38).

herbicide A pesticide designed specifically to kill plants.

herd immunity The resistance of a population to the spread of an infectious agent based on the immunity of a high portion of individuals.

home health care Care that is provided in the patient's residence for the purpose of promoting, maintaining, or restoring health.

home health care services Health care services provided in the patient's place of residence (home or apartment).

homebound A person unable to leave home for normal activities such as shopping, meals, or other activities.

hospice "Is a cluster of special services for the dying. It blends medical, spiritual, legal, financial, and family support services" (see Chapter 13, reference 21).

Hospital Survey and Construction Act of 1946 (Hill-Burton Act) Federal legislation that provided substantial funds for hospital construction.

host A person or other living animal that affords subsistence or lodgment to a communicable agent under natural conditions.

hypercholesterolemia High levels of cholesterol in the blood.

hypertension Systolic pressure equal to or greater than 140 mm of mercury (Hg) and/or diastolic pressure equal to or greater than 90 mm Hg for extended periods of time.

illegal alien An individual who entered this country without permission.

illicit (illegal) drugs Drugs that cannot be legally manufactured, distributed, bought, or sold and that lack recognized medical value.

immigrant Individuals who migrate to this country from another country for the purpose of seeking permanent residence.

impact evaluation Focuses on immediate observable effects of a program.

impairments Defects in the functioning of one's sense organs or limitations in one's mobility or range of motion.

implementation Putting a planned program into action.

incidence rate The number of new health-related events or cases of a disease in a population exposed to that risk during a particular period of time, divided by the total number in that same population.

incubation period The period of time between exposure to an infectious agent and the onset of symptoms.

independent practice associations (IPAs) Legal entities separate from the HMO that are physician organizations composed of community-based independent physicians in solo or group practices that provide services to HMO members.

independent providers Health care professionals with the education and legal authority to treat any health problem.

Indian Health Service (IHS) An operating division of the Department of Health and Human Services whose goal is to raise the health status of the American Indian and Alaska Native to the highest possible level by providing a comprehensive health services delivery system.

indirect transmission Communicable disease transmission involving an intermediate step; for example, airborne, vehicleborne, or vectorborne transmission.

industrial hygienist A health professional concerned with health hazards in the workplace, including such things as problems with ventilation, noise, and lighting; also responsible for measuring air quality and recommending plans for improving the healthiness of work environments.

industrial smog Smog formed primarily by sulfur dioxide and suspended particles from the burning of coal, also known as gray smog.

infant death (infant mortality) Death of a child under 1 year of age.

infant mortality rate The number of deaths of children under 1 year of age per 1,000 live births.

infection The lodgment and growth of a virus or microorganism in a host organism.

infectious disease See *communicable disease*.

infectivity The ability of a pathogen to lodge and grow in a host.

informal caregiver One who provides unpaid care or assistance to one who has some physical, mental, emotional, or financial need that limits his or her independence.

inhalants Breathable substances that produce mind-altering effects; for example, glue.

injury Physical harm or damage to the body resulting from an exchange, usually acute, of mechanical, chemical, thermal, or other environmental energy that exceeds the body's tolerance.

injury prevention (control) An organized effort to prevent injuries or to minimize their severity.

injury prevention education The process of changing people's health-directed behavior in such a way as to reduce unintentional injuries.

inpatient care facilities Any in which a patient stays overnight, such as a hospital.

insecticides Pesticides designed specifically to kill insects.

instrumental activities of daily living (IADLs) Measure of more complex tasks such as handling personal finances, preparing meals, shopping, doing homework, traveling, using the telephone, and taking medications.

intensity Cardiovascular workload measured by heart rate.

intentional injury An injury that is judged to have been purposely inflicted, either by the victim or another.

intern A first-year resident.

intervention An activity or activities designed to create change in people.

intimate partner violence (IPV) Rape, physical assault, or stalking perpetrated by current or former dates, spouses, or cohabiting partners, with cohabiting meaning living together at least some of the time as a couple.

ionizing radiation High-energy radiation that can knock an electron out of orbit creating an ion and can thereby damage living cells and tissues (UV radiation, gamma rays, X-rays, alpha and beta particles).

isolation The separation of infected persons from those who are susceptible.

Joint Commission The predominant organization responsible for accrediting health care facilities.

labor-force ratio A ratio of the total number of those individuals who are not working (regardless of age) to the number of those who are.

lag phase Initial phase of the population growth S-curve, when growth is slow.

law enforcement The application of federal, state, and local laws to arrest, jail, bring to trial, and sentence those who break drug laws or break laws because of drug use.

leachates Liquids created when water mixes with wastes and removes soluble constituents from them by percolation.

lead A naturally occurring mineral element found throughout the environment and used in large quantities for industrial products, including batteries, pipes, solder, paints, and pigments.

licensed practical nurse (LPN) Those prepared in 1- to 2-year programs to provide nontechnical bedside nursing care under the supervision of physicians or registered nurses.

life expectancy The average number of years a person from a specific cohort is projected to live from a given point in time.

limited (restricted) care providers Health care providers who provide care for a specific part of the body; for example, dentists.

limited-service hospitals Hospitals that offer only the specific services needed by the population served.

litigation The process of seeking justice for injury through courts.

lobotomy Surgical severance of nerve fibers of the brain by incision.

long-term care   Different kinds of help that people with chronic illnesses, disabilities, or other conditions need to deal with the circumstances that limit them physically or mentally.

low-birth-weight infant   An infant that weighs less than 2,500 grams, or 5.5 pounds, at birth.

Lyme disease   A systematic, bacterial, tickborne disease with symptoms that include dermatologic, arthritic, neurologic, and cardiac abnormalities.

mainstream smoke   Tobacco smoke inhaled and exhaled by the smoker.

major depression   An affective disorder characterized by a dysphoric mood, usually depression, or loss of interest or pleasure in almost all usual activities or pastimes.

majority   Those with characteristics that are found in more than 50% of a population.

malignant neoplasm   Uncontrolled new tissue growth resulting from cells that have lost control over their growth and division.

managed care   "A system of health care delivery that (1) seeks to achieve efficiency by integrating the basic functions of health care delivery, (2) employs mechanisms to control utilization of medical services, and (3) determines the price at which the services are purchased and how much the providers get paid" (see Chapter 13, reference 1).

marijuana   Dried plant parts of *Cannabis sativa.*

maternal, infant, and child health   The health of women of childbearing age from pre-pregnancy, through pregnancy, labor and delivery, and the postpartum period and the health of the child prior to birth through adolescence.

maternal mortality   The death of a woman while pregnant or within 42 days of termination of pregnancy, irrespective of the duration and the site of the pregnancy, from any cause related to or aggravated by the pregnancy or its management but not from accidental or incidental causes.

maternal mortality rate   Number of mothers dying per 100,000 live births in a given year.

Meals on Wheels program   A community-supported nutrition program in which prepared meals are delivered to elders in their homes, usually by volunteers.

median age   The age at which half of the population is older and half is younger.

Medicaid   A national federal-state health insurance program for low-income Americans.

medical preparedness   "The ability of the *health care system* to prevent, protect against, quickly respond to, and recover from health emergencies, particularly those whose scale, timing, or unpredictability threatens to overwhelm routine capabilities" (see Chapter 13, reference 53).

medically indigent   Those lacking the financial ability to pay for their own medical care.

Medicare   A national health insurance program for people 65 years of age and older, certain younger disabled people, and people with permanent kidney failure.

Medigap   Private health insurance to supplement Medicare benefits—that is, to fill in the gaps of Medicare.

mental disorders   Health conditions characterized by alterations in thinking, mood, or behavior (or some combination thereof) associated with distress and/or impaired functioning.

mental health   Emotional and social well-being, including one's psychological resources for dealing with the day-to-day problems of life.

mental illness   A collective term for all mental disorders.

Mental Retardation Facilities and Community Mental Health Centers (CMHC) Act   A law that made the federal government responsible for assisting in the funding of mental health facilities and services.

metastasis   The spread of a disease, such as cancer, by the transfer of cells by means of the blood or lymphatics.

methamphetamine   The amphetamine drug most widely abused.

methaqualone   An illicit depressant drug.

methcathinone (cat)   An illicit, synthetic drug, similar to the amphetamines, that first appeared in the United States in 1991.

middle old   Those 75 to 84 years of age.

migration   Movement of people from one country to another.

minority groups   Subgroups of the population that consist of fewer than 50% of the population.

minority health   The morbidity and mortality of American Indians/Alaska Natives, Asian Americans and Pacific Islanders, black Americans, and Americans of Hispanic origin in the United States.

mixed model HMO   A hybrid form of a health maintenance organization.

model for unintentional injuries   The public health triangle (host, agent, and environment) modified to indicate energy as the causative agent of injuries.

modern era of public health   The era of American public health that began in 1850 and continues today.

modifiable risk factor Factors contributing to the development of a noncommunicable disease that can be altered by modifying one's behavior or environment; for example, cigarette smoking is a modifiable risk factor for coronary heart disease.

moral treatment Treatment for mental illness based on belief that mental illness was caused by moral decay.

morbidity rate The rate of illness in a population.

mortality (fatality) rate The rate of deaths in a population.

multicausation disease model A visual representation of the host, together with various internal and external factors that promote and protect against disease.

multiplicity The number of activities that make up the intervention.

municipal solid waste (MSW) Waste generated by individual households, businesses, and institutions located within municipalities.

narcotics Drugs similar to morphine that reduce pain and induce a stuporous state.

natality (birth) rate The rate of births in a population.

National Alliance on Mental Illness (NAMI) A national self-help group that supports the belief that major mental disorders are brain diseases that are of genetic origin and biological in nature and are diagnosable and treatable with medications.

National Ambient Air Quality Standards (NAAQSs) Standards created by the EPA for allowable concentration levels of outdoor air pollutants.

National Electronic Telecommunications System (NETS) The electronic reporting system by which state health departments send health records to the Centers for Disease Control and Prevention (CDC).

National Institute of Mental Health (NIMH) The nation's leading mental health research agency, housed in the National Institutes of Health.

National Institute for Occupational Safety and Health (NIOSH) A research body within the Centers for Disease Control and Prevention, Department of Health and Human Services, that is responsible for developing and recommending occupational safety and health standards.

National Institute on Drug Abuse (NIDA) The federal government's lead agency for drug abuse research; part of the National Institutes of Health.

National Institutes of Health (NIH) The research division of the Department of Health and Human Services. It is part of the Public Health Service.

National Mental Health Association (NMHA) A national voluntary health association that advocates for mental health and for those with mental illnesses; it has 600 affiliates in 43 states.

natural disaster A natural hazard that results in substantial loss of life or property.

natural hazards Naturally occurring phenomena or events that produce or release energy in amounts that exceed human endurance, causing injury, disease, or death (such as radiation, earthquakes, tsunamis, volcanic eruptions, hurricanes, tornados, and floods).

needs assessment The process of collecting and analyzing information to develop an understanding of the issues, resources, and constraints of the priority population, as related to the development of health promotion programs.

neonatal deaths (neonatal mortality) Deaths occurring during the first 28 days after birth.

neonatologist A medical doctor who specializes in the care of newborns from birth to 2 months of age.

net migration The population gain or loss resulting from migration.

network model HMO A type of HMO that contracts with more than one medical group practice.

neuroleptic drugs Drugs that reduce nervous activity; another term for antipsychotic drug.

nonallopathic providers Independent providers who provide nontraditional forms of health care.

noncommunicable disease (noninfectious disease) A disease not caused by a communicable agent, and that thus cannot be transmitted from infected host to susceptible host.

nonphysician practitioners (NPPs) Clinical professionals who practice in many of the areas similar to those in which physicians practice, but who do not have an MD or DO degree (see Chapter 13, reference 1).

nonpoint source pollution All pollution that occurs through the runoff, seepage, or falling of pollutants into the water.

nontarget organisms All other susceptible organisms in the environment, for which a pesticide was not intended.

notifiable diseases Infectious diseases for which health officials request or require reporting for public health reasons.

observational study An analytic, epidemiological study in which an investigator or investigators observe the natural course of events, noting exposed and unexposed subjects and disease development.

occupational disease Any abnormal condition or disorder, other than one resulting from an occupational injury, caused by an exposure to environmental factors associated with employment.

occupational health nurse (OHN) A registered nurse whose primary responsibilities include prevention of illness and promotion of health in the workplace.

occupational injury An injury that results from exposure to a single incident in the work environment (e.g., cut, fracture, sprain, amputation).

occupational physician (OP) or occupational medical practitioner (OMP) A medical practitioner (doctor) whose primary concern is preventive medicine in the workplace.

Occupational Safety and Health Act of 1970 (OSHAct) Comprehensive federal legislation aimed at assuring safe and healthful working conditions for working men and women.

Occupational Safety and Health Administration (OSHA) The federal agency located within the Department of Labor and created by the OSHAct that is charged with the responsibility of administering the provisions of the OSHAct.

odds ratio A probability statement about the association between a particular disease and a specific risk factor, often the outcome of a retrospective (case/control) study.

Office of National Drug Control Policy (ONDCP) The headquarters of America's drug control effort, located in the executive branch of the federal government, and headed by a director appointed by the president.

official health agency See *governmental health agency*.

old Those 65 years of age and older.

old-age dependency ratio The dependency ratio that includes only the old.

old old Those 85 years of age and older.

Older Americans Act of 1965 (OAA) Federal legislation to improve the lives of elders.

operationalize (operational definition) To provide working definitions.

osteopathic providers Independent health care providers whose remedies emphasize the interrelationships of the body's systems in prevention, diagnosis, and treatment.

outcome evaluation Focuses on the end result of the program.

outpatient care facilities Any facility in which the patient receives care and does not stay overnight.

over-the-counter (OTC) drugs (nonprescription drugs) Drugs (except tobacco and alcohol) that can be legally purchased without a physician's prescription (e.g., aspirin).

ownership A feeling that one has a stake in or "owns" the object of interest.

ozone O_3, an inorganic molecule considered to be a pollutant in the atmosphere because it harms human tissue, but considered beneficial in the stratosphere because it screens out UV radiation.

packaged pricing Several related health services are included in one price.

pandemic An outbreak of disease over a wide geographical area, such as a continent.

parity The concept of equality in health care coverage for people with mental illness and those with other medical illnesses or injuries.

passive smoking The inhalation of environmental tobacco smoke by nonsmokers.

pathogenicity The capability of a communicable agent to cause disease in a susceptible host.

peer counseling programs School-based drug education programs in which students discuss alcohol and other drug-related problems with other students.

pest Any organism—multicelled animal or plant, or microbe—that has an adverse effect on human interests.

pesticides Synthetic chemicals developed and manufactured for the purpose of killing pests.

pharmaceuticals and personal care products (PPCPs) Synthetic chemicals found in everyday consumer health care products and cosmetics.

phasing in Implementation of an intervention with small groups prior to its implementation with the entire priority population.

philanthropic foundation An endowed institution that donates money for the good of humankind.

photochemical smog The visible, photochemical smog also known as brown smog.

physical dependence Drug dependence in which discontinued use results in the onset of physical illness.

pilot test Presentation of the intervention to just a few individuals, who are either from the intended priority population or from a very similar population.

placebo A blank treatment (e.g., a sugar pill).

pneumoconiosis Fibrotic lung disease caused by the inhalation of dusts, especially mineral dusts.

point-of-service (POS) option An option of a health maintenance organization plan that allows enrollees to be at least partially reimbursed for selecting a health care provider outside the plan.

point source epidemic curve An epidemic curve depicting a distribution of cases that can all be traced to a single source of exposure.

point source pollution Pollution that can be traced to a single identifiable source.

polydrug use Concurrent use of multiple drugs.

population at risk Those in the population who are susceptible to a particular disease or condition.

population health The health status of people who are not organized and have no identity as a group or locality and the actions and conditions to promote, protect, and preserve their health.

population-based public health practice Incorporates interventions aimed at disease prevention and health promotion, specific protection, and case findings.

postneonatal deaths (postneonatal mortality) Deaths that occur between 28 days and 365 days after birth.

pre-existing condition A medical condition that had been diagnosed or treated usually within 6 months before the date a health insurance policy goes into effect.

preferred provider organization (PPO) An organization that buys fixed-rate (discount) health services from providers and sells them (via premiums) to consumers.

premature infant One born following a gestation period of 38 weeks or less, or one born at a low birth weight.

prenatal health care (prenatal care) One of the fundamentals of a safe motherhood program, which includes three major components: risk assessment, treatment for medical conditions or risk reduction, and education. Prenatal health care should begin before pregnancy when a couple is considering having a child and continue throughout pregnancy.

prepaid health care A method of paying for covered health care services on a per-person premium basis for a specific period of time prior to service being rendered. Also referred to as capitation.

preplacement examination A physical examination of a newly hired or transferred worker to determine medical suitability for placement in a specific position.

prevalence rate The number of new and old cases of a disease in a population in a given period of time, divided by the total number of that population.

prevention The planning for and taking of action to forestall the onset of a disease or other health problem before the occurrence of undesirable health events.

preventive care Care given to healthy people to keep them healthy.

primary care "Is clinical preventive services, first-contact treatment services, and ongoing care for commonly encountered medical conditions" (see Chapter 13, reference 19).

primary pollutants Air pollutants emanating directly from transportation, power and industrial plants, and refineries.

primary prevention Preventive measures that forestall the onset of illness or injury during the prepathogenesis period.

priority population (audience) Those whom a program is intended to serve.

private (proprietary) or investor-owned hospitals For-profit hospitals.

pro-choice A medical/ethical position that holds that women have a right to reproductive freedom.

pro-life A medical/ethical position that holds that performing an abortion is an act of murder.

problem drinker One for whom alcohol consumption results in personal, economic, medical, social, or any other type of problem.

professional nurse A registered nurse holding a bachelor of science degree in nursing (BSN).

program planning A process by which an intervention is planned to help meet the needs of a priority population.

propagated epidemic curve An epidemic curve depicting a distribution of cases traceable to multiple sources of exposure over time.

proportionate mortality ratio (PMR) The percentage of overall mortality in a population that can be assigned to a particular cause or disease.

prospective reimbursement "Uses pre-established criteria to determine in advance the amount of reimbursement" (see Chapter 13, reference 1).

prospective study An epidemiological study that begins in the present and continues into the future for the purpose of observing the development of disease (e.g., cohort study).

providers Health care facilities or health professionals that provide health care services.

psychiatric rehabilitation Intensive, individualized services encompassing treatment, rehabilitation, and support delivered by a team of providers over an indefinite period to individuals with severe mental disorder to help them maintain stable lives in the community.

psychoactive drugs Mind-altering drugs; drugs that affect the central nervous system.

psychological dependence A psychological state characterized by an overwhelming desire to continue use of a drug.

psychopharmacological therapy Treatment for mental illness that involves medications.

psychotherapy A treatment that involves verbal communication between the patient and a trained clinician.

public health Actions that society takes collectively to ensure that the conditions in which people can be healthy can occur.

public health preparedness "The ability of the *public health system, community, and individuals* to prevent, protect against, quickly respond to, and recover from health emergencies, particularly those in which scale, timing, or unpredictability threatens to overwhelm routine capabilities" (see Chapter 1, reference 53).

public health professional A health care worker who works in a public health organization.

Public Health Service (PHS) An agency in the Department of Health and Human Services (HHS) that comprises 8 of the 11 operating divisions of HHS.

public health system The organizational mechanism of those activities undertaken within the formal structure of government and the associated efforts of private and voluntary organizations and individuals.

public hospitals Hospitals that are supported and managed by governmental jurisdictions.

public policy The guiding principles and courses of action pursued by governments to solve practical problems affecting society.

quality management and utilization review The analysis of provided health care for its appropriateness by someone other than the patient and provider.

quarantine Limitation of freedom of movement of those who have been exposed to a disease and may be incubating it.

quasi-governmental health organizations Organizations that have some responsibilities assigned by the government but operate more like voluntary agencies; for example, the American Red Cross.

radiation A process in which energy is emitted as particles or waves.

radon A naturally occurring, colorless, tasteless, odorless, radioactive gas formed during the radioactive decay of uranium-238.

rate The number of events (cases of disease) that occur in a given period of time.

recovery Outcome sought by most people with mental illness; includes increased independence, effective coping, supportive relationships, community participation, and sometimes gainful employment.

recycling The collecting, sorting, and processing of materials that would otherwise be considered waste into raw materials for manufacturing new products, and the subsequent use of those new products.

reform phase of public health The period of public health from 1900 to 1920, characterized by social movements to improve health conditions in cities and in the workplace.

refugee A person who flees one area or country to seek shelter or protection from danger in another.

registered environmental health specialists (REHSs) (sanitarians) Environmental workers responsible for the inspection of restaurants, retail food outlets, public housing, and other sites to ensure compliance with public health codes.

registered nurse (RN) One who has successfully completed an accredited academic program and a state licensing examination.

regulation The enactment and enforcement of laws to control conduct.

rehabilitation center A facility in which restorative care is provided following injury, disease, or surgery.

reimbursement Payments made by the third-party payers to providers.

relative risk A statement of the relationship between the risk of acquiring a disease when a specific risk factor is present and the risk of acquiring that same disease when the risk factor is not present.

resident A physician who is training in a specialty.

resource-based relative value scale Reimbursement to physicians according to the relative value of the service provided.

Resource Conservation and Recovery Act of 1976 (RCRA) The federal law that sets forth guidelines for the proper handling and disposal of solid and hazardous wastes.

respite care Planned short-term care, usually for the purpose of relieving a full-time informal caregiver.

restorative care Care provided to patients after a successful treatment or when the progress of a incurable disease has been arrested.

retirement communities Residential communities that have been specifically developed for those in their retirement years.

retrospective study An epidemiological study that looks into the past for clues to explain the present distribution of disease.

risk factors Factors that increase the probability of disease, injury, or death.

Roe v. Wade A 1973 Supreme Court decision that made it unconstitutional for state laws to prohibit abortions.

Rohypnol (flunitrazepam) A depressant in the benzodiazepine group that has achieved notoriety as a date rape drug.

rollover protective structures (ROPS) Factory-installed or retrofitted reinforced framework on a cab to protect the operator of a tractor in case of a rollover.

runoff Water that flows over land surfaces (including paved surfaces), typically from precipitation.

Safe Drinking Water Act (SDWA) The federal law that regulates the safety of public drinking water.

safety engineer A health and safety professional, sometimes with an engineering background, employed by a company for the purpose of reducing unintentional injuries in the workplace.

safety programs Those parts of the workplace health and safety program aimed at reducing unintentional injuries on the job.

sanitary landfills Waste disposal sites on land suited for this purpose and on which waste is spread in thin layers, compacted, and covered with a fresh layer of clay or plastic foam each day.

sanitation The practice of establishing and maintaining healthy or hygienic conditions in the environment.

school health coordinator A professional at the district (or school) level responsible for management and coordination of all school health policies, activities, and resources.

school health council Individuals from a school or school district and its community who work together to provide advice on aspects of the school health program.

school health education The development, delivery, and evaluation of a planned curriculum, kindergarten through grade 12.

school health policies Written statements that describe the nature and procedures of a school health program.

school health services Health services provided by school health workers to appraise, protect, and promote the health of students and school personnel.

scope Part of the curriculum that outlines what will be taught.

secondary medical care Specialized attention and ongoing management for common and less frequently encountered medical conditions, including support services for people with special challenges due to chronic or long-term conditions.

secondary pollutants Air pollutants formed when primary air pollutants react with sunlight and other atmospheric components to form new harmful compounds.

secondary prevention Preventive measures that lead to early diagnosis and prompt treatment of a disease or injury to limit disability and prevent more severe pathogenesis.

secondhand smoke Environmental tobacco smoke.

self-funded insurance program One that pays the health care costs of its employees with the premiums collected from the employees and the contributions made by the employer.

self-help groups Groups of concerned members of the community who are united by a shared interest, concern, or deficit not shared by other members of the community (Alcoholics Anonymous, for example).

senior centers Facilities where elders can congregate for fellowship, meals, education, and recreation.

septic tank A watertight concrete or fiberglass tank that holds sewage; one of two main parts of a septic system.

sequence Part of the curriculum that states in what order the content will be taught.

sick building syndrome A term to describe a situation in which the air quality in a building produces generalized signs and symptoms of ill health in the building's occupants.

sidestream tobacco smoke The smoke that comes off the end of burning tobacco products.

silicosis Acute or chronic lung disease caused by the inhalation of free crystalline silica; those affected include workers in mines, stone quarries, sand and gravel operations, and abrasive blasting operations.

sliding scale fee A fee based on ability to pay.

sludge A semiliquid mixture of solid waste that includes bacteria, viruses, organic matter, toxic metals, synthetic organic chemicals, and solid chemicals.

smokeless tobacco (spit tobacco) Includes oral snuff, loose leaf chewing tobacco, plug chewing tobacco, and nasal snuff.

social capital "Relationships and structures within a community that promote cooperation for mutual benefit" (see Chapter 5, reference 1).

Social Security Administration (SSA) An independent federal agency that administers programs that provide financial support to special groups of Americans.

socioeconomic status A demographic term which takes into consideration the combination of social and economic factors.

solid waste Solid refuse from households, agriculture, and businesses.

solid waste management (integrated waste management) The collection, transportation, and disposal of solid waste.

sound-level meter Instrument used to measure sound.

source reduction A waste management approach involving the reduction or elimination of use of materials that produce an accumulation of solid waste.

Special Supplemental Food Program for Women, Infants, and Children See *WIC*.

specialty hospital   A hospital that provides mainly one type of medical service, is for-profit, and is owned at least in part by the physicians who practice in it.

specific rate   A rate of a specific disease in a population or the rate of events in a specific population (e.g., cause-specific death rate, age-specific death rate).

spectrum of health care delivery   The array of types of care—from preventive to continuing, or long-term, care. It comprises four levels of care.

spiritual era of public health   A time during the Middle Ages when the causation of communicable disease was linked to spiritual forces.

staff model HMO   A health maintenance organization that hires its own staff of health care providers.

standard of acceptability   A comparative mandate, value, norm, or group.

stimulant   A drug that increases the activity of the central nervous system; for example, methamphetamine.

student assistance programs (SAPs)   School-based drug education programs to assist students who have alcohol or other drug problems.

Substance Abuse and Mental Health Services Administration (SAMHSA)   An operating division of the Department of Health and Human Services whose stated mission is the reduction of the incidence and prevalence of alcohol and other drug abuse and mental disorders, the improvement of treatment outcomes, and the curtailment of the consequences of mental health problems for families and communities.

sudden infant death syndrome (SIDS)   Sudden unanticipated death of an infant in whom, after examination, there is no recognized cause of death.

summative evaluation   The evaluation that determines the impact of a program on the priority population.

Superfund legislation   See *Comprehensive Environmental Response, Compensation, and Liability Act (CERCLA)*.

Supplemental Security   Program of the Social Security Administration that provides cash benefits to elderly, blind, and disabled Americans with minimal resources.

surface water   Precipitation that does not infiltrate the ground or return to the atmosphere by evaporation; the water in streams, rivers, and lakes.

Synar Amendment   A federal law that requires states to set the minimum legal age for purchasing tobacco products at 18 years and that requires states to enforce this law.

synesthesia   Impairment of mind (by hallucinogens) characterized by a sensation that senses are mixed (e.g., seeing sounds and hearing images).

tardive dyskinesia   Irreversible condition of involuntary and abnormal movements of the tongue, mouth, arms, and legs, which can result from long-term use of certain antipsychotic drugs (such as chlorpromazine).

target organism (target pest)   The organism (or pest) for which a pesticide is applied.

task force   "A self-contained group of 'doers' that is not ongoing, but rather brought together due to a strong interest in an issue and for a specific purpose" (see Chapter 5, reference 14).

terrorism   Calculated use of violence (or threat of violence) against civilians to attain goals that are political or religious in nature.

tertiary medical care   Specialized and technologically sophisticated medical and surgical care for those with unusual or complex conditions (generally no more than a few percent of the need in any service category).

tertiary prevention   Measures aimed at rehabilitation following significant pathogenesis.

thermal inversion   Condition that occurs when warm air traps cooler air at the surface of the earth.

third-party payment system   A health insurance term indicating that bills will be paid by the insurer (the government or private insurance company) and not the patient (first party) or the health care provider (the second party).

Thorazine   See *chlorpromazine*.

Title X   A portion of the Public Health Service Act of 1970 that provides funds for family planning services for low-income people.

tolerance   Physiological and enzymatic adjustments that occur in response to the chronic presence of drugs, reflected in the need for ever-increasing doses to achieve a previous level of effect.

top-down funding   A method of funding in which funds are transmitted from the federal or state government to the local level.

total dependency ratio   The dependency ratio that includes both youth and old.

transinstitutionalization   Transferring patients from one type of public institution to another, usually as a result of policy change.

treatment   An activity or activities designed to create change in people.

ultraviolet (UV) radiation   Radiation energy with wavelengths 0 to 400 nanometers.

unintentional injury An injury judged to have occurred without anyone intending that harm be done.

unmodifiable risk factors Factors contributing to the development of a noncommunicable disease that cannot be altered by modifying one's behavior or environment.

unsafe act Any behavior that would increase the probability of an injury occurring.

unsafe condition Any environmental factor or set of factors (physical or social) that would increase the probability of an injury occurring.

U.S. Census The enumeration of the population of the United States that is conducted every 10 years; begun in 1790.

vector A living organism, usually an arthropod, that can transmit a communicable disease agent to a susceptible host (e.g., mosquitoes, ticks, lice, fleas).

vectorborne disease A communicable disease transmitted by insects or other arthropods; for example, St. Louis encephalitis.

vectorborne disease outbreak (VBDO) An occurrence of an unexpectedly large number of cases of disease caused by an agent transmitted by insects or other arthropods.

vehicle An inanimate material or object, such as clothes, bedding, toys, hypodermic needles; or nonliving biological materials such as food, milk, water, blood, serum or plasma, tissues or organs, that can serve as a source of infection.

vehicleborne disease A communicable disease transmitted by nonliving objects; for example, typhoid fever can be transmitted by water.

visitor services A community social service involving one individual taking time to visit with another who is unable to leave his or her residence.

vital statistics Statistical summaries of vital records—records of major life events, such as births, deaths, marriages, divorces, and infant deaths.

volatile organic compounds (VOCs) Compounds that exist as vapors over the normal range of air pressures and temperatures.

voluntary health agency A nonprofit organization created by concerned citizens to deal with health needs not met by governmental health agencies.

voluntary hospital A nonprofit hospital administered by a religious, fraternal, or other charitable community organization.

wastewater The aqueous mixture that remains after water has been used or contaminated by humans.

wastewater treatment The process of improving the quality of wastewater (sewage) to the point that it can be released into a body of water without seriously disrupting the aquatic environment, causing health problems in humans, or causing nuisance conditions.

water pollution Any physical or chemical change in water that can harm living organisms or make the water unfit for other uses.

waterborne disease A disease that is transmitted through contamination of water.

waterborne disease outbreak (WBDO) A disease in which at least two persons experience a similar illness after the ingestion of drinking water or after exposure to water used for recreational purposes and epidemiological evidence implicates water as the probable source of the illness.

watershed The area of land from which all of the water that is under it or drains from it goes into the same place and drains in one point; for example, the Mississippi River watershed drains and collects all the water from the land extending from east of the Rocky Mountains to the Appalachian Mountains and from the upper Midwest all the way south to the Gulf of Mexico.

WIC (also known as the Special Supplemental Food Program for Women, Infants, and Children) A federal program sponsored by the United States Department of Agriculture designed to provide supplemental foods, nutrition and health education, and referrals for health and social services to improve the health of at-risk, economically disadvantaged women who are pregnant or are caring for infants and children under age 5.

workers' compensation laws A set of federal laws designed to compensate those workers and their families who suffer injuries, disease, or death from workplace exposure.

worksite health promotion (WHP) programs Workplace-based, employer-sponsored programs provided to employees and aimed at improving the health of employees through changes in behavior and lifestyle.

World Health Assembly Body of delegates of the member nations of the World Health Organization.

World Health Organization (WHO) Most widely recognized international governmental health organization today. Created in 1948 by representatives of United Nations countries.

years of potential life lost (YPLL) The number of years lost when death occurs before the age of 65 or 75.

young old Those 65 to 74 years of age.

youth dependency ratio The dependency ratio that includes only youth.

youth gang   A self-formed association of peers, bound together by mutual interests, with identifiable leadership and well-defined lines of authority, who act in concert to achieve a specific purpose and whose acts generally include illegal activity and control over a territory or an enterprise.

zero population growth (ZPG)   A state in which the birth and death rates for a given population are equal.

zoonosis   A communicable disease transmissible under natural conditions from vertebrate animals to humans.

Index

PHOTO CREDITS

Unit Openers Hannus Design Associates

Chapter 1

1.2 © Rubberball Productions/Getty Images; **1.3** © Weldon Schloneger/ShutterStock, Inc.; **1.4** © Styve Reineck/ShutterStock, Inc.; **1.5** Courtesy of Dr. John Noble, Jr./CDC; **1.7** Courtesy of Library of Congress, Prints & Photographs Division, [reproduction number LC-USZ62-7386]; **1.8** © coka/ShutterStock, Inc.; **1.9** © Reuters/Kai Pfaffenbach/Landov

Chapter 2

2.1 © PR Newswire/AP Photos; **2.3** Courtesy of James Gathany/CDC; **2.7** © National Library of Medicine; **2.8** © Keystone/Laurent Gillieron/AP Photos; **2.9** © Suzanne Tucker/ShutterStock, Inc.

Chapter 3

3.1 Courtesy of The National Archives; **3.7** Photographed by Lloyd Wolf for the U.S. Census Bureau, Public Information Office (PIO); **3.8** Courtesy of CDC

Chapter 4

4.1 Photographs by the U.S. Census Bureau, Public Information Office (PIO).; **4.4** © Custom Medical Stock Photo; **4.5** Courtesy of Scott Bauer/USDA; **4.11** © Gustau Nacarino/Thomson Reuters; **4.12** © Photodisc

Chapter 5

5.1 © Divanir4a/Dreamstime.com; **5.4** © Jack Hollingsworth/Photodisc/Getty Images; **5.5** Courtesy of U.S. Surgeon General's Office; **5.8** © GoGo Images/age fotostock

Chapter 6

6.1 (photo) © Photodisc; **6.2** © Steve Miller/AP Photos; **6.3** © auremar/ShutterStock, Inc.; **6.4** © Bill Aron/PhotoEdit, Inc.; **6.5** © Michael Newman/PhotoEdit, Inc.; **6.6** © Jonathan Ross/Dreamstime.com; **6.7** © Chitose Suzuki/AP Photos

Chapter 7

7.1 © Anthony Harris/ShutterStock, Inc.; **7.12** © Joe Marquette/AP Photos; **7.13** © Monkey Business Images/Dreamstime.com; **7.21** © Kitti/ShutterStock, Inc.; **7.25** © A. Ramey/PhotoEdit, Inc.

Chapter 8

8.4 © corepics/ShutterStock, Inc.; **8.9** © Bilderbuch/age fotostock

Chapter 9

9.1 © Lisa F. Young/Dreamstime.com ; **9.2** © AP Photos; **9.3** © Glenda M. Powers/ShutterStock, Inc.; **9.7** © rj lerich/ShutterStock, Inc.; **9.8** © Elena Elisseeva/ShutterStock, Inc.; **9.9** © Brisbane/ShutterStock, Inc.; **9.10** © Lisa F. Young/Fotolia.com; **9.11** © The Centers for Medicare & Medicaid Services; **9.12** © Ken Hammond/USDA

Chapter 10

10.1 © Richard Gunion/Dreamstime.com

Chapter 11

11.2 © Gerald Bernard/ShutterStock, Inc., Inc.; **11.4** Courtesy of Cpl. Brian Reimers/U.S. Marines; **11.6, 11.7** © National Library of Medicine, **11.8** Courtesy of Department of Social and Health Services, Washington State; **11.9** © AP Photos; **11.11** © James Shaffer/PhotoEdit, Inc.; **11.12** © Photos.com; **11.13** © Tim Harman/ShutterStock, Inc.; **11.14** © David Buffington/Photodisc/Getty Images

Chapter 12

12.2 © Monkey Business/Fotolia.com; **12.4** © BananaStock/age fotostock; **12.5** © Mark Humphrey/AP Photos; **12.6** © Tiburon Studios/ShutterStock, Inc.; **12.7** © Kyle Carter/The Meridian Star/AP Photos; **12.9** © Netea Mircea Valentin/ShutterStock, Inc.; **12.12** Courtesy of Gerald L. Nino/U.S. Customs and Border Protection, **12.13** © Lisa C. McDonald/ShutterStock, Inc.

Chapter 13

13.1 © Reuters/Brian Snyder/Landov; **13.2** © Kimberly White/Bloomberg News/Landov; **13.3** © Reuters/Jason Reed/Landov; **13.4** © Stuart Pearce/Pixtal/age fotostock; **13.5** © Rob Marmion/ShutterStock, Inc.; **13.7** © Susan Van Etten/PhotoEdit, Inc.; **13.10** © Photos.com; **13.14** © SuperStock/age fotostock

Chapter 14

14.1 © Aaron Kohr/ShutterStock, Inc.; **14.5** © Mike Wintroath/AP Photos; **14.8** © Robert Malota/Dreamstime.com; **14.10** Courtesy of USGS; **14.11** © Jaimie Duplass/ShutterStock, Inc.; **14.12** Courtesy of U.S. Food and Drug Administration; **Box 14.6 (photo)** © michael ledray/ShutterStock, Inc.; **14.15** © Visions of America, LLC/Alamy Images; **14.17** © Tony Freeman/PhotoEdit, Inc.; **14.20** © Eduardo Munoz/Reuters/Landov; **14.23** © Gulnara Samoilova/AP Photos; **14.24** Courtesy of Patsy Lynch/FEMA

Chapter 15

15.1 © Gala_Kan/ShutterStock, Inc.; **15.9** © Dedyukhin Dmitry/ShutterStock, Inc.; **15.11** © Ingram Publishing/Index Stock Imagery, Inc.; **15.13** © Yuri Arcurs/ShutterStock, Inc.; **15.18** © Joyfull/Dreamstime.com; **15.23** © Blend Images/Alamy Images; **15.25** © Charlie Hutton/ShutterStock, Inc.

Chapter 16

16.1 Courtesy of Library of Congress, Prints & Photographs Division, National Child Labor Committee Collection [reproduction number LC-DIG-nclc-01640]; **16.2** Courtesy of Library of Congress, Prints & Photographs Division, National Child Labor Committee Collection [reproduction number LC-DIG-nclc-01137]; **16.3** © National Library of Medicine; **16.12** © Steve Helber/AP Photos; **16.14** © David R. Photolibrary, Inc./Alamy Images; **16.15** © Reuters/Landov; **16.16** © Rubberball Productions/Creatas; **16.17** © Photos.com; **16.18** © Blaj Gabriel/ShutterStock, Inc.

Unless otherwise indicated, all photographs and illustrations are under copyright of Jones & Bartlett Learning, or have been provided by the authors.